Yòng Yào Xīn Dé Shí Jiang

Ten Lectures on the Use of

MEDICINALS

from the Personal Experience of

JIĀO SHÙ-DÉ

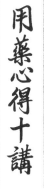

D1737664

JIĀO SHÙ-DÉ

Translated by Craig Mitchell, Nigel Wiseman,
Marnae Ergil, and Shelly Ochs

Edited by Nigel Wiseman and Andrew Ellis

PARADIGM PUBLICATIONS

Brookline, Massachusetts · Taos, New Mexico

2003

Ten Lectures on the Use of Medicinals

From the Personal Experience of

Jiāo Shù-Dé

焦树德著

用药心得十讲

Translated by Craig Mitchell, Shelley Ochs,
Marnae Ergil, and Nigel Wiseman. Annotated by Andrew Ellis.

Copyright © Paradigm Publications
44 Linden Street
Brookline, MA 02445 USA

Library of Congress Cataloging-in-Publication Data

Jiao, Shude
    [Yong yao xin de shi jiang. English]
    Ten Lectures on the Use of Chinese Medicinals / by Jiao Shu-De = Yong yao xin de shi
  jiang / Jiao Shude chu ; translated by Craig Mitchell . . . [et al.]
         p. ; cm.
    Includes index.
    ISBN 0-912111-62-3 (alk. paper)
    1. Herbs—Therapeutic use. 2. Medicine, Chinese. I. Title: Yong yao xin de shi jiang.
  II. Title.
    [DNLM: 1. Pharmaceutical preparations. 2. Medicine, Chinese Traditional. QV 55 J61y
  2001a]
    RM666.H33 J5313 2001
    615'.321'0951–dc21

                                                                         2001021009

Council of Oriental Medical Publishers (C.O.M.P.) Designation: Whole-text translation of Chinese 用药心得十讲 *Yòngyào Xīndé Shí Jiǎng* by 焦树德 *Jiāo Shù-Dé*, with addition of notes approved by author. English terminology from *Practical Dictionary of Chinese Medicine*, Wiseman and Féng, Paradigm Publications, Brookline MA, 1998.

Library of Congress Number: 2001021009
International Standard Book Number (ISBN): 0-912111-62-3
Printed in the United States of America

Contents

Publisher's Foreword
出版者的话

In his *Ten Lectures in the Use of Medicinals*, Comrade Jiāo Shù-Dé of the Academy of Traditional Chinese Medicine gives his personal experience in the clinical use of Chinese medicinals. After its appearance as a lecture series in the *Barefoot Doctors' Journal*, it won great acclaim among readers, especially barefoot doctors. At the request of readers, we have combined the lectures into a single volume for the benefit of barefoot doctors and rural grass-roots medical workers. Before publication, the author edited the text thoroughly so as to give barefoot doctors and comrades who have learned Chinese medicine a better grasp of the basic theory of Chinese medicine, and therefore enhance their skill in the use of Chinese medicinals.

This book was first published in 1977, and for this second edition, the author has once more edited the text, added new materials, and changed the weights to metric units.

People's Medical Publishing
May 1979

Translators' Preface
译者的序

Over recent years, the Western interest in Chinese medicine, once almost exclusively confined to acupuncture, has extended to the method of healing much more common in China, medicinal therapy. To the considerable collection of medicinal literature that has assembled on the bookshelves in Western countries, we proudly add a work by the acclaimed PRC physician, Professor Jiāo Shù-Dé.

As the Publisher's Foreword states, the present work originally took the form of lectures published in the *Barefoot Doctors' Journal.* In this lies its principal distinguishing feature: the book was originally intended for health-care workers possessing a rudimentary knowledge of Chinese medicine. By comparison with much Chinese literature on medicinal therapy, it is both more concise in its content and clearer in its presentation. Professor Jiāo's work does not, however, pale by comparison with other modern masters, either in scope or in depth. Its lasting popularity in China is attributable to the fact that it has won the acclaim of practitioners and scholars as well as that of barefoot doctors. It is for this reason that we consider this work as being eminently suitable in the initial transmission of Chinese medical knowledge. We are confident that the clarity of its presentation will gain it the appreciation of English-speakers studying Chinese medicinal therapy, and that the comprehensiveness and depth of its content will win it the lasting place in the West that it has already attained in China.

The present volume comprises a complete translation of the original work. We have liberally inserted headings for easier reference. We have added copious notes clarifying points in the original text, explaining concepts with which readers may be unfamiliar, and discussing the identification and availability of medicinals, and protected species. In a few cases, parentheses in the original text have been relegated to the footnotes for easier reading. All such additions and changes have been instituted with the knowledge and consent of Professor Jiāo. To the index of medicinals contained in the original Chinese text we have added the names of diseases and signs appearing in the text to make the text all the more useful for the reader.

Over 170 terms are explained in the Glossary of Terms contained in the Appendix. Other terms readers may be unfamiliar with can in most cases be accessed in *A Practical Dictionary of Chinese Medicine* (Wiseman and Féng, 1998).

For the convenience of readers, underlined superscript numerals have been placed after certain mentions of terms and names of medicinals. These numerals refer to the pages in the Glossary of Terms and in the body of the text on which useful information can be found. The underlining distinguishes these references from superscripts referring to footnotes.

Acknowledgements
志　谢

We thank Professor Jiāo for not only giving us the honor of translating his most valuable work, but also for his untiring helpfulness in making sure we understood the text correctly. Our special thanks also go to Professor Zhèng Jīn-Shēng (郑金生) of the China Academy of Traditional Chinese Medicine (中国中医研究院) for his help in arranging the publication. Not least, we thank Dr. Féng Yè (冯晔) of Chang Gung University for kindly reviewing the text and Michael Helme for his careful editing of it.

Lecture One
What To Pay Attention To
用药需注意什么？

1. Pay Attention to the Principle of Pattern Identification as the Basis of Determining Treatment: The medicine of our country progressed steadily over thousands of years, giving rise to the treatment system of *pattern identification as the basis of determining treatment* (辨证论治 *biàn zhèng lùn zhì*). This includes the concepts of principles, methods, formulas, and medicinals (理、法、方、药; *lǐ、 fǎ、 fāng、 yào*). When using medicinals in clinical practice, prescriptions must be composed in such a way as to conform to the requirements of the treatment method. The establishment of the treatment method must rely on the guidance provided by the principle of pattern identification as the basis of determining treatment. Therefore, principles, methods, formulas, and medicinals are inseparably connected. In order to make correct use of the principle of pattern identification as the basis of determining treatment, it is necessary to master specific theoretical knowledge.

Physicians of the past accumulated abundant experience in the clinical use of medicine. To provide some examples, *fù zǐ* (aconite) and *gān jiāng* (dried ginger) are hot-natured medicinals, but their heat is different; *shí gāo* (gypsum) and *huáng lián* (coptis) are both cold-natured medicinals, but their coldness is different; *guì zhī* (cinnamon twig) and *má huáng* (ephedra) are both effusing-dissipating medicinals, but their effusing-dissipating actions are different; *mài dōng* (ophiopogon) and *dì huáng* (rehmannia) both enrich yīn, but their yīn-enriching actions are different; *shú dì huáng* (cooked rehmannia) and *ròu guì* (cinnamon bark) are both kidney-supplementing medicinals, but one supplements kidney yīn, while the other supplements kidney yáng. One and the same *chái hú* (bupleurum) is used in one formula to effuse and dissipate and to harmonize, while in another formula it is used to upbear. We can see another example in *dà huáng* (rhubarb), which in different formulas can have very different actions depending on the accompanying medicinals, the processing, and the dosage. We must study and make use of this invaluable theory and experience to help raise the efficacy of our treatments.

In recent years, reports of experiments on animals have made it possible to explain such things. For example, it is effective to use medicinals that enrich yīn and subdue yáng in the treatment of animals with neurogenic hypertension, but yīn-enriching and yáng-subduing medicinals administered separately have a much less powerful action to reduce hypertension. Furthermore, for neurogenic hypertension, *guì fù bā wèi wán* (Cinnamon Bark and Aconite Eight-Ingredient Pill) has no effect, whereas in cases of hypertension related to the kidney, this formula is very effective. The use of *liù wèi dì huáng tāng* (Six-Ingredient Rehmannia Decoction) alone can also be effective, but to use only *fù zǐ* (aconite) and *ròu guì* (cinnamon bark) is ineffective.

Another example is the use of *sì wù tāng* (Four Agents Decoction) and *bā zhēn tāng* (Eight-Gem Decoction) in the treatment of animals with acute anemia. These formulas both increase the production of red blood cells, and in the latter formula this effect is particularly marked. This illustrates the rationale of "dual supplementation of qì and blood" and "when yáng arises, yīn grows."

Other researchers have tested *bǔ zhōng yì qì tāng* (Center-Supplementing Qì-Boosting Decoction) and demonstrated that it has a selective action to contract the uterus and its peripheral tissue. It also regulates peristalsis in the small intestine and restores normal tension to the intestines, which has a direct influence on the nutritional absorption in the intestines. With regard to the action of stimulating intestinal function and promoting nutritional absorption, this is identical to the Chinese medical concept of "supplementing the center and boosting the qì" (补中益气 *bǔ zhōng yì qì*). So, if one wishes to avoid the sort of methodology in which no distinction is made between hot- and cold-natured medicinals, no attention is paid to dosage or the changes of combining medicinals, neither vacuity, repletion, heat, or cold of the symptoms, nor the transformations or transmutations are taken into consideration, and in which medicinals are used in a formulaic fashion, care must be taken to apply the principle of pattern identification as the basis of determining treatment when using medicinals.

2. Pay Attention to Transformations Occurring in Medicinal Combinations and in Different Dosages: Combining Chinese medicinals causes multiple interactions. The appropriateness of medicinal combinations in prescriptions has a direct effect on the efficacy of the treatment. For example, *má huáng* (ephedra) is fundamentally a sweat-promoting medicinal, but by combining it with an appropriate amount of *shēng shí gāo* (crude gypsum) its sweat-promoting effect is reduced, and its roles of diffusing the lung and calming panting as well as opening the lung and disinhibiting water come into play. *Jīng jiè* (schizonepeta) belongs to the category of exterior-resolving medicinals. When combined with *fáng fēng* (saposhnikovia) and *sū yè* (perilla leaf), it acts as a warm, acrid, exterior-resolving medicinal, but when combined with *bò hé* (mint) and *jú huā* (chrysanthemum), it acts as a cool, acrid, exterior-resolving medicinal. *Fáng fēng* (saposhnikovia) treats headache: combined with *bái zhǐ* (Dahurian angelica), it tends to treat anterior headache; combined with *qiāng huó* (notopterygium), it tends to treat posterior headache; combined with *chuān xiōng* (chuanxiong) and *màn jīng zǐ* (vitex), it tends to treat bilateral headache. Furthermore, *huáng lián* (coptis) with *ròu guì* (cinnamon bark) treats insomnia from noninteraction of the heart and kidney; *bàn xià* (pinellia) with *shú mǐ* (broomcorn millet) treats insomnia from stomach disharmony; *dà huáng* (rhubarb) with *gān cǎo* (licorice) treats vomiting that occurs immediately after eating. When looking at formula composition, modifying just one or two medicinals often strengthens the therapeutic effect. For example, *sì jūn zǐ tāng* (Four Gentlemen Decoction)[1] contains *rén shēn* (ginseng), *bái zhú* (white atractylodes), *fú líng* (poria), and *gān cǎo* (licorice); it fortifies the spleen and supplements the qì. When the spleen's function of movement and transformation is reduced, the formula can give rise to many side-effects such as oppression in the chest and fullness in the stomach. Qiān Yǐ 钱乙, a famous Sòng Dynasty physician, added *chén pí* (tangerine peel) to this formula to rectify qì and harmonize the center, and thereby prevent such side-effects. The modified version is called *wǔ wèi yì gōng sǎn* (Five-Ingredient Special Achievement Powder), which has become a commonly used formula. Furthermore, investigation of *bǔ zhōng yì qì tāng* (Center-Supplementing Qì-Boosting Decoction) in animals has demonstrated that *shēng má* (cimicifuga) and *chái hú* (bupleurum) have a pronounced coordinating effect, strengthening the effects of the other medicinals, particularly with regard to intestinal peristalsis. If one removes these two medicinals, the formula has a significantly reduced action on peristalsis, but these two medicinals used alone have no effect on peristalsis. Scientists have also conducted animal studies with *yīn chén hāo tāng* (Virgate Wormwood Decoction). They have found that *yīn chén* (virgate wormwood), *zhī zǐ* (gardenia), and *dà huáng* (rhubarb) used singly do not have a gallbladder-disinhibiting action. When used together as a formula, however, these three medicinals (which form *yīn chén hāo tāng* (Virgate Wormwood Decoction)) can stimulate a qualitative and quantitative increase in bile excretion. Another study investigating 55 formulas that each included *huáng lián* (coptis) concluded that when used in combination with a suitable formula it reduced the development of drug resistance, elevated bacterial suppression, strengthened toxin-resolving action, and reduced the toxicity and side-effects associated with single medicinals. Through these examples we can see the importance of the interactions resulting from medicinal combinations.

The dosage of medicinals also has a very important relationship to therapeutic effect. For example, in *guì zhī tāng* (Cinnamon Twig Decoction), the dosage of *guì zhī* (cinnamon twig) and *bái sháo* (white peony) is equal, resulting in the actions of harmonizing the construction and defense and resolving the flesh. Nevertheless, in *guì zhī jiā sháo yào tāng* (Cinnamon Twig Decoction Plus Peony), the dosage of *bái sháo* (white peony) is double that of *guì zhī* (cinnamon twig), and the formula is inappropriate for greater yáng (*tài yáng*) disease, being used instead for greater yīn (*tài yīn*) disease with abdominal fullness and periodic pain. In *xiǎo jiàn zhōng tāng* (Minor Center-Fortifying Decoction), the dosage of *bái sháo* (white peony) is increased to double that of *guì zhī* (cinnamon twig), and *yí táng* (malt sugar) is added, so that the formula is able to warm and fortify the center burner and to relieve pain in the abdomen. *Hòu pò* (official magnolia bark), *dà huáng* (rhubarb), and *zhǐ shí* (unripe bitter orange) are the only ingredients in *hòu pò sān wù tāng* (Officinal Magnolia Bark Three-Agent Decoction), *xiǎo chéng qì tāng* (Minor Qì-

---

[1]In the original text, this formula *sì jūn zǐ tāng* (Four Gentlemen Decoction),is called *sì wèi bǔ qì tāng* (Four-Ingredients Qì-Supplementing Decoction). In the People's Republic of China, the names of certain formulas with feudal connotations were at one time renamed. In recent periods of liberalized policies, the traditional names have been readopted. In all such cases throughout this text we have used the traditional names. (Ed.)

Coordinating Decoction), and *hòu pò dà huáng tāng* (Officinal Magnolia Bark and Rhubarb Decoction), yet because the dosage of these three ingredients varies in the three formulas, the names of the formulas and the patterns they treat are different. In addition, the original prescription for *qīng wēn bài dú yǐn* (Scourge-Clearing Toxin-Vanquishing Beverage) includes the following quantitative variations:

> *Qīng wēn bài dú yǐn* (Scourge-Clearing Toxin-Vanquishing Beverage)
>> *shēng shí gāo* (生石膏 crude gypsum, Gypsum Fibrosum Crudum): large pack 6–8 liǎng, medium pack 2–4 liǎng, small pack 8 qián–1 liǎng 2 qián.
>> *shēng dì huáng* (生地黄 dried/fresh rehmannia, Rehmanniae Radix Exsiccata seu Recens): large pack 6 qián–1 liǎng, medium pack 3–5 qián, small pack 2–4 qián.
>> *chuān huáng lián* (川黄连 Sìchuān coptis, Coptidis Rhizoma Sichuanense): large pack 4–6 qián, medium pack 2–4 qián, small pack 1–1.5 qián.

The prescription continues:

> When the six pulses are deep, fine, and rapid, use a large pack; when deep and rapid, use a medium pack; when floating, large, and rapid, use a small pack.

Thus we can see the importance of the interactions caused by changes in dosage within a prescription.

Also, medicinal dosage is intimately related to the patient's age, the patient's weight, the strength of the evil, the strength of the constitution, and the local temperature and weather.

When using medicinals in clinical practice, failure to consider the interactions caused by varying combinations and dosages invariably results in a prescription whose effect is less than ideal or nonexistent, even though the principle and methodology behind it are in theory correct.

3. Pay Attention to the Differences Between Processed and Raw Medicinals: Medicinal processing has a 2000-year history in Chinese medicine. Throughout this history, there has been continual development of methods and the accumulation of extensive experience in processing and use. Although there are specialists in the techniques of medicinal processing, clinical physicians must fully understand the effects that medicinal processing has on medicinal actions to make appropriate choices in prescriptions. For example, *shēng jiāng* (fresh ginger) dissipates wind-cold, harmonizes the center, and checks retching; *gān jiāng* (dried ginger) warms the stomach and spleen, and returns yáng and stems counterflow; *pào jiāng* (blast-fried ginger) warms the channels and stanches bleeding, and dispels cold evils around the umbilicus and the smaller abdomen; *wēi jiāng* (roasted ginger) is mainly used to harmonize the center and check retching—compared to *shēng jiāng* (fresh ginger) it is not dissipating and compared to *gān jiāng* (dried ginger) it is not drying. Also, *dāng guī* (Chinese angelica) washed with wine moves and quickens the blood; when char-fried, it stanches bleeding. Similarly, *shí gāo* (gypsum) is used in crude form to clear heat and drain fire, and used in processed form (cooked) to close sores and relieve itching. *Dì huáng* (rehmannia) used raw is cold and sweet, and it cools the blood, nourishes yīn, and clears heat; when cooked, it becomes sweet and warm, and supplements the kidney, enriches yīn, and replenishes essence. *Yǐ mǐ* (coix) used raw tends to disinhibit dampness, but stir-fried it tends to fortify the spleen. *Dà huáng* (rhubarb) used raw has the greatest draining power and it is appropriate for emergency precipitation to preserve yīn; when steamed, its draining power is moderated, so it is appropriate for the elderly or those in weak health; when charred, its draining power is markedly reduced, and instead it checks descent of blood with the stool. *Jīng jiè* (schizonepeta) used raw is a wind-dissipating exterior-resolving medicinal; when used charred, it is effective for postpartum blood dizziness and uterine bleeding. *Mǔ lì* (oyster shell) is used in crude form to calm the liver and subdue yáng, soften hardness and dissipate binds, and disperse scrofula; it is used calcined to constrain sweat, astringe essence, and check vaginal discharge. These few examples illustrate the difference in actions between raw and processed medicinals. When writing a prescription, it is important to pay attention to this fact and to choose flexibly on the basis of the actual situation.

4. Pay Attention to Decoction and Administration Methodologies: Physicians of the past accumulated a great amount of experience with regard to decoction and administration methodologies. We should pay attention to this valuable experience. For example, the decoction and administration methodology used in the *Shāng Hán Lùn* (伤寒论 "On Cold Damage") for *guì zhī tāng* (Cinnamon Twig Decoction) is as follows:

> ...use seven cups of water for one pack of medicinals. Boil over a mild flame to get three cups. Remove the dregs and take one cup warm. About a half hour later, drink approximately one cup of hot, thin gruel to reinforce the strength of the medicinals. Cover with a blanket and lie down for about two hours. Ideally, the whole body should become moist from slight sweating. One cannot allow a great dripping sweat. Great sweating will not eliminate the disease. If after one cup the disease is completely better, do not take the remaining two cups. If after one cup mild sweating is absent reduce the time between doses and give another cup according to the previous method. The three cups can be finished in about half a day. If the disease is severe, take it throughout a whole day and night. After finishing one pack, if the disease signs are still evident, take another pack. If sweating is difficult, one can take up to two or three packets.

The decoction and administration method for *dà chéng qì tāng* (Major Qì-Coordinating Decoction) is as follows:

> Use ten teacups of clear water and first cook *zhǐ shí* (unripe bitter orange) and *hòu pò* (officinal magnolia bark) until five cups remain. Remove the medicinal dregs and add *dà huáng* (rhubarb). Decoct until two cups remain and remove the medicinal dregs. Add *máng xiāo* (mirabilite) and boil once or twice over a low flame. Divide into two doses. After stool draining precipitation has occurred, cease taking the decoction.

The decoction and administration methodology for *dà bàn xià tāng* (Major Pinellia Decoction), which contains *bàn xià* (pinellia), *rén shēn* (ginseng), and *bái mì* (honey), is as follows:

Mix the honey into about 10 cups of water and stir with a spoon 240 times. Use this honey-water to cook the medicinals until two-and-a-half cups remain. Take one cup warm and divide the remaining one-and-a-half cups into two doses.

The decoction and administration methodology for *dà wū tóu jián* (Major Wild Aconite Brew) is as follows:

Place five pieces of large *wū tóu* (wild aconite) in three cups of water and decoct to get one cup. Remove the medicinal dregs and add two cups of *fēng mì* (honey).[2] Decoct again until the vapor ceases and there are two cups left. [Use] 0.7 cups for strong people and 0.5 cups for weak people. If there is no effect, take another dose the following day. One should not take two doses in one day.

Another example is the decoction and administration methodology for *yín qiáo sǎn* (Lonicera and Forsythia Powder) from *Wēn Bìng Tiáo Biàn* (温病条辨 "Systematized Identification of Warm Diseases"):

. . . make into a powder, taking six qián each time. Decoct the medicinals with a decoction of fresh *lú gēn* (phragmites) only until one smells a strong medicinal flavor. One should not cook it for too long. For severe diseases, take once about every four hours, taking it three times during the day and once at night. If the disease does not resolve, take the original prescription again.

A further example is *jī míng sǎn* (Cockcrow Powder), which must be taken in the early morning around 4 A.M. to produce an effect. Many such examples could be cited.

From these examples, we can see that decoction and administration methodologies have an important influence on the therapeutic effect. Therefore, to achieve beneficial effects, it is important to pay attention not only to medicinal processing, combination of medicinals, and formula composition, but also to the decoction and administration methodology. In general, it is appropriate to use a high flame for exterior-resolving medicinals, and not to cook them too long (about 15–20 minutes). These formulas should be taken every two to four hours, and administration of the formula is stopped as soon as the patient recovers. It is appropriate to use a low flame for supplementing and boosting medicinals, cooking them longer (about 30–40 minutes). These formulas should be taken once in the morning and once at night, and they are taken for a longer period of time. Medicinals for offensive precipitation should be taken on an empty stomach. Medicinals that treat diseases of the upper burner should be taken after meals. Medicinals that treat diseases of the lower burner should be taken before meals. Medicinals that treat diseases of the center burner should be taken between meals. In acute or urgent cases, speed is essential so one need not pay close attention to the time of day. These statements

---

[2] The thick honey drink causes the *wū tóu* (wild aconite) to remain in the center burner. Hence, it achieves the aim of warming the center. (Ed.)

are generalities, and the actual methods of decoction and administration must be decided on the basis of the specific disease pattern. In summary, we must carefully analyze the pathocondition, follow any requirements of the medicinal prescription that we have created, and provide detailed instructions to the patient's family on how to brew the medicinals. Which ingredients should be precooked? Which should be added at the end? Should the medicine be taken before or after meals? Approximately how many hours should be allowed between doses? How many doses should be taken in total? One must not ignore these questions and inflexibly instruct patients to take their formula once in the morning and once at night, regardless of whether it is a pattern of external contraction or internal damage. If one does, one will frequently find that even if the formula suits the pathocondition, because the decoction or administration method is wrong, the treatment is ineffectual. If physicians encounter such a situation and fail to understand the reason for it, they may prescribe a different formula and prolong the course of the disease.

5. Pay Attention to Varying Formulas in Accordance with Signs: During their long history of treatment experience, physicians of the past not only accumulated abundant experience about the natures, flavors, and actions of individual medicinals, but they also created many effective formulas. Through the composition of formulas and by using medicinals in specific combinations, they were able to improve therapeutic effects. The content, theory, and composition of these formulas is the precious legacy of traditional Chinese medicine. We must continue this tradition and its development, but while using the formulas of past physicians, it is important to pay attention to varying formulas in accordance with signs. One must not use formulas inflexibly or mechanically. For example, some physicians do not dare to change even one medicinal from the original formula when writing a prescription for *sì wù tāng* (Four Agents Decoction) to regulate menstruation. For advanced menstruation with copious bleeding, for example, they do not dare to reduce the dosage of *chuān xiōng* (chuanxiong) or even to remove it and add *ài yè tàn* (charred mugwort); for delayed menstruation where in severe cases periods may only arrive once every two months, they do not dare to increase the dosage of *chuān xiōng* (chuanxiong) or add *hóng huā* (carthamus); in patterns of blood aspect vacuity heat, they do not dare to change *shú dì huáng* (cooked rehmannia) to *shēng dì huáng* (dried/fresh rehmannia). Also, there are those who write a prescription for *bā zhèng sǎn* (Eight Corrections Powder) and who do not dare to alter the dosage of *dà huáng* (rhubarb) or even to remove it, so that the patient not only fails to be relieved of the **strangury disease**[564] (淋病 *lín bìng*), but also experiences diarrhea. In extreme cases, some people do not even dare to alter the dosages of three pieces of *shēng jiāng* (fresh ginger) or four pieces of *dà zǎo* (jujube). When used in this way, the prescription's therapeutic effect cannot be optimal. Physicians of the past criticized this situation, describing it as *having a formula without medicinals* (有方 无药 *yǒu fāng wú yào*). The idea is that although one may have found an effective classical formula, it will not be effective unless the ingredients are varied on the basis of the specific patient condition.

Another situation is one in which practitioners do not refer to a classical formula or principle when writing a prescription and instead choose medicinals on a purely symptomatic basis. For example, to address the patient's headache, they might use *chuān xiōng* (chuanxiong) and *jú huā* (chrysanthemum); for the leg pain, they add *niú xī* (achyranthes) and *mù guā* (chaenomeles); if the patient also has some flowery vision they add *cǎo jué míng* (fetid cassia) and *shí jué míng* (abalone shell); if the patient also has mild indigestion, they add *jiāo sān xiān* (scorch-fried three immortals)[555]; and if there is also abdominal distention, they further add *mù xiāng* (costusroot) and *bīng láng* (areca). On the basis of symptoms, they prescribe eight or ten medicinals, but between these there is no organic relationship. There is no differentiation between chief medicinals and assistants, no recognition of the interactions that occur when combining medicinals, no organization to allow for complementarity between medicinals, no combinations that incline the formula in a particular direction, no process of pattern identification, no principle or methodology. In short, although there is an absence of any theoretical coherence, they consider it a prescription. This type of prescription will not yield ideal results. Physicians of the past criticized this as *having medicinals without a formula* (有药 无方 *yǒu yào wú fāng*). The idea is that by using various medicinals that treat the head for a headache or that treat the leg for leg pain with no organizing principle for the formula or without using an effective classical formula for reference, the therapeutic effect will not be good.

Optimally, one should choose an effective prescription according to the requirements of pattern identification and methodology. Then, on the basis of the patient's actual condition, one analyzes the medicinals in the formula. If there are some that do not suit the current condition, these should be removed. If it is necessary to add one or two medicinals, choose those that suit the patient's requirements based on pattern identification and methodology. One must choose medicinals that complement each other when combined, so as to strengthen the therapeutic effect without negatively influencing the original structure of the formula. Physicians of the past referred to this as *having medicinals and a formula* (有药有方 *yǒu yào yǒu fāng*). The idea is that the prescription should suit the requirements of pattern identification and methodology. Furthermore, the formula should be organized using an effective classical formula for reference or according to the principles of formula composition, on the basis of the requirements of principle and methodology. The additional medicinals must also be suitable, and there must be an organic relationship between these individual medicinals. This type of prescription will produce a satisfactory effect. For example, when one identifies a lesser yáng (*shào yáng*) pattern, the principle and method is to harmonize the lesser yáng. The formula of choice is *xiǎo chái hú tāng* (Minor Bupleurum Decoction). When writing the formula, one must consider if thirst is pronounced, in which case one should remove *bàn xià* (pinellia) and add *tiān huā fěn* (trichosanthes root) to engender the fluids; if there is heat vexation in the chest and no retching, remove *bàn xià* (pinellia) and *rén shēn* (ginseng) and add *guā lóu* (trichosanthes) to flush depressed heat; if there is pain in the abdomen, reduce *huáng qín* (scutellaria) and add *bái sháo* (white peony) to boost the center and dispel pain; if thirst is absent and if there is mild heat in the exterior, remove *rén shēn* (ginseng) and add *guì zhī* (cinnamon twig) to resolve the fleshy exterior. When the condition is more severe, the dosage should be larger; when the condition is milder, the dosage can be reduced. In summer, the dosage of *shēng jiāng* (fresh ginger) can be reduced, whereas in winter it can be increased. With all of these modifications, however, the composition of the formula never breaks away from the requirements of principle and methodology of harmonizing the lesser yáng and abating evil in the half-interior half-exterior.

In summary, Chinese medicinals should be used in formulas that are organized according to definite principles. Formulas should be used flexibly with variations according to the pattern. Of course, this flexible use does not permit vagueness as regards therapeutic goals, and should meet the requirements of pattern identification and the rigor of methodology. At the same time, disease progression is characterized by unceasing transformations and transmutations. During one period, one may need to use certain modifications, but during another period, different modifications may be required. Therefore, when using Chinese medicinals it is important to pay attention to formula interactions and to variation of the medicinals in accordance with the signs observed. This methodology greatly helps to increase clinical efficacy.

6. Pay Attention to Incorporating the Findings of Modern Scientific Research: Things develop; history advances. Modern scientific research on Chinese medicinals continues to produce ever more findings. We must use these findings in clinical practice to endow the principle of pattern identification as the basis of determining treatment with new content, advance the development of integrated Chinese-Western medicine, and raise the level of therapeutic efficacy. For example, *jīn yín huā* (lonicera), *lián qiáo* (forsythia), *yú xīng cǎo* (houttuynia), *pú gōng yīng* (dandelion), *dì dīng* (violet), *huáng lián* (coptis), *zhī zǐ* (gardenia), and *huáng bǎi* (phellodendron) all have a pronounced antibacterial effect; *huáng qí* (astragalus) strengthens and protects the liver; *lù róng* (velvet deerhorn) contains male hormones that strengthen the entire body; *bái sháo* (white peony) and *mǎ chǐ xiàn* (purslane) have a strong antibacterial effect that fights the bacterium that causes dysentery (*Bacillus dysenteriae*); *bèi wǔ jiā pí* (periploca) has an effect similar to that of strophanthin; *rén shēn* (ginseng) and *wǔ wèi zǐ* (schisandra) have an adaptogenic effect.[3] When we write prescriptions, we can, depending on the condition, consider these research findings to choose medicinals that will ensure maximum clinical efficacy. At the same time, it is important when making our choices to apply the principle of deciding treatment in accordance with the pattern identified. Treatments should not be applied mechanically. For example, in vacuity cold dysentery, using *huáng lián* (coptis), *bái sháo* (white peony), and *mǎ chǐ xiàn* (purslane) alone to control the bacteria *Bacillus dysenteriae* will invariably have an effect that is not ideal. If one simultaneously uses the treatment principle appropriate to "vacuity cold" and also uses *gān jiāng* (dried ginger), *wú yú* (evodia), *fù zǐ* (aconite), *bái zhú* (white atractylodes), and *dǎng shēn* (codonopsis) to warm and supplement the spleen and kidney, it is easy to achieve a desirable effect. Also, using a powder preparation of *wǔ wèi zǐ* (schisandra) can return elevated G.P.T. levels in hepatitis patients to normal. Two or three weeks after ceasing ingestion, however, many experience elevation again. If one applies pattern identification as

---

[3]The adaptogenic effect strengthens the nonspecific defensive power of the organism. (Ed.)

the basis of determining treatment to choose a decoction that suits the condition, then the therapeutic effect will be stable and there will be no further elevation. Therefore, we should actively make use of this clinical research and must also pay attention to mastering pattern identification as the basis of determining treatment. We should act in accordance with the teachings of Chairman Máo: "Make the past serve the present; make foreign things serve China," and "Weed through the old to bring forth the new." It is only by integrating the strong points of both Chinese and Western medicine that we can enhance therapeutic efficacy, achieve a higher standard of treatment based on pattern identification, and advance the development of traditional Chinese medicine to create a new medicine as early as possible.

7. Know as Much About Chinese Medicinal Decocting Pieces as Possible: Chinese medicinals that have been processed for use in dispensaries are known as "decocting pieces" (饮片 *yǐn piàn*). A clinical physician should make an effort to know about one or two hundred varieties of decocting pieces. During the process of learning to recognize these decocting pieces, one should pay attention to increasing one's understanding of medicinals' shapes, processing methods, qualities, growing locations, qì, and flavors. This provides significant benefit when one is choosing medicinals for a prescription. There are examples where failure to sufficiently understand such qualities of Chinese medicinals has led to errors. For example, prescribing a pair of *gé jiè* (gecko) in a decoction medicine; writing a prescription for a branch or a pair of *líng yáng jiǎo* (antelope horn) or even prescribing 10–15 g/ 3–5 qián; some believe that *hǎi piāo xiāo* (cuttlefish bone) is a bone and therefore very heavy and so prescribe 30–60 g/1–2 liǎng; some do not understand how heavy *dài zhě shí* (hematite) is or how light *hǎi fú shí* (costazia bone/pumice) is and so use a nonstandard dosage; an extreme example are those who take *hú lú bā* (fenugreek), the seed of a plant, to be the stalk of *hú lú* (bottle gourd); or who send the patient's family out to look for old window paper thinking that is *pò gù zhǐ* (psoralea).[4]

In summary, things are all related to each other. Clinical physicians cannot simply write prescriptions and get ideal results. They must pay attention to the proper combinations and grasp all the important points in order to achieve good clinical effects. Here, I have set out some of the important points to which everyone should pay attention.

---

[4]The Chinese name literally means "ripped old paper." In China, paper rather than glass was used in windows. This medicinal is more commonly called *bǔ gǔ zhī* 补骨脂 (literally "bone-supplementing fat"). (Ed.)

Lecture Two
Effusing & Dissipating Medicinals
发散药 *Fā Sàn Yào*

This lecture introduces medicinals that promote sweating and that resolve and dissipate exterior evils. The majority of these medicinals are acrid and because acridity effuses and dissipates they resolve exterior evils through the outward movement of the sweat. Bear in mind effusing and dissipating medicinals should not be cooked for too long; generally, 15–20 minutes is sufficient.

---

1. 麻黄 Má Huáng   Ephedrae Herba
Ephedra

Má huáng (ephedra) has four chief actions: 1) to promote sweating and dissipate cold; 2) to diffuse the lung and calm panting[559] (喘 *chuǎn*); 3) to move water and disperse swelling; 4) to dissipate yīn flat-abscesses[569] (阴疽 *yīn jū*) and disperse concretions and binds. Since in clinical practice it is most commonly used to promote sweating with warmth and acridity, it is usually classified among wind-cold effusing and dissipating medicinals.

Besides promoting sweating with warmth and acridity, and resolving the exterior and dissipating cold, *má huáng* also has a pronounced lung-diffusing panting-calming action. One can use it to treat any case of externally contracted panting and cough due to invasion of wind-cold that fetters the interstices and prevents normal perfusion of lung qì. One can continue to use it even if the exterior pattern has already resolved and yet panting and cough remain. In such cases, one uses *zhì má huáng* (mix-fried ephedra).[1] *Shēng má huáng* (raw ephedra) strongly promotes sweating and resolves the exterior; *zhì má huáng* (mix-fried ephedra) is less strong in this action but more effective in calming panting and suppressing cough.

When using *má huáng* to treat panting and cough it is best to combine it with *xìng rén* (apricot kernel). *Má huáng* calms panting and suppresses cough by diffusing lung qì; *xìng rén* (apricot kernel) calms panting and suppresses cough by

---

[1] *Zhì má huáng* (炙麻黄, mix-fried ephedra): Mix-fried means heated in a wok with a relatively small amount of liquid such as honey, fat, or vinegar. In the case of *má huáng* (ephedra), this means mix-fried with honey. See mix-fried[557] (炙 *zhì*) in the Glossary of Terms. (Ed.)

downbearing qì and transforming phlegm. *Má huáng* is harsh in nature, whereas *xìng rén* (apricot kernel) is mild and moistening. When combined, these two medicinals more powerfully calm panting and suppress cough; thus in clinical practice it is said that "*xìng rén* is *má huáng*'s helping hand."[2]

When patients with panting and cough display a lung heat pattern (thick yellow phlegm, dry throat, hot breath from the nose and mouth, exacerbation of the panting and cough on exposure to heat, yellow tongue fur, rapid pulse, etc.), it is necessary to add medicinals such as *shēng shí gāo* (crude gypsum), or *huáng qín* (scutellaria) and *zhī mǔ* (anemarrhena) to clear lung heat and calm panting. Commonly used formulas include *má xìng shí gān tāng* (Ephedra, Apricot Kernel, Gypsum, and Licorice Decoction) and *dìng chuǎn tāng* (Panting-Stabilizing Decoction).[3]

Besides resolving the exterior and calming panting, *má huáng* also moves water and disperses swelling. It mainly treats: 1) pronounced upper body **water swelling**[567] (水肿 *shuǐ zhǒng*); 2) water swelling of the head, face, and limbs; or 3) acute water swelling concurrent with an exterior pattern. *Má huáng* warms and diffuses lung qì, and opens the interstices; it helps diffuse and transform upper burner water qì to move water and disperse swelling. When *má huáng* is used to treat water swelling, one of the following situations can occur through which the swelling will disperse: a) the water resolves through sweating; b) urination increases; c) watery diarrhea occurs; or d) slight sweating occurs and urination increases markedly. These actions are related to the theories that "the lung governs the skin and [body] hair," "the lung distributes the fluids and transports them down to the bladder," "the lung and large intestine stand in interior-exterior relationship," and "water swelling disease has its root in the kidney and its tip in the lung." On the basis of clinical experience, variations of *yuè bì jiā zhú tāng* (Spleen-Effusing Decoction Plus White Atractylodes), which is given below, have been found to be very effective in the treatment of the edema of nephritis.

Yuè bì jiā zhú tāng 越婢加术汤   Spleen-Effusing Decoction Plus White Atractylodes

---

má huáng (麻黄 ephedra, Ephedrae Herba)
shēng shí gāo (生石膏 crude gypsum, Gypsum Fibrosum Crudum)

---

[2] *Má huáng* (麻黄, ephedra) with *xìng rén* (杏仁, apricot kernel) is a useful pairing on account of both the similarities and differences between the two. Both are bitter and downbearing, which mutually reinforces the pair's ability to downbear lung qì in the treatment of cough and panting. *Má huáng* (ephedra), however, is also acrid and drying; this tendency can be moderated by the sweet flavor and moistening quality of *xìng rén* (apricot kernel). This mutual assistance allows the combination to powerfully downbear lung qì while not damaging that delicate viscus. (Ed.)

[3] *Dìng chuǎn tāng* (Panting-Stabilizing Decoction) is an example of *má huáng* (ephedra) combined with *huáng qín* (scutellaria), and *má xìng shí gān tāng* (Ephedra, Apricot Kernel, Gypsum, and Licorice Decoction) is an example of it combined with *shēng shí gāo* (crude gypsum). *Dìng chuǎn tāng* includes several medicinals to diffuse and downbear lung qì, calm panting, and transform phlegm; thus it is stronger in those functions than *má xìng shí gān tāng*. *Má xìng shí gān tāng*, on the other hand, is better able to clear heat than *dìng chuǎn tāng*. Both formulas are suitable for exterior patterns of wind-cold fettering the lung and giving rise to heat in the lung, panting, and cough. Both formulas are given in Chapter 9; see page 431. (Ed.)

cāng zhú (苍术 atractylodes, Atractylodis Rhizoma)

gān cǎo (甘草 licorice, Glycyrrhizae Radix)

shēng jiāng (生姜 fresh ginger, Zingiberis Rhizoma Recens)

dà zǎo (大枣 jujube, Jujubae Fructus)

COMBINATIONS

Má huáng combined with *shú dì huáng* (cooked rehmannia), *bái jiè zǐ* (white mustard), and *dāng guī* (Chinese angelica) dissipates yīn flat-abscesses[569] (阴疽 *yīn jū*) and disperses concretions and binds. Being warming, freeing, effusing, and dissipating in nature and having a clear and light flavor and qì, it acts in the exterior to diffuse and outthrust from the interstices, and in the interior to penetrate accumulated phlegm and congealed blood. Thus the *Shén Nóng Běn Cǎo Jīng* (神农本草经 "The Divine Husbandman's Herbal Foundation Canon") records it as being capable of "breaking concretions, hardness, accumulations, and gatherings." The formula *yáng hé tāng* (Harmonious Yáng Decoction) given in *Wài Kē Zhèng Zhì Quán Shēng Jí* (外科证治全生集 "Life-For-All Compendium of External Medicine, Patterns, and Treatment") best exemplifies the use of *má huáng* (1.5 g/ 5 fēn) combined with *shú dì huáng* (cooked rehmannia) (30 g/1 liǎng) to dissipate and disperse yīn flat-abscesses[569] (阴疽 *yīn jū*), phlegm nodes, streaming sores, and lumps.

Yáng hé tāng 阳和汤   Harmonious Yáng Decoction

má huáng (麻黄 ephedra, Ephedrae Herba)

shú dì huáng (熟地黄 cooked rehmannia, Rehmanniae Radix Praeparata)

bái jiè zǐ (白芥子 white mustard, Sinapis Albae Semen)

lù jiǎo jiāo (鹿角胶 deerhorn glue, Cervi Cornus Gelatinum)

pào jiāng tàn (炮姜炭 blast-fried ginger, Zingiberis Rhizoma Praeparatum)

ròu guì (肉桂 cinnamon bark, Cinnamomi Cortex)

gān cǎo (甘草 licorice, Glycyrrhizae Radix)

Practice has shown that *"má huáng* with *shú dì huáng* (cooked rehmannia) frees the network vessels, but does not treat the exterior, while *shú dì huáng* (cooked rehmannia) with *má huáng* supplements the blood, but is not slimy and clogging."

On the basis of clinical experience, I myself have successfully treated Raynaud's disease and obliterating phlebitis[4] by combining *má huáng* with medicinals such as the following, varied in accordance with signs:

shú dì huáng (熟地黄 cooked rehmannia, Rehmanniae Radix Praeparata)

---

[4]Obliterating phlebitis and Raynaud's disease display symptoms similar to those of flat-abscesses in many ways. They are painful, deep-lying lesions that are not hot or red. For this reason, modern practitioners treat these conditions as flat abscesses. *Yáng hé tāng* (Harmonious Yáng Decoction) is the representative formula for treating flat-abscesses. It invigorates yáng and thus breaks through the yīn mist and disperses the internal collection of toxin that lies trapped in the flesh by yīn-cold. The formula also treats classical disease categories such as crane's-knee wind (鹤膝风 *hè xī fēng*), streaming sores (流注 *liú zhù*), and bone-clinging flat-abscesses (附骨疽 *fù gǔ jū*), as well as modern disease categories such as tubercular lymphadenitis and deep-lying cysts. (Ed.)

bái jiè zǐ (白芥子 white mustard, Sinapis Albae Semen)

guì zhī (桂枝 cinnamon twig, Cinnamomi Ramulus)

hóng huā (红花 carthamus, Carthami Flos)

lù jiǎo shuāng (鹿角霜 degelatinated deerhorn, Cervi Cornu Degelatinatum)

zhì shān jiǎ (炙山甲 mix-fried pangolin scales, Manis Squama cum Liquido Fricta)

Dosage

The dosage of *má huáng* is generally 2–9 g/7–8 fēn up to 3 qián. To treat water swelling, a larger dose is generally used, from 10 g/3 qián up to as much as 15 g/ 5 qián, or, when used singly, even 20–25 g/7–8 qián. For this use, one combines it with 20–45 g/7 qián–1.5 liǎng of *shēng shí gāo* (crude gypsum), or in proportions of about 3 : 1, to reduce *má huáng*'s sweat-promoting effect and achieve the action of diffusing the lung and disinhibiting urine.

Caution

Má huáng should not be used for panting due to lung vacuity, externally contracted wind-heat, **simple drum distention**[563] (单臌胀 *dān gǔ zhàng*), **welling-abscesses**[567] (痈 *yōng*),[5] and **boils**[543] (疖 *jié*).

---

2. 桂枝 **Guì Zhī**   Cinnamomi Ramulus
Cinnamon Twig

Warm in nature and acrid in flavor,[6] *guì zhī* (cinnamon twig) dissipates cold and resolves the exterior. It is often combined with *má huáng* (ephedra) to treat common colds due to wind-cold characterized by absence of sweating, and it helps *má huáng* promote sweating and resolve the exterior. *Guì zhī* is also combined with *bái sháo* (white peony) to treat common cold due to wind-cold characterized by the presence of sweating; it has the effects of harmonizing construction and defense, and of resolving the flesh and checking sweating.

Combinations

Guì zhī also warms the channels, dispels wind-cold, quickens blood, and frees the network vessels. a) Combined with medicinals such as *dāng guī* (Chinese angelica), *chì bái sháo* (red/white peony), *chuān xiōng* (chuanxiong), *hóng huā* (carthamus), and *táo rén* (peach kernel), it treats delayed menstruation, menstrual block, abdominal pain during menstruation, and concretion lumps (癥块 *zhēng kuài*) in the

---

[5]The implication is that although *má huáng* (ephedra) is appropriate for flat-abscesses, which are cold and yīn in nature, it is inappropriate for welling-abscesses, which are hot and yáng. In addition, most modern books discourage giving *má huáng* to patients who have hypertension and older texts caution about excessive or continued use of this medicinal. (Ed.)

[6]Many modern books indicate that *guì zhī* (cinnamon twig) is sweet as well as acrid. The moderating action of the sweet flavor reduces its acrid, dispersing power, making it less effective for exterior resolving than a purely acrid medicinal such as *jīng jiè* (schizonepeta). With its moderated acrid-dispersing flavor, *guì zhī* is the ideal medicinal for exterior patterns that occur with sweating. (Ed.)

abdomen. b) Combined with *piàn jiāng huáng* (sliced turmeric) and *fáng fēng* (saposhnikovia), it treats pain in the shoulder and arm that arises when wind-cold obstructs the network vessels and impedes the flow of qì and blood. c) Combined with *chì sháo* (red peony), *hóng huā* (carthamus), and *shēn jīn cǎo* (ground pine), it treats pain in the limbs and hypertonicity of the joints that makes stretching difficult. d) With medicinals such as *qiāng huó* (notopterygium), *dú huó* (pubescent angelica), *fáng fēng* (saposhnikovia), *wēi líng xiān* (clematis), *dāng guī* (Chinese angelica), and *fù piàn* (sliced aconite), it treats joint pain and pain in the limbs due to wind, cold, and dampness. It is often used to treat pain due to rheumatic arthritis.

Guì zhī also assists heart yáng and warms and transforms water-rheum. a) Combined with *fú líng* (poria), *zhū líng* (polyporus), *bái zhú* (white atractylodes), *zé xiè* (alisma), *sū zǐ* (perilla fruit), *sāng pí* (mulberry root bark), and *zhì gān cǎo* (mix-fried licorice), it treats palpitations, **fearful throbbing**[549] (怔忡 *zhēng zhōng*), and **puffy swelling**[560] (浮肿 *fú zhǒng*) due to **water-rheum intimidating the heart**[567] (水饮凌心 *shuǐ yǐn líng xīn*). b) Combined with *guā lóu* (trichosanthes), *xiè bái* (Chinese chive), *hóng huā* (carthamus), and *wǔ líng zhī* (squirrel's droppings), it treats devitalized heart yáng causing **chest impediment**[543] (胸痹 *xiōng bì*) and heart pain. On the basis of traditional experience, it is now used to treat cardiac insufficiency, angina pectoris, myocardial infarction, and so forth. Nevertheless, it is important to pay attention to the principle of determining treatment in accordance with patterns identified; *guì zhī* cannot be used for heat patterns.

A special characteristic of *guì zhī* is that it moves transversely to the limbs and joints, enabling all medicinals to reach the shoulders, arms, and fingers. Thus it is a channel-conducting medicinal for diseases of the upper limbs.

Dosage

The dosage is generally 3–9 g/1–3 qián. Under special circumstances, one can use up to 15–30 g/5 qián–1 liǎng.[7]

Caution

Guì zhī must not be given to patients suffering from yīn blood vacuity or who suffer from bleeding.[8] Similarly, it should not be used when there is absence of external cold evil or if yáng qì is exuberant in the interior.

3. 荆芥 Jīng Jiè
Schizonepeta

Schizonepetae
Herba

Acrid in flavor and slightly warm in nature, *jīng jiè* (schizonepeta) promotes sweating and resolves the exterior. a) Combined with *fáng fēng* (saposhnikovia) and *sū*

---

[7]This large dosage (15–30 g) is usually reserved for treatment of wind-cold impediment patterns. (Ed.)

[8]*Běn Cǎo Gāng Mù* (本草纲目 "The Comprehensive Herbal Foundation") states: "*Guì zhī* (cinnamon twig) is acrid and dispersing, it unblocks the uterus and breaks blood." Practitioners regard this as a warning not to use this medicinal if there is excessive menstrual bleeding. (Ed.)

yè (perilla leaf), it resolves the exterior with warmth and acridity. b) Combined with *bò hé* (mint), *jīn yín huā* (lonicera), and *sāng yè* (mulberry leaf), it has a cool acrid exterior-resolving action. c) Combined with *fáng fēng* (saposhnikovia), *dāng guī* (Chinese angelica), *chuān xiōng* (chuanxiong), and *sū gěng* (perilla stem), it treats postpartum contraction of wind. *Jīng jiè* differs from other warm acrid exterior-resolving medicinals in that it is used for both wind-cold and wind-heat exterior patterns.

Jīng jiè can also outthrust papules, relieve itching, and treat skin diseases. a) Combined with medicinals such as *chán tuì* (cicada molting), *gé gēn* (pueraria), and *bò hé* (mint), it can treat inhibited outthrust of measles.[9] b) Combined with *chì sháo* (red peony), *cāng zhú* (atractylodes), *huáng bǎi* (phellodendron), *bái xiān pí* (dictamnus), and *kǔ shēn* (flavescent sophora), it treats **wind papules**[568] (风疹 *fēng zhěn*), eczema, **scab**[561] (疥 *jiè*), **lichen**[556] (癣 *xiǎn*), and other skin lesions.

Jīng jiè also clears latent heat in the blood-aspect and it rectifies the blood and stanches bleeding. a) Combined with *dì yú* (sanguisorba) and *huái huā tàn* (charred sophora flower), it treats bloody stool. b) Combined with *ǒu jié* (lotus root node), *hēi shān zhī* (charred gardenia), and *bái máo gēn* (imperata), it treats **spontaneous external bleeding**[564] (衄血 *nǜ xuè*). c) Combined with *dāng guī* (Chinese angelica), *yì mǔ cǎo* (leonurus), *zōng tàn* (charred trachycarpus), and *xù duàn tàn* (charred dipsacus), it treats profuse menstruation, **flooding and spotting**[550] (崩漏 *bēng lòu*), and postpartum loss of blood. d) Combined with *hóng huā* (carthamus), it moves **malign blood**[556] (恶血 *è xuè*). When used to stanch bleeding, it should be char-fried.

Comparisons

The stalks and spikes cut together and used raw are called *jīng jiè* (schizonepeta); when only the spikes are used, it is called *shēng jiè suì* (raw schizonepeta spike); char-fried, it is called *jīng jiè tàn* (charred schizonepeta) or *jiè suì tàn* (charred schizonepeta spike).[10] *Jīng jiè* dissipates wind evil in the whole body; *shēng jiè suì* dissipates wind evil from the head. The char-fried forms stanch bleeding and treat excessive postpartum blood loss and **blood dizziness**[542] (血晕 *xuè yūn*). One should specify clearly on prescriptions which form is to be used.

Jīng jiè eliminates wind from the blood, so it is a commonly used medicinal for wind diseases, blood diseases, sores, and postpartum diseases.

Whereas *jīng jiè* is best for treating wind evil "**outside the membrane within the skin**"[559] (皮里膜外 *pí lǐ mó wài*) and in the blood vessels, *fáng fēng* (saposhnikovia)[17] excels in treating wind evil in the bones and flesh.

Dosage

The dosage is generally 3–9 g/1–3 qián. To treat postpartum bleeding and blood dizziness, use 30 g/1 liǎng of *jiè suì tàn* (charred schizonepeta spike) as a single medicinal in a water decoction.

---

[9]This method of treatment is used to promote the eruption of macules in the initial stage of measles or other pox diseases, particularly when the macules have failed to erupt normally. (Ed.)

[10] *Jīng jiè* (荆芥, schizonepeta) that is exported is usually just the spikes, i.e., *shēng jiè suì* (生芥穗, raw schizonepeta spike). (Ed.)

CAUTION

Patients taking *jīng jiè* should not eat fish, crabs, globefish, or donkey meat.[11]

---

4. 防风 **Fáng Fēng**   Saposhnikoviae Radix
Saposhnikovia

Fáng fēng (saposhnikovia) is the most commonly used warm acrid sweat-promoting medicinal. It is combined with *jīng jiè* (schizonepeta) and *sū yè* (perilla leaf) to treat exterior patterns of wind-cold causing common cold. Compared to *jīng jiè*, *fáng fēng* more powerfully dispels wind and resolves the exterior to treat generalized pain; however, *jīng jiè* more effectively dispels wind, resolves the exterior, and promotes sweating.[12] In clinical practice, the two are often used together.

COMBINATIONS

Fáng fēng eliminates wind and dampness in the channels and network vessels and in the sinews and bones. It is used to treat wind-cold-damp impediment[552] (痹 *bì*), generalized joint pain, stiff neck and spine pain, and hypertonicity of the limbs. For this purpose it is combined with medicinals such as the following:

qiāng huó (羌活 notopterygium, Notopterygii Rhizoma et Radix)

dú huó (独活 pubescent angelica, Angelicae Pubescentis Radix)

dāng guī (当归 Chinese angelica, Angelicae Sinensis Radix)

yǐ mǐ (苡米 coix, Coicis Semen)[13]

wēi líng xiān (威灵仙 clematis, Clematidis Radix)

shēn jīn cǎo (伸筋草 ground pine, Lycopodii Herba)

jī xuè téng (鸡血藤 spatholobus, Spatholobi Caulis)

Fáng fēng is markedly effective in dispelling wind and resolving tetany[565] (痉 *jìng*). It is used to treat grinding of the teeth, hoisted eyes[552] (吊眼 *diào yǎn*), convulsions of the limbs and arched-back rigidity[542] (角弓反张 *jiǎo gōng fǎn zhāng*) caused by liver wind stirring internally or wind-phlegm harassing the upper body and for lockjaw[556] (破伤风 *pò shāng fēng*). For this purpose it is used with *quán xiē* (scorpion) since it can strengthen the latter's effect of dispelling wind and checking tetany[565] (痉 *jìng*). It is also combined with medicinals such as *gōu téng* (uncaria), *wú gōng* (centipede), *bái jiāng cán* (silkworm), and *bái fù zǐ* (typhonium).

Fáng fēng also enters the qì aspect of the liver channel; therefore it treats abdominal pain and diarrhea due to liver depression damaging the spleen. It is often

---

[11]According to the author, the caution about donkey meat is based on an incident reported in the literature in which accidental simultaneous ingestion of the two substances resulted in a toxic reaction. (Ed.)

[12]*Jīng jiè* (schizonepeta), being purely acrid, is excellent for resolving the exterior. *Fáng fēng* (saposhnikovia), on the other hand, is acrid and sweet and thus is less adept at resolving the exterior. From the earliest texts to the present time authors have extolled this medicinal's ability to dispel wind and relieve pain. Because of its moderate nature and flavor, it can be taken for the long periods of time necessary to treat an entrenched disorder such as impediment. (Ed.)

[13]*yǐ mǐ* 苡米 is another name for *yì yǐ rén* 薏苡仁.

combined with medicinals such as *bái zhú* (white atractylodes) and *bái sháo* (white peony). For example, *tòng xiè yào fāng* (Essential Formula for Painful Diarrhea)[14] is a formula used for this kind of illness.

Tòng xiè yào fāng 痛泻要方   Essential Formula for Painful Diarrhea

---

fáng fēng (防风 saposhnikovia, Saposhnikoviae Radix)

bái zhú (白术 white atractylodes, Atractylodis Macrocephalae Rhizoma)

bái sháo (白芍 white peony, Paeoniae Radix Alba)

chén pí (陈皮 tangerine peel, Citri Reticulatae Pericarpium)

Fáng fēng has the special effect of addressing bloody stool due to intestinal wind. In former times, persistent, recurrent descent of blood with the stool was attributed to wind evil in the large intestine. When treating this, the inclusion of *fáng fēng* (saposhnikovia) in the prescription invariably produces good results. It is often combined with *dì yú tàn* (charred sanguisorba), *huái jiǎo tàn* (charred sophora fruit), and *chǎo huái huā* (stir-fried sophora flower).

Fáng fēng is combined with *fù zǐ* (aconite) to reduce the toxicity of the latter. *Fáng fēng* is also combined with *huáng qí* (astragalus) to strengthen the effect of the latter.

Dosage

The dosage is generally 6–9 g/2–3 qián.

Caution

Inappropriate for headache due to yīn vacuity stirring fire.

---

5. 紫苏 Zǐ Sū   Perillae Folium,
Perilla   Caulis et Calyx

Including

  ▷ *Sū yè* (苏叶 perilla leaf, Perillae Folium)

  ▷ *Sū gěng* (苏梗 perilla stem, Perillae Caulis)

Zǐ sū (perilla) is warm and acrid; its qì is aromatic. It is mainly used to resolve the exterior and dissipate cold, but it also aromatically rectifies qì, and harmonizes the stomach and checks vomiting. It is often used to treat wind-cold common cold with vomiting, oppression in the chest, and stomach discomfort (commonly referred to in Chinese as 停食着凉 *tíng shí zháo liáng*, "catching a chill with food stoppage"). *Zǐ sū* is often combined with medicinals such as *huò xiāng* (agastache),

---

[14] This formula is from *Dān Xī Xīn Fǎ* (丹溪心法 "Dan Xī's Experiential Methods"). Zhū Dān-Xī (朱丹溪) recommends it for treating diarrhea accompanied by abdominal pain and suggests adding *shēng má* (cimicifuga) for chronic cases. In the original formula all the medicinals are stir-fried (*chǎo*) except *fáng fēng* (saposhnikovia). In modern clinical practice it is used to treat both chronic and acute enteritis. Note that this formula is also called *bái zhú sháo yào sǎn* (White Atractylodes and Peony Powder). (Ed.)

jīng jiè (schizonepeta), *fáng fēng* (saposhnikovia), *chén pí* (tangerine peel), and *shén qū* (medicated leaven), as in *huò xiāng zhèng qì sǎn* (Agastache Qì-Righting Powder). On the basis of modern clinical experience, this medicinal is often used to treat acute gastroenteritis.

COMPARISONS

Sū yè (perilla leaf) is used to resolve the exterior and dissipate cold. *Sū gěng* (perilla stem) is used to move qì and loosen the center. *Zǐ sū* (perilla) stem and leaf are used together to harmonize the stomach and check vomiting. *Sū zǐ* (perilla fruit)[216] is used to downbear qì and disperse phlegm (lightly stir-fry and crush).

Sū gěng (perilla stem) also has the effect of rectifying qì and quieting the fetus, and it is often used for vomiting or for abdominal distention in pregnancy.

Zǐ sū, which has aromatic qì, aromatically repels foulness, dispels summerheat and transforms turbidity, and resolves the toxin of fish and crabs; therefore it is also often used for summerheat-damp foul turbidity or poisoning from fish and crabs that results in oppression in the chest, vomiting, and abdominal pain.

Sū zǐ[216] has a strong qì-precipitating and phlegm-dispersing action and is effective in treating panting counterflow and phlegm cough. Nevertheless, it is contraindicated in cases of spleen-stomach qì vacuity with frequent diarrhea.

COMBINATIONS

Zǐ sū combined with *dú huó* (pubescent angelica), *cāng zhú* (atractylodes), and *bīng láng* (areca) treats **leg qì**[556] (脚气 *jiǎo qì*). Combined with *shēng shí gāo* (crude gypsum) and *bái zhǐ* (Dahurian angelica), it treats bad breath. Combined with *xiāng fù* (cyperus) and *má huáng* (ephedra), it promotes sweating and resolves the exterior.

DOSAGE

The usual dosage is 6–9 g/2–3 qián. When *sū yè* (perilla leaf) is included in a prescription, it is customary to specify "**add at end**"[542] (后下 *hòu xià*).

---

6. 羌活 Qiāng Huó
Notopterygium

Notopterygii Rhizoma
et Radix

Qiāng huó (notopterygium) has three main actions: 1) it resolves the exterior with warmth and acridity; 2) it dispels wind and overcomes dampness; and 3) it upbears the yáng qì of the greater yáng (*tài yáng*) channel and the governing vessel.

Qiāng huó is often used to treat exterior patterns of common cold due to wind-cold. It is markedly effective for cold body,[15] absence of sweating, and headache. Because it also overcomes dampness, it is effective for common cold complicated by dampness evil, which has signs such as aversion to cold, **heat effusion**[551] (发热 *fā rè*, i.e., fever), heavy body, joint pain, somnolence, and no desire to turn over in bed.

---

[15]Cold body, 身冷 *shēn lěng*: A subjective feeling of cold in the patient. To the physician, the body may feel hot. (Ed.)

Besides being used as a warm-acrid exterior-resolving medicinal, a major characteristic of *qiāng huó* is that it dispels wind-damp. It treats wind and dampness contending with each other that causes generalized joint pain, pain in the nape and neck, and pain and stiffness in the spine and back with excellent results. On the basis of experience, in modern practice it has been successfully used to treat rheumatic arthritis, rheumatic fever, and rheumatoid arthritis, often in combination with medicinals such as the following:

dú huó (独活 pubescent angelica, Angelicae Pubescentis Radix)

guì zhī (桂枝 cinnamon twig, Cinnamomi Ramulus)

chì sháo (赤芍 red peony, Paeoniae Radix Rubra)

hóng huā (红花 carthamus, Carthami Flos)

wēi líng xiān (威灵仙 clematis, Clematidis Radix)

fáng fēng (防风 saposhnikovia, Saposhnikoviae Radix)

fù zǐ (附子 aconite, Aconiti Radix Lateralis Praeparata)

zhī mǔ (知母 anemarrhena, Anemarrhenae Rhizoma)

yǐ mǐ (苡米 coix, Coicis Semen)

sōng jié (松节 knotty pine wood, Pini Nodi Lignum)

COMPARISONS

The wind-damp–dispelling action of *qiāng huó* is different from that of *dú huó* (pubescent angelica). *Qiāng huó* is often used for upper body wind-damp, being effective for pain in the spine, nape, head, and back. *Dú huó*,[447] on the other hand, tends to be used for lower body wind-damp, being effective for pain in the lumbus, thighs, lower legs, and feet.

Qiāng huó and *guì zhī* (cinnamon twig)[14] both dispel wind and dissipate cold. Nevertheless, *qiāng huó* more effectively dissipates wind-cold from the head, nape, spine, and back, while *guì zhī* more effectively dispels wind-cold from the shoulders, arms, and fingers.

COMBINATIONS

Combinations vary according to purpose: a) Combined with *piàn jiāng huáng* (sliced turmeric) and *guì zhī* (cinnamon twig), *qiāng huó* (notopterygium) treats wind-damp pain in the shoulder, arm, and hand. b) Combined with *jīng jiè* (schizonepeta) and *fáng fēng* (saposhnikovia), it treats wind-cold common cold with headache and absence of sweating; it is even more effective for pronounced pain in the back of the head. c) Combined with *cāng zhú* (atractylodes), it treats headache that feels as if the head were tightly wrapped (头痛如裹 *tóu tòng rú guǒ*). d) Combined with *jú huā* (chrysanthemum), *bái jí lí* (tribulus), and *màn jīng zǐ* (vitex), it treats red eyes due to contraction of wind.

Qiāng huó is also often used as a channel conductor to treat pain in the upper body or back of the head.

DOSAGE

The normal dose is 3–9 g/1–3 qián.

Caution

Qiāng huó is acrid, warm, drying, and harsh. It is contraindicated for generalized empty pain and for weakness and lack of strength due to blood vacuity.

7. 独活 Dú Huó Pubescent Angelica	Angelicae Pubescentis Radix

Dú huó (pubescent angelica)[16] is another warm, acrid, effusing, and dissipating medicinal. It treats headache, aversion to cold, heat effusion (fever), generalized pain, and aching pain in the lumbus and legs due to wind-cold common cold. Nevertheless, because it has the pronounced effect of dispelling wind and overcoming dampness, it is most commonly used for its wind-damp–dispelling effect in the treatment of impediment pain (痹痛 *bì tòng*), for which it is combined with medicinals such as:

wēi líng xiān (威灵仙 clematis, Clematidis Radix)

fáng fēng (防风 saposhnikovia, Saposhnikoviae Radix)

qín jiāo (秦艽 large gentian, Gentianae Macrophyllae Radix)

xī xiān cǎo (豨莶草 siegesbeckia, Siegesbeckiae Herba)

sōng jié (松节 knotty pine wood, Pini Nodi Lignum)

tòu gǔ cǎo (透骨草 speranskia/balsam, Speranskiae seu Impatientis Herba)

I often use it combined with medicinals such as *sāng jì shēng* (mistletoe), *xù duàn* (dipsacus), *bǔ gǔ zhī* (psoralea), *wēi líng xiān* (clematis), *niú xī* (achyranthes), *zé lán* (lycopus), *hóng huā* (carthamus), and *fù piàn* (sliced aconite) for effective treatment of rheumatic arthritis that manifests in vacuity cold. It is especially effective for lumbar and leg pain. The common method of use is as follows: *qiāng huó* (notopterygium)[19] for pronounced upper body pain; *dú huó* for lower body pain; *qiāng huó* and *dú huó* (pubescent angelica) combined for generalized pain. *Dú huó* is less effective than *qiāng huó* in effusing, dissipating, and resolving the exterior. Animal experiments have demonstrated the analgesic and anti-arthritic effects of this medicinal.

Combinations

Other important combinations are as follows: a) Combined with *xì xīn* (asarum), *dú huó* treats lesser yīn (*shào yīn*) headache, i.e., headache accompanied by dizzy vision and pain radiating into the teeth and cheeks, or pain on exposure to wind. b) Combined with *niú xī* (achyranthes), *mù guā* (chaenomeles), *cāng zhú* (atractylodes), *dì lóng* (earthworm), *wǔ jiā pí* (acanthopanax), and *xù duàn* (dipsacus), it treats wind-damp pain and limpness in the legs that makes walking difficult. c) Combined with *huáng bǎi tàn* (charred phellodendron), *xù duàn tàn* (charred dipsacus), and *sāng jì shēng* (mistletoe), it is also used to treat uterine bleeding.

---

[16]See more about *dú huó* (pubescent angelica) in Chapter 9, Miscellaneous Medicinals, page 447. (Ed.)

Dosage

The usual dosage is 6–9 g/2–3 qián; for strong individuals suffering from severe illness, one can use 12 g/4 qián. Used externally as a **steam-wash**[564] (熏洗剂 *xūn xǐ jì*) for wind-damp pain and joint pain, one can use up to 15–30 g/5 qián–1 liǎng. For this purpose it is often combined with medicinals such as:

guì zhī (桂枝 cinnamon twig, Cinnamomi Ramulus)

tòu gǔ cǎo (透骨草 speranskia/balsam, Speranskiae seu Impatientis Herba)

wū tóu (乌头 wild aconite, Aconiti Kusnezoffii Radix)

dāng guī (当归 Chinese angelica, Angelicae Sinensis Radix)

hóng huā (红花 carthamus, Carthami Flos)

fáng fēng (防风 saposhnikovia, Saposhnikoviae Radix)

shēng ài yè (生艾叶 raw mugwort, Artemisiae Argyi Folium Crudum)

Caution

This medicinal is inappropriate for blood vacuity headache, kidney vacuity lumbar pain, and insufficiency of yīn-liquid.

---

8. 白芷 Bái Zhǐ
Dahurian Angelica
Angelicae Dahuricae Radix

Bái zhǐ (dahurian angelica) is warm in nature and acrid in flavor. It has five major actions: 1) dissipating wind, 2) eliminating dampness, 3) freeing the orifices, 4) expelling pus, and 5) relieving pain.

1. Dissipating Wind: *Bái zhǐ* is a warm, acrid, effusing, and dissipating medicine that treats wind-cold common cold, especially with pronounced headache. It also treats itchy wind papules that come and go.

2. Eliminating Dampness: *Bái zhǐ* is aromatic, dry, and harsh. Being dry, it can overcome dampness; hence it has the effect of eliminating dampness. It is used to treat white vaginal discharge due to downpour of cold-damp. For this it is often combined with medicinals such as *cāng zhú* (atractylodes), *chǎo yǐ mǐ* (stir-fried coix), *fú líng* (poria), *shū bái pí* (ailanthus root bark), and *bái jī guān huā* (white cockscomb). It is also effective for treating enduring diarrhea due to spleen vacuity with exuberant dampness, for which it is combined with medicinals such as *ròu dòu kòu* (nutmeg), *hē zǐ* (chebule), *fú líng* (poria), and *qiàn shí* (euryale).

3. Freeing the Orifices: *Bái zhǐ* is acrid and aromatic, **mobile and penetrating**[557] (走窜 *zǒu cuàn*). It aromatically opens the orifices and is often used to free the nasal orifices for nasal congestion and for runny nose with fishy-smelling purulent nasal mucus (a condition traditionally called "**deep-source runny nose**,"[546] 鼻渊 *bí yuān*); it is frequently combined with medicinals such as *xì xīn* (asarum), *cāng ěr zǐ* (xanthium), *xīn yí* (magnolia flower), and *bò hé* (mint). In clinical practice, these medicinals are commonly varied in accordance with signs for various forms of acute and chronic sinusitis and rhinitis, and they always produce good results.

4. Expelling Pus: *Bái zhǐ* also disperses toxin and expels pus, engenders flesh, eliminates putridity, and engenders the new. It is combined with medicinals such as *dān pí* (moutan), *dōng guā zǐ* (wax gourd seed), *bài jiàng cǎo* (patrinia), *hóng téng* (sargentodoxa), and *shēng dà huáng* (raw rhubarb) to treat intestinal welling-abscess, i.e., conditions including acute appendicitis. Combined with *guā lóu* (trichosanthes), it treats mammary welling-abscess[557] (乳痈 *rǔ yōng*). It is often combined with medicinals such as *chì sháo* (red peony), *hóng huā* (carthamus), *pú gōng yīng* (dandelion), *dì dīng* (violet), *yě jú huā* (wild chrysanthemum flower), and *jīn yín huā* (lonicera) to treat welling-abscess (*yōng*) swellings and sores. A well-known formula for external medical conditions that includes *bái zhǐ* (Dahurian angelica) among its ingredients is *xiān fāng huó mìng yǐn* (Immortal Formula Life-Giving Beverage).[17]

Xiān fāng huó mìng yǐn 仙方活命饮   Immortal Formula Life-Giving Beverage

---

jīn yín huā (金银花 lonicera, Lonicerae Flos)

fáng fēng (防风 saposhnikovia, Saposhnikoviae Radix)

chì sháo (赤芍 red peony, Paeoniae Radix Rubra)

bèi mǔ (贝母 fritillaria, Fritillariae Bulbus)

shān jiǎ (山甲 pangolin scales, Manis Squama)

tiān huā fěn (天花粉 trichosanthes root, Trichosanthis Radix)

gān cǎo (甘草 licorice, Glycyrrhizae Radix)

rǔ xiāng (乳香 frankincense, Olibanum)

bái zhǐ (白芷 Dahurian angelica, Angelicae Dahuricae Radix)

mò yào (没药 myrrh, Myrrha)

zào jiǎo cì (皂角刺 gleditsia thorn, Gleditsiae Spina)

dāng guī wěi (当归尾 Chinese angelica tail, Angelicae Sinensis Radicis Extremitas)

chén pí (陈皮 tangerine peel, Citri Reticulatae Pericarpium)

5. Relieving Pain: *Bái zhǐ* is effective in treating various forms of headache, especially anterior headache or pain in the eyebrow bone. In addition to treating headache, it also treats toothache, stomach pain, and painful sores. Nevertheless, it is important to apply the principle of determining treatment in accordance with patterns identified and to vary medicinals according to signs.

Both *bái zhǐ* and *xì xīn* (asarum)[24] can relieve toothache, but *xì xīn* (asarum) tends to be used for pain in the tooth marrow or for toothache at night, while *bái zhǐ* treats pain and swelling of the gums stretching into the cheek.[18]

---

[17]This formula is also known as *zhēn rén huó mìng yǐn* (True Human Life-Giving Beverage). Modern texts ascribe this formula the following functions: clearing heat, resolving toxin, moving qì, quickening blood, dispersing swelling, and dispersing concretions. (Ed.)

[18]Because *xì xīn* (asarum) enters the kidney channel and the kidney governs the marrow, this medicinal is used for pain deep within the tooth. The gums, being fleshy, are governed by the yáng brightness (*yáng míng*) and therefore *bái zhǐ* (Dahurian angelica), which enters the yáng brightness (*yáng míng*), is used for pain in the gum or cheek. (Ed.)

In modern practice, *bái zhǐ* has been used to treat stomach pain due to ulcers. Besides relieving pain, it can engender flesh, eliminate putridity, and engender the new. Further investigation and observation is required to determine whether it is effective for stomach ulcers.

According to modern reports, this medicinal has an antibacterial and antimycotic effect. In small amounts, it can stimulate the medulla oblongata and the spinal nerves.

DOSAGE

The normal dosage is 3–9 g/1–3 qián.

CAUTION

Contraindicated in blood vacuity with heat or effulgent yīn vacuity fire. To avoid damaging qì and blood, it is generally not used for welling- or flat-abscesses (痈疽 *yōng jū*) that have already ruptured.

---

9. 藁本 Gǎo Běn   Ligustici Rhizoma
Chinese Lovage

Warm, acrid, effusing, and dissipating, *gǎo běn* (Chinese lovage) is mainly used for vertex headache in common cold due to wind-cold.

Gǎo běn dissipates governing vessel wind-cold, and since the vertex lies on the path of the governing vessel, this medicinal is effective in treating vertex headache. Other medicinals treat pain in other parts of the head: *qiāng huó* (notopterygium) dissipates greater yáng (*tài yáng*) channel wind-cold and is effective in treating posterior headache; *bái zhǐ* (Dahurian angelica) dissipates yáng brightness (*yáng míng*) channel wind-cold and is effective in treating anterior headache; *chuān xiōng* (chuanxiong) tracks down lesser yáng (*shào yáng*) channel wind evil, resolves lesser yáng (*shào yáng*) channel blood depression, and hence is effective in treating bilateral headache.

Gǎo běn goes directly to the vertex; thus it is a channel conductor for diseases of the vertex. Nevertheless, because the governing vessel and the kidney channel are connected, it also treats cold pain in the lumbar spine due to wind-cold invading the lumbus.

DOSAGE

The dosage is generally 1.5–10 g/5 fēn–3 qián.

---

10. 细辛 Xì Xīn   Asari Herba
Asarum

Warm and acrid, *xì xīn* (asarum) dissipates wind-cold. It is used for wind-cold common cold characterized by headache, aversion to cold, heat effusion (fever), and generalized joint pain. It is frequently combined with medicinals such as *jīng jiè* (schizonepeta), *fáng fēng* (saposhnikovia), *qiāng huó* (notopterygium), and *sū yè* (perilla leaf). This medicinal is upbearing and floating in nature; therefore it treats all wind diseases of the head and face.

The main action of *xì xīn* is to penetrate and outthrust stagnation. Acridity opens and frees, and *xì xīn* opens stagnant qì in the chest, unblocks the orifices of the lung, and frees the joints. It treats cough and counterflow qì ascent, cold phlegm panting and cough, tearing on exposure to wind, nasal congestion inhibiting the sense of smell, wind-cold impediment pain, and other related symptoms. Its acridity frees lung qì; hence it is also said to have the effect of "disinhibiting the waterways" (利水道 *lì shuǐ dào*).

COMBINATIONS

Xì xīn enters the heart, kidney, lung, and liver channels. a) Combined with *guì zhī* (cinnamon twig), *xiè bái* (Chinese chive), *dāng guī* (Chinese angelica), and *dān shēn* (salvia), it treats **chest impediment**[543] (胸痹 *xiōng bì*) and heart pain. b) With *dú huó* (pubescent angelica), *sāng jì shēng* (mistletoe), *xù duàn* (dipsacus), *wū yào* (lindera), and *dāng guī* (Chinese angelica), it treats pain in the lumbus, knees, and abdomen. c) With *gān jiāng* (dried ginger), *wǔ wèi zǐ* (schisandra), *bàn xià* (pinellia), *má huáng* (ephedra), and *xìng rén* (apricot kernel), it treats cough and panting due to cold rheum invading the lung.[19] d) With *dāng guī* (Chinese angelica), *chì sháo* (red peony), *chuān xiōng* (chuanxiong), *hóng huā* (carthamus), *bái zhǐ* (Dahurian angelica), and *guā lóu* (trichosanthes), it treats binding, pain, and distention in the breasts and absence of menstruation. e) With *cǎo jué míng* (fetid cassia), *shí jué míng* (abalone shell), *yáng gān* (goat's or sheep's liver), *mù zéi cǎo* (equisetum), and *xià kū cǎo* (prunella), it treats eye pain, itchy eyes, and tearing.

COMPARISONS

Cán shā (silkworm droppings) also frees congestion and stagnation, but it is used to dispel wind-damp stagnating in the flesh and causing pain. On the other hand, *xì xīn* mainly tracks down wind, damp, and cold evil stagnating in the liver and kidney, resulting in sinew and bone pain. It often produces good results in the treatment of chronic pain when added to appropriate formulas.

Dú huó (pubescent angelica) tracks down latent wind in the qì aspect of the kidney channel. *Xì xīn* tracks down wind-cold in the blood aspect of the liver-kidney.[20]

DOSAGE

The normal dosage of *xì xīn* is 1–3 g/3 fēn–1 qián, and generally no more than 3.2 g/1 qián. There is an old saying that "*xì xīn* should not exceed one qián" (3.125 g). Nevertheless, this really only applies to *xì xīn* taken on its own. When combined with other medicinals, the amount to be used depends on the presenting

---

[19]The combination just given is seen in *xiǎo qīng lóng tāng* (Minor Green-Blue Dragon Decoction).

[20]The references to wind in the qì aspect and the blood aspect are meant to illustrate that *xì xīn* (asarum) penetrates to a deeper level in the body than *dú huó* (pubescent angelica). (Ed.)

condition. In clinical practice, there are prescriptions that use up to 1.5 g/0.5 qián, 6 g/2 qián, or even 9 g/3 qián. However, one must decide the dosage only after careful evaluation of the patient's condition. One should not use large doses without careful consideration.

---

11. 辛夷 Xīn Yí   Magnoliae Flos
Magnolia Flower

Having an acrid flavor and warm qì, *xīn yí* (magnolia flower) dispels wind and frees the orifices and is particularly effective for freeing the nose and dispelling wind-cold. It is therefore often used to free the nasal orifices and is an important medicinal for treating diseases of the nose. For example, to treat nasal congestion due to wind-cold common cold, it is combined with *xì xīn* (asarum), *jīng jiè* (schizonepeta), *fáng fēng* (saposhnikovia), and *cāng ěr zǐ* (xanthium). For rhinitis or sinusitis, it is combined with *bái zhǐ* (Dahurian angelica), *xì xīn* (asarum), *cāng ěr zǐ* (xanthium), *chuān xiōng* (chuanxiong), *jú huā* (chrysanthemum), and *jīn yín huā* (lonicera). In clinical practice, it is used in accordance with signs to treat **deep-source runny nose**[546] 鼻渊 *bí yuān*), **sniveling nose**[564] (鼻鼽 *bí qiú*), **nose piles**[559] (鼻窒 *bí zhì*), sores in the nose, or general nasal congestion and runny nose.

Comparisons

Cāng ěr zǐ (xanthium)[27] also treats diseases of the nose, but tends to dissipate wind-damp from the head and treat headache due to head wind, whereas *xīn yí* (magnolia flower) tends to dissipate upper burner wind-cold and open and diffuse the orifices of the lung.

Xì xīn (asarum) is also an acrid, freeing, mobile, and penetrating medicinal that frees the qì of the whole body, but it tends to enter the heart and kidney channels. In contrast, *xīn yí*[26] mainly frees the qì of the upper burner, but combined with medicinals such as *sāng zhī* (mulberry twig), *guì zhī* (cinnamon twig), *sōng jié* (knotty pine wood), and *hóng huā* (carthamus), it also frees the joints.

Bái zhǐ (dahurian angelica)[22] is also an aromatic orifice-freeing medicinal, but it mainly dissipates wind-cold in the head, and treats anterior headache and nasal congestion. *Xīn yí* is effective in dissipating upper burner wind-cold, diffusing the lung, and freeing the nasal orifices.

Special Uses

Xīn yí combined with *é bù shí cǎo* (centipeda), *cāng ěr zǐ* (xanthium), *bái zhǐ* (Dahurian angelica), *bò hé* (mint), and *méi piàn* (borneol), ground to a fine powder, and placed into the nose in small quantities treats conditions such as nasal congestion inhibiting the sense of smell, rhinitis, and sinusitis.[21]

---

[21] This combination of medicinals is often wrapped in gauze and placed in the nose (usually alternating nostrils on alternate nights). Alternatively, the powder can be dabbed directly into the vestibule of the nose. (Ed.)

Dosage

For internal use, the dosage for *xīn yí* (magnolia flower) is generally 6–10 g/ 2–3 qián.

Caution

Contraindicated in effulgent yīn vacuity fire.

12. 苍耳子 Cāng Ěr Zǐ   Xanthii Fructus
Xanthium

Sweet in flavor and warm in nature, *cāng ěr zǐ* (xanthium) dispels wind, frees the orifices, and dissipates binds. In clinical practice, it is commonly used for the three purposes below.

1. Dispelling Wind-Damp: *Cāng ěr zǐ* treats **generalized impediment**[551] (周 痹 *zhōu bì*) and hypertonicity of the limbs due to wind-damp. For this it is often combined with medicinals such as *qiāng huó* (notopterygium), *tòu gǔ cǎo* (speranskia/balsam), *wēi líng xiān* (clematis), and *yǐ mǐ* (coix). This medicinal is effective for freeing the vertex and the brain; therefore it is also effective for wind-damp headache.

2. Freeing the Orifices of the Lung: *Cāng ěr zǐ* is used to treat nasal congestion, rhinitis, sinusitis, and incessantly runny nose. For this it is frequently combined with:

xīn yí (辛夷 magnolia flower, Magnoliae Flos)
bái zhǐ (白芷 Dahurian angelica, Angelicae Dahuricae Radix)
xì xīn (细辛 asarum, Asari Herba)
chuān xiōng (川芎 chuanxiong, Chuanxiong Rhizoma)
jú huā (菊花 chrysanthemum, Chrysanthemi Flos)

3. Skin Diseases: *Cāng ěr zǐ* dispels wind, relieves itching, and dissipates binds. It is used to treat all forms of **scab**[561] (疥 *jiè*), **lichen**[556] (癣 *xiǎn*), **itchy papules**[554] (痒疹 *yǎng zhěn*), and **numbing wind**[559] (麻风 *má fēng*, i.e., leprosy).

In addition, *cāng ěr zǐ* that is freshly harvested in the autumn with its stems and leaves can be cut up and boiled in water to make a paste, which is strained off, smeared on cloth, and applied to the umbilicus and fontanel gate (anterior fontanel) regions; this treats child gān disease characterized by an enlarged abdomen, yellowing, emaciation, lack of spirit in the eyes, and indigestion. The plaster is also applied to scrofula, boils, and **toxin swellings**[566] (肿毒 *zhǒng dú*), because it disperses scrofula, swellings (as in tuberculosis of the lymph nodes), and sore-toxin.

Dosage

The dosage is generally 6–9 g/2–3 qián. This medicinal possesses minor toxicity and should not be used in large quantities.

13. 香薷 Xiāng Rú
Mosla
Moslae Herba

Acrid in flavor and slightly warm in nature, *xiāng rú* (mosla) resolves the exterior, dispels summerheat and transforms dampness, and disinhibits water and disperses swelling. It mainly treats exterior patterns of summer colds and summerheat-damp with signs such as aversion to cold and heat effusion (fever), headache, absence of sweating, generalized pain, or abdominal pain, and vomiting and diarrhea. It is often combined for this purpose with medicinals such as *hé yè* (lotus leaf), *bái biǎn dòu* (lablab), *pèi lán* (eupatorium), and *huò xiāng* (agastache). It also treats water-damp, puffy swelling, and inhibited urination (e.g., edema of acute nephritis). For this it is often combined with *bái zhú* (white atractylodes).

Comparisons

Xiāng rú dispels summerheat by disinhibiting damp turbidity. In comparison, *bái biǎn dòu* (lablab)[104] disperses summerheat by fortifying the spleen and transforming dampness, and *hé yè* (lotus leaf) disperses summerheat by upbearing and outthrusting clear qì.

Má huáng (ephedra)[11] resolves the exterior in the treatment of exterior patterns due to cold damage in winter, whereas *xiāng rú* resolves the exterior in the treatment of exterior patterns due to summerheat damage in summer.

Dosage

The dosage is generally 3–6 g/1–2 qián. One can use up to 9 g/3 qián for severe illness in strong patients.

Caution

Contraindicated in patients with a weak constitution who are susceptible to vacuity sweating.

14. 生姜 Shēng Jiāng
Fresh Ginger
Zingiberis Rhizoma Recens

Including
  ▷ *Shēng jiāng zhī* (生姜汁 ginger juice, Zingiberis Rhizomatis Succus)
  ▷ *Shēng jiāng pí* (生姜皮 ginger skin, Zingiberis Rhizomatis Cortex)
  ▷ *Wēi jiāng* (煨姜 roasted ginger, Zingiberis Rhizoma Tostum)
See also
  ▷ *Gān jiāng* (干姜 dried ginger, Zingiberis Rhizoma)[348]

Acrid in flavor and slightly warm in nature, *shēng jiāng* (fresh ginger) is often used for wind-cold common cold in formulas that resolve the exterior, promote sweating, and dissipate wind-cold. It is combined with medicinals such as *má huáng* (ephedra), *jīng jiè* (schizonepeta), *guì zhī* (cinnamon twig), and *sū yè* (perilla leaf).

Shēng jiāng is also used on its own, sliced or crushed, and boiled with an appropriate quantity of *hóng táng* (brown sugar) to treat wind-cold common cold. Physicians of former times said *shēng jiāng* "moves in the yáng aspect, effuses the exterior, and dissipates cold; it diffuses lung qì, resolves depression and regulates the center; it stimulates the appetite, opens phlegm, and makes food go down." This description is worth bearing in mind.

Shēng jiāng combined with *bàn xià* (pinellia) has a distinct capacity to harmonize the stomach and check vomiting; moreover, the toxicity of *bàn xià* is resolved by this combination. *Shēng jiāng* also resolves the toxin of *tiān nán xīng* (arisaema).

Shēng jiāng combined with *dà zǎo* (jujube) boosts the spleen and stomach and original qì, as well as warming the center and dispelling dampness. Combined with *bái sháo* (white peony), it restrains the latter's coldness, warms the channels, and relieves pain.

Comparisons

Shēng jiāng zhī (生姜汁, ginger juice) transforms phlegm and checks retching. It is used for wind-phlegm clenched jaw preventing speech and for hemiplegia from wind-phlegm obstructing the channels and network vessels. For this purpose, it is often combined with *zhú lì zhī* (bamboo sap). Add 31 g/1 liǎng of *zhú lì zhī* to six or seven drops of *shēng jiāng zhī* (ginger juice) and divide into two doses.[22]

Gān jiāng (dried ginger)[348] warms the center and dispels cold, and warms the lung and transforms rheum. *Pào jiāng* (炮姜, blast-fried ginger)[23] warms the channels and stanches bleeding. *Shēng jiāng* (fresh ginger) dissipates wind-cold and checks retching. *Wēi jiāng* (roasted ginger)[24] treats abdominal pain due to stomach cold; it harmonizes the center and checks retching, but is not as drying as *gān jiāng* and not as dissipating as *shēng jiāng*. It is important to select the right form for each condition.

Shēng jiāng pí (生姜皮, ginger skin) moves water qì to disperse puffy swelling. For this purpose it is combined with medicinals such as *dōng guā pí* (wax gourd rind), *dà fù pí* (areca husk), *sāng bái pí* (mulberry root bark), *zhū líng* (polyporus), and *fú líng* (poria).

Dosage

The dosage of *shēng jiāng* (fresh ginger) is generally two or three slices, or 3–9 g/ 1 qián–3 qián. The dosage for each of *gān jiāng* (dried ginger), *wēi jiāng* (roasted ginger), and *pào jiāng* (blast-fried ginger) is generally 1.5–6 g/5 fēn–2 qián. Under special circumstances, one can use 9–12 g/3–4 qián. The dosage for *shēng jiāng pí*

---

[22] *Zhú lì zhī* (竹沥汁, bamboo sap), which is a liquid, is not readily available in the West. It can be found in China packaged in vials. *Tiān zhú huáng* (天竹黄, bamboo sugar) is the most common substitute. (Ed.)

[23] *Pào jiāng* (炮姜, blast-fried ginger) is made by stir-frying *gān jiāng* (dried ginger) vigorously in an iron wok over a fierce fire until the decocting pieces give off smoke and their surfaces become scorched, swollen, and cracked. (Ed.)

[24] *Wēi jiāng* (煨姜, roasted ginger) is prepared by wrapping *shēng jiāng* (fresh ginger) in paper and placing it in glowing embers. When the paper is charred, the wrapped *shēng jiāng* is withdrawn from the embers, the paper removed, and the ginger sliced. (Ed.)

(ginger skin) is 1–4.5 g/3 fēn–1.5 qián. The dosage for *shēng jiāng* should not be excessive since it can stimulate the kidney and cause inflammation.

---

15. 薄荷 Bò Hé
Mint   Menthae Herba

Bò hé (mint) is chiefly used as a cool, acrid, exterior-resolving medicinal. Cool in nature and acrid in flavor, it promotes sweating and is often used to treat wind-heat common cold with symptoms such as dizzy head, headache, and sore swollen throat. It is often combined with medicinals such as:

jīng jiè (荆芥 schizonepeta, Schizonepetae Herba)

jīn yín huā (金银花 lonicera, Lonicerae Flos)

sāng yè (桑叶 mulberry leaf, Mori Folium)

jú huā (菊花 chrysanthemum, Chrysanthemi Flos)

The wind-heat–dissipating action of *bò hé* makes it effective for wind papules, itchy papules, and measles caused by wind-heat. For this purpose it is often combined with medicinals such as:

lián qiáo (连翘 forsythia, Forsythiae Fructus)

chì sháo (赤芍 red peony, Paeoniae Radix Rubra)

bái xiǎn pí (白藓皮 dictamnus, Dictamni Cortex)

kǔ shēn (苦参 flavescent sophora, Sophorae Flavescentis Radix)

chán tuì (蝉蜕 cicada molting, Cicadae Periostracum)

Bò hé also clears the liver and **brightens the eyes**[543] (明目 *míng mù*). It is used for symptoms such as sore red swollen eyes, blurred vision, headache, and dizzy head caused by liver depression transforming into fire. For this purpose it is frequently combined with medicinals such as *jú huā* (chrysanthemum) and *dōng sāng yè* (frostbitten mulberry leaf).[25]

Most people are aware that the main effects of *bò hé* are to dissipate wind-heat, and to clear the liver and brighten the eyes, but fail to observe that it disperses food and precipitates qì, disperses distention, and treats sudden turmoil (cholera) with vomiting and diarrhea. In these situations it is frequently combined with medicinals such as *mù xiāng* (costusroot), *bīng láng* (areca), *dà fù pí* (areca husk), *jiāo sān xiān* (scorch-fried three immortals),[26] and *cǎo dòu kòu* (Katsumada's galangal seed).

COMBINATIONS

Bò hé combined with *dì gǔ pí* (lycium root bark), *yín chái hú* (stellaria), and *qín jiāo* (large gentian) abates steaming bone consumptive heat (fever); combined

---

[25] *Dōng sāng yè* 冬桑叶 (literally, winter mulberry leaf) refers to the leaves that are picked just after the first frost. This medicinal is sometimes called *shuāng sāng yè* 霜桑叶 (literally, frost mulberry leaf). (Ed.)

[26] The three immortals are *mài yá* (barley sprout), *shén qū* (medicated leaven), and *shān zhā* (crataegus). (Ed.)

with *sāng bái pí* (mulberry root bark), it drains lung heat; combined with *sì wù tāng* (Four Agents Decoction), it regulates menstruation and normalizes qì.

Sì wù tāng 四物汤	Four Agents Decoction

dì huáng (地黄 rehmannia, Rehmanniae Radix)

dāng guī (当归 Chinese angelica, Angelicae Sinensis Radix)

bái sháo (白芍 white peony, Paeoniae Radix Alba)

chuān xiōng (川芎 chuanxiong, Chuanxiong Rhizoma)

In *xiāo yáo sǎn* (Free Wanderer Powder), *bò hé* helps to dissipate depression and regulate qì.

Xiāo yáo sǎn 逍遥散	Free Wanderer Powder

chái hú (柴胡 bupleurum, Bupleuri Radix)

bái zhú (白术 white atractylodes, Atractylodis Macrocephalae Rhizoma)

fú líng (茯苓 poria, Poria)

dāng guī (当归 Chinese angelica, Angelicae Sinensis Radix)

bái sháo (白芍 white peony, Paeoniae Radix Alba)

zhì gān cǎo (炙甘草 mix-fried licorice, Glycyrrhizae Radix cum Liquido Fricta)

chén pí (陈皮 tangerine peel, Citri Reticulatae Pericarpium)

bò hé (薄荷 mint, Menthae Herba)

wēi jiāng (煨姜 roasted ginger, Zingiberis Rhizoma Tostum)

Comparisons

Sāng yè (mulberry leaf) and *bò hé* are both often used as wind-coursing and heat-clearing medicinals, but *sāng yè* (mulberry leaf) tends to cool the blood and clear heat and to course wind and brighten the eyes, while *bò hé* tends to enter the qì aspect and has a powerful cool-acrid resolving and dissipating action.

Bò hé (mint) is not used in enduring illness or after major illness since it can cause incessant sweating.

Dosage

Generally the dosage is 1.5–6 g/5 fēn–2 qián. In severe illness, one can use 9 g/3 qián.

16. 菊花 Jú Huā   Chrysanthemi Flos
Chrysanthemum

Sweet, bitter, and slightly cold, *jú huā* (chrysanthemum) courses wind and dissipates heat. It is often used at the onset of wind-warmth or for wind-heat common cold with symptoms such as headache and red eyes.

Jú huā is a commonly used medicinal in opthalmology. It is used to treat liver channel wind-heat with sore, red, and swollen eyes, clouded and flowery vision, tearing on exposure to wind, and **nebulous eye screens**[558] (目生云翳 *mù shēng yún yì*), for which it has the effect of clearing and disinhibiting the head and eyes. It is often combined with medicinals such as the following:

huáng qín (黄芩 scutellaria, Scutellariae Radix)

mì méng huā (密蒙花 buddleia, Buddleja Flos)

cǎo jué míng (草决明 fetid cassia, Cassiae Semen)

qīng xiāng zǐ (青葙子 celosia, Celosiae Semen)

mù zéi cǎo (木贼草 equisetum, Equiseti Hiemalis Herba)

sāng yè (桑叶 mulberry leaf, Mori Folium)

chán tuì (蝉蜕 cicada molting, Cicadae Periostracum)

It is also effective for dizzy head and headache due to ascendant hyperactivity of liver yáng and liver wind harassing the upper body. For this it is often combined with medicinals such as:

shēng shí jué míng (生石决明 crude abalone shell, Haliotidis Concha Cruda)

bái jí lí (白蒺藜 tribulus, Tribuli Fructus)

shēng dì huáng (生地黄 dried/fresh rehmannia, Rehmanniae Radix Exsiccata seu Recens)

bái sháo (白芍 white peony, Paeoniae Radix Alba)

màn jīng zǐ (蔓荆子 vitex, Viticis Fructus)

COMPARISON

Both *jú huā* and *bò hé* (mint)[30] dissipate wind-heat and clear the head and eyes, but *bò hé* tends to effuse and dissipate, and its cool, acrid sweat-promoting action is greater than that of *jú huā*. *Jú huā* tends to clear liver heat and dispel liver wind as well as to nourish the liver and brighten the eyes; it can therefore be frequently used. *Bò hé*, however, has no liver-nourishing effect, and should not be taken for extended periods.

MISCELLANEOUS

Jú huā also has a heat-clearing, toxin resolving action that makes it suitable for the treatment of swollen clove sores and sore-toxin; it is commonly used in external medicine. It is generally combined with medicinals such as *jīn yín huā* (lonicera), *lián qiáo* (forsythia), *pú gōng yīng* (dandelion), and *dì dīng* (violet). In this application, *yě jú huā* (wild chrysanthemum flower) is often used.[27]

DOSAGE

The dosage for *jú huā* is generally 6–9 g/2–3 qián. Under special circumstances one can use up to 12 g/4 qián or 15 g/5 qián.

---

[27]This application of *yě jú huā* (wild chrysanthemum flower) is usually in the form of a wash or compress. (Ed.)

17. 牛蒡子 Niú Bàng Zǐ   Arctii Fructus
Arctium

Acrid and bitter in flavor and cool in nature, *niú bàng zǐ* (arctium) dissipates wind and eliminates heat, diffuses the lung and outthrusts papules, and clears heat and resolves toxin.

Niú bàng zǐ combined with medicinals such as *sāng yè* (mulberry leaf), *jú huā* (chrysanthemum), *jīn yín huā* (lonicera), and *bò hé* (mint) treats exterior patterns at the onset of wind-heat common cold and warm disease, especially when they manifest in cough, sore throat, and itchy throat.

In children suffering from measles, signs of depressed heat in the lung channel, such as cough, red sore throat, and noneruption of measles papules, can be treated with *niú bàng zǐ* to diffuse the lung and outthrust papules. For this purpose it is commonly combined with medicinals such as:

jīng jiè (荆芥 schizonepeta, Schizonepetae Herba)

lú gēn (芦根 phragmites, Phragmitis Rhizoma)

huáng qín (黄芩 scutellaria, Scutellariae Radix)

chán tuì (蝉蜕 cicada molting, Cicadae Periostracum)

gé gēn (葛根 pueraria, Puerariae Radix)

jié gěng (桔梗 platycodon, Platycodonis Radix)

bò hé (薄荷 mint, Menthae Herba)

Niú bàng zǐ clears heat and resolves toxin. It is often used for sore, red, swollen throat, as in conditions such as acute tonsillitis, laryngitis, and pharyngitis. For this it can be combined with medicinals such as *shān dòu gēn* (bushy sophora), *xuán shēn* (scrophularia), *jié gěng* (platycodon), *gān cǎo* (licorice), and *huáng qín* (scutellaria). It is also combined with medicinals such as *jīn yín huā* (lonicera), *lián qiáo* (forsythia), *kǔ shēn* (flavescent sophora), *dāng guī wěi* (Chinese angelica tail), and *chì sháo* (red peony) to treat swelling and sore-toxin and to accelerate dispersion of welling-abscesses.

Niú bàng zǐ is also known for its effect of disinhibiting congealed stagnant qì in the lumbus and knees. It is combined with *xù duàn* (dipsacus) and *niú xī* (achyranthes) for migratory pain in the lumbus and knees due to qì stagnation.

DOSAGE

The normal dosage is 3–9 g/1–3 qián.

CAUTION

This medicinal should not be used in patients with spleen-stomach vacuity cold who normally suffer from diarrhea.

18. 蔓荆子 Màn Jīng Zǐ   Viticis Fructus
Vitex

Cool in nature and acrid in flavor, *màn jīng zǐ* (vitex) is mainly used to dissipate wind and clear heat, to cool the liver and brighten the eyes, and to treat headache.

Màn jīng zǐ combined with medicinals such as *jīng jiè* (schizonepeta), *bò hé* (mint), *jú huā* (chrysanthemum), and *niú bàng zǐ* (arctium) treats symptoms such as headache, heat effusion (fever), eye pain, and swollen face due to contraction of wind-heat, for which it has a cool acrid heat-dissipating effect.

This medicinal dissipates wind-heat in the upper body. It therefore treats any sign due to wind-heat invading the upper body, such as headache, red eyes, or clouded vision. For this purpose it is combined with medicinals such as:

sāng yè (桑叶 mulberry leaf, Mori Folium)

jú huā (菊花 chrysanthemum, Chrysanthemi Flos)

cǎo jué míng (草决明 fetid cassia, Cassiae Semen)

qīng xiāng zǐ (青葙子 celosia, Celosiae Semen)

bò hé (薄荷 mint, Menthae Herba)

The greatest feature of *màn jīng zǐ* is its ability to dissipate wind-heat in the head and treat headache. It is especially effective for pain near the Greater Yáng point (太阳穴 *tài yáng xuè*, i.e., in the region of the temples). In clinical practice, it is often combined with *jīng jiè* (schizonepeta), *fáng fēng* (saposhnikovia), *jú huā* (chrysanthemum), and *bái jí lí* (tribulus). Used singly and steeped in liquor to make a medicinal wine, it treats chronic headache. Combined with medicinals that nourish the blood and dispel wind, such as *dāng guī* (Chinese angelica), *chuān xiōng* (chuanxiong), *bái sháo* (white peony), *shú dì huáng* (cooked rehmannia), *qiāng huó* (notopterygium), and *fáng fēng* (saposhnikovia), it is also used to treat head-wind headache.

Comparisons

Gǎo běn (Chinese lovage)[24] is often used to treat wind-cold headache and *bái zhǐ* (Dahurian angelica)[22] is often used to treat wind-damp headache. *Màn jīng zǐ* is often used to treat wind-heat headache.

Bái jí lí (tribulus)[474] tends to be used to treat dizziness and headache due to upward harassment of liver wind. *Màn jīng zǐ* tends to be used for upward attack of wind-heat that results in heaviness, clouding, and oppression of the head, as well as headache.

Dosage

4.5–9 g/1.5 qián–3 qián.

Caution

Contraindicated for headache or eye pain due to blood vacuity.

19. 浮萍 Fú Píng   Spirodelae Herba
Duckweed

Fú píng (duckweed)[28] is a cold, acrid medicinal that promotes sweating. It is light, floating, upbearing, and dissipating and can be used for wind-heat exterior patterns characterized by heat effusion (fever), headache, absence of sweating, thirst, sore pharynx, and a rapid floating pulse, especially when ordinary cool, acrid, exterior-resolving formulas fail to promote sweating. To this end, it is combined with medicinals such as *bò hé* (mint), *huáng qín* (scutellaria), *jīng jiè* (schizonepeta), *xìng rén* (apricot kernel), and *dàn dòu chǐ* (fermented soybean (unsalted)). Because *fú píng* courses wind and dissipates heat, and outthrusts the fleshy exterior, it is often used to treat heat evil depressed in the fleshy exterior causing noneruption of measles. For this it is combined with medicinals such as *niú bàng zǐ* (arctium), *chán tuì* (cicada molting), *bò hé* (mint), and *gé gēn* (pueraria). It is also used to treat wind-heat **dormant papules**[546] (癮疹 *yǐn zhěn*).

Besides dissipating heat with cold and acridity, *fú píng* also diffuses the lung and disinhibits water to disperse water swelling. It is suitable for generalized water swelling with heat effusion (fever), as observed in acute nephritis, for example.

Dosage
The normal dosage is 1.5–6 g/5 fēn–2 qián. In severe illness, one can use up to 9 g/3 qián. Fresh *fú píng*[29] is used in dosages of 9–15 g/3–5 qián and is added to the decoction at the end.

Caution
Contraindicated in patients with weak constitution and spontaneous sweating.

20. 蝉蜕 Chán Tuì   Cicadae Periostracum
Cicada Molting

Also called *chán yī* 蝉衣. *Chán tuì* (cicada molting) is salty and cold, and has the following four major actions.

1. **Dissipating Wind-Heat:** *Chán tuì* (cicada molting) is suitable for externally contracted wind-heat and the initial stage of warm disease. For this purpose it is often combined with medicinals such as *jīn yín huā* (lonicera), *lián qiáo* (forsythia), *bò hé* (mint), and *jú huā* (chrysanthemum). It is particularly effective when there is concurrent loss of voice or sore throat, for which it is combined

---

[28]The correct plant is *Spirodela polyrrhiza*. It is the small round leaf (2–5 mm in diameter) found floating on the surface of many ponds and lakes. Often in the West this medicinal is substituted for by the large-leafed (2–10 cm long) plant *Pistia stratiotes*. Another substitute that closely resembles *Spirodela polyrrhiza* is *Lemna minor*, which is brownish in color and has only one root descending from the leaf, whereas *Spirodela polyrrhiza* is green and has many fine root hairs descending into the water from the leaf.

[29]Fresh duckweed in this context means the freshly-picked plant.

with medicinals such as *jié gěng* (platycodon), *pàng dà hài* (sterculia), and *shè gān* (belamcanda).

2. **Outthrusting Measles:** *Chán tuì* is suitable for measles in children with heat effusion (fever) and noneruption of papules. It dissipates heat and outthrusts papules, and prevents heat toxin from falling inward. For this purpose it is often combined with medicinals such as:

niú bàng zǐ (牛蒡子 arctium, Arctii Fructus)

jīn yín huā (金银花 lonicera, Lonicerae Flos)

bò hé (薄荷 mint, Menthae Herba)

lú gēn (芦根 phragmites, Phragmitis Rhizoma)

gé gēn (葛根 pueraria, Puerariae Radix)

Combined with medicinals such as *fáng fēng* (saposhnikovia), *jīng jiè* (schizonepeta), *fú píng* (duckweed), *bái xiǎn pí* (dictamnus), and *chì sháo* (red peony), it is also used to treat wind papules (urticaria).

3. **Dispelling Wind and Resolving Tetany**[565]: *Chán tuì* is suitable for lockjaw, high fever with fright reversal, and facial paralysis (Bell's palsy). In such cases it dispels wind and stops convulsions, and relieves spasm. For this it is often combined with medicinals such as *quán xiē* (scorpion), *gōu téng* (uncaria), *wú gōng* (centipede), and *bái jiāng cán* (silkworm). It is also often used for wind strike with loss of voice. It is added to formulas that eliminate wind, quicken the network vessels, and open the orifices.

4. **Abating Screens and Brightening the Eyes:** This medicinal is suitable for wind-heat attacking the eyes, causing red eyes, clouded vision, or **nebulous eye screens**[558] (目生云翳 *mù shēng yún yì*). For this purpose it is often combined with medicinals such as:

jú huā (菊花 chrysanthemum, Chrysanthemi Flos)

mù zéi cǎo (木贼草 equisetum, Equiseti Hiemalis Herba)

sāng yè (桑叶 mulberry leaf, Mori Folium)

cǎo jué míng (草决明 fetid cassia, Cassiae Semen)

màn jīng zǐ (蔓荆子 vitex, Viticis Fructus)

COMPARISONS

Chán tuì is effective in dissipating wind-heat, eliminating eye screens, outthrusting papules, and in dispelling wind and resolving **tetany**[565] (痉 *jìng*). *Shé tuì* (snake slough), which possesses minor toxicity, is effective in eliminating wind evil and abating eye screens. It is mostly used for skin diseases such as **scab**[561] (疥 *jiè*), **lichen**[556] (癣 *xiǎn*), and itching.

SPECIAL USES

This medicinal also has the effect of stopping night crying in infants. I frequently add 1.5–6 g/5 fēn–3 qián to formulas that harmonize the stomach, disperse food, and clear heat, and it is invariably effective for incessant night crying in infants.

DOSAGE

Generally the dosage is 2.5–6 g/8 fēn–2 qián. Strong patients with exuberant evil are given up to 10 g/3 qián. For lockjaw, one can use up to 25–30 g/8 qián–1 liǎng, or even more. One must consider the specific situation and decide.

Caution

Chán tuì should not be used in vacuity patterns, pregnancy,[30] or the absence of wind-heat.

---

21. 柴胡 Chái Hú   Bupleuri Radix
Bupleurum

Bitter in flavor and neutral in nature,[31] *chái hú* (bupleurum) harmonizes the lesser yáng (*shào yáng*) (effuses the exterior and harmonizes the interior), courses the liver and resolves depression, and abates heat and upbears yáng. It is often used in the following applications:

1. **Harmonizing the Lesser Yáng:** *Chái hú* causes externally contracted evils that have penetrated midway from the exterior into the interior to pass out through the exterior. This effect is called "effusing the exterior and harmonizing the interior" (发表和里 *fā biǎo hé lǐ*). Since the position half-interior half-exterior corresponds to the lesser yáng (*shào yáng*) among the channels, this effect is also, and more commonly, called "harmonizing the lesser yáng (*shào yáng*)" (和解少阳 *hé jiě shào yáng*). The classical signs observed when the evil is half in the interior and half in the exterior are **alternating cold and heat**[542] (寒热往来 *hán rè wǎng lái*, i.e., the patient subjectively feels hot for a time and then cold), fullness in the chest and rib-side, bitter taste in the mouth and dry pharynx, poor appetite, vexation with desire to vomit, a thin white tongue fur, and a stringlike pulse. When one sees these signs, use *chái hú* in formulas such as *xiǎo chái hú tāng* (Minor Bupleurum Decoction).

Xiǎo chái hú tāng 小柴胡汤   Minor Bupleurum Decoction

chái hú (柴胡 bupleurum, Bupleuri Radix)

huáng qín (黄芩 scutellaria, Scutellariae Radix)

bàn xià (半夏 pinellia, Pinelliae Rhizoma)

dǎng shēn (党参 codonopsis, Codonopsis Radix)

gān cǎo (甘草 licorice, Glycyrrhizae Radix)

shēng jiāng (生姜 fresh ginger, Zingiberis Rhizoma Recens)

dà zǎo (大枣 jujube, Jujubae Fructus)

---

[30]The prohibition against *chán tuì* being used during pregnancy can be traced to the Táng Dynasty. In the *Míng Yī Bié Lù* (名医别录 "Other Records of Famous Physicians"), this medicinal is recommended as one for helping the fetus to descend during a difficult delivery. Later texts do not mention this function, but do include a caution about using it during pregnancy. (Ed.)

[31]Some texts describe *chái hú* as being slightly cold and slightly acrid. This places it in the category of cool-acrid exterior-resolving medicinals. There are several species of *Bupleurum* used medicinally; this may help to explain why authors differ about its flavor and nature. (Ed.)

For patients with thirst, remove *bàn xià* (pinellia) and add *tiān huā fěn* (trichosanthes root). For strong patients who have not been ill for long and whose right qì is not yet vacuous, remove *dǎng shēn* (codonopsis). For cough, remove *dǎng shēn* (codonopsis) and add *wǔ wèi zǐ* (schisandra) and *gān jiāng* (dried ginger). For dry mouth and tongue with scant liquid, add *shēng shí gāo* (crude gypsum), and so forth.

In acute febrile diseases, such as influenza, acute urinary infection, acute tonsillitis, and lobar pneumonia, when I observe alternating cold and heat, fullness in the chest and rib-side, bitter taste in the mouth and dry pharynx, vexation and frequent retching, and a stringlike pulse, I usually use *xiǎo chái hú tāng* (Minor Bupleurum Decoction) varied according to signs. In flu, for example, I remove the *dǎng shēn* (codonopsis) and add *jīng jiè* (schizonepeta), *bò hé* (mint), and *jīn yín huā* (lonicera). For acute urinary infections, I remove the *dǎng shēn* (codonopsis), *shēng jiāng* (fresh ginger), and *dà zǎo* (jujube) and add:

> *huáng bǎi* (黄柏 phellodendron, Phellodendri Cortex)
> *zhū líng* (猪苓 polyporus, Polyporus)
> *zé xiè* (泽泻 alisma, Alismatis Rhizoma)
> *mù tōng* (木通 trifoliate akebia, Akebiae Trifoliatae Caulis)

In acute tonsillitis, I remove *dǎng shēn* (codonopsis), *shēng jiāng* (fresh ginger), and *dà zǎo* (jujube) and add:

> *shān dòu gēn* (山豆根 bushy sophora, Sophorae Tonkinensis Radix)
> *shè gān* (射干 belamcanda, Belamcandae Rhizoma)
> *bò hé* (薄荷 mint, Menthae Herba)
> *jīn yín huā* (金银花 lonicera, Lonicerae Flos)
> *jǐn dēng lóng* (锦灯笼 lantern plant calyx, Physalis Calyx seu Fructus)[32]
> *xuán shēn* (玄参 scrophularia, Scrophulariae Radix)[33]

When treating lobar pneumonia, I remove *dǎng shēn* (codonopsis) and add *jīng jiè* (schizonepeta), *bò hé* (mint), *jīn yín huā* (lonicera), and *lián qiáo* (forsythia). I invariably get good results with these variations.

2. Coursing the Liver and Resolving Depression: When liver qì is depressed and the normal upbearing and downbearing flow of yīn and yáng, qì and blood is upset, this gives rise to upper-body signs including headache, distention in the chest, and rib-side pain, and to lower-body signs including abdominal pain, umbilical pain, qì binding in the abdomen, and menstrual block. *Chái hú* enters the hand and foot lesser yáng (*shào yáng*) and reverting yīn (*jué yīn*) channels (i.e., the liver, gallbladder, pericardium, and triple burner channels). Within the channels, it governs qì to outthrust yáng qì, whereas within the viscera it governs blood to outthrust yīn qì. *Chái hú* (bupleurum) diffuses qì and blood and rotates the pivot[34];

---

[32] *Jǐn dēng lóng* 锦灯笼 is discussed in a later chapter on cold and cool medicinals (see page 271). It clears heat, resolves toxin, disperses fire, and dissipates swelling in the treatment of sore swollen throat. (Ed.)

[33] *Xuán shēn* 玄参 is often referred to as *xuán shēn* 玄参.[129] (Ed.)

[34] Rotates the pivot, 旋转枢机 *xuán zhuǎn shū jī*: The lesser yáng (*shào yáng*) is said to be the pivot. It is at the pivotal point between the greater yáng (*tài yáng*) in the exterior (opening)

it disinhibits depressed yáng and transforms stagnant yīn; and it courses the liver and resolves depression. For this purpose it is often combined with medicinals such as:

dāng guī (当归 Chinese angelica, Angelicae Sinensis Radix)

bái sháo (白芍 white peony, Paeoniae Radix Alba)

bái zhú (白术 white atractylodes, Atractylodis Macrocephalae Rhizoma)

fú líng (茯苓 poria, Poria)

bò hé (薄荷 mint, Menthae Herba)

xiāng fù (香附 cyperus, Cyperi Rhizoma)

chuān xiōng (川芎 chuanxiong, Chuanxiong Rhizoma)

zhǐ qiào (枳壳 bitter orange, Aurantii Fructus)

Below are examples of formulas that serve this function:

Xiāo yáo sǎn 逍遥散   Free Wanderer Powder

chái hú (柴胡 bupleurum, Bupleuri Radix)

dāng guī (当归 Chinese angelica, Angelicae Sinensis Radix)

bái sháo (白芍 white peony, Paeoniae Radix Alba)

bái zhú (白术 white atractylodes, Atractylodis Macrocephalae Rhizoma)

fú líng (茯苓 poria, Poria)

gān cǎo (甘草 licorice, Glycyrrhizae Radix)

shēng jiāng (生姜 fresh ginger, Zingiberis Rhizoma Recens)

bò hé (薄荷 mint, Menthae Herba)

Chái hú shū gān sǎn 柴胡疏肝散   Bupleurum Liver-Coursing Powder

chái hú (柴胡 bupleurum, Bupleuri Radix)

bái sháo (白芍 white peony, Paeoniae Radix Alba)

zhǐ qiào (枳壳 bitter orange, Aurantii Fructus)

gān cǎo (甘草 licorice, Glycyrrhizae Radix)

chuān xiōng (川芎 chuanxiong, Chuanxiong Rhizoma)

xiāng fù (香附 cyperus, Cyperi Rhizoma)

3. Uplifting Yáng Qì: *Chái hú* conducts clear qì upward to treat downward fall of clear yáng characterized by spleen-stomach vacuity, shortness of breath, sagging in the abdomen, persistent diarrhea, sagging in the anus, heaviness in the lumbus and abdomen, profuse menstruation, frequent urination, prolapse of the internal organs, and prolapse of the uterus. For this it is combined with medicinals such as:

zhì huáng qí (炙黄芪 mix-fried astragalus, Astragali Radix cum Liquido Fricta)

bái zhú (白术 white atractylodes, Atractylodis Macrocephalae Rhizoma)

shēng má (升麻 cimicifuga, Cimicifugae Rhizoma)

---

and the yáng brightness (*yáng míng*) in the interior (closing). "Rotate the pivot" means to free the lesser yáng. (Ed.)

fáng fēng (防风 saposhnikovia, Saposhnikoviae Radix)

gé gēn (葛根 pueraria, Puerariae Radix)

dǎng shēn (党参 codonopsis, Codonopsis Radix)

Below are examples of formulas that serve this function:

Bǔ zhōng yì qì tāng 补中益气汤   Center-Supplementing Qì-Boosting Decoction

---

zhì huáng qí (炙黄芪 mix-fried astragalus, Astragali Radix cum Liquido Fricta)

dǎng shēn (党参 codonopsis, Codonopsis Radix)

gān cǎo (甘草 licorice, Glycyrrhizae Radix)

bái zhú (白术 white atractylodes, Atractylodis Macrocephalae Rhizoma)

chén pí (陈皮 tangerine peel, Citri Reticulatae Pericarpium)

dāng guī (当归 Chinese angelica, Angelicae Sinensis Radix)

chái hú (柴胡 bupleurum, Bupleuri Radix)

shēng má (升麻 cimicifuga, Cimicifugae Rhizoma)

Shēng yáng yì wèi tāng 升阳益胃汤   Yáng-Upbearing Stomach-Boosting
Decoction

---

zhì huáng qí (炙黄芪 mix-fried astragalus, Astragali Radix cum Liquido Fricta)

bàn xià (半夏 pinellia, Pinelliae Rhizoma)

gān cǎo (甘草 licorice, Glycyrrhizae Radix)

dǎng shēn (党参 codonopsis, Codonopsis Radix)

bái sháo (白芍 white peony, Paeoniae Radix Alba)

qiāng huó (羌活 notopterygium, Notopterygii Rhizoma et Radix)

dú huó (独活 pubescent angelica, Angelicae Pubescentis Radix)

fáng fēng (防风 saposhnikovia, Saposhnikoviae Radix)

bái zhú (白术 white atractylodes, Atractylodis Macrocephalae Rhizoma)

chén pí (陈皮 tangerine peel, Citri Reticulatae Pericarpium)

fú líng (茯苓 poria, Poria)

zé xiè (泽泻 alisma, Alismatis Rhizoma)

chái hú (柴胡 bupleurum, Bupleuri Radix)

huáng lián (黄连 coptis, Coptidis Rhizoma)

shēng jiāng (生姜 fresh ginger, Zingiberis Rhizoma Recens)

dà zǎo (大枣 jujube, Jujubae Fructus)

Shēng tí tāng 升提汤   Upraising Decoction

▷ From *Fù Qīng Zhǔ Nǚ Kē* (傅青主女科 "Fù Qīng-Zhǔ's Gynecology")

shú dì huáng (熟地黄 cooked rehmannia, Rehmanniae Radix Praeparata)

shān zhū yú (山茱萸 cornus, Corni Fructus)

bā jǐ tiān (巴戟天 morinda, Morindae Officinalis Radix)

gǒu qǐ zǐ (枸杞子 lycium, Lycii Fructus)

bái zhú (白术 white atractylodes, Atractylodis Macrocephalae Rhizoma)

huáng qí (黄芪 astragalus, Astragali Radix)

dǎng shēn (党参 codonopsis, Codonopsis Radix)

chái hú (柴胡 bupleurum, Bupleuri Radix)

Note that when *chái hú* is used to upbear yáng, the dosage should be small.

4. Treating Heat Entering the Blood Chamber: When women have heat effusion (fever) due to an external contraction around the time of menstruation, the external evil can enter the blood chamber. If the period has just finished, the external evil exploits the emptiness of the blood chamber and invades, giving rise to alternating cold and heat. In extreme cases, high fever and delirious speech may develop at night time, these being signs of heat entering the blood chamber. For this, *chái hú* is added to a formula appropriate to the pattern identified because it works by opening the internal heat evil block and by lifting the evil qì from the blood out to the qì. Alternatively, one can use *xiǎo chái hú tāng* (Minor Bupleurum Decoction) varied according to signs. In my own practice, I always use *xiǎo chái hú tāng* (Minor Bupleurum Decoction) varied according to signs and achieve good results.

5. Treating Malaria: Malaria[556] (疟疾 *nüè jí*) is marked by "alternating cold and heat." Physicians in former times therefore advocated treating malaria by harmonizing the lesser yáng (*shào yáng*), using *chái hú* (bupleurum) formulas varied according to signs. For example, if there is first aversion to cold and then heat effusion, and if the cold and heat occur with fixed periodicity, one can use *xiǎo chái hú tāng* (Minor Bupleurum Decoction) varied according to signs. If there is more cold than heat, or only cold, one can use *xiǎo chái hú tāng* (Minor Bupleurum Decoction) together with *guì zhī tāng* (Cinnamon Twig Decoction) varied according to the signs. If there is more heat than cold, or only heat, one can use *xiǎo chái hú tāng* (Minor Bupleurum Decoction) together with *bái hǔ tāng* (White Tiger Decoction) varied according to accompanying signs. To these formulas I add *cháng shān* (dichroa), *cǎo guǒ* (tsaoko), and *bīng láng* (areca) and usually get good results. Modern research has demonstrated that *chái hú* (bupleurum) has an antimalarial effect and can inhibit and eliminate malarial parasites. However, malaria as spoken of in Chinese medicine is defined by signs, and is not necessarily the disease spoken of in modern Western medicine as being caused by malarial parasites. As long as the signs are present, the treatment is effective.

Chái hú (bupleurum) enters the liver and gallbladder and courses qì and blood. I often use the following formula:

Xiè shū tāng 燮枢汤	Pivot-Harmonizing Decoction

chái hú (柴胡 bupleurum, Bupleuri Radix) 9–15 g/3–5 qián

huáng qín (黄芩 scutellaria, Scutellariae Radix) 9–12 g/3-4 qián

chǎo chuān liàn zǐ (炒川楝子 stir-fried toosendan, Toosendan Fructus Frictus) 9–12 g/3-4 qián

bàn xià (半夏 pinellia, Pinelliae Rhizoma) 10 g/3 qián

hóng huā (红花 carthamus, Carthami Flos) 9 g/3 qián

zào jiǎo cì (皂角刺 gleditsia thorn, Gleditsiae Spina) 3–5 g/1–2 qián

bái jí lí (白蒺藜 tribulus, Tribuli Fructus) 9–12 g/3–4 qián

piàn jiāng huáng (片姜黄 sliced turmeric, Curcumae Longae Rhizoma Sectum)
    9 g/3 qián

liú jì nú (刘寄奴 anomalous artemisia, Artemisiae Anomalae Herba) 9 g/3 qián

zé xiè (泽泻 alisma, Alismatis Rhizoma) 9–12 g/3–4 qián

jiāo sì xiān (焦四仙 scorch-fried four immortals, Quattuor Immortales Usti)
    (barley sprout, medicated leaven, crataegus, and areca)

chǎo lái fú zǐ (炒莱菔子 stir-fried radish seed, Raphani Semen Frictum) 10 g/3 qián

If there is a thick white tongue fur, then I add 10 g/3 qián of *dòu kòu* (Katsumada's galangal seed). This formula, which I have named *xiè shū tāng* (Pivot-Harmonizing Decoction),[35] can be varied according to signs. I generally find it effective for chronic hepatitis patients whose liver function has been abnormal for a long time and who exhibit signs such as dull pain in the right rib-side (or pain in both rib-sides), persistent oppression in the stomach duct, abdominal distention, yellow urine, ungratifying defecation, poor appetite, fur on the tongue that is either white or yellow, and a pulse that is stringlike and slippery. According to modern research reports, *chái hú* is effective in healing experimental damage to the liver in white rats.

Chái hú is used in various combinations. Combined with *huáng qín* (scutellaria), it clears and dissipates bound heat in the qì aspect of the liver and gallbladder. Combined with *huáng lián* (coptis), it clears and dissipates depressed heat in the blood aspect of the heart channel. Combined with *bái sháo* (white peony) and *dāng guī* (Chinese angelica), it harmonizes the blood and regulates menstruation, to treat abdominal pain.

COMPARISONS

Different sorts of *chái hú* are distinguished in clinical practice. *Nán chái hú* (southern bupleurum), which comes from *Bupleurum chinense*, has relatively mild medicinal strength that makes it suitable for coursing the liver and resolving depression. *Yín chái hú* (stellaria) is cool, in comparison, and is suitable for abating vacuity heat and treating steaming bone. *Zhú yè chái hú* (bamboo-leaf bupleurum), which is the tender twigs, leaves, stems, and roots of *Bupleurum scorzonerifolium* that are cut transversely to be used as medicine, has the mildest medicinal strength, and is used only for mild qì depression. *Běi chái hú* (northern bupleurum), which is from mature *Bupleurum scorzonerifolium*, harmonizes the lesser yáng (*shào yáng*), abates heat and upbears yáng, courses the liver, and treats malaria. If one sim-

---

[35]According to the *Sù Wèn* (素问 "Elementary Questions"), opening (开 *kāi*), closing (合 *hé*), and pivot (枢 *shú*) are interior-exterior levels in the channel system. "Opening" means open to the exterior; "closing" means confined in the interior; "pivot" means located between opening and closing. Among the yáng channels, greater yáng (*tài yáng*) governs the opening, yáng brightness (*yáng míng*) governs the closing, and lesser yáng (*shào yáng*) governs the pivot. Among the yīn channels, greater yīn (*tài yīn*) governs opening, reverting yīn (*jué yīn*) governs closing, and lesser yīn (*shào yīn*) governs the pivot. In the name Pivot-Harmonizing Decoction, "pivot" of course refers to the lesser yáng. (Ed.)

ply writes *chái hú* (bupleurum) on a prescription, the pharmacist gives *běi chái hú* (northern bupleurum).[36]

Chái hú first downbears and then upbears, diffusing qì and dissipating binds, to open depression and regulate menstruation. *Qián hú* (peucedanum) first upbears and then downbears, precipitating qì and downbearing fire, to transform phlegm and suppress cough.

Dosage

The dosage is generally 0.9–9 g/3 fēn–3 qián. To abate heat and treat malaria, use 10–15 g/3–5 qián. For particularly severe conditions, use up to 30 g/1 liǎng.[37]

Caution

Contraindicated for patients with yīn vacuity internal heat in whom yáng qì is susceptible to upbearing and stirring.

---

[36]*Běi chái hú* (northern bupleurum) can be differentiated from the southern variety by observation. The northern species is more flexible and less apt to break when the root is bent. Further, the root of the northern variety divides into several smaller roots but not into root hairs, whereas the lower roots of the southern variety do not divide and end in fine root hairs. Note that the root hairs are often removed during processing, thus careful examination is required for accurate identification. Although *Bupleurum chinensis* is the variety of *chái hú* most commonly seen in the West, identification is complicated by other species such as *hēi chái hú* (black bupleurum) that have entered into trade. (Ed.)

[37]The primary use of large doses (30 g) of *chái hú* (bupleurum) is to treat high fever. (Ed.)

Lecture Three
Draining & Disinhibiting Medicinals
泻利药 *Xiè Lì Yào*

This lecture discusses draining precipitation medicinals, urine-disinhibiting and dampness-dispelling medicinals, joint-freeing medicinals, and water-expelling medicinals. Cold natured fire-draining medicinals are placed within a later lecture entitled Cold and Cool Medicinals.

1. 大黄 Dà Huáng Rhubarb	Rhei Radix et Rhizoma

Dà huáng (rhubarb) is bitter and cold. It drains blood-aspect repletion heat, precipitating gastrointestinal accumulations and eliminating the old to allow the new to arrive. Therefore, clinically it is often used to free the stool and drain fire, to disperse welling-abscesses and dissipate swellings, to clear heat and dry dampness, and to quicken the blood and free the channels. Nevertheless, it is most commonly used as a **draining precipitation**[546] medicinal.

In patients with acute febrile disease for 5 or 6 days, or an inability to defecate for 7 or 8 days, there may be symptoms such as unabating high fever, stronger fever in the afternoon, bouts of sweating, clouded spirit, delirious speech at night, picking at bedclothes, abdominal distention and fullness, hard **glomus**[551] (痞 *pǐ*) that refuses pressure, thick yellow tongue fur or rough yellow and scorched black tongue fur, and a pulse that is forceful with heavy pressure. This is a pattern of fire-heat accumulating and binding in the intestines and stomach. In this situation, *shēng dà huáng* (raw rhubarb), *máng xiāo* (mirabilite), *hòu pò* (officinal magnolia bark), and *zhǐ shí* (unripe bitter orange) are used for offensive precipitation and to drain fire. When the patient has had one or two thin bowel movements, the heat [effusion] (fever) generally abates and the pathocondition is eliminated.

For patients with intense stomach fire, mouth and tongue sores, thirst, dry pharynx, painful swollen gums, bound stool, or nosebleed or vomiting of blood, give 3–6 g/1–2 qián of *shēng dà huáng* steeped in boiled water for 20–30 minutes. The decoction should be taken once every day. After only two or three days of use it will free the stool, drain fire, and cure the disease. One can use this method when it is necessary to free the stool in any repletion pattern in which the stool is dry or several days have passed without a bowel movement.

At the onset of heat dysentery, when there is gastrointestinal damp-heat accumulation with tenesmus and ungratifying defecation, use *shēng dà huáng* accompanied by medicinals such as *huáng lián* (coptis), *mù xiāng* (costusroot), and *bīng láng* (areca) to drain and eliminate gastrointestinal accumulation and check dysentery. This is called the method of **treating the unstopped by unstopping**[566] (通因通用 *tōng yīn tōng yòng*).

Dà huáng also has the effect of dissipating swelling and dispersing welling-abscesses. In all cases of welling-abscess with swelling, heat, and pain that do not disperse, use *dà huáng* to drain interior toxic heat, to push forward congestion and stagnation, and to disperse swelling and dissipate welling-abscess. In this situation it is commonly used in combination with medicinals such as the following:

> *chì sháo* (赤芍 red peony, Paeoniae Radix Rubra)
> *dāng guī wěi* (当归尾 Chinese angelica tail, Angelicae Sinensis Radicis Extremitas)
> *jīn yín huā* (金银花 lonicera, Lonicerae Flos)
> *lián qiáo* (连翘 forsythia, Forsythiae Fructus)
> *dān pí* (丹皮 moutan, Moutan Cortex)

For example: a) *Dà huáng* made into pills with *bái zhǐ* (Dahurian angelica) and taken internally treats toxic welling-abscess on the back of the head and on the back. b) Combined with medicinals such as *dān pí* (moutan), *táo rén* (peach kernel), *máng xiāo* (mirabilite), *dōng guā zǐ* (wax gourd seed), and *chì sháo* (red peony), it treats intestinal welling-abscess (appendicitis). In recent years, acute appendicitis has been treated effectively with a modified *dà huáng mǔ dān pí tāng* (Rhubarb and Moutan Decoction).[305]

Dà huáng is also used to clear heat and eliminate dampness. For example, when treating jaundice (yáng jaundice), besides using *yīn chén* (virgate wormwood), *zhī zǐ* (gardenia), *chē qián zǐ* (plantago seed), and *huáng bǎi* (phellodendron), a suitable addition of *dà huáng* speeds the actions of clearing heat, eliminating dampness, and abating jaundice. Furthermore, external application of *dà huáng* powder is used to treat symptoms such as **yellow-water sores**[568] (黄水疮 *huáng shuǐ chuāng*) and eczema.

For women with static blood in the interior causing signs such as **menstrual block**[557] (经闭 *jīng bì*), dry skin lacking in luxuriance, emaciation, reduced eating, fullness in the smaller abdomen, dull blue-green eyeballs, and night sweating (commonly called dry-blood consumption), use *dà huáng zhè chóng wán* (Rhubarb and Ground Beetle Pill). This is an old empirical formula that has been made into a ready-prepared medicine. Take one pill two times per day.

Dà huáng zhè chóng wán 大黄蟅虫丸   Rhubarb and Ground Beetle Pill

---

dà huáng (大黄 rhubarb, Rhei Radix et Rhizoma)

huáng qín (黄芩 scutellaria, Scutellariae Radix)

gān cǎo (甘草 licorice, Glycyrrhizae Radix)

táo rén (桃仁 peach kernel, Persicae Semen)

xìng rén (杏仁 apricot kernel, Armeniacae Semen)

chì sháo (赤芍 red peony, Paeoniae Radix Rubra)

shēng dì huáng (生地黄 dried/fresh rehmannia, Rehmanniae Radix Exsiccata seu Recens)

gān qī (干漆 lacquer, Toxicodendri Resina)

méng chóng (虻虫 tabanus, Tabanus)

shuǐ zhì (水蛭 leech, Hirudo)

qí cáo (蛴螬 June beetle grub, Holotrichiae Vermiculus) (scarab larva)

zhè chóng (蟅虫 ground beetle, Eupolyphaga seu Steleophaga)[1]

Dà huáng enters the blood aspect; it sinks, downbears, and moves downward. Therefore, in women with menstrual block caused by blood stasis, one can add *dà huáng* to menstruation-regulating medicinals in order to quicken the blood and free the channels.

In addition, *dà huáng* combined with *gān cǎo* (licorice) checks vomiting. I have obtained satisfactory results treating neurogenic vomiting using *shēng dà huáng* combined with *shēng gān cǎo* (raw licorice), as in *dà huáng gān cǎo tāng* (Rhubarb and Licorice Decoction), together with *shēng dài zhě shí* (crude hematite), *xuán fù huā* (inula flower), *bàn xià* (pinellia), *dǎng shēn* (codonopsis), and *bīng láng* (areca).

Comparisons

Hēi bái chǒu (morning glory)[86] drains and precipitates; it possesses minor toxicity and primarily attacks and expels water accumulation in the abdomen. *Dà huáng* also drains precipitation, but it mainly flushes gastrointestinal accumulation and stagnation and heat bind.

Bā dòu (croton)[51] and *dà huáng* both are drastic draining medicinals. Nevertheless, *bā dòu* is hot in nature, while *dà huáng* is cold in nature.

When *dà huáng* is used raw, it is a fierce draining precipitant (so offensive precipitation formulas often use *shēng dà huáng*, while invariably noting "add at end"[542] 后下 *hòu xià*). When stir-fried with wine (or steeped in wine, or washed with wine), it reaches the upper part of the body and expels heat with downward movement. Washing with wine also helps its draining power, making it suitable for symptoms such as red eyes, toothache, mouth sores, and burning heat in the chest. When decocted, its draining power is harmonious and moderate, making it suitable for elderly people with weak health. Char-fried, it is used for accumulation and stagnation in the large intestine accompanied by descent of blood with the stool because it has a blood-stanching effect.

---

[1] *Zhè chóng* (ground beetle) is also called *dì biē* 地鳖 in Chinese. (Au.)

a) When *dà huáng* and *máng xiāo* (mirabilite)[48] are used together, it makes the draining precipitation stronger and faster.

b) When used with *huáng qín* (scutellaria) and *zhī zǐ* (gardenia),[252] it drains lung fire.

c) When used with *huáng lián* (coptis),[246] it drains heart fire.

d) When used with *lóng dǎn cǎo* (gentian),[281] it drains liver fire.

e) When used with *shēng shí gāo* (crude gypsum),[243] it drains stomach fire.

Dosage

The dosage is generally 1.5–9 g/5 fēn–3 qián. Nevertheless, in certain disease conditions, one can use 12–15 g/4–5 qián.

Caution

Dà huáng is inappropriate for patients with insufficiency of original qì, stomach vacuity blood weakness, disease in the qì aspect, or dry stool from yīn vacuity.

Some patients loathe taking decoctions and vomit each time a decoction is taken. In such cases, after decocting the medicine, boil *dà huáng* 1 g/3 fēn and *gān cǎo* (licorice) 1 g/3 fēn in a cup of water. This should be drunk slowly; then, after 15–20 minutes, if there is no vomiting, take the original decoction and there should not be vomiting. This is effective with most people.

---

2. 芒硝 Máng Xiāo   Natrii Sulfas
Mirabilite

Máng xiāo (mirabilite) is bitter, salty, and cold; it is a salty draining precipitant. It is primarily used to treat bound stool caused by intense heat evil and is often used along with *dà huáng* (rhubarb). This medicinal causes the fluid in the intestine to increase, softening hardness and moistening dryness. *Dà huáng*[45] flushes accumulation and stagnation. When the two are used together, the draining power is strengthened and the offensive precipitation action is speedier.

Besides being a draining precipitant, *máng xiāo* (mirabilite) also softens hardness and breaks the blood. To treat blood stasis menstrual block, it can be combined with medicinals such as:

dāng guī (当归 Chinese angelica, Angelicae Sinensis Radix)
hóng huā (红花 carthamus, Carthami Flos)
táo rén (桃仁 peach kernel, Persicae Semen)
chuān xiōng (川芎 chuanxiong, Chuanxiong Rhizoma)

To treat concretions, conglomerations, and accumulation lumps in the abdomen, it can be combined with medicinals such as:

cāng zhú (苍术 atractylodes, Atractylodis Rhizoma)
bái zhú (白术 white atractylodes, Atractylodis Macrocephalae Rhizoma)
sān léng (三棱 sparganium, Sparganii Rhizoma)

é zhú (莪术 curcuma rhizome, Curcumae Rhizoma)

mǔ lì (牡蛎 oyster shell, Ostreae Concha)

yù jīn (郁金 curcuma, Curcumae Radix)

dān shēn (丹参 salvia, Salviae Miltiorrhizae Radix)

shān zhā hé (山楂核 crataegus pit, Crataegi Endocarpium et Semen)

Decocted in water and used as an external wash, *máng xiāo* treats conditions such as red eyes and hemorrhoids. Combined with *péng shā* (borax) and *bīng piàn* (borneol) and ground into a fine powder, it is applied topically to treat mouth and tongue sores or used as a **laryngeal insufflation**[556] (吹喉 *chuī hòu*) to treat sore swollen throat.[2]

When *máng xiāo* and *lái fú* (radish) are decocted together, filtered, and cooled, it results in the formation of crystals. These crystals undergo efflorescence to produce a fine white powder that is called *yuán míng fěn* (refined mirabilite).[3] Compared to *máng xiāo*, the draining precipitation effect of *yuán míng fěn* is more moderate, but its treatment effect is, for the most part, the same. It is primarily used for situations where the heat is relatively mild and the body is relatively weak.

DOSAGE

The dosage for *máng xiāo* is 3–6 g/1–2 qián. For *yuán míng fěn* the dosage is 3–9 g/1–3 qián. Both are **taken drenched**[565] (冲服 *chōng fú*) with a decoction.

CAUTION

Contraindicated in the absence of stagnant heat evil and in patients with debility from old age.

---

3. 番泻叶 Fān Xiè Yè   Sennae Folium
Senna

Fān xiè yè (senna) is sweet and bitter in flavor and cold or cool in nature. It is a precipitating medicinal that is very convenient to use. To treat constipation due to fire-heat binding internally, steep 5–7 g/2–2.5 qián of this medicinal in hot water for approximately half an hour. Divide the resulting juice into two doses and take once every 4–5 hours. (If after the first dose draining precipitation is achieved (i.e., there is a bowel movement), then do not take the second.) Those with habitual constipation can take a daily dose before sleep or in the morning.

Small amounts of *fān xiè yè* clear and eliminate stomach heat, open the stomach, and increase food intake. An appropriate amount is used for draining precipitation

---

[2]This combination is called *bīng péng sǎn* (Borneol and Borax Powder). Equal parts of *máng xiāo* (mirabilite) and *péng shā* (borax) are ground to a fine powder and combined with a small amount of *bīng piàn* (borneol). In earlier times *zhū shā* (cinnabar) was also included. Note that, for internal use, natural *bīng piàn* must be used. Natural *bīng piàn* is grayish in color and quite expensive; it is usually referred to as *méi piàn* 梅片. (Ed.)

[3] *Yuán míng fěn* (元明粉, refined mirabilite), being the most refined form of mirabilite, is also used for external application to sensitive areas such as the eyes. (Ed.)

to free the stool. Too much can give rise to nausea and, in severe cases, vomiting. To free the stool and drain precipitation, 3–7 g/1–2.5 qián is generally used, either steeped in water or in a decoction.

CAUTION

The draining precipitation effect of *fān xiè yè* enters the breast milk and causes diarrhea in nursing children. This medicinal also enters the lower body and causes hyperemia. Therefore, it is contraindicated for nursing women and is unsuitable for menstruating women, pregnant women, and for those with hemorrhoids.

---

4. 芦荟 Lú Huì   Aloe
Aloe

Lú huì is bitter in flavor and cold in nature. It has a draining precipitation effect, but it also cools the liver, brightens the eyes, disperses gān accumulation, clears heat, and kills worms.

Lú huì enters the blood aspect of the liver channel and frees menstruation. It can be combined with medicinals such as *dāng guī* (Chinese angelica), *chuān xiōng* (chuanxiong), *shú dì huáng* (cooked rehmannia), *qiàn cǎo* (madder), and *hóng huā* (carthamus) to treat menstrual block. Being able to cool the liver and **brighten the eyes**[543] (明目 *míng mù*), it is combined with medicinals such as *cǎo jué míng* (fetid cassia), *qīng xiāng zǐ* (celosia), *shēng dì huáng* (dried/fresh rehmannia), *bái sháo* (white peony), *yè míng shā* (bat's droppings), and *shí hú* (dendrobium) to treat blood heat clouded vision.

Lú huì combined in a pill preparation with medicinals such as *hú huáng lián* (picrorhiza), *jiāo sān xiān* (scorch-fried three immortals), *shǐ jūn zǐ* (quisqualis), *cāng zhú* (atractylodes), *bái zhú* (white atractylodes), *jī nèi jīn* (gizzard lining), *fú líng* (poria), *bīng láng* (areca), *huáng qín* (scutellaria), and *dǎng shēn* (codonopsis) treats **child gān accumulation**[543] (小儿疳积 *xiǎo ér gān jī*) and worm accumulation with signs such as yellow face and emaciation, enlarged abdomen with green-blue veins, and postmeridian low-grade fever.

On the basis of past experience, it is believed that *lú huì* has the fastest action to cause medicinals to enter the liver. In recent years, chronic hepatitis has been treated with approximately 0.3 g/1 fēn of *lú huì* (aloe) ground to a powder, packed in capsules, and taken with a pattern-appropriate decoction such as the following:

> *chái hú* (柴胡 bupleurum, Bupleuri Radix)
> *huáng qín* (黄芩 scutellaria, Scutellariae Radix)
> *bàn xià* (半夏 pinellia, Pinelliae Rhizoma)
> *jiāo sān xiān* (焦三仙 scorch-fried three immortals, Tres Immortales Usti)
> *bīng láng* (槟榔 areca, Arecae Semen)
> *bái jí lí* (白蒺藜 tribulus, Tribuli Fructus)
> *zào jiǎo cì* (皂角刺 gleditsia thorn, Gleditsiae Spina)
> *hóng huā* (红花 carthamus, Carthami Flos)

cǎo dòu kòu (草豆蔻 Katsumada's galangal seed, Alpiniae Katsumadai Semen)

chǎo lái fú zǐ (炒莱菔子 stir-fried radish seed, Raphani Semen Frictum)

This has a definite effect in aiding recovery of liver function and decreasing symptoms. For hepatitis in children, when liver function fails to recover for a long time, use *lú huì* combined with medicinals such as:

hú huáng lián (胡黄连 picrorhiza, Picrorhizae Rhizoma)

chái hú (柴胡 bupleurum, Bupleuri Radix)

huáng qín (黄芩 scutellaria, Scutellariae Radix)

huáng lián (黄连 coptis, Coptidis Rhizoma)

jiāo sān xiān (焦三仙 scorch-fried three immortals, Tres Immortales Usti)

cāng zhú (苍术 atractylodes, Atractylodis Rhizoma)

bīng láng (槟榔 areca, Arecae Semen)

chǎo jī nèi jīn (炒鸡内金 stir-fried gizzard lining, Galli Gigeriae Endothelium Corneum Frictum)

hóng huā (红花 carthamus, Carthami Flos)

qiàn cǎo (茜草 madder, Rubiae Radix)

bàn xià (半夏 pinellia, Pinelliae Rhizoma)

zhǐ shí (枳实 unripe bitter orange, Aurantii Fructus Immaturus)

This formula, made into a honey pill and taken for 2–3 months, will gradually bring about improvement.

DOSAGE

When used in formulas as a draining precipitant to treat heat binding in the intestines and stomach, approximately 0.6–1.5 g/2–5 fēn of *lú huì* will cause precipitation, although for some as little as 0.3 g/1 fēn will be effective. For this reason, dosage should be determined on the basis of a careful appreciation of the patient's condition. When used in formulas to free menstruation, cool the blood, disperse gān, and kill worms, approximately 0.2 g/0.5 fēn will suffice. A child's dosage must be reduced still further. Because this medicinal is extremely bitter in flavor, it is commonly ground into a fine powder, put into a capsule, and swallowed after taking the decoction medicine. It is generally not decocted. For children it is generally used in pills.

CAUTION

Lú huì has a blood-breaking effect and is therefore contraindicated in pregnancy.

---

5. 巴豆 Bā Dòu　　Crotonis Fructus
Croton

Bā dòu is acrid, hot, and toxic. It drains cold accumulation and expels phlegm aggregation in drastic draining formulas. It is used for cold-phlegm accumulations and gatherings, for food accuumlations with distention and fullness, or for any glomus, aggregations, concretions, and bindings in the abdomen that need to be expelled through the stool by the draining method.

When taken internally, *bā dòu shuāng* (croton frost) is generally used (*bā dòu* that has been processed to remove the oil[4]) in pills or powder preparations. Each time use approximately several lí (around 0.06–0.25 g); do not use more than this. If after taking *bā dòu shuāng* there is incessant diarrhea, quickly taking cold gruel or cold water may resolve it. Note that if this occurs, one should not eat hot gruel or drink hot water, because the more heat that is consumed, the stronger the draining power will become.

Other than its draining precipitation effect, *bā dòu* also disperses and eliminates accumulation lumps. To treat hepatosplenomegaly due to early-stage cirrhosis of the liver, I use 1.5–2.5 g/5–8 fēn of *bā dòu shuāng* mixed together with a powder of the following medicinals:

> *huáng lián* (黄连 coptis, Coptidis Rhizoma) 24 g/8 qián
>
> *hòu pò* (厚朴 officinal magnolia bark, Magnoliae Officinalis Cortex) 18 g/6 qián
>
> *wú yú* (吴萸 evodia, Evodiae Fructus) 9 g/3 qián
>
> *zé xiè* (泽泻 alisma, Alismatis Rhizoma) 9 g/3 qián
>
> *bái zhú* (白术 white atractylodes, Atractylodis Macrocephalae Rhizoma) 9 g/3 qián
>
> *zhǐ shí* (枳实 unripe bitter orange, Aurantii Fructus Immaturus) 12 g/4 qián
>
> *huáng qín* (黄芩 scutellaria, Scutellariae Radix) 9 g/3 qián
>
> *yīn chén* (茵陈 virgate wormwood, Artemisiae Scopariae Herba) 9 g/3 qián
>
> *gān jiāng* (干姜 dried ginger, Zingiberis Rhizoma) 4.5 g/1.5 qián
>
> *shā rén* (砂仁 amomum, Amomi Fructus) 6 g/2 qián
>
> *dǎng shēn* (党参 codonopsis, Codonopsis Radix) 9 g/3 qián
>
> *fú líng* (茯苓 poria, Poria) 9 g/3 qián
>
> *chuān wū* (川乌 aconite root, Aconiti Radix) 9 g/3 qián
>
> *chuān jiāo* (川椒 zanthoxylum, Zanthoxyli Pericarpium) 9 g/3 qián
>
> *táo rén* (桃仁 peach kernel, Persicae Semen) 9 g/3 qián
>
> *hóng huā* (红花 carthamus, Carthami Flos) 9 g/3 qián
>
> *xiāng fù* (香附 cyperus, Cyperi Rhizoma) 12 g/4 qián
>
> *sān léng* (三棱 sparganium, Sparganii Rhizoma) 9 g/3 qián
>
> *é zhú* (莪术 curcuma rhizome, Curcumae Rhizoma) 9 g/3 qián
>
> *zào jiǎo cì* (皂角刺 gleditsia thorn, Gleditsiae Spina) 3 g/1 qián
>
> *shēng mǔ lì* (生牡蛎 crude oyster shell, Ostreae Concha Cruda) 12 g/4 qián
>
> *zhì shān jiǎ* (炙山甲 mix-fried pangolin scales, Manis Squama cum Liquido Fricta) 6 g/2 qián
>
> *kūn bù* (昆布 kelp, Laminariae/Eckloniae Thallus) 12 g/4 qián

---

[4] *Bā dòu shuāng* (croton frost) is made by crushing this medicinal and boiling it in water briefly five times (changing the water each time) to remove toxins. It is then oven dried, ground to a powder, and pressed between absorbent paper to remove its oils. The paper is changed and pressing continued until no more oil is evident. The medicinal is then ground to a very fine powder and stored for use. (Ed.)

hǎi piāo xiāo (海螵蛸 cuttlefish bone, Sepiae Endoconcha) 6 g/2 qián

shān zhā hé (山楂核 crataegus pit, Crataegi Endocarpium et Semen)
    9 g/3 qián

guì zhī (桂枝 cinnamon twig, Cinnamomi Ramulus) 9 g/3 qián

liàn mì (炼蜜 processed honey, Mel Praeparatum)

This is blended with honey and formed into pills that each weigh 3 g/1 qián. Twice a day, swallow 1/2 pill to 2 pills (the correct dosage will cause mild diarrhea) with warm water. From reviewing many different cases, it is clear that this pill has a definite effect on hepatomegaly. Some patients experience immediate dispersion after taking this preparation once, while others require three or four courses. The amount of *bā dòu shuāng* and the other medicinals can be varied according to the signs. Case examples of this treatment are too few; therefore, it is provided for reference only.

Bā dòu shuāng is a precipitating medicinal that when used in very small dosages causes precipitation. At the same time, it disperses gān and transforms accumulations, so it is often used in pills and powders for children. For example, it is used in *bǎo chì sǎn* (Infant-Safeguarding Red Powder) and *tiě wá sǎn* (Iron Baby Powder), which are both commercially available.

Bā dòu (without the husk), accompanied by medicinals such as *hú táo rén* (walnut), *dà fēng zǐ* (hydnocarpus), and *shuǐ yín* (mercury), pounded like a mud plaster and applied externally, treats scab sores[561] (疥疮 *jiè chuāng*). Note that *bā dòu* is toxic, so after touching it one should not rub the eyes, because it will cause swelling of the eyelid.

6. 火麻仁 Huǒ Má Rén   Cannabis Fructus
Cannabis Fruit

Also called *má rén* 麻仁. *Huǒ má rén* (cannabis fruit) is sweet in nature and neutral in flavor. Because it contains fatty oils, it is enriching and moistening and it lubricates the intestines to free the stool. It is suitable for dry bound stool caused by an insufficiency of fluids in elderly people, people recovering from febrile diseases, and postpartum women. It is often used with medicinals such as:

yù lǐ rén (郁李仁 bush cherry kernel, Pruni Semen)

táo rén (桃仁 peach kernel, Persicae Semen)

guā lóu rén (瓜蒌仁 trichosanthes seed, Trichosanthis Semen)

shú dà huáng (熟大黄 cooked rhubarb, Rhei Radix et Rhizoma Conquiti)

fēng mì (蜂蜜 honey, Mel)

Comparisons

Hēi zhī má (black sesame)[141] and *huǒ má rén* both free the stool by moistening. *Hēi zhī má* tends to enrich and supplement the liver and kidney and to nourish the blood and boost essence, and thereby moisten dryness, but *huǒ má rén* tends to relax the spleen, engender liquid, increase humor, and moisten the intestines, and thereby free the stool.

DOSAGE

The dosage is generally 9–15 g/3–5 qián. When the dryness bind is severe, use 20–25 or 30 g/7–8 qián or 1 liǎng.

---

7. 郁李仁 **Yù Lǐ Rén**   Pruni Semen
Bush Cherry Kernel

Acrid and bitter in flavor and neutral in nature, *yù lǐ rén* (bush cherry kernel) opens bound qì of the pylorus,[5] moistens dryness of the large intestine, and moves qì to moisten dryness and free the intestines. It also disinhibits water and disperses swelling.

Yù lǐ rén is combined with *huǒ má rén* (cannabis fruit), *quán guā lóu* (trichosanthes), and *fān xiè yè* (senna), ground to a powder, and made into honey pills for habitual constipation. Each pill should be about 10 g/3 qián and 1–2 pills should be taken each time.

Because *yù lǐ rén* moves qì and disinhibits water, it is used for ascites accompanied by constipation.

COMPARISONS

Huǒ má rén (cannabis fruit)[53] tends to enter the blood aspect of the spleen and large intestine, engender liquid and moisten dryness, and increase humor and relax the spleen to lubricate the intestines and free the stool. *Yù lǐ rén* tends to enter the qì aspect of the spleen and large intestine, free the pylorus and dissipate binds and move large intestine qì to abduct stagnation and moisten the intestines.

SPECIAL USES

In addition, if there is insomnia due to fright and taking a typical sleep-quieting formula has no effect, then one can, according to the principle of pattern identification as the basis for determining treatment, add 10–15 g /3–5 qián of wine-soaked *yù lǐ rén* (*yù lǐ rén* soaked for ten minutes in *huáng jiǔ* (yellow wine), after which the wine is removed). This addition is invariably effective.

DOSAGE

The dosage is generally 6–12 g/2–4 qián. Under special conditions, one can use up to 30 g/1 liǎng.

---

[5]The pylorus is called the "dark gate," 幽门 *yōu mén*, in Chinese. (Ed.)

---

8. 蜂蜜 Fēng Mì   Mel
Honey

Sweet in flavor and cool in nature, *fēng mì* (honey) moistens the intestines and frees the stool. It is used for dry bound stool in elderly patients, in weak patients, and in those with a fluid insufficiency or with dry stagnation in the intestines. Use 1–3 soup spoons of *fēng mì* taken with water 2–3 times per day.

After heating, *fēng mì* is no longer very cool and it supplements the center. It is a very good product for enriching and nourishing and is used to regulate and nourish after illness.

COMPARISONS

Yí táng (malt sugar), *fēng mì* (honey), and *dà zǎo* (jujube)[105] are all sweet in flavor and supplement the center. *Yí táng* is slightly warm in nature and primarily enters the spleen. It relaxes tension and relieves abdominal pain, but its ability to enrich, moisten, and lubricate the intestines is not as great as *fēng mì*. *Fēng mì* moistens the lung and treats cough from lung dryness. *Dà zǎo* is sweet and warm and it supplements the center. It primarily supplements the spleen and stomach, but it has no strength to moisten the intestines and free the stool.

---

9. 木通 Mù Tōng   Akebiae
Trifoliate Akebia   Trifoliatae Caulis

Cold in nature and bitter in flavor, *mù tōng* (trifoliate akebia)[6] disinhibits water and frees strangury, and causes heat to move downward, as well as freeing menstruation and freeing milk. In clinical practice, it is most commonly used to disinhibit urine and treat strangury.

Mù tōng downbears and drains heart fire. It abducts heart channel damp-heat out through the urine. Accompanied by *shēng dì huáng* (dried/fresh rehmannia), *zhú yè* (lophatherum), and *shēng gān cǎo shāo* (raw fine licorice root), which together constitute *dǎo chì sǎn* (Red-Abducting Powder), it addresses inhibited uri-

---

[6]The name *mù tōng* 木通 can refer to different botanical entities. Originally, *Akebia Fruit quinata* (or *Akebia Fruit trifoliata*) was the preferred plant, although it is seldom used today. Most of what we see in modern times is either 川木通 *chuān mù tōng* (*Clematis armandii* or *Clematis montana*) or 关木通 *guān mù tōng* (*Aristolochia kaempferi* or *Aristolochia moupinensis*). Since the latter contains aristolochic acid, which is currently suspected of causing ill effects, most distributors in the West now carry only *chuān mù tōng*. It is easy to distinguish *chuān mù tōng* from *guān mù tōng* through visual inspection. The outer surface of a slice of *guān mù tōng* is very smooth, making a nice oval or circle if traced on paper. *Chuān mù tōng*'s circumference, on the other hand, is quite jagged. Interestingly, in the *Shén Nóng Běn Cǎo* (神农本草 "The Divine Husbandman's Herbal Foundation"), *mù tōng* was referred to as 通草 *tōng cǎo*. Later when *tōng cǎo* (the pith of *Tetrapanax papyriferi*, the rice-paper plant[57]) entered common use, what had hitherto been known as *tōng cǎo* came to be known as *mù tōng* to avoid confusion between the two medicinals. (Ed.)

nation, pain in the urethra, red-tipped tongue, and other signs caused by exuberant heart fire with damp-heat pouring downward. *Mù tōng* has a pronounced capacity to disinhibit water and clear heat. It treats patterns such as heat strangury or blood strangury caused by binding heat in the bladder. For this purpose it is often combined with medicinals such as *chē qián zǐ* (plantago seed), *zhī zǐ* (gardenia), *qū mài* (dianthus), *biǎn xù* (knotgrass), *huá shí* (talcum), and *dà huáng* (rhubarb). Combined with these medicinals and varied in accordance with signs, it treats acute urinary tract infections.

Mù tōng also diffuses and frees the blood vessels, frees milk, and disinhibits the joints. Combined with medicinals such as *chuān xiōng* (chuanxiong), *dāng guī* (Chinese angelica), *hóng huā* (carthamus), *chì sháo* (red peony), and *táo rén* (peach kernel), it treats menstrual block. Decocted with *zhū tí* (pig's trotter), it treats scant postpartum breast milk.[7] Combined with medicinals such as *sāng zhī* (mulberry twig), *fáng jǐ* (fangji), *sōng jié* (knotty pine wood), *wēi líng xiān* (clematis), *qiāng huó* (notopterygium), and *dú huó* (pubescent angelica), it treats inhibited movement of the joints, and sinew and bone pain.

COMPARISONS

Mù tōng and *zé xiè* (alisma)[62] both disinhibit urine and dispel dampness. Nevertheless, *zé xiè* tends to drain and disinhibit liver and kidney channel damp-heat, whereas *mù tōng* tends to drain and disinhibit heart and small intestine channel damp-heat.

Mù tōng differs from other urine-disinhibiting medicinals in that it not only frees urine, but also frees stool. This is a special characteristic of *mù tōng*.

RESEARCH

According to modern reports, *mù tōng* has an obvious diuretic and cardiotonic effect. Combined with medicinals such as *fú líng* (poria), *zhū líng* (polyporus), *sāng pí* (mulberry root bark), *sū zǐ* (perilla fruit), and *zé xiè* (alisma), it treats cardiac insufficiency and the resulting signs such as inhibited urination, puffy swelling of both feet, generalized puffy swelling, vexation, oppression, and hasty panting. Nevertheless, remember that the accompanying medicinals should be varied according to the fundamental principle of pattern identification as the basis of determining treatment.

DOSAGE

The dosage is generally 3–9 g/1–3 qián.

CAUTION

This medicinal is contraindicated in the absence of interior damp-heat. It is also contraindicated if there is **seminal efflux**[562] (滑精 *huá jīng*), weak qì, or pregnancy.

---

[7]The folk medicine of China is replete with recipes for postpartum soups. Pig's trotters are the common denominator of these remedies, often combined with peanuts. (Ed.)

10. 通草 Tōng Cǎo
Rice-Paper Plant Pith
Tetrapanacis Medulla

Tōng cǎo (rice-paper plant pith) is sweet and bland in flavor and slightly cold in nature. It disinhibits urine, frees milk, drains lung heat, and soothes stomach qì.

Tōng cǎo has a light and soft quality. Its bland flavor percolates dampness and disinhibits urine. Its cold nature clears heat and downbears fire.

a) To treat water swelling and inhibited urination, it can be combined with medicinals such as:

fáng jǐ (防己 fangji, Stephaniae Tetrandrae Radix)

fú líng (茯苓 poria, Poria)

zhū líng (猪苓 polyporus, Polyporus)

dà fù pí (大腹皮 areca husk, Arecae Pericarpium)

b) To treat heat strangury and inhibited urination, *tōng cǎo* can be combined with medicinals such as:

mù tōng (木通 trifoliate akebia, Akebiae Trifoliatae Caulis)

qū mài (瞿麦 dianthus, Dianthi Herba)

lián qiáo (连翘 forsythia, Forsythiae Fructus)

zhú yè (竹叶 lophatherum, Lophatheri Herba)

c) To treat damp-heat brewing internally with signs such as generalized heaviness and pain, thick white tongue fur, absence of thirst, oppression in the chest, absence of hunger, postmeridian generalized heat [effusion] (fever), and inhibited urination, *tōng cǎo* is combined with medicinals such as:

xìng rén (杏仁 apricot kernel, Armeniacae Semen)

kòu rén (蔻仁 nutmeg, Myristicae Semen)

yǐ rén (苡仁 coix, Coicis Semen)

huá shí (滑石 talcum, Talcum)

hòu pò (厚朴 officinal magnolia bark, Magnoliae Officinalis Cortex)

bàn xià (半夏 pinellia, Pinelliae Rhizoma)

zhú yè (竹叶 lophatherum, Lophatheri Herba)

d) To treat symptoms such as lung heat cough, inhibited urination, vexing thirst, and other signs attributable to an exterior pattern accompanied by dampness, *tōng cǎo* is combined with medicinals such as:

xìng rén (杏仁 apricot kernel, Armeniacae Semen)

huáng qín (黄芩 scutellaria, Scutellariae Radix)

yǐ rén (苡仁 coix, Coicis Semen)

sāng yè (桑叶 mulberry leaf, Mori Folium)

dà dòu juǎn (大豆卷 dried soybean sprout, Sojae Semen Germinatum)

e) To free milk and treat **scant breast milk**[561] (乳汁少 *rǔ zhī shǎo*), *tōng cǎo* is decocted to make a beverage. For this purpose it is combined with medicinals such as:

> *chuān shān jiǎ* (穿山甲 pangolin scales, Manis Squama)
> *chuān xiōng* (川芎 chuanxiong, Chuanxiong Rhizoma)
> *gān cǎo* (甘草 licorice, Glycyrrhizae Radix)
> *zhū tí* (猪蹄 pig's trotter, Suis Pes)

COMPARISONS

Mù tōng (trifoliate akebia)[22] downbears heart fire, conducts heat downward, and disinhibits water. Within its downbearing nature, there is also freeing: it frees the blood vessels, frees the stool, and frees and disinhibits the joints. *Tōng cǎo* drains lung heat, assists downbearing of the qì, and disinhibits water. Within its downbearing nature, there is also upbearing: it causes the stomach qì to reach the upper burner and free milk.

Dēng xīn cǎo (juncus) clears heart heat, conducts heat qì downward, and disinhibits water. *Tōng cǎo* downbears lung qì, percolates dampness and clears heat, and disinhibits water.

Wáng bù liú xíng (vaccaria)[411] and *mù tōng* (trifoliate akebia) mainly move the blood vessels and free stasis and stagnation to free milk. *Tōng cǎo* mainly causes stomach qì to ascend in order to free milk.

DOSAGE

The dosage is generally 3–9 g/1–3 qián. Nevertheless, in some formulas that free milk one can use up to 15–18 g/5–6 qián or even 30 g/1 liǎng.

CAUTION

Contraindicated during pregnancy.

---

11. 茯苓 Fú Líng   Poria
Poria

Including
> ▷ *Bái fú líng* (白茯苓 white poria, Poria Alba)
> ▷ *Chì fú líng* (赤茯苓 red poria, Poria Rubra)
> ▷ *Fú shén* (茯神 root poria, Poria cum Pini Radice)
> ▷ *Fú shén mù* (茯神木 pine root in poria, Poriae Pini Radix)

Fú líng is sweet and bland in flavor and neutral in nature. It has three main actions: a) disinhibiting water to eliminate dampness; b) quieting the heart and spirit; c) boosting the spleen and checking diarrhea.

Fú líng disinhibits dampness through bland percolation and it disinhibits urine and disperses water swelling. It is used to treat symptoms of collected water, affecting any of the five viscera and six bowels, appearing anywhere in the body. Here are some examples:

1) To treat generalized puffy swelling caused by spleen vacuity collected dampness, it can be combined with medicinals such as:

dǎng shēn (党参 codonopsis, Codonopsis Radix)

bái zhú (白术 white atractylodes, Atractylodis Macrocephalae Rhizoma)

bàn xià (半夏 pinellia, Pinelliae Rhizoma)

chén pí (陈皮 tangerine peel, Citri Reticulatae Pericarpium)

zhū líng (猪苓 polyporus, Polyporus)

zé xiè (泽泻 alisma, Alismatis Rhizoma)

sāng pí (桑皮 mulberry root bark, Mori Cortex)

dōng guā pí (冬瓜皮 wax gourd rind, Benincasae Exocarpium)

2) To treat collected phlegm and abiding water in the region of the stomach and chest, causing fullness, oppression, and inability to eat, it can be combined as in *fú líng yǐn* (Poria Beverage):

Fú líng yǐn 茯苓饮   Poria Beverage

---

fú líng (茯苓 poria, Poria)

dǎng shēn (党参 codonopsis, Codonopsis Radix)

bái zhú (白术 white atractylodes, Atractylodis Macrocephalae Rhizoma)

zhǐ shí (枳实 unripe bitter orange, Aurantii Fructus Immaturus)

jú pí (橘皮 tangerine peel, Citri Reticulatae Pericarpium)

shēng jiāng (生姜 fresh ginger, Zingiberis Rhizoma Recens)

3) To treat collected water (suspended rheum) in the chest and rib-side area, it can be combined with medicinals such as:

guā lóu (瓜蒌 trichosanthes, Trichosanthis Fructus)

chuān jiāo mù (川椒目 zanthoxylum seed, Zanthoxyli Semen)

sāng pí (桑皮 mulberry root bark, Mori Cortex)

sū zǐ (苏子 perilla fruit, Perillae Fructus)

tíng lì zǐ (葶苈子 lepidium/descurainia, Lepidii/Descurainiae Semen)

jú hóng (橘红 red tangerine peel, Citri Reticulatae Exocarpium Rubrum)

guì zhī (桂枝 cinnamon twig, Cinnamomi Ramulus)

zhū líng (猪苓 polyporus, Polyporus)

zé xiè (泽泻 alisma, Alismatis Rhizoma)

bái jí lí (白蒺藜 tribulus, Tribuli Fructus)

Fú líng (poria) is sweet in flavor and boosts the spleen; it assists splenic movement and transformation of water-damp, thereby achieving the effect of fortifying the spleen. To treat spleen vacuity with exuberant dampness that results in watery diarrhea, for example, *fú líng* can be combined with medicinals such as:

dǎng shēn (党参 codonopsis, Codonopsis Radix)

bái zhú (白术 white atractylodes, Atractylodis Macrocephalae Rhizoma)

zhū líng (猪苓 polyporus, Polyporus)

zé xiè (泽泻 alisma, Alismatis Rhizoma)

huò xiāng (藿香 agastache, Agastaches Herba)

chē qián zǐ (车前子 plantago seed, Plantaginis Semen)

chǎo qiàn shí (炒芡实 stir-fried euryale, Euryales Semen Frictum)

fú lóng gān (伏龙肝 oven earth, Terra Flava Usta)

Combined with *dǎng shēn* (codonopsis), *bái zhú* (white atractylodes), and *gān cǎo* (licorice), *fú líng* treats spleen vacuity and weak qì.

In the treatment of chaotic intestinal function (manifesting as spleen vacuity with non-transformation of water-dampness in the center burner causing indigestion and unformed stool), one can achieve definite results using an appropriate variation of *líng guì zhú gān tāng* (Poria, Cinnamon Twig, White Atractylodes, and Licorice Decoction).

Líng guì zhú gān tāng 苓桂术甘汤   Poria, Cinnamon Twig, White Atractylodes, and Licorice Decoction

---

fú líng (茯苓 poria, Poria)

guì zhī (桂枝 cinnamon twig, Cinnamomi Ramulus)

bái zhú (白术 white atractylodes, Atractylodis Macrocephalae Rhizoma)

gān cǎo (甘草 licorice, Glycyrrhizae Radix)

To this can be added medicinals such as:

chǎo bái sháo (炒白芍 stir-fried white peony, Paeoniae Radix Alba Fricta)

mù xiāng (木香 costusroot, Aucklandiae Radix)

wú zhū yú (吴茱萸 evodia, Evodiae Fructus)

ròu dòu kòu (肉豆蔻 nutmeg, Myristicae Semen)

Fú líng (poria) quiets the heart and spirit; thus it treats insomnia and forgetfulness. It is mainly used for patterns of dual vacuity of the heart and spleen with disquieted heart spirit, insomnia, and forgetfulness. For this purpose it is often combined with medicinals such as:

dāng guī (当归 Chinese angelica, Angelicae Sinensis Radix)

bái zhú (白术 white atractylodes, Atractylodis Macrocephalae Rhizoma)

bǎi zǐ rén (柏子仁 arborvitae seed, Platycladi Semen)

yuǎn zhì (远志 polygala, Polygalae Radix)

suān zǎo rén (酸枣仁 spiny jujube, Ziziphi Spinosi Semen)

zhū shā (朱砂 cinnabar, Cinnabaris) 0.6–0.9 g/2–3 fēn (take drenched)

Comparisons

The ability of *zhū líng* (polyporus)[61] to disinhibit water is greater than that of *fú líng*, but it does not have a supplementing nature. It is generally used to dispel evils and it is not used to supplement the right. *Fú líng*, by contrast, disinhibits dampness through bland percolation, boosts the spleen and quiets the heart; yet it does have a supplementing nature. It dispels evil and supports the right and it is commonly used in supplementing formulas.

In speaking of *fú líng* generally one means *bái fú líng* (white poria). When its color is pale red, it is called *chì fú líng* (red poria), which tends to clear heat and disinhibit dampness. When it grows wrapped around *sōng gēn* (pine root), it is called *fú shén* (root poria), which tends to quiet the heart and quiet the spirit. The skin of the outer aspect of *fú líng* is called *fú líng pí* (poria skin), which tends to disinhibit water and disperse swelling. The *sōng gēn* within *fú shén* is called *fú shén mù* (pine root in poria) and it tends to soothe the sinews and relieve hypertonicity. *Fú shén mù* treats pulling heart pain, spirit fright, and forgetfulness; it also calms the liver and dispels wind. When treating angina pectoris in coronary heart disease with formulas that loosen the chest, free *yáng*, quicken the blood, and open the orifices, add 15–30 g/5 qián–1 liǎng of *fú shén mù*; this addition will sometimes relieve pain.

DOSAGE

The dosage is generally 9–12 g/3–4 qián. For *fú líng pí* or *fú shén mù*, use 15–30 g/5 qián–1 liǎng.

CAUTION

Inappropriate if there is yīn vacuity with lack of fluids and dessication. Also, use with care if there is seminal efflux.

12. 猪苓 Zhū Líng   Polyporus
Polyporus

Zhū líng (polyporus) is sweet and bland in flavor and neutral in nature. Its primary function is to disinhibit water and percolate dampness. It is used for any patho-condition including symptoms such as water swelling, scant urine, diarrhea from exuberant damp, **strangury-turbidity**[565] (淋浊 *lín zhuó*), and jaundice.

a) To treat watery diarrhea with scant urine, combine with *bái zhú* (white atractylodes) and *fú líng* (poria).

b) For spleen dampness with swelling and fullness, and oppression and distention in the stomach duct, combine with the following:

cāng zhú (苍术 atractylodes, Atractylodis Rhizoma)

bái zhú (白术 white atractylodes, Atractylodis Macrocephalae Rhizoma)

hòu pò (厚朴 officinal magnolia bark, Magnoliae Officinalis Cortex)

shā rén (砂仁 amomum, Amomi Fructus)

chén pí (陈皮 tangerine peel, Citri Reticulatae Pericarpium)

fú líng (茯苓 poria, Poria)

c) For heat strangury and painful inhibited urination, combine with medicinals such as:

biǎn xù (萹蓄 knotgrass, Polygoni Avicularis Herba)

qū mài (瞿麦 dianthus, Dianthi Herba)

mù tōng (木通 trifoliate akebia, Akebiae Trifoliatae Caulis)

huáng bǎi (黄柏 phellodendron, Phellodendri Cortex)

huá shí (滑石 talcum, Talcum)

d) For jaundice (yáng jaundice), combine with medicinals such as:

yīn chén (茵陈 virgate wormwood, Artemisiae Scopariae Herba)

chē qián zǐ (车前子 plantago seed, Plantaginis Semen)

huáng bǎi (黄柏 phellodendron, Phellodendri Cortex)

zhī zǐ (栀子 gardenia, Gardeniae Fructus)

dà huáng (大黄 rhubarb, Rhei Radix et Rhizoma)

e) To treat heat effusion (fever), thirst, inhibited urination, and a floating pulse, *zhū líng* can be combined with *zé xiè* (alisma), *huá shí* (talcum), and *ē jiāo* (ass hide glue), which together form *zhū líng tāng* (Polyporus Decoction).

Zhū líng and *zé xiè* (alisma) disinhibit water more effectively when they are used together.

COMPARISONS

Chē qián zǐ (plantago seed)[64] disinhibits water and does not damage yīn; it also clears heat. *Zhū líng* specifically disinhibits water.

DOSAGE

The dosage is generally 6–12 g/2–4 qián. In special circumstances, use up to 20–25 g or 30 g/7–8 qián or 1 liǎng.

CAUTION

Contraindicated for yīn vacuity with clouded vision, in the absence of dampness, and when there is thirst.

---

13. 泽泻 Zé Xiè   Alismatis Rhizoma
Alisma

Zé xiè (alisma) is sweet, bland, and slightly salty in flavor and cold in nature. It has two main uses: a) draining fire from the liver and kidney channels; b) expelling water from the bladder and triple burner. In clinical practice it is mainly used as a urine-disinhibiting, dampness-dispelling, and heat-clearing medicinal.

a) To treat water swelling, distention and fullness, and inhibited urination, it can be combined with medicinals such as:

chē qián zǐ (车前子 plantago seed, Plantaginis Semen)

tōng cǎo (通草 rice-paper plant pith, Tetrapanacis Medulla)

sāng pí (桑皮 mulberry root bark, Mori Cortex)

zhū líng (猪苓 polyporus, Polyporus)

b) For **turbid unctuous urine**[566] (小便浑浊如膏 *xiǎo biàn hún zhuó rú gāo*), combine it with medicinals such as:

fú líng (茯苓 poria, Poria)

hǎi jīn shā (海金沙 lygodium spore, Lygodii Spora)

huá shí (滑石 talcum, Talcum)

bì xiè (萆薢 fish poison yam, Dioscoreae Hypoglaucae seu Semptemlobae Rhizoma)

c) For heat strangury, painful urination, and inhibited urination, combine with medicinals such as:

shēng dì huáng (生地黄 dried/fresh rehmannia, Rehmanniae Radix Exsiccata seu Recens)

mù tōng (木通 trifoliate akebia, Akebiae Trifoliatae Caulis)

zhū líng (猪苓 polyporus, Polyporus)

huáng bǎi (黄柏 phellodendron, Phellodendri Cortex)

shí wéi (石韦 pyrrosia, Pyrrosiae Folium)

d) For water swelling during pregnancy, combine with medicinals such as

sāng pí (桑皮 mulberry root bark, Mori Cortex)

zhǐ qiào (枳壳 bitter orange, Aurantii Fructus)

sāng jì shēng (桑寄生 mistletoe, Taxilli Herba)

fú líng (茯苓 poria, Poria)

dà fù pí (大腹皮 areca husk, Arecae Pericarpium)

e) For urinary calculus, combine with medicinals such as:

hǎi jīn shā (海金沙 lygodium spore, Lygodii Spora)

jīn qián cǎo (金钱草 moneywort, Lysimachiae Herba)

niú xī (牛膝 achyranthes, Achyranthis Bidentatae Radix)

zé lán (泽兰 lycopus, Lycopi Herba)

dōng kuí zǐ (冬葵子 mallow seed, Malvae Semen)

zhū líng (猪苓 polyporus, Polyporus)

fú líng (茯苓 poria, Poria)

chì sháo yào (赤芍药 red peony, Paeoniae Radix Rubra)

f) *Zé xiè* clears and disinhibits liver and gallbladder damp-heat to treat signs such as red eyes, rib-side pain, vomiting, nausea, reduced eating, jaundice, and reddish urine. For this purpose it is combined with medicinals such as:

lóng dǎn cǎo (龙胆草 gentian, Gentianae Radix)

huáng qín (黄芩 scutellaria, Scutellariae Radix)

chái hú (柴胡 bupleurum, Bupleuri Radix)

yīn chén (茵陈 virgate wormwood, Artemisiae Scopariae Herba)

qīng dài (青黛 indigo, Indigo Naturalis)

chē qián zǐ (车前子 plantago seed, Plantaginis Semen)

In clinical practice *zé xiè* is often combined with kidney-supplementing medicinals. With *zé xiè* as an assistant, supplementing medicinals can be prevented from engendering heat and causing kidney fire. *Zé xiè* is the first medicinal chosen for treating the kidney, bladder, or liver when there is fire evil or damp-heat in the kidney.

Zé xiè combined with *bái zhú* (white atractylodes), as in *zé xiè tāng* (Alisma Decoction), treats **propping rheum**[560] (支饮 *zhī yǐn*) and rheum collecting in the stomach (胃内停引 *wèi nèi tíng yǐn*) resulting in dizzy head and vision.

COMPARISONS

Zé xiè disinhibits urine and disperses water swelling. It is suitable for dispersing ascites from water drum distention. *Zé lán* (lycopus)[412] moves blood and disperses water swelling. It is suitable for dispersing ascites from blood drum distention.

DOSAGE

The dosage is generally 6–9 g/2–3 qián. When the disease condition requires, one can use 15–18 g or up to 30 g/5–6 qián or up to 1 liǎng.

CAUTION

Contraindicated for yīn vacuity without damp-heat and kidney vacuity with clouded vision.

---

14. 车前子 Chē Qián Zǐ   Plantaginis Semen
Plantago Seed

Including

▷ *Chē qián cǎo* (车前草 plantago, Plantaginis Herba)

Chē qián zǐ (plantago seed) is sweet in flavor and cold in nature. It disinhibits water, clears heat, frees strangury, boosts the liver and kidney, and brightens the eyes.

1. **Dispersing Water Swelling:** *Chē qián zǐ* disinhibits water and disperses swelling. For this purpose it is often combined with medicinals such as *fú líng* (poria), *zé xiè* (alisma), and *dōng guā pí* (wax gourd rind) and used to treat all forms of water swelling.

2. **Freeing Strangury and Urinary Block:** *Chē qián zǐ* is sweet, cold, disinhibiting, and lubricating; its nature is good for downbearing and draining, so it disinhibits damp and clears heat. It is used for damp-heat pouring downward and heat bind in the bladder and small intestine with signs such as strangury, rough inhibited urination, desire but inability to urinate, spontaneous dribbling with inability to urinate, urethral pain, and, possibly in severe cases, dribbling urinary block or dribbling with difficult urination. For this purpose, *chē qián zǐ* is often combined with medicinals such as:

fú líng (茯苓 poria, Poria)

zé xiè (泽泻 alisma, Alismatis Rhizoma)

huá shí (滑石 talcum, Talcum)

mù tōng (木通 trifoliate akebia, Akebiae Trifoliatae Caulis)

qū mài (瞿麦 dianthus, Dianthi Herba)

huáng bǎi (黄柏 phellodendron, Phellodendri Cortex)

biǎn xù (萹蓄 knotgrass, Polygoni Avicularis Herba)

3. Treating Eye Diseases: *Chē qián zǐ* is sweet and cold and it clears heat and brightens the eyes. It is used for liver fire flaming upward with signs such as red eyes, swollen eyes, and eye pain, as in acute eye diseases. It is often used with medicinals that clear fire or dissipate wind-heat, such as:

jú huā (菊花 chrysanthemum, Chrysanthemi Flos)

sāng yè (桑叶 mulberry leaf, Mori Folium)

cǎo jué míng (草决明 fetid cassia, Cassiae Semen)

huáng lián (黄连 coptis, Coptidis Rhizoma)

huáng qín (黄芩 scutellaria, Scutellariae Radix)

màn jīng zǐ (蔓荆子 vitex, Viticis Fructus)

jīn yín huā (金银花 lonicera, Lonicerae Flos)

mì méng huā (密蒙花 buddleia, Buddleja Flos)

Chē qián zǐ nourishes yīn and enriches the liver and kidney. It is used for liver-kidney yīn vacuity that results in dim cloudy vision and loss of visual acuity. It is often used with medicinals that enrich and supplement the liver and kidney such as:

shēng dì huáng (生地黄 dried/fresh rehmannia, Rehmanniae Radix Exsiccata seu Recens)

shú dì huáng (熟地黄 cooked rehmannia, Rehmanniae Radix Praeparata)

tù sī zǐ (菟丝子 cuscuta, Cuscutae Semen)

shí hú (石斛 dendrobium, Dendrobii Herba)

gǒu qǐ zǐ (枸杞子 lycium, Lycii Fructus)

4. Checking Diarrhea: For exuberant damp causing watery diarrhea, the method of "separating and disinhibiting" (分利 *fēn lì*) is commonly used to check diarrhea. This refers to using urine-disinhibiting medicinals to cause water-damp to be expelled through the urine, so as to reach the goal of checking diarrhea. For this purpose, *chē qián zǐ* is combined with medicinals such as:

zhū líng (猪苓 polyporus, Polyporus)

fú líng (茯苓 poria, Poria)

yǐ rén (苡仁 coix, Coicis Semen)

zhú yè (竹叶 lophatherum, Lophatheri Herba)

bái zhú (白术 white atractylodes, Atractylodis Macrocephalae Rhizoma)

chǎo bái biǎn dòu (炒白扁豆 stir-fried lablab, Lablab Semen Album Frictum)

chǎo shān yào (炒山药 stir-fried dioscorea, Dioscoreae Rhizoma Frictum)

For diarrhea in children during the summer with stool like thin water that continues incessantly for several days, add *chē qián zǐ* 3–9 g/1–3 qián and *jié gěng* (platycodon) 0.9–1.5 g/3–5 fēn to *wǔ wèi yì gōng sǎn* (Five-Ingredient Special Achievement Powder), which contains *dǎng shēn* (codonopsis), *bái zhú* (white atractylodes), *gān cǎo* (licorice), *fú líng* (poria), and *chén pí* (tangerine peel). This combination invariably produces a quite satisfactory effect.

Comparisons

Chē qián zǐ (plantago seed)[64] disinhibits water, clears heat, brightens the eyes, and checks diarrhea. *Chē qián cǎo* (plantago) disinhibits dampness, clears heat, and additionally it cools the blood and stanches bleeding. It is used for bloody urine, blood ejection (吐血 *tù xuè*), and nosebleed.

Huá shí (talcum) and *chē qián zǐ* (plantago seed) both disinhibit water, but *huá shí* also dispels summerheat, whereas *chē qián zǐ* also boosts the liver and kidney and brightens the eyes.

Research

Modern experiments have demonstrated that *chē qián zǐ* truly has a distinct diuretic effect. Not only does it increase the water that is expelled, but at the same time it increases the amount of urea, uric acid, and sodium chloride that is expelled. In addition, it has a definite hypotensive effect. It is used for hypertension with signs such as clouded vision, red eyes, yellow urine, and scant urine.

Note

Chē qián zǐ is generally used in decoction medicine. Because it contains a large amount of a mucous-like substance, it should be wrapped in gauze for decocting.

Dosage

The dosage is generally 3–9 g/1–3 qián. In special cases, use up to 15–30 g/ 5 qián–1 liǎng.

---

15. 滑石 Huá Shí   Talcum
Talcum

Huá shí (talcum) is sweet and bland in flavor and cold in nature. It disinhibits water, dispels dampness, frees strangury, lubricates the urinary orifice (lubricates and disinhibits the urethra), clears summerheat, and allays thirst. It is often used to treat heat strangury, blood strangury, or sand strangury that result in signs such as urethral pain and inhibited urination (see **strangury**[564] 淋 *lín*). It is used together with medicinals such as:

zhū líng (猪苓 polyporus, Polyporus)

zé xiè (泽泻 alisma, Alismatis Rhizoma)

chē qián zǐ (车前子 plantago seed, Plantaginis Semen)

qū mài (瞿麦 dianthus, Dianthi Herba)

hǎi jīn shā (海金沙 lygodium spore, Lygodii Spora)

dōng kuí zǐ (冬葵子 mallow seed, Malvae Semen)

biǎn xù (萹蓄 knotgrass, Polygoni Avicularis Herba)

The blandness of *huá shí* percolates damp, and its cold nature clears heat; therefore, it is suitable for treating summerheat-heat disease (generalized fever, vexation, thirst, inhibited urination, spontaneous sweating, and a soggy slippery pulse) and for damp warm disease (generalized fever that is not very high but does not abate for several days, generalized heaviness, somnolence, indifferent expression, poor appetite, thick white slimy tongue fur, and a slippery moderate pulse).

a) To treat summerheat-heat disease, *huá shí* is often used together with medicinals such as *gān cǎo* (licorice) (as in *liù yī sǎn* (Six-to-One Powder)), *bái biǎn dòu* (lablab), *biǎn dòu huā* (lablab flower), *zhú yè* (lophatherum), *hé yè* (lotus leaf), and *lǜ dòu yī* (mung bean seed-coat).

b) To treat damp warm disease, *huá shí* is often used together with medicinals such as:

yǐ mǐ (苡米 coix, Coicis Semen)

tōng cǎo (通草 rice-paper plant pith, Tetrapanacis Medulla)

pèi lán (佩兰 eupatorium, Eupatorii Herba)

bái dòu kòu (白豆蔻 cardamom, Amomi Fructus Rotundus)

dà dòu juǎn (大豆卷 dried soybean sprout, Sojae Semen Germinatum)

c) To treat **summerheat stroke**[565] (中暑 *zhòng shǔ*) with symptoms such as vomiting and diarrhea, it is used together with medicinals such as:

huò xiāng (藿香 agastache, Agastaches Herba)

pèi lán (佩兰 eupatorium, Eupatorii Herba)

zhú rú (竹茹 bamboo shavings, Bambusae Caulis in Taenia)

bàn xià qū (半夏曲 pinellia leaven, Pinelliae Massa Fermentata) and

fú líng (茯苓 poria, Poria)

Huá shí fěn (talcum powder) is applied topically to moisten the skin, clear heat, and dispel dampness. It is used for **prickly heat**[560] (痱子 *fèi zi*), eczema, and damp itch of the toes. It is used singly or combined with medicinals such as *shí gāo* (gypsum), *kū fán* (calcined alum), and *bò hé* (mint).[8]

Comparisons

Dōng kuí zǐ (mallow seed)[72] and *huá shí* both disinhibit urine and open orifices, but *dōng kuí zǐ* also frees milk, whereas *huá shí* also clears summerheat-heat.

Tōng cǎo (rice-paper plant pith),[57] *mù tōng* (trifoliate akebia),[22] and *huá shí* all disinhibit urine. *Tōng cǎo* leads lung heat downward and disinhibits urine. *Mù tōng* abducts heart fire downward and disinhibits urine. *Huá shí* eliminates bladder damp-heat and disinhibits urine. Thus there are similarities and differences between them.

Dosage

The dosage is generally 9–30 g/3 qián–1 liǎng.

Caution

Contraindicated for spleen-stomach vacuity cold, seminal efflux, or copious urination.

---

[8]Powdered combinations for external use are prepared by grinding the medicinals together and sifting the powder through a fine sieve. *Huá shí* (talcum) is sometimes powdered through a method known as water grinding. This involves working the *huá shí* in a mortar and pestle and putting the resulting powder in water. After the precipitate has settled, the water is poured off and reserved. The dregs are collected and ground again and the process is repeated until a good deal of *huá shí* has disappeared into the collected poured off water. That collected water is evaporated and the fine powdered residue the water leaves behind is known as *shuǐ fēi huá shí* (水飞滑石, water-ground talcum). (Ed.)

---

16. 石韦 Shí Wéi   Pyrrosiae Folium
Pyrrosia

Shí wéi (pyrrosia) is bitter in flavor and slightly cold in nature. Its main actions are clearing lung-channel qì-aspect heat, disinhibiting bladder damp-heat, and disinhibiting water and freeing strangury. It is used for dribbling urinary block, heat strangury, blood strangury, and sand and stone strangury caused by failure of the lung qì to clear [heat] and damp-heat in the bladder. It is often combined with medicinals such as *huá shí* (talcum), *qū mài* (dianthus), *biǎn xù* (knotgrass), *mù tōng* (trifoliate akebia), and *hǎi jīn shā* (lygodium spore). Combined with medicinals such as *xiǎo jì* (field thistle), *xiān hè cǎo* (agrimony), and *bái máo gēn* (imperata), it treats bloody urine. Combined with medicinals such as *bīng láng* (areca) and *zhī mǔ* (anemarrhena), it is used for cough caused by lung qì heat.

COMPARISONS

Hǎi jīn shā (lygodium spore)[70] and *shí wéi* both clear and disinhibit bladder damp-heat and treat strangury. Yet *hǎi jīn shā* tends to enter the blood aspect, while *shí wéi* tends to enter the qì aspect. *Hǎi jīn shā* is generally used for sand and stone strangury, while *shí wéi* is generally used for damp-heat strangury.

According to the findings of modern experiments and research, when chemotherapy or radiation therapy causes a drop in white blood cells, this medicinal has the effect of increasing the white blood cell count.

DOSAGE

The dosage is generally 6–9 g/2–3 qián. In special circumstances, use 15–30 g/ 5 qián–1 liǎng.

---

17. 萹蓄 Biǎn Xù   Polygoni
Knotgrass   Avicularis Herba

Bitter in flavor and neutral in nature, *biǎn xù* (knotgrass) clears and disinhibits bladder damp-heat. It is mainly used to treat heat strangury and inhibited urination. It is often used together with medicinals such as:

zhū líng (猪苓 polyporus, Polyporus)

fú líng (茯苓 poria, Poria)

zé xiè (泽泻 alisma, Alismatis Rhizoma)

mù tōng (木通 trifoliate akebia, Akebiae Trifoliatae Caulis)

huá shí (滑石 talcum, Talcum)

qū mài (瞿麦 dianthus, Dianthi Herba)

Biǎn xù disinhibits dampness and clears heat; thus it is also used to treat damp-heat depression that results in jaundice (yáng jaundice). For this purpose it is combined with medicinals such as:

yīn chén (茵陈 virgate wormwood, Artemisiae Scopariae Herba)

chē qián zǐ (车前子 plantago seed, Plantaginis Semen)

huáng qín (黄芩 scutellaria, Scutellariae Radix)

huáng bǎi (黄柏 phellodendron, Phellodendri Cortex)

To treat eczema, it is used together with medicinals such as:

cāng zhú (苍术 atractylodes, Atractylodis Rhizoma)

huáng bǎi (黄柏 phellodendron, Phellodendri Cortex)

bái xiǎn pí (白藓皮 dictamnus, Dictamni Cortex)

kǔ shēn (苦参 flavescent sophora, Sophorae Flavescentis Radix)

Because *biǎn xù* has a special ability to treat heat strangury, it has been found in modern clinical practice to be effective in the treatment of urinary infection. For this purpose it is often combined with medicinals such as *huáng bǎi* (phellodendron), *mù tōng* (trifoliate akebia), *fú líng* (poria), *zé xiè* (alisma), *qū mài* (dianthus), and *shí wéi* (pyrrosia). According to reports of modern experiments, this medicinal has an inhibitory effect on *Staphylococcus aureus*, *Bacillus dysenteriae*, *Pseudomonas pyocyanea*, *Bacillus typhosus*, and skin fungi.

Biǎn xù stir-fried with vinegar treats roundworm. It is used for pain in the upper abdomen caused by roundworm. For this purpose it is combined with medicinals such as:

wū méi (乌梅 mume, Mume Fructus)

chuān jiāo (川椒 zanthoxylum, Zanthoxyli Pericarpium)

huáng lián (黄连 coptis, Coptidis Rhizoma)

shǐ jūn zǐ (使君子 quisqualis, Quisqualis Fructus)

wú yú (吴萸 evodia, Evodiae Fructus)

DOSAGE

The dosage is generally 6–15 g/2–5 qián.

---

18. 瞿麦 Qū Mài   Dianthi Herba
Dianthus

Bitter in flavor and cold in nature, *qū mài* (dianthus) clears heart heat and disinhibits damp-heat in the small intestine and bladder. It is mainly used for heat strangury, blood strangury, sand strangury, bloody urine, and inhibited urination. It is often used together with medicinals such as:

zé xiè (泽泻 alisma, Alismatis Rhizoma)

huá shí (滑石 talcum, Talcum)

mù tōng (木通 trifoliate akebia, Akebiae Trifoliatae Caulis)

biǎn xù (萹蓄 knotgrass, Polygoni Avicularis Herba)

zhū líng (猪苓 polyporus, Polyporus)

fú líng (茯苓 poria, Poria)

A special characteristic of *qū mài* is that it enters the blood aspect and clears blood heat; therefore, it is often used to treat blood strangury with bloody urine. In general, it is used together with medicinals such as *chǎo zhī zǐ* (stir-fried gardenia), *huáng bǎi tàn* (charred phellodendron), *hǎi jīn shā* (lygodium spore), *bái máo gēn* (imperata), and *dēng xīn tàn* (charred juncus). At the same time, it quickens the blood and dispels stasis; thus, combined with medicinals such as *dāng guī* (Chinese angelica), *chuān xiōng* (chuanxiong), *hóng huā* (carthamus), *táo rén* (peach kernel), and *niú xī* (achyranthes), it is used to treat conditions such as menstrual block or menstruation with purple black clots.

RESEARCH

According to modern reports, *qū mài* is effective in the treatment of ascites from schistosomiasis.

COMPARISON

Because *qū mài suì* (dianthus flower) disinhibits urine better than the stem, it is more commonly used for that purpose than the stem.

Biǎn xù (knotgrass)[68] primarily clears and disinhibits damp-heat in the bladder, and also treats jaundice and eczema. *Shí wéi* (pyrrosia) primarily clears damp-heat from the lung and bladder, tends to enter the qì aspect, and is generally used for damp-heat strangury. In contrast, *qū mài* primarily clears damp-heat from the heart, small intestine, and bladder; it tends to enter the blood aspect and is generally used for blood strangury.

DOSAGE

The dosage is generally 4.5–10 g/1.5–3 qián.

CAUTION

Inappropriate for use in pregnancy.

---

19. 海金沙 Hǎi Jīn Shā   Lygodii Spora
Lygodium Spore

Hǎi jīn shā (lygodium spore) is sweet and bland in flavor and cold in nature. It disinhibits urine, and clears and disinhibits damp-heat in the small intestine and bladder. It is mainly used for various forms of **strangury disease**[564] (淋病 *lín bìng*) and is combined with different medicinals depending on the type of strangury.

a) For heat strangury it is combined with medicinals such as the following:

shí wéi (石韦 pyrrosia, Pyrrosiae Folium)

biǎn xù (萹蓄 knotgrass, Polygoni Avicularis Herba)

mù tōng (木通 trifoliate akebia, Akebiae Trifoliatae Caulis)

zhū líng (猪苓 polyporus, Polyporus)

fú líng (茯苓 poria, Poria)

zé xiè (泽泻 alisma, Alismatis Rhizoma)

huáng bǎi (黄柏 phellodendron, Phellodendri Cortex)

b) For sand or stone strangury it is combined with medicinals such as:

dōng kuí zǐ (冬葵子 mallow seed, Malvae Semen)

jīn qián cǎo (金钱草 moneywort, Lysimachiae Herba)

huá shí (滑石 talcum, Talcum)

chē qián zǐ (车前子 plantago seed, Plantaginis Semen)

zhū líng (猪苓 polyporus, Polyporus)

shí wéi (石韦 pyrrosia, Pyrrosiae Folium)

c) For blood strangury it is combined with medicinals such as *huáng bǎi tàn* (charred phellodendron), *bái máo gēn* (imperata), *zé xiè* (alisma), and *qū mài* (dianthus).

RESEARCH

On the basis of experience in recent years, using *hǎi jīn shā* combined with medicinals such as *dōng kuí zǐ* (mallow seed), *niú xī* (achyranthes), *jīn qián cǎo* (moneywort), *zé xiè* (alisma), *zé lán* (lycopus), *chì sháo* (red peony), *bīng láng* (areca) (or *chén xiāng* (aquilaria)), and *wáng bù liú xíng* (vaccaria) produces highly satisfactory results in the treatment of urinary calculus. I have encountered 2 or 3 cases, verified by X-ray, of urethral calculi being expelled through the ureter. When lumbar pain is pronounced, *hǎi jīn shā* is combined with medicinals such as *sāng jì shēng* (mistletoe), *xù duàn* (dipsacus), *gǒu jǐ* (cibotium), *dù zhòng* (eucommia), *rǔ xiāng* (frankincense), and *mò yào* (myrrh).

COMPARISONS

Qū mài (dianthus),[69] *bì xiè* (fish poison yam), and *hǎi jīn shā* are all used to treat strangury. While *qū mài* is generally used to treat blood strangury, *bì xiè* is used to treat unctuous strangury (膏淋 *gāo lín*) and *hǎi jīn shā* is used to treat stone strangury.

DOSAGE

The dosage is generally 3–9 g/1–3 qián. When using this medicinal singly, use 15–30 g/5 qián–1 liäng.

CAUTION

Contraindicated when there is constitutional vacuity with frequent urination or when damp-heat is absent.

---

20. 金钱草 Jīn Qián Cǎo   Lysimachiae Herba
Moneywort

Sweet and bitter in flavor and slightly cold in nature, *jīn qián cǎo* (moneywort) disinhibits water and expels stones, and clears and disinhibits damp-heat in the liver, gallbladder, bladder, and kidney channels. It is mainly used to disinhibit urine and free strangury (stone strangury) and to expel stones (biliary calculi, renal calculi, urethral calculi, and bladder calculi).

When combined with medicinals such as *chái hú* (bupleurum), *huáng qín* (scutellaria), *bàn xià* (pinellia), *zhǐ shí* (unripe bitter orange), *bīng láng* (areca), *dà huáng* (rhubarb), *yuán míng fěn* (refined mirabilite), and *yīn chén* (virgate wormwood), it treats biliary calculi. When combined with medicinals such as *zhū líng* (polyporus), *fú líng* (poria), *dōng kuí zǐ* (mallow seed), *huá shí* (talcum), *niú xī* (achyranthes), *bīng láng* (areca), *hǎi jīn shā* (lygodium spore), *zé lán* (lycopus), and *zé xiè* (alisma), it is used for urinary calculus.

Care should be taken to apply the principle of pattern identification as the basis of determining treatment and to vary the medicinals depending on the presence of vacuity or repletion and cold or heat. For example, in a case of biliary calculi, if the patient presents with liver depression and qì stagnation signs (such as ribside pain and distention, oppression in the chest, stomach duct blockage, essence-spirit depression, and tendency to frequent sighing), it should be combined with liver-soothing and qì-rectifying medicinals such as *mù xiāng* (costusroot), *xiāng fù* (cyperus), *chǎo chuān liàn zǐ* (stir-fried toosendan), and *yù jīn* (curcuma). If ribside pain or right lateral epigastric pain of fixed location is observed and stasis macules are visible on the tongue, then *jīn qián cǎo* should be combined with medicinals such as *wǔ líng zhī* (squirrel's droppings), *shēng pú huáng* (raw typha pollen), *yán hú suǒ* (corydalis), *rǔ xiāng* (frankincense), *mò yào* (myrrh), *dān shēn* (salvia), and *hóng huā* (carthamus) to quicken the blood and transform stasis. If there is habitual constipation, a large dose of *dà huáng* (rhubarb) and *yuán míng fěn* (refined mirabilite) should be used. If urinary calculus manifests with such signs as kidney vacuity lumbar pain and lack of strength in the knees, *jīn qián cǎo* should be combined with kidney-boosting medicinals such as *sāng jì shēng* (mistletoe), *xù duàn* (dipsacus), *gǒu qǐ zǐ* (lycium), and *tóng jí lí* (complanate astragalus seed). If there is lesser abdominal pain that likes warmth and that may spread to the testicles or perineum, *jīn qián cǎo* should be combined with medicinals that warm the liver and kidney and move qì, such as *chǎo chuān liàn zǐ* (stir-fried toosendan), *chǎo xiǎo huí xiāng* (stir-fried fennel), *wú yú* (evodia), *wū yào* (lindera), and *lì zhī hé* (litchee pit). If there is rough voiding of reddish urine, urethral pain, or, possibly in severe cases, bloody urine, then it should be combined with medicinals such as *huáng bǎi* (phellodendron), *mù tōng* (trifoliate akebia), *qū mài* (dianthus), *shēng dì huáng* (dried/fresh rehmannia), and *biǎn xù* (knotgrass). Note that the more appropriately the formula is tailored to the signs, the more effective it is.

DOSAGE

The dosage is generally about 30 g/1 liǎng. When this medicinal is used singly, then 60–90 g/2–3 liǎng is used.

---

21. 冬葵子 Dōng Kuí Zǐ   Malvae
Mallow Seed   Verticillatae Semen

Dōng kuí zǐ (mallow seed) is sweet in flavor, cold in nature, lubricating, and disinhibiting. It disinhibits urine, lubricates the intestines, and frees milk. Combined with medicinals such as *chē qián zǐ* (plantago seed), *zhū líng* (polyporus), *fú líng* (poria), *qū mài* (dianthus), *biǎn xù* (knotgrass), and *huá shí* (talcum), it is used for signs such as painful urinary strangury, scant urine, and frequent urination accompanied by dry, bound stool. Combined with medicinals such as *tōng cǎo* (rice-paper plant pith), *wáng bù liú xíng* (vaccaria), and *zhì shān jiǎ* (mix-fried pangolin scales), it is used for **breast milk stoppage**[543] (乳汁不通 *rǔ zhī bù tōng*). Combined with medicinals such as *lòu lú* (rhaponticum), *guā lóu* (trichosanthes), *bái zhǐ* (Dahurian angelica), and *chì sháo* (red peony), it is used for the onset of mammary welling-abscess.

In modern clinical practice, this medicinal has been proven effective in the treatment of urinary calculi in combination with medicinals such as *jīn qián cǎo* (moneywort), *hǎi jīn shā* (lygodium spore), *niú xī* (achyranthes), *zé lán* (lycopus), and *zé xiè* (alisma) because of its ability to lubricate and disinhibit the orifices. For example, a patient who for two days had been passing stones and suffering from lower abdominal pain that radiated to the lower back and urinary tract, short painful urination with reddish urine, dry stool, a yellow tongue fur, and a slippery rapid pulse was diagnosed as having damp-heat strangury and sand and stone strangury. The Western medical diagnosis was urinary calculus. I used the following formula:

> *dōng kuí zǐ* (冬葵子 mallow seed, Malvae Semen) 15 g/5 qián
> *niú xī* (牛膝 achyranthes, Achyranthis Bidentatae Radix) 15 g/5 qián
> *zé lán* (泽兰 lycopus, Lycopi Herba) 12 g/4 qián
> *huáng bǎi* (黄柏 phellodendron, Phellodendri Cortex) 12 g/4 qián
> *zé xiè* (泽泻 alisma, Alismatis Rhizoma) 9 g/3 qián
> *zhū líng* (猪苓 polyporus, Polyporus) 15 g/5 qián
> *fú líng* (茯苓 poria, Poria) 15 g/5 qián
> *jīn qián cǎo* (金钱草 moneywort, Lysimachiae Herba) 30 g/1 liǎng
> *biǎn xù* (萹蓄 knotgrass, Polygoni Avicularis Herba) 12 g/4 qián
> *shēng dà huáng* (生大黄 raw rhubarb, Rhei Radix et Rhizoma Crudi)
>   6 g/2 qián
> *wū yào* (乌药 lindera, Linderae Radix) 6 g/2 qián
> *qū mài* (瞿麦 dianthus, Dianthi Herba) 12 g/4 qián
> *huáng qín* (黄芩 scutellaria, Scutellariae Radix) 10 g/3 qián

This formula was taken decocted with water. Altogether, two packets were taken before two small black and brown stones, about the size of grains of rice, were expelled in the urine. The patient then recovered completely.

COMPARISONS

Chē qián zǐ (plantago seed)[64] clears heat and disinhibits dampness so as to free strangury. It also disinhibits dampness so as to check diarrhea. *Dōng kuí zǐ* is slippery and disinhibits the orifices so as to free strangury. It also lubricates the intestines and frees the stool.

Wáng bù liú xíng (vaccaria)[411] frees milk by freeing and moving the blood vessels, whereas *dōng kuí zǐ* frees milk by disinhibiting and eliminating stagnation.

Dosage

The dosage is generally 6–9 g/2–3 qián. In special conditions, use up to 15–30 g/ 5 qián–1 liǎng.

This medicinal is a disinhibiting and freeing substance; therefore, it is inappropriate for pregnant women and in the absence of a repletion evil.

---

22. 薏苡仁 Yì Yǐ Rén   Coicis Semen

Coix

Also called 苡仁 *yǐ rén* or 苡米 *yǐ mǐ* in Chinese. *Yì yǐ rén* (coix) is sweet and bland in flavor and slightly cold in nature. It has four main actions: a) disinhibiting dampness; b) fortifying the spleen; c) expelling pus; and d) soothing the sinews. Use it raw to disinhibit dampness, expel pus, and soothe the sinews; use it stir fried to fortify the spleen and stomach.

1. Disinhibiting Dampness: *Shēng yǐ mǐ* (raw coix) disinhibits water and dispels dampness. It is often combined with medicinals such as *chē qián zǐ* (plantago seed), *zhū líng* (polyporus), *fú líng* (poria), and *zé xiè* (alisma) to treat water swelling and inhibited urination. Combined with medicinals such as *mù guā* (chaenomeles), *niú xī* (achyranthes), *fáng jǐ* (fangji), *zǐ sū* (perilla), and *bīng láng* (areca), it is used for pain and swelling of the knee and foot and for **damp leg qi**[545] (湿脚气 *shī jiǎo qì*).

2. Fortifying the Spleen: *Chǎo yǐ mǐ* (stir-fried coix) fortifies the spleen and eliminates dampness. It is often combined with medicinals such as *bái zhú* (white atractylodes), *fú líng* (poria), *chǎo shān yào* (stir-fried dioscorea), *chǎo bái biǎn dòu* (stir-fried lablab), and *qiàn shí* (euryale) to treat spleen vacuity diarrhea. When there is spleen vacuity with exuberant dampness, *shēng yǐ mǐ* (raw coix) and *shú yǐ mǐ* (cooked coix) are often used together to fortify the spleen and disinhibit dampness.

3. Expelling Pus: *Shēng yǐ mǐ* (raw coix) not only disinhibits dampness, it also clears heat and expels pus. For example, combined with medicinals such as *dōng guā zǐ* (wax gourd seed), *táo rén* (peach kernel), and *lú gēn* (phragmites), it is used for pulmonary welling-abscess (肺痈 *fèi yōng*, equivalent to pulmonary abscess in Western medicine). Combined with medicinals such as *jié gěng* (platycodon) and *bái jí* (bletilla), it is used for pulmonary welling-abscess that has already ruptured, with spitting of great quantities of pus and blood, and it assists in expelling the pus. Combined with medicinals such as *jīn yín huā* (lonicera), *dāng guī* (Chinese angelica), *shēng dì huáng* (dried/fresh rehmannia), *xuán shēn* (scrophularia), *shēng dì yú* (raw sanguisorba), *huáng qín* (scutellaria), *gān cǎo* (licorice), *shēng dà huáng* (raw rhubarb), and *dān pí* (moutan), it is used for acute appendicitis. Combined with medicinals such as *fù zǐ* (aconite) and *bài jiàng cǎo* (patrinia), it is used for appendicitis that has already suppurated, perforated, and formed an abscess that has persisted for several days.

4. Soothing the Sinews: *Shēng yǐ mǐ* (raw coix) also soothes the sinews, disinhibits the joints, and relieves impediment pain. Combined with medicinals such as *wēi líng xiān* (clematis), *fáng jǐ* (fangji), *qiāng huó* (notopterygium), *dú huó* (pubescent angelica), *sāng zhī* (mulberry twig), *chì sháo* (red peony), *dāng guī* (Chinese angelica), and *fù piàn* (sliced aconite), it is used for wind-damp impediment pain, tension of the sinews and hypertonicity, and inability of the limbs to extend and stretch. When there is chronic wind-damp impediment, hypertonicity of the sinews, and deformity of the joints and limbs, then add to the combination mentioned above medicinals such as *gǔ suì bǔ* (drynaria), *shēn jīn cǎo* (ground pine), *zhì shān jiǎ* (mix-fried pangolin scales), *hóng huā* (carthamus), *dì lóng* (earthworm), *hǔ gǔ* (tiger bone) (or *bào gǔ*), *xù duàn* (dipsacus), and *mù guā* (chaenomeles). These additions quicken the blood and free the network vessels, and soothe the sinews and strengthen the bones. In such cases, use *shēng yǐ mǐ* and *shú yǐ mǐ* together to disinhibit dampness and soothe the sinews, as well as to fortify the spleen and boost the stomach.

COMPARISONS

Mù guā (chaenomeles)[78] and *yǐ mǐ* both soothe the sinews. Nevertheless, *mù guā* tends to treat damp-cold that results in tension of the sinews and leg cramps, whereas *yǐ rén* tends to treat damp-heat causing hypertonicity of the sinews and difficulty in stretching the limbs.

Bái biǎn dòu (lablab)[104] and *yǐ mǐ* both fortify the spleen. Nevertheless, *bái biǎn dòu* tends to disperse summerheat and eliminate dampness to fortify the spleen, whereas *yǐ mǐ* tends to disinhibit dampness through bland percolation to fortify the spleen.

DOSAGE

The dosage is generally 10–20 g/3–6 qián. However, this medicinal is bland in flavor and moderate in strength, so if the disease is severe, it is often necessary to use a larger dose, such as 30–60 g/1–2 liǎng, and to take it over a long period of time.

This medicinal is inappropriate if there is seminal efflux or copious urination. It is contraindicated in pregnancy.

---

23. 防己 Fáng Jǐ   Stephaniae
Fangji   Tetrandrae Radix

Main Types

  ▷ *hàn fáng jǐ* (汉防己 mealy fangji, Stephaniae Tetrandrae Radix)
  ▷ *Guǎng fáng jǐ* (广防己 southern fangji, Aristolochiae Fangchi Radix)
  ▷ *Mù fáng jǐ* (木防己 woody fangji, Cocculi Radix)

Fáng jǐ (fangji) is extremely bitter, acrid, and cold. It disinhibits water and dispels wind, frees and moves the channels and network vessels, and drains lower burner blood-aspect damp-heat.

Combined with medicinals such as *huáng qí* (astragalus), *guì zhī* (cinnamon twig), *bái zhú* (white atractylodes), and *fú líng* (poria), *fáng jǐ* treats **wind water**[568] (风水 *fēng shuǐ*), which is characterized by puffy swelling of the head, face, and extremities, aversion to wind, bone joint pain, and a floating pulse, and **skin water**[563] (皮水 *pí shuǐ*) characterized by water swelling in the extremities. Listed below are two formulas that illustrate this use.

Fáng jǐ huáng qí tāng 防己黄芪汤   Fangji and Astragalus Decoction

fáng jǐ (防己 fangji, Stephaniae Tetrandrae Radix)

huáng qí (黄芪 astragalus, Astragali Radix)

bái zhú (白术 white atractylodes, Atractylodis Macrocephalae Rhizoma)

gān cǎo (甘草 licorice, Glycyrrhizae Radix)

shēng jiāng (生姜 fresh ginger, Zingiberis Rhizoma Recens)

dà zǎo (大枣 jujube, Jujubae Fructus)

Fáng jǐ fú líng tāng 防己茯苓汤   Fangji and Poria Decoction

fáng jǐ (防己 fangji, Stephaniae Tetrandrae Radix)

huáng qí (黄芪 astragalus, Astragali Radix)

fú líng (茯苓 poria, Poria)

guì zhī (桂枝 cinnamon twig, Cinnamomi Ramulus)

gān cǎo (甘草 licorice, Glycyrrhizae Radix)

For these patterns, it may be appropriate to add *má huáng* (ephedra), *sāng pí* (mulberry root bark), and *dōng guā pí* (wax gourd rind) in order to diffuse the lung and disinhibit water.

Combined with medicinals such as *wēi líng xiān* (clematis), *yǐ mǐ* (coix), *qiāng huó* (notopterygium), *dú huó* (pubescent angelica), *hóng huā* (carthamus), and *chì sháo* (red peony), *fáng jǐ* is used for symptoms such as painful swollen joints and limb hypertonicity occurring in wind-damp impediment. Combined with *mù guā* (chaenomeles), *yǐ rén* (coix), *dì lóng* (earthworm), *niú xī* (achyranthes), *bīng láng* (areca), and *fú líng* (poria), it is used for depressed damp-heat causing symptoms such as puffy swelling of the legs, pain and swelling of the feet, and **damp leg qì**[545] (湿脚气 *shī jiǎo qì*). Combined with medicinals such as *mù tōng* (trifoliate akebia), *zé xiè* (alisma), and *zhū líng* (polyporus), it is used for pathoconditions such as damp-heat in the bladder and inhibited urination.

Comparisons

There are two main types of *fáng jǐ*: *hàn fáng jǐ* (mealy fangji) and *mù fáng jǐ* (woody fangji), whose effects are basically the same.[9] Nevertheless, with careful discrimination, there are small differences. It is generally said that *hàn fáng jǐ*

---

[9]The PRC Pharmacopoeia considers *hàn fáng jǐ* to be the main type, and hence represents the Chinese pharmaceutical term by the Latin *Radix Stephaniae Tetrandrae*. In addition to *hàn fáng jǐ* (汉防己, mealy fangji, Stephaniae Tetrandrae Radix), and *mù fáng jǐ* (木防己, woody fangji, Cocculi Radix) mentioned by Prof. Jiāo, there is also *guǎng fáng jǐ* (广防己, southern fangji, Aristolochiae Fangchi Radix), *Guǎng fáng jǐ* belongs to the genus *Aristolochia*

tends to dispel dampness and is suitable for lower burner damp-heat, lower body water swelling, and **damp leg qi**[545] (湿脚气 *shī jiǎo qì*). *Mù fáng jǐ* tends to dispel wind, free the network vessels, and relieve pain. It is suitable for upper body water swelling and wind-damp pain. If "*fáng jǐ* 防己" is written on a prescription, the pharmacy will generally give *hàn fáng jǐ* 汉防己. When one wishes to use *mù fáng jǐ* 木防己, it is necessary to specify.

Tōng cǎo (rice-paper plant pith),[57] sweet and bland, expels qì-aspect damp-heat. *Fáng jǐ*, bitter and cold, drains blood-aspect damp-heat.

Mù guā (chaenomeles)[78] is sour and warm; it transforms dampness, soothes the sinews, and quickens the network vessels. It is effective for hypertonicity of the sinews and wilting of the legs. *Fáng jǐ* is bitter and cold; it disinhibits water, frees the network vessels, and drains heat. It is effective for water swelling and **leg qi**[556] (脚气 *jiǎo qì*).

RESEARCH

According to modern reports, *mù fáng jǐ* treats all forms of neuralgia. It is used for conditions such as intercostal neuralgia, tubercular chest pain, all forms of muscular pain, frozen shoulder, **wrenching and contusion**[568] (闪挫 *shǎn cuò*), stomach pain, and menstrual pain.

DOSAGE

The dosage is generally 3–9 g/1–3 qián. This medicinal is very bitter and very cold; thus it is inappropriate to use large doses because it may damage the stomach and the center burner. Modern reports suggest that small amounts of *hàn fáng jǐ* cause an increase in urine volume, but that large amounts cause urine volume to decrease.

CAUTION

This medicinal is very moving in nature, and so is contraindicated for yīn vacuity or in the absence of damp-heat repletion evil. It also is inappropriate for qì-aspect heat.

---

and contains aristolochic acid. While the correct species for this medicinal is considered to be *Aristolochia fangchi*, there are many species of the genus Aristolochia that are substituted for this medicinal, including *Aristolochia tagala*, *Aristolochia austroszechuanica*, *Aristolochia heterophylla*, and *Aristolochia moupinensis*. It is very difficult to distinguish between these species visually and unfortunately it is also difficult to tell some of these species from plants that contain no aristolochic acid such as *hàn fáng jǐ* and *mù fáng jǐ*. *Hàn fáng jǐ* (Stephania tetrandra) is the most commonly prescribed form of *fáng jǐ*. Only a negative test for the presence of aristolochic acid and a positive test for tetradrine insure the correct identification of this medicinal. *Mù fáng jǐ* is *Cocculus trilobus*; it contains no aristolochic acid. It is sometimes mistakenly sold as *hàn fáng jǐ*. (Ed.)

24. 木瓜 Mù Guā   Chaenomelis Fructus
Chaenomeles

Mù guā (chaenomeles) is sour in flavor and warm in nature. It mainly disinhibits dampness and rectifies the spleen, and soothes the sinews and quickens the network vessels.

1. Disinhibiting Dampness and Rectifying the Spleen: *Mù guā* disinhibits dampness and warms the spleen and stomach. It is used for exuberant dampness in the center burner that results in symptoms such as vomiting, diarrhea, and abdominal distention. For this purpose it is often used together with medicinals such as *zǐ sū* (perilla), *wú yú* (evodia), *huí xiāng* (fennel), *pèi lán* (eupatorium), and *gān cǎo* (licorice). It is also commonly used for dampness evil streaming into the lower leg and upper surface of the foot resulting in **damp leg qi**[545] (湿脚气 *shī jiǎo qì*). For this purpose it is often used together with medicinals such as *zǐ sū* (perilla), *wú yú* (evodia), *jié gěng* (platycodon), *bīng láng* (areca), *jú pí* (tangerine peel), and *shēng jiāng* (fresh ginger) (as in *jī míng sǎn* (Cockcrow Powder)).

2. Soothing the Sinews and Quickening the Network Vessels: *Mù guā* treats diseases of the sinews. It relaxes sinew tension and tightens slack sinews. In clinical practice it is used for summerheat-damp damaging the center, engendering incessant vomiting and diarrhea that causes spasms of the gastrocnemius of both legs (traditionally called 霍乱转筋 *huò luàn zhuǎn jīn*, "cholera cramps"). For this pattern it is commonly used together with medicinals such as *huò xiāng* (agastache), *pèi lán* (eupatorium), *bái biǎn dòu* (lablab), *dǎng shēn* (codonopsis), *wú yú* (evodia), *bái sháo* (white peony), and *gān cǎo* (licorice). For invasion of damp evil causing disharmony of the channels and network vessels, slack sinews, inhibited joints, swelling, distention, and deep pain (damp impediment), it is often used in combination with medicinals such as *hǔ gǔ* (tiger bone), *niú xī* (achyranthes), *wǔ jiā pí* (acanthopanax), *dāng guī* (Chinese angelica), *chuān xiōng* (chuanxiong), *chuān wū* (aconite root), *wēi líng xiān* (clematis), and *hǎi fēng téng* (kadsura pepper stem).

Bái sháo (white peony) treats diseases of the sinews. It primarily **emolliates the liver**[548] (柔肝 *róu gān*) and relaxes tension to nourish the sinews. *Mù guā* also treats diseases of the sinews, but it chiefly disinhibits dampness and warms the liver to soothe the sinews.

Dosage
The dosage is generally 6–12 g/2–4 qián.

Caution
This medicinal is sour in flavor; used singly, it has an astringent effect. Therefore, when the tendons and joints are inhibited and at the same time urination is inhibited, it is inappropriate for single use and it must be combined with water-disinhibiting medicinals.

25. 五加皮 Wǔ Jiā Pí
Acanthopanax
Acanthopanacis
Cortex

Acrid and bitter in flavor and warm in nature, *wǔ jiā pí* (acanthopanax) disinhibits dampness and disperses swelling, strengthens the lumbus and knees, and strengthens sinew and bone. It is used for conditions such as wind-damp impediment pain, limp legs, aching lumbus and knees, and puffy swelling of the legs. It is commonly used together with medicinals such as:

niú xī (牛膝 achyranthes, Achyranthis Bidentatae Radix)

yǐ rén (苡仁 coix, Coicis Semen)

bì xiè (萆薢 fish poison yam, Dioscoreae Hypoglaucae seu Semptemlobae Rhizoma)

mù guā (木瓜 chaenomeles, Chaenomelis Fructus)

dú huó (独活 pubescent angelica, Angelicae Pubescentis Radix)

Wǔ jiā pí, combined with *mù guā* (chaenomeles) and *niú xī* (achyranthes), ground to a powder, is given to children with limp legs and an inability to walk. According to modern research, it has been shown that *nán wǔ jiā pí* (acanthopanax) is rich in vitamins A and B, and volatile oils (acanthopanax oil); therefore, it is used for various diseases caused by vitamin A or B deficiency. Combined with medicinals such as *fú líng pí* (poria skin), *sāng pí* (mulberry root bark), *dōng guā pí* (wax gourd rind), *chén pí* (tangerine peel), and *má huáng* (ephedra), it is used for acute nephritis with lumbar pain and water swelling. Combined with medicinals such as *fú líng* (poria), *zhū líng* (polyporus), *zé xiè* (alisma), and *guì zhī* (cinnamon twig), it is used for cardiac insufficiency causing puffy swelling of the legs. According to research reports, *běi wǔ jiā pí* (periploca) has actions similar to K-strophanthin and so has a cardiotonic effect. Applying modern discoveries within the framework of pattern identification as the basis of determining treatment can increase therapeutic efficacy.

When this medicinal is steeped in liquor, it is called *wǔ jiā pí jiǔ* (acanthopanax wine). It dispels wind-damp, strengthens sinew and bone, strengthens the lumbus and knees, and is used wherever necessary according to the signs.

Wǔ jiā pí is also applied topically. For example, combined with medicinals such as *huáng bǎi* (phellodendron), *shé chuáng zǐ* (cnidium seed), *fáng fēng* (saposhnikovia), and *kǔ shēn* (flavescent sophora), decocted in water, and used as a topical wash, it treats symptoms such as scrotal damp itch and eczema.

COMPARISON

Wǔ jiā pí is also called *nán wǔ jiā pí* 南五加皮, literally "southern *wǔ jiā pí*," in distinction to *běi wǔ jiā pí* 北五加皮 "northern *wǔ jiā pí*," which botanically comes from the plant of a different genus, *Periploca sepium*. Although their effects are for the most part the same, there are minor differences. *Běi wǔ jiā pí* (periploca) is generally used to disinhibit dampness and treat water swelling. *Wǔ jiā pí* (acanthopanax) is generally used to strengthen sinew and bone and to treat limp legs.[10]

DOSAGE

The dosage is generally 3–9 g/1–3 qián.

CAUTION

Cease *běi wǔ jiā pí* (periploca) if the pulse is found to become slower (less than 60 beats per minute).

---

26. 冬瓜皮 Dōng Guā Pí	Benincasae
Wax Gourd Rind	Exocarpium

Including
 ▷ *Dōng guā zǐ* (冬瓜子 wax gourd seed, Benincasae Semen)

Dōng guā pí (wax gourd rind), sweet in flavor and cold in nature, disinhibits urine and is mainly used to treat various forms of water swelling. For this purpose it is often combined with medicinals such as *sāng pí* (mulberry root bark), *fú líng pí* (poria skin), *zhū líng* (polyporus), *zé xiè* (alisma), and *chē qián zǐ* (plantago seed). To mitigate its cold nature, it is often combined with warm medicinals such as *shēng jiāng* (fresh ginger), *jiāng pí* (ginger skin), and *chén pí* (tangerine peel).

Dōng guā zǐ (wax gourd seed) is sweet in flavor and slightly cold in nature; it expels pus and disinhibits dampness, downbears phlegm and clears the lung, and moistens dryness and abducts stagnation. For these reasons, it is used for pulmonary welling-abscess, intestinal welling-abscess, cough due to lung heat and copious phlegm, and dry stool. To treat pulmonary welling-abscess, it is often combined with medicinals such as *táo rén* (peach kernel), *jié gěng* (platycodon), *shēng yǐ mǐ* (raw coix), and *lú gēn* (phragmites). To treat intestinal welling-abscess (appendicitis), it is often combined with medicinals such as *shēng dà huáng* (raw rhubarb), *dān pí* (moutan), *yǐ rén* (coix), *lián qiáo* (forsythia), *chì sháo* (red peony), and *bài jiàng cǎo* (patrinia). To treat lung heat with copious phlegm, it is often combined with medicinals such as *zhī mǔ* (anemarrhena), *bèi mǔ* (fritillaria), *guā lóu* (trichosanthes), and *xìng rén* (apricot kernel).

DOSAGE

The dosage of *dōng guā pí* (wax gourd rind) is generally 15–30 g/5 qián–1 liǎng. If the disease is severe, use up to 60 g/2 liǎng. The dosage of *dōng guā zǐ* is generally 9–15 g/3–5 qián. To treat lung or intestinal welling-abscess, use up to 30 g/1 liǎng.

CAUTION

Inappropriate for spleen-stomach vacuity cold or sloppy soft stool.

---

[10]*Běi wǔ jiā pí* (*Periploca sepium*) is sometimes substituted for *wǔ jiā pí* (*Acanthopanacis gracilistylus*). The former has a stronger aroma than the latter and so is also known by the name 香加皮 *xiāng jiā pí*, which means "fragrant (*wǔ*) *jiā pí*." In modern times this medicinal has been found to have a cardiotonic effect. *Běi wǔ jiā pí* is considered to be slightly toxic. (Ed.)

27. 茵陈 Yīn Chén
Virgate Wormwood

Artemisiae
Virgate Wormwood
Herba

Also called *yīn chén hāo* 茵陈蒿. Bitter in flavor and slightly cold in nature, *yīn chén* (virgate wormwood) clears heat, disinhibits dampness, and abates jaundice. Combined with medicinals such as *zhī zǐ* (gardenia), *huáng bǎi* (phellodendron), *dà huáng* (rhubarb), and *chē qián zǐ* (plantago seed), it is used for yáng jaundice (damp-heat jaundice). Combined with medicinals such as *fù zǐ* (aconite), *gān jiāng* (dried ginger), *bái zhú* (white atractylodes), *fú líng* (poria), and *zé xiè* (alisma), it is used for yīn jaundice (cold-damp jaundice). When there is dampness in the exterior, it effuses sweat mildly; when there is dampness in the interior, it disinhibits urine and dispels dampness. Therefore, one can use it for yáng jaundice, yīn jaundice, exterior dampness, or interior dampness. In modern clinical practice, jaundice due to infectious hepatitis (which generally corresponds to yáng jaundice in Chinese medicine) has been treated with a combination of *yīn chén* (virgate wormwood), *zhī zǐ* (gardenia), *huáng bǎi* (phellodendron), *chē qián zǐ* (plantago seed), *chái hú* (bupleurum), *huáng qín* (scutellaria), and *dà huáng* (rhubarb). This formula, varied appropriately in accordance with the signs, has a pronounced jaundice-abating effect.

Yīn chén is also used for damp-warmth or the onset of summerheat-warmth in which there are symptoms such as alternating cold and heat, bitter taste in the mouth, oppression in the chest, dry retching, dizzy head, rib-side pain, no thought of food and drink, or hearing loss.   For this purpose it is often combined with medicinals such as *huáng qín* (scutellaria), *zhú rú* (bamboo shavings), *chén pí* (tangerine peel), *bàn xià* (pinellia), *zhǐ qiào* (bitter orange), *bái dòu kòu* (cardamom), and *yǐ rén* (coix).

Yīn chén disinhibits the gallbladder and also suppresses bacteria. Combined with medicinals such as *jīn yín huā* (lonicera), *lián qiáo* (forsythia), *zhǐ shí* (unripe bitter orange), *chái hú* (bupleurum), *jiāo sān xiān* (scorch-fried three immortals), *bīng láng* (areca), *chì sháo* (red peony), and *lái fú zǐ* (radish seed), it is used for infection of the biliary tract. Combined with *kǔ liàn zǐ* (chinaberry seed), or *kǔ liàn pí* (chinaberry bark), as well as *wū méi* (mume), *shǐ jūn zǐ* (quisqualis), *bīng láng* (areca), *chuān jiāo* (zanthoxylum), *dà huáng* (rhubarb), and *yán hú suǒ* (corydalis), it is used for biliary tract ascariasis.

DOSAGE

The dosage is generally 9–15 g/3–5 qián. When the disease is severe, use 25–30 g/8 qián–1 liǎng. In specific conditions, up to 60 g/2 liǎng can be used.

---

28. 玉米须 Yù Mǐ Xū   Mays Stylus
Corn Silk

Sweet in flavor and neutral in nature, *yù mǐ xū* (corn silk) disinhibits urine and disperses water swelling. Combined with medicinals such as *sāng pí* (mulberry root bark), *fú líng pí* (poria skin), and *chén pí* (tangerine peel), it is used for nephritis with water swelling. Combined with medicinals such as *yīn chén* (virgate wormwood), *huáng bǎi* (phellodendron), and *zhī zǐ* (gardenia), it is used for jaundice in infectious hepatitis. But it is most commonly used to treat all forms of water swelling when used singly, brewed in water, and taken internally.

According to the findings of modern experimental research, this medicinal is a cholagogue and hypotensive. It is used together with medicinals such as *yīn chén* (virgate wormwood), *jīn qián cǎo* (moneywort), *yán hú suǒ* (corydalis), and *lú gēn* (phragmites) to treat cholecystitis and gallstones (sandy calculi or small stones).

Cooked singly, this medicinal is also used for treatment of hypertension and diabetes mellitus.

Dosage

The dosage is 15–30 g/5 qián–1 liǎng. When used alone, the dosage is 45–60 g/ 1.5–2 liǎng.

---

29. 抽葫芦 Chōu Hú Lú   Lagenariae
Bottle Gourd   Depressae Fructus

Sweet in flavor and neutral in nature, *chōu hú lú* (bottle gourd) disinhibits urine and disperses swelling. It treats **water drum distention**[566] (水臌 *shuǐ gǔ* i.e., ascites) and water swelling. It is used as a single medicinal, but is also used in urine-disinhibiting formulas. For example, combined with medicinals such as *dà fù pí* (areca husk), *fú líng pí* (poria skin), *chē qián zǐ* (plantago seed), and *chē qián cǎo* (plantago), it is used for ascites. Combined with medicinals such as *bái zhú* (white atractylodes), *fú líng* (poria), *huáng qí pí* (astragalus root bark), and *dōng guā pí* (wax gourd rind), it is used for generalized puffy swelling.

For ascites in cirrhosis of the liver, I have achieved satisfactory results in several cases using *hú lú* in combination with medicinals such as:

chái hú (柴胡 bupleurum, Bupleuri Radix)

huáng qín (黄芩 scutellaria, Scutellariae Radix)

fú líng (茯苓 poria, Poria)

zé xiè (泽泻 alisma, Alismatis Rhizoma)

dōng guā pí (冬瓜皮 wax gourd rind, Benincasae Exocarpium)

dà fù pí (大腹皮 areca husk, Arecae Pericarpium)

chē qián zǐ (车前子 plantago seed, Plantaginis Semen)

chǎo lái fú zǐ (炒莱菔子 stir-fried radish seed, Raphani Semen Frictum) *bái jí lí* (白蒺藜 tribulus, Tribuli Fructus)

shuǐ hóng huā zǐ (水红花子 prince's-feather, Polygoni Orientalis Fructus)

chén xiāng (沉香 aquilaria, Aquilariae Lignum Resinatum)

Dosage

In decoction, the dosage is generally 12–30 g/4 qián–1 liǎng. When used as a single medicinal brew, use 30–60 g/1–2 liǎng. Also, this medicinal can be stone-baked and ground to a fine powder. It is then taken in 9 g/3 qián doses, three times per day with warm water. In this form, it is used for about 10 days.

---

30. 甘遂 Gān Suì
Kansui
Kansui Radix

Bitter in flavor, cold in nature, and toxic, *gān suì* (kansui) drains and expels water-rheum. It is a fierce water expellant. *Gān suì* is used for severe repletion patterns of ascites, hydrothorax, and water swelling. For example, combined with medicinals such as *huáng qín* (scutellaria), *mù xiāng* (costusroot), and *shā rén* (amomum), *gān suì* is used for water drum distention (conditions such as cirrhosis of the liver with ascites or ascites from schistosomiasis). Combined with medicinals such as *yuán huā* (genkwa), *tíng lì zǐ* (lepidium/descurainia), and *xìng rén* (apricot kernel), it is used for collection of water-rheum in the chest and rib-side (hydrothorax). Combined with *máng xiāo* (mirabilite) and *dà huáng* (rhubarb), it is used for external contraction of evil heat and internal amassment of water-rheum binding and gathering between the chest, rib-side, stomach duct, and abdomen (**chest bind**[543] 结胸 *jié xiōng*). Combined with *qiān niú zǐ* (morning glory), it is used for water swelling and abdominal fullness (kidney-type water swelling).

Gān suì enters three channels: the lung, spleen, and kidney. It expels and drains water evil phlegm-rheum from the upper, center, and lower burners by causing the water to be drained through the stool. It is used singly and in combination with other medicinals.

The active constituents in this medicinal do not dissolve in water; therefore, it is generally used as a powder preparation or as a pill preparation.

The effect of *shēng gān suì* (raw kansui) is stronger and its toxicity is greater than *wēi gān suì* (roasted kansui). Mix-frying with vinegar reduces and moderates the draining precipitation effect and the toxicity. *Gān suì* (kansui) clashes[11] with *gān cǎo* (licorice); thus, when it is used together with *gān cǎo* the toxicity increases.

Dosage

The dosage of *shēng gān suì* (raw kansui) is 0.3–1 g/1–3 fēn. The dosage of *wēi gān suì* (roasted kansui) or *gān suì* (kansui) that has been mix-fried with vinegar is 1.5–3 g/0.5–1 qián. One should begin with a small amount and then gradually increase the dosage according to need.

---

[11]Clashing, 反 *fǎn*: One of the **seven relations**[562] (七情). (Ed.)

Caution

This medicinal is a drastic precipitating water-expelling medicinal and its draining power is fierce. It is contraindicated for vacuity patterns, patients with a weak constitution, and pregnant women.

| **31. 大戟 Dà Jǐ** | Euphorbiae seu |
| Euphorbia/Knoxia | Knoxiae Radix |

Dà jǐ (euphorbia/knoxia) is bitter in flavor, cold in nature, and toxic. It offensively drains water-rheum and fiercely expels water. It is used for serious conditions such as distention and fullness from water swelling, water accumulation in the chest and abdomen, and cirrhosis giving rise to ascites. According to modern reports, it also is used for ascites in advanced schistosomiasis. It is used singly and in combinations. For example, combined with *yuán huā* (genkwa), *gān suì* (kansui), and *dà zǎo* (jujube) (*shí zǎo tāng* (Ten Jujubes Decoction)), it is used for water accumulation in the chest and rib-side (thoracic fluid accumulation). Combined with *gān suì* (kansui) and *bái jiè zǐ* (white mustard), as in *kòng xián dān* (Drool-Controlling Elixir), it is used for accumulation of phlegm turbidity water-rheum causing glomus and oppression in the chest and stomach duct, with symptoms such as aversion to water with no desire for fluids, palpitations, and shortness of breath. Combined with *gān suì* (kansui) and *tíng lì zǐ* (lepidium/descurainia), it is used for ascites in advanced schistosomiasis.

Comparisons

Dà jǐ drains and expels water from the upper, center, and lower burners, and from the bowels and viscera. *Gān suì* (kansui)[83] drains and expels water from the triple burner channel tunnels. The two medicinals are often used together to expel water evil amassment in the bowels and viscera and the channel tunnels. *Dà jǐ* also disperses swelling and dissipates binds, and treats swelling and toxicity of welling-abscess and sores, as in *zǐ jīn dān* (Purple Gold Elixir), which is also called *yù shū dān* (Jade Pivot Elixir).[517]

Dosage

The dosage is generally 0.6–1.5 g/2–5 fēn. In special circumstances it may be increased. Use as a powder or a pill.

Caution

This medicinal is toxic, and it has a drastic draining effect. It is contraindicated for patients with a weak constitution or who are pregnant. Cease using it if signs of poisoning appear, such as swelling in the throat, vomiting, dizziness, and spasm. This medicinal clashes with (反 *fǎn*) *gān cǎo* (licorice); thus the two should not be used together.

32. 芫花 Yuán Huā
Genkwa

Genkwa
Flos

Yuán huā (genkwa) is warm, acrid, and highly toxic. It is a drastic precipitant and water expellant and it also eliminates phlegm-rheum. Used in the pill formula *zhōu chē wán* (Boats and Carts Pill), it treats severe cases of acute edema, ascites, or hydrothorax occurring in patients with replete constitution and qì.

Zhōu chē wán 舟车丸   Boats and Carts Pill

---

yuán huā (芫花 genkwa, Genkwa Flos)

gān suì (甘遂 kansui, Kansui Radix)

dà jǐ (大戟 euphorbia/knoxia, Euphorbiae seu Knoxiae Radix)

qiān niú zǐ (牵牛子 morning glory, Pharbitidis Semen)

bīng láng (槟榔 areca, Arecae Semen)

qīng fěn (轻粉 calomel, Calomelas)

jú hóng (橘红 red tangerine peel, Citri Reticulatae Exocarpium Rubrum)

qīng pí (青皮 unripe tangerine peel, Citri Reticulatae Pericarpium Viride)

mù xiāng (木香 costusroot, Aucklandiae Radix)

Combined with *dà huáng* (rhubarb) and *tíng lì zǐ* (lepidium/descurainia), it also is used for phlegm turbidity water-rheum that results in cough, counterflow panting, and fullness.

Yuán huā is often used together with *dà jǐ* (euphorbia/knoxia)[480] and *gān suì* (kansui). Comparing the three medicinals, *yuán huā* is the most toxic, followed by *gān suì*, and then *dà jǐ*. Using it mix-fried with vinegar reduces its toxicity. These three medicinals all clash with *gān cǎo* (licorice); thus, if used together, the toxicity increases.

According to modern reports, this medicinal is used for conditions such as hepatitis-induced ascites, ascites in advanced schistosomiasis, and thoracic water accumulation.

DOSAGE

The dosage is generally 0.5–1.5 g/1 fēn–5 fēn. When the disease is severe and the body is strong, the dosage may be slightly increased.

CAUTION

Contraindicated for patients with a weak constitution or who are pregnant.

---

33. 商陆 **Shāng Lù**   Phytolaccae Radix
Phytolacca

Shāng lù (phytolacca) is bitter, cold, and toxic. It disinhibits urine and expels water, and clears heat and downbears qì. Nevertheless, clinically it is primarily used as a water-expelling medicinal to treat all forms of serious water swelling. For example, combined with *lǐ yú* (carp) and decocted (*lǐ yú tāng* (Carp Soup)), it is used for all forms of water swelling (such as nephrotic edema and cardiac edema) because it disinhibits urine and disperses swelling. Combined with medicinals such as *bīng láng* (areca), *dà fù pí* (areca husk), *fú líng pí* (poria skin), *chuān jiāo mù* (zanthoxylum seed), *chì xiǎo dòu* (rice bean), *mù tōng* (trifoliate akebia), *zé xiè* (alisma), and *dù zhòng* (eucommia), it is used for conditions such as water swelling and **water drum distention**[566] (水臌 *shuǐ gǔ*, ascites in hepatitis), abdominal distention, and inhibited urine and stool.

This medicinal has a stimulating effect on the stomach and intestines, and it is more effective when taken after meals.

Shāng lù, ground to a powder, made into a water paste (or mixed with a little vinegar), and applied topically, is used for the swelling and toxicity of welling-abscess and sores, because it disperses swelling and draws out toxins.

Dosage

The dosage is 1.5–4.5 g/5 fēn–1.5 qián when used in decoction. If it is used as a single medicinal in powder form, the dosage is generally 0.4–1.5 g/2–5 fēn. This medicinal is toxic so the dosage should not be excessive because it can cause poisoning or a contrary reaction in which the volume of urine decreases. After using a dosage of this medicinal, the volume of urine should visibly increase. I once encountered a case in which, after use of this medicinal, a urine test indicated cylindruria before any marked increase in urination. Whether this was related to the toxicity is unclear.

Caution

Contraindicated for those in weak health and for pregnant women.

---

34. 牵牛子 **Qiān Niú Zǐ**   Pharbitidis Semen
Morning Glory

Qiān niú zǐ (morning glory), also called *hēi bái chǒu* 黑白丑 in Chinese, is cold in nature, bitter in flavor, and mildly toxic. It **precipitates qì**[559] (下气 *xià qì*), frees the stool and urine, and expels water and disperses swelling. It is often used for water swelling with symptoms such as ascites, constipation (caused by binding depression of damp-heat), panting, and distention. To treat the fullness and distention of ascites (for example, hepatitis with ascites), *qiān niú zǐ* is often combined with medicinals such as *dà jǐ* (euphorbia/knoxia), *yuán huā* (genkwa), *gān suì* (kansui), *qīng pí* (unripe tangerine peel), *chén pí* (tangerine peel), and *qīng fěn* (calomel), as in *zhōu chē wán* (Boats and Carts Pill).[85] This makes use of its draining precipitation effect to expel water, precipitate qì, and disperse distention. Combined with medicinals such as *zhǐ shí* (unripe bitter orange), *bīng láng* (areca), *jiāo sān xiān* (scorch-fried three immortals), and *mù xiāng* (costusroot), it is used for triple burner qì stagnation, damp-heat binding depression, and the constipation and abdominal distention of gastrointestinal accumulation. Combined with medicinals such as *dà huáng* (rhubarb), *bīng láng* (areca), *xióng huáng* (realgar), and *shǐ jūn zǐ* (quisqualis), it is used for abdominal pain, abdominal distention, and dry stool caused by worm accumulation.

When used as a single medicinal, grind 3–9 g/1–3 qián of this medicinal to a fine powder.[12] Half of this should be raw and half stir-fried. Each time take 1–2.5 g/ 3–8 fēn and swallow with warm water. Take once a day, once every other day, or once every three days (determine the dosage based on whether the constitution is strong or weak). This method drains water and disinhibits urine; thus it is used for conditions such as water swelling and ascites.

Qiān niú zǐ is often used in pills or powders and is very rarely used in decoctions. In addition to *zhōu chē wán* (Boats and Carts Pill), I would like to present my experience with an empirical formula that expels water, *xiāo shuǐ dān* (Water-Dispersing Elixir).

Xiāo shuǐ dān 消水丹	Water-Dispersing Elixir

qiān niú zǐ (牵牛子 morning glory, Pharbitidis Semen) 250 g/8 liǎng

chén xiāng (沉香 aquilaria, Aquilariae Lignum Resinatum) 60 g/2 liǎng

hǔ pò (琥珀 amber, Succinum) 30 g/1 liǎng

gān suì (甘遂 kansui, Kansui Radix) 250 g/8 liǎng

Grind these medicinals to a fine powder, and make pills with water about the size of a *lǜ dòu* (mung bean). If the patient is relatively weak, use 10 to 20 pills per dose; if the patient is strong, use 30 to 60 pills per dose.

Take every other day with water or once every three or four days. In the beginning, use a small dosage; later, gradually increase the dosage, and continue use for 20 days to one month. After each use, the patient will pass thin stool several times and there will be an increase in urination. After the water swelling has diminished, one should take food and drink that is easy to digest, rich in nutrients, and low in salt. Nourish the body well for several days to allow the body to recover.

This medicinal drains precipitation and expels water, as well as disinhibits urine. It also precipitates qì, disperses accumulations, and kills worms. It is different from the other water-expelling medicinals discussed above.

---

[12]Unprocessed *qiān niú zǐ* (morning glory) is bitter, cold, and toxic. It drains water, disperses swelling, and kills worms (parasites). It is used to treat water swelling and parasite accumulation. Stir-fried, it is less bitter and cold and it is only slightly toxic. This form is best for expelling phlegm. It is often used to treat phlegm-related coughing and panting. The black seeds are considered to be stronger than the light-colored seeds. (Ed.)

DOSAGE

The dosage is generally 2–4.5 g/7 fēn–1.5 qián. Observe the circumstances of the body to determine the dosage, but begin with a small dosage.

CAUTION

Contraindicated for patients with a weak constitution or who are pregnant.

Although water-expelling medicinals such as *gān suì* (kansui), *dà jǐ* (euphorbia/knoxia), *yuán huā* (genkwa), *shāng lù* (phytolacca), and *qiān niú* (morning glory) expel water and disperse swelling, in the final analysis they are attacking-expellants and drastic-draining medicinals. They should only be used for patients with strong constitutions and exuberant evil. In addition, it is important to pay attention not to use them in excessive amounts or for excessively long periods, because any of these will damage the right. These medicinals are products that treat the tip; thus after the water evil has abated, it is important to pay attention to supporting the right.

Finally, *mù tōng* (trifoliate akebia), *yǐ mǐ* (coix), *tōng cǎo* (rice-paper plant pith), *fáng jǐ* (fangji), *mù guā* (chaenomeles), and *wǔ jiā pí* (acanthopanax), besides disinhibiting urine and dispelling dampness, also soothe the sinews and free the joints. This is a point of differentiation from other general urine-disinhibiting and dampness-dispelling medicinals. The medicinals that dispel wind-damp and treat joint pain will be discussed later (Lecture 9).

Lecture Four
Supplementing Medicinals
补益药 *Bǔ Yì Yào*

This lecture introduces more than simply medicinals that supplement qì, supplement the blood, supplement yīn, and supplement yáng. To overcome the limits of individual categories, spirit-quieting and securing and astringing medicinals, which are similiar to supplementing medicinals in that they are of benefit to right qì, have also been included in this lecture.

1. 人参 Rén Shēn
Ginseng
Ginseng Radix

Rén shēn (ginseng) is sweet and slightly bitter in flavor. Raw, it is neutral in nature; cooked, it is warm in nature. It supplements the five viscera, quiets the spirit, fortifies the spleen and supplements the lung, boosts qì and engenders liquid, and greatly supplements the original qì of the body. It is often used in the following situations.

1. **Stemming Vacuity Desertion:** In all patterns of enduring illness with qì vacuity, major loss of blood, or acute fulminant disease resulting in sudden faintness of breath verging on expiration, **reversal cold of the limbs**[561] (四肢厥冷 *sì zhī jué lěng*), dripping vacuity sweating, clouded spirit without speech, a pulse that is faint and dissipated as if present but not present, and other critical signs of qì desertion, brew 15–30 g/5 qián–1 liǎng of *rén shēn* with water and pour the decoction into the mouth as an emergency treatment to greatly supplement original qì and stem vacuity desertion. This formula is called *dú shēn tāng* (Pure Ginseng Decoction). If the icy cold feeling in the limbs is pronounced, add 9–12 g/ 3–4 qián of *fù piàn* (sliced aconite) to strengthen the effect of returning yáng and stemming counterflow. This is called *shēn fù tāng* (Ginseng and Aconite Decoction). If vacuity sweating is profuse, add *mài dōng* (ophiopogon) and *wǔ wèi zǐ* (schisandra) to boost qì and nourish yīn, check sweating and stem desertion. This formula is called *shēng mài sǎn* (Pulse-Engendering Powder). In recent years, *dú shēn tāng*

(Pure Ginseng Decoction), *shēn fù tāng* (Ginseng and Aconite Decoction), and *shēng mài sǎn* (Pulse-Engendering Powder) have often been used satisfactorily as emergency formulas for various forms of shock, and the latter two formulas have, in some places, been made into injection fluid.

2. Treating Qì Vacuity: The spleen is the root of later heaven; it is the source of qì engenderment for the body. The lung governs the qì of the whole body; it is the sea of the true qì of the body. Spleen-lung qì vacuity is marked by shortness of breath, laziness to speak, low voice, fatigued limbs, poor appetite, bright white complexion, listlessness of essence-spirit, panting on physical exertion, and a vacuous forceless pulse. When treating this, *rén shēn* can be used to supplement the qì of the spleen and lung to address the qì vacuity. For this purpose it is frequently combined with *bái zhú* (white atractylodes), *fú líng* (poria), *gān cǎo* (licorice), *huáng qí* (astragalus), *shān yào* (dioscorea), and *wǔ wèi zǐ* (schisandra). Examples of this use are:

Sì jūn zǐ tāng[1] 四君子汤   Four Gentlemen Decoction

---

rén shēn (人参 ginseng, Ginseng Radix)
bái zhú (白术 white atractylodes, Atractylodis Macrocephalae Rhizoma)
fú líng (茯苓 poria, Poria)
zhì gān cǎo (炙甘草 mix-fried licorice, Glycyrrhizae Radix cum Liquido Fricta)

Bǔ fèi tāng 补肺汤   Lung-Supplementing Decoction

---

rén shēn (人参 ginseng, Ginseng Radix)
huáng qí (黄芪 astragalus, Astragali Radix)
shú dì huáng (熟地黄 cooked rehmannia, Rehmanniae Radix Praeparata)
wǔ wèi zǐ (五味子 schisandra, Schisandrae Fructus)
zǐ wǎn (紫菀 aster, Asteris Radix)
sāng pí (桑皮 mulberry root bark, Mori Cortex)

Given that the "root of the qì is in the kidney," for lung-kidney qì vacuity with shortness of breath and panting, difficulty inhaling, and forceless cough, *rén shēn* can be used together with *gé jiè* (gecko), as in *shēn jiè sǎn* (Ginseng with Gecko Powder).

3. Supporting the Right and Dispelling the Evil: *Rén shēn* supplements (and boosts) the right qì and strengthens the body's ability to fight disease; therefore, for patterns with vacuity of the right qì and exuberance of the evil qì, adding *rén shēn* to an evil-dispelling prescription will support right and dispel evil. For example, *rén shēn* combined with *zǐ sū* (perilla), *qián hú* (peucedanum), *jié gěng* (platycodon), and *zhǐ qiào* (bitter orange), which forms *shēn sū yǐn* (Ginseng and Perilla Beverage), treats common cold and cough in individuals with weak health

---

[1]*Sì jūn zǐ tāng* (Four Gentlemen Decoction) was called *sì wèi bǔ qì tāng* (Four-Ingredient Qì-Supplementing Decoction) in the original text. See footnote on page 3 on term changes in the People's Republic of China. (Ed.)

and qì vacuity. Combined with *shēng shí gāo* (crude gypsum), *zhī mǔ* (anemarrhena), and *gēng mǐ* (non-glutinous rice), forming *rén shēn bái hǔ tāng* (Ginseng White Tiger Decoction), it treats qì-aspect high fever, heat evil damaging the right, and vacuity of the right with exuberant heat.

I generally use *dǎng shēn* (codonopsis) as a substitute for this medicinal, as described under *dǎng shēn* (codonopsis).[92] Nonetheless, in emergency situations or urgent patterns (such as vacuity desertion and shock) or to treat severe diseases, *rén shēn* is more suitable.

Rén shēn is currently commercially available in wild and cultivated forms. The wild type is referred to as *yě shān shēn* (wild ginseng) or *lǎo shān shēn* (old mountain ginseng). The cultivated type is divided into *hóng rén shēn* (red ginseng), *bái rén shēn* (white ginseng), and *shēng shài shēn* (sun-dried ginseng). *Rén shēn* produced in Korea is called *gāo lì shēn* (Korean ginseng).

Hóng rén shēn (红人参, red ginseng) supplements qì with an unyielding, fortifying, warming, and drying nature. It vitalizes yáng qì and so is suitable for returning yáng. *Shēng shài shēn* is more neutral in nature, being neither warm nor drying. It supplements qì and also nourishes liquid, and so is suitable for supporting right and dispelling evil. *Bái rén shēn* (白人参, white ginseng), also called *táng shēn* 糖参, is the most neutral in nature, but it is not as powerful as the others. It is suitable for fortifying the spleen and boosting the lung. *Gāo lì shēn* (高丽参, Korean ginseng) is also divided into red, white, and sun-dried varieties. The comparisons between these types is the same as above. *Yě shān shēn* (野山参, wild ginseng) greatly supplements original qì, yet is neither warm nor drying. Within supplementing qì, it also nourishes yīn liquid. Nevertheless, because it is scarce, *yě shān shēn* is more expensive and thus less commonly used.

Tài zǐ shēn (pseudostellaria) boosts qì and fortifies the spleen, but its supplementing power is weak. It is suitable for insufficiency of qì and blood, vacuity following illness, and dry mouth from lack of liquid.

Rén shēn lú (ginseng top) is bitter in flavor and has an ascending nature that can cause vomiting. For patients in weak health who need to be treated by the method of ejection, *rén shēn lú* (ginseng top) can be used as a substitute for *guā dì* (melon stalk). In addition, for vacuity patients with prolapse of the rectum, adding 0.3–0.6 g/1–2 fēn of *rén shēn lú* (ginseng top) to an appropriate formula has an upraising effect.

Dosage

The dosage is generally 1.5–9 g/5 fēn–3 qián. Nevertheless, when using a formula such as *dú shēn tāng* (Pure Ginseng Decoction) for emergency revival, use 9–30 g/3 qián–1 liǎng.

Caution

Contraindicated in congestion of lung qì marked by oppression in the chest with a suffocating sensation, in the presence of an unresolved exterior evil, as well as in all repletion patterns and heat patterns.

This medicinal clashes with *lí lú* (veratrum) and fears *wǔ líng zhī* (squirrel's droppings).

If the patient experiences severe abdominal distention after taking *rén shēn* (ginseng), this can be resolved with *lái fú zǐ* (radish seed) and *shān zhā* (crataegus).

RESEARCH

According to findings of modern scientific research, *rén shēn* strengthens the intensity and adaptability of cerebral cortex excitation. It enhances the ability to analyze complex stimuli and therefore strengthens conditioned reflexes. It has a tonic effect that increases the body's ability to resist various types of pathogens. It improves appetite and sleep, increases body weight, and reduces fatigue. It also strengthens the heart and promotes gonad function in both men and women. Finally, it decreases blood sugar, fights toxicity, and increases tolerance to hypoxia. These actions can be taken into consideration when applying pattern identification as the basis for determining treatment.

---

2. 党参 Dǎng Shēn   Codonopsis Radix
Codonopsis

Sweet and neutral in flavor and nature, *dǎng shēn* (codonopsis) supplements qì and fortifies the spleen. It is frequently used in place of *rén shēn* (ginseng) to treat qì vacuity patterns.

1. Fortifying the Spleen and Stomach: Insufficiency of qì in the spleen and stomach can give rise to symptoms such as fatigued cumbersome limbs, shortness of breath and lack of strength, poor appetite, and sloppy soft stool. *Dǎng shēn* strengthens spleen-stomach function and boosts qì. It is frequently combined with medicinals such as *bái zhú* (white atractylodes), *fú líng* (poria), *gān cǎo* (licorice), and *chén pí* (tangerine peel) to form *wǔ wèi yì gōng sǎn* (Five-Ingredient Special Achievement Powder), or with *bái zhú* (white atractylodes), *shān yào* (dioscorea), *bái biǎn dòu* (lablab), *qiàn shí* (euryale), *lián ròu* (lotus seed), *yǐ mǐ* (coix), and *fú líng* (poria) to form *shēn líng bái zhú sǎn* (Ginseng, Poria, and White Atractylodes Powder).

2. Boosting Qì and Supplementing the Blood: In patterns of dual vacuity of qì and blood (shortness of breath, laziness and fatigue, white face, pale tongue, possibly vacuity obesity in severe cases, and a fine weak pulse), *dǎng shēn* can be used in combination with *bái zhú* (white atractylodes), *fú líng* (poria), *gān cǎo* (licorice), *dāng guī* (Chinese angelica), *shú dì huáng* (cooked rehmannia), *bái sháo* (white peony), and *chuān xiōng* (chuanxiong) to form *bā zhēn tāng* (Eight-Gem Decoction), which achieves dual supplementation of qì and blood. Furthermore, according to the experience of past physicians, boosting qì promotes blood supplementation and fortifying the spleen helps to engender blood. Because of this, when treating blood vacuity patterns, *dǎng shēn* is commonly included to boost qì and fortify the spleen, thereby helping to supplement the blood. An example of this use is *rén shēn yǎng róng tāng* (Ginseng Construction-Nourishing Decoction).

Rén shēn yǎng róng tāng 人参养荣汤   Ginseng Construction-Nourishing Decoction

---

bái zhú (白术 white atractylodes, Atractylodis Macrocephalae Rhizoma)

fú líng (茯苓 poria, Poria)

gān cǎo (甘草 licorice, Glycyrrhizae Radix)

dāng guī (当归 Chinese angelica, Angelicae Sinensis Radix)

shú dì huáng (熟地黄 cooked rehmannia, Rehmanniae Radix Praeparata)

bái sháo (白芍 white peony, Paeoniae Radix Alba)

yuǎn zhì (远志 polygala, Polygalae Radix)

wǔ wèi zǐ (五味子 schisandra, Schisandrae Fructus)

chén pí (陈皮 tangerine peel, Citri Reticulatae Pericarpium)

dǎng shēn (党参 codonopsis, Codonopsis Radix), replacing *rén shēn* (ginseng)

Another example is *guī pí tāng* (Spleen-Returning Decoction).

Guī pí tāng 归脾汤   Spleen-Returning Decoction

---

dǎng shēn (党参 codonopsis, Codonopsis Radix)

huáng qí (黄芪 astragalus, Astragali Radix)

bái zhú (白术 white atractylodes, Atractylodis Macrocephalae Rhizoma)

dāng guī (当归 Chinese angelica, Angelicae Sinensis Radix)

bái sháo (白芍 white peony, Paeoniae Radix Alba)

chén pí (陈皮 tangerine peel, Citri Reticulatae Pericarpium)

lóng yǎn ròu (龙眼肉 longan flesh, Longan Arillus)

mù xiāng (木香 costusroot, Aucklandiae Radix)

yuan zhì (远志 polygala, Polygalae Radix)

These two formulas are frequently used to boost qì and supplement the blood. According to the findings of modern research, *dǎng shēn* increases hematochrome and red blood cells by stimulating the spleen. In recent years, *dǎng shēn* has often been combined with medicinals such as *dāng guī* (Chinese angelica), *bái sháo* (white peony), *shēng dì huáng* (dried/fresh rehmannia), and *shú dì huáng* (cooked rehmannia) to treat various forms of anemia.

    3. **Treating Cough and Panting from Qì Vacuity:** Because the lung governs qì, qì is not governed when the lung is in a state of vacuity. The result is shortness of breath and hasty panting, feeble enunciation, a weak, low coughing sound, spontaneous sweating, fear of wind, susceptibility to cold and flu, and forceless expectoration of phlegm. For qì vacuity cough and panting, *dǎng shēn* is frequently combined with:

mài dōng (麦冬 ophiopogon, Ophiopogonis Radix)

wǔ wèi zǐ (五味子 schisandra, Schisandrae Fructus)

huáng qí (黄芪 astragalus, Astragali Radix)

gān jiāng (干姜 dried ginger, Zingiberis Rhizoma)

bèi mǔ (贝母 fritillaria, Fritillariae Bulbus)

gān cǎo (甘草 licorice, Glycyrrhizae Radix)

4. Substituting Ginseng in Pure Ginseng Decoction: In emergency vacuity desertion patterns, I generally use a decoction of *rén shēn* (ginseng), which is known as *dú shēn tāng* (Pure Ginseng Decoction). Nevertheless, if *rén shēn* is unavailable, use 30–50 g/1–1.5 liǎng of *dǎng shēn* with 6–9 g/2–3 qián of *fù zǐ* (aconite), and 15–30 g/5 qián–1 liǎng of *shēng bái zhú* (raw white atractylodes); decoct and administer quickly as a substitute for *dú shēn tāng* (Pure Ginseng Decoction).

COMPARISONS

Huáng qí (astragalus)[95] supplements qì; it not only upbears and supplements spleen qì but also boosts the lung and secures the exterior. By contrast, *dǎng shēn* supplements qì, but only fortifies the spleen and supplements qì; it has no strength to secure the exterior. Yet *dǎng shēn* also boosts qì and engenders liquid, whereas *huáng qí* has no capacity to engender liquid. *Huáng qí* also disinhibits water, whereas *dǎng shēn* has no capacity to disinhibit water.

Bái zhú (white atractylodes) primarily supplements spleen qì, but also fortifies the spleen and dries dampness. *Dǎng shēn* supplements both spleen and lung qì, but its strength to dry dampness does not approach that of *bái zhú* (white atractylodes).

Huáng jīng (polygonatum) supplements qì, and also moistens the lung and heart, replenishes essence and marrow, and assists the sinews and bones. However, being neutral and harmonious in nature, it is slow in producing its effects, and so is effective only when taken over a long period of time. *Dǎng shēn* (codonopsis) supplements qì and also is rapidly effective.

Because of different cultivation areas, *dǎng shēn* falls into two types: *tái dǎng shēn* (Tàishān codonopsis) (or *tái shēn* 台参) and *lù dǎng shēn* (Lù'ān codonopsis). Their effects are very similar and pharmacies currently make no distinction.

DOSAGE

The dosage is generally 3–9 g/1–3 qián. In severe or emergency cases, use 15–30 g/5 qián–1 liǎng, or even much more.

CAUTION

The contraindications and points for attention are the same as for *rén shēn* (ginseng).

RESEARCH

According to modern research, *dǎng shēn* has a tonic effect. It strengthens the resistance of the body, increases red blood cells, and reduces white blood cells. It causes dilation of the peripheral blood vessels and lowers blood pressure. It also inhibits excitation of the adrenal glands. These actions can be taken into consideration when applying pattern identification as the basis for determining treatment.

3. 黄芪 Huáng Qí
Astragalus
Astragali Radix

Huáng qí (astragalus) is sweet in flavor and slightly warm in nature. It aids defense qì, secures the skin and exterior, supplements center qì, upbears clear qì, expresses the toxin of sores, and disinhibits urine.

1. Securing the Exterior and Checking Sweating: In constitutionally weak people or after severe or enduring illness, exterior vacuity with insecurity of defense qì frequently causes spontaneous sweating and susceptibility to wind-cold common cold. To treat exterior vacuity spontaneous sweating, *huáng qí* is used to secure the exterior and check sweating. For this purpose it is frequently combined with *fú xiǎo mài* (light wheat), *má huáng gēn* (ephedra root), *wǔ wèi zǐ* (schisandra), *duàn lóng gǔ* (calcined dragon bone), and *duàn mǔ lì* (calcined oyster shell). For vacuity defense qì patterns, with symptoms such as tendency to sweat and susceptibility to cold and flu, *huáng qí* is used to help the defense qì and to secure the skin and exterior. For this purpose it is frequently combined with medicinals such as *bái zhú* (white atractylodes), *fáng fēng* (saposhnikovia) (as in *yù píng fēng sǎn* (Jade Wind-Barrier Powder)), *guì zhī* (cinnamon twig), and *bái sháo* (white peony).

2. Supplementing the Center and Boosting Qì: When spleen-stomach vacuity and insufficiency of center qì causes fatigued limbs, laziness to speak, poor appetite, enduring sloppy stool, yellow face, and shortness of breath, possibly accompanied by sagging heaviness in the lumbus and abdomen, or by prolapse of the rectum, use *huáng qí* to supplement center qì and upraise clear qì. It is frequently combined with medicinals such as *dǎng shēn* (codonopsis), *bái zhú* (white atractylodes), *dāng guī* (Chinese angelica), *chén pí* (tangerine peel), *shēng má* (cimicifuga), and *chái hú* (bupleurum) as in *bǔ zhōng yì qì tāng* (Center-Supplementing Qì-Boosting Decoction).[40] *Huáng qí* is combined with *dǎng shēn* (codonopsis) (or *rén shēn*), *shēng má* (cimicifuga), *bái zhú* (white atractylodes), and *gān cǎo* (licorice) to form *jǔ yuán jiān* (Origin-Lifting Brew), which treats spleen yáng vacuity and center qì fall that result in shortness of breath, sagging of the abdomen, enduring diarrhea, prolapse of the rectum, and **flooding and spotting**[550] (崩漏 *bēng lòu*).

3. Dispersing Water Swelling: *Huáng qí* also disinhibits urine. It is often used to treat water swelling of the head and face or of the limbs, for which it is combined with *fáng jǐ* (fangji), *bái zhú* (white atractylodes) (or *cāng zhú* (atractylodes)), *gān cǎo* (licorice), and *jiāng pí* (ginger skin), as in *fáng jǐ huáng qí tāng* (Fangji and Astragalus Decoction). Alternatively, *huáng qí* combined with *fú líng* (poria), *guì zhī* (cinnamon twig), *gān cǎo* (licorice), and *fáng jǐ* (fangji) to form *fáng jǐ fú líng tāng* (Fangji and Poria Decoction), is used for water swelling affecting the skin of the whole body and the limbs that is accompanied by a sensation of fear of wind. According to recent reports, using this medicinal singly in a daily dose of 60–90 g/ 2–3 liǎng, taken in a concentrated decoction, is effective for water swelling associated with nephritis. *Huáng qí* also helps with proteinuria, for which it is combined with:

> *dǎng shēn* (党参 codonopsis, Codonopsis Radix)
>
> *fú líng* (茯苓 poria, Poria)
>
> *bì xiè* (萆薢 fish poison yam, Dioscoreae Hypoglaucae seu Semptemlobae Rhizoma)
>
> *shān yào* (山药 dioscorea, Dioscoreae Rhizoma)
>
> *yǐ mǐ* (苡米 coix, Coicis Semen)

Combined with *běi wǔ jiā pí* (periploca), *guì zhī* (cinnamon twig), *zhū líng* (polyporus), and *fú líng* (poria), it is effective for cardiac edema. Nonetheless, attention should be paid to appropriate pattern identification as the basis for determining treatment. According to experimental research, when it is used as a diuretic, the dosage should not be too large; approximately 9 g/3 qián is appropriate.

4. Supplementing Qì and Engendering Blood: Qì and blood are rooted in each other. In cases of major blood loss that result in blood vacuity and qì desertion, which manifest in signs such as white face, sweating, shortness of breath, and a fine rapid pulse, use 60–120 g/2–4 liǎng of *huáng qí* and 9–15 g/3–5 qián of *dāng guī* (Chinese angelica), decocted as an emergency treatment to supplement qì and thereby engender blood.[2] If the manifestations are reversal cold of the limbs, generalized cold sweating, and an acute drop in blood pressure, add *rén shēn* (ginseng), *fù zǐ* (aconite), *mài dōng* (ophiopogon), and *wǔ wèi zǐ* (schisandra) to the decoction as an emergency treatment to save the patient.

5. Expressing Toxin and Expelling Pus: In qì and blood vacuity patients with sores, an insufficiency of right qì impairs the body's ability to express toxin outward, so that pus is not transformed and toxin is not expelled, causing thin, watery pus and sores that fail to close. Use *shēng huáng qí* (raw astragalus) combined with *dǎng shēn* (codonopsis), *bái zhǐ* (Dahurian angelica), *fáng fēng* (saposhnikovia), *dāng guī* (Chinese angelica), *chuān xiōng* (chuanxiong), *guì xīn* (shaved cinnamon bark), *hòu pò* (officinal magnolia bark), *jié gěng* (platycodon), *wǔ wèi zǐ* (schisandra), and *gān cǎo* (licorice), as in *tuō lǐ shí bǔ sǎn* (Internal Expression Ten Supplements Powder) and *tuō lǐ huáng qí sǎn* (Internal Expression Astragalus Powder). According to modern research, *huáng qí* increases capillary resistance, dilates blood vessels, improves blood circulation, and allows chronically damaged myocytes to return to normal activity. Thus it treats chronic, ulcerating sores, and welling- and flat-abscesses.

Used raw, *huáng qí* moves in the exterior, secures the exterior and checks sweating, expels pus, and closes sores; used mix-fried its emphasis is on the interior, where it supplements the center and boosts qì, upraises the clear qì of the center burner, supplements qì and engenders blood, and disinhibits urine.

---

[2]This medicinal combination is known as *dāng guī bǔ xuè tāng* (Chinese Angelica Blood-Supplementing Decoction).

Huáng qí pí (astragalus root bark) has similar actions to those of *huáng qí*, but it tends to move in the exterior and is used to secure the exterior and check sweating or for qì vacuity water swelling.

DOSAGE

The dosage is generally 3–10 g/1–3 qián. In severe diseases, use as much as 30–120 g/1–4 liǎng.

CAUTION

Should not be used in patterns with oppression in the chest and fullness in the stomach, exterior repletion and exuberant evil, or qì repletion with irascibility.

RESEARCH

According to modern reports, *huáng qí* protects the liver, strengthens the heart, lowers blood pressure, and suppresses bacteria. It also has effects similar to reproductive hormones.

---

4. 白术 Bái Zhú White Atractylodes	Atractylodis Macrocephalae Rhizoma

Including

> *Cāng zhú* (苍术 atractylodes, Atractylodis Rhizoma)

Sweet and bitter in flavor and slightly warm in nature, *bái zhú* (white atractylodes) fortifies the spleen and dries dampness, boosts qì and engenders blood, and harmonizes the center and quiets the fetus. It is often used as a qì-supplementing medicinal, but when combined with blood-supplementing medicinals it also supplements the blood (when center burner movement and transformation is healthy, qì and blood are automatically engendered).

1. **Fortifying the Spleen and Drying Dampness:** In spleen-stomach vacuity, when the center burner fails to move and transform, food is not digested properly, water-damp fails to transform, and the appetite is poor, signs such as oppression in the stomach duct, abdominal distention, sloppy soft stool, vomiting, water flood (phlegm-rheum or water swelling), and fatigued limbs are often observed. For these signs of spleen vacuity and damp turbidity failing to transform, *bái zhú* is used to fortify the spleen and dry dampness and thereby assist movement and transformation in the center burner. It is frequently combined with medicinals such as *dǎng shēn* (codonopsis), *fú líng* (poria), *chén pí* (tangerine peel), *bàn xià* (pinellia), *mù xiāng* (costusroot), and *cǎo dòu kòu* (Katsumada's galangal seed). When spleen vacuity, failure of movement and transformation, and exuberant dampness in the center burner give rise to spleen vacuity diarrhea, use *bái zhú* combined with the following medicinals to fortify the spleen and check diarrhea.

dǎng shēn (党参 codonopsis, Codonopsis Radix)

fú líng (茯苓 poria, Poria)

zhū líng (猪苓 polyporus, Polyporus)

chē qián zǐ (车前子 plantago seed, Plantaginis Semen)

chǎo shān yào (炒山药 stir-fried dioscorea, Dioscoreae Rhizoma Frictum)

chǎo qiàn shí (炒芡实 stir-fried euryale, Euryales Semen Frictum)

chǎo bái biǎn dòu (炒白扁豆 stir-fried lablab, Lablab Semen Album Frictum)

2. Boosting Qì and Engendering Blood: The spleen and stomach are the root of later heaven; they represent the source of blood and qì formation in the body. This medicinal is especially able to fortify the spleen, boost qì, and supplement the center burner; thus it boosts qì and engenders blood. For this purpose, *bái zhú* is frequently combined with the following:

dǎng shēn (党参 codonopsis, Codonopsis Radix)

fú líng (茯苓 poria, Poria)

gān cǎo (甘草 licorice, Glycyrrhizae Radix)

dāng guī (当归 Chinese angelica, Angelicae Sinensis Radix)

bái sháo (白芍 white peony, Paeoniae Radix Alba)

shú dì huáng (熟地黄 cooked rehmannia, Rehmanniae Radix Praeparata)

chuān xiōng (川芎 chuanxiong, Chuanxiong Rhizoma)

Examples of this use include *bā zhēn tāng* (Eight-Gem Decoction) and *rén shēn yǎng róng tāng* (Ginseng Construction-Nourishing Decoction). In recent years, on the basis of theory and accumulated experience, these formulas have often been used to treat various forms of anemia.

3. Harmonizing the Center and Quieting the Fetus: During pregnancy, a great amount of blood is required to nourish the fetus. This increases the burden of the center burner, which is the source of blood, and sometimes causes abnormalities of movement and transformation in the center burner, such as impaired harmonious downbearing of the stomach and counterflow ascent of stomach qì, resulting in signs such as retching counterflow, dizziness, oppression in the chest, and inability to eat. This is referred to in Chinese medicine as "malign obstruction" (恶阻 *è zǔ*), and in colloquial English as "morning sickness." *Bái zhú* is used to fortify the spleen and transform dampness and to harmonize the center and quiet the fetus, for which it is combined with medicinals such as:

chén pí (陈皮 tangerine peel, Citri Reticulatae Pericarpium)

zhú rú (竹茹 bamboo shavings, Bambusae Caulis in Taenia)

sū gěng (苏梗 perilla stem, Perillae Caulis)

fú líng (茯苓 poria, Poria)

huò xiāng (藿香 agastache, Agastaches Herba)

shēng jiāng (生姜 fresh ginger, Zingiberis Rhizoma Recens)

If there is also fetal heat (rapid pulse, heat vexation, yellow tongue fur, and desire for cold food and drink), add *huáng qín* (scutellaria), *zhī zǐ* (gardenia), and *bái sháo* (white peony). If there is also blood vacuity (withered-yellow complexion, pale lips, flusteredness, shortness of breath, and a fine pulse), add *dāng guī* (Chinese angelica), *bái sháo* (white peony), and *shēng dì huáng* (dried/fresh rehmannia). If there is kidney vacuity and insecurity of the fetal origin (aching lumbus and sagging abdomen, weak legs, habitual miscarriage, and a weak cubit pulse), add:

sāng jì shēng (桑寄生 mistletoe, Taxilli Herba)

xù duàn (续断 dipsacus, Dipsaci Radix)

shān yào (山药 dioscorea, Dioscoreae Rhizoma)

shān yú ròu (山萸肉 cornus, Corni Fructus)

shú dì huáng (熟地黄 cooked rehmannia, Rehmanniae Radix Praeparata)

wǔ wèi zǐ (五味子 schisandra, Schisandrae Fructus)

huáng qí (黄芪 astragalus, Astragali Radix)

dǎng shēn (党参 codonopsis, Codonopsis Radix)

Once the center qì is fortified and the liver and kidney qì and blood are sufficient, the fetal origin will naturally be secure.

In addition to being used for the patterns described above, *bái zhú* is also combined with *zhū líng* (polyporus), *fú líng pí* (poria skin), *dōng guā pí* (wax gourd rind), *chē qián zǐ* (plantago seed), and *guì zhī* (cinnamon twig) to treat spleen vacuity water swelling. Combined with *huáng qí* (astragalus), *fáng fēng* (saposhnikovia), and *fú xiǎo mài* (light wheat), it treats qì vacuity spontaneous sweating. Combined with *zhǐ shí* (unripe bitter orange), *é zhú* (curcuma rhizome), *shén qū* (medicated leaven), *mài yá* (barley sprout), *shān zhā hé* (crataegus pit), *shēng mǔ lì* (crude oyster shell), *táo rén* (peach kernel), and *dān shēn* (salvia), it treats abdominal masses, such as concretion, bind, and aggregation lumps in the abdomen.

COMPARISONS

Dǎng shēn (codonopsis)[92] and *rén shēn* (ginseng)[89] both supplement qì, tending to supplement the spleen, lung, and original qì. They are suitable for supplementing vacuity and for emergency revival. *Bái zhú* also supplements qì, tending to fortify the spleen and supplement center qì in order to engender qì. It is suitable for engendering qì and blood to treat vacuity patterns.

Cāng zhú (atractylodes) and *bái zhú* (white atractylodes) both fortify the spleen and dry dampness. However, *cāng zhú* is aromatic, bitter, and warm and has a dry and harsh nature. It upbears yáng, dissipates depression, and dries dampness. It has a stronger upbearing and dissipating action than *bái zhú*, but its ability to fortify the spleen, supplement qì, and engender blood is weaker.

Shēng bái zhú (raw white atractylodes) is suitable for boosting qì and engendering blood. *Chǎo bái zhú* (stir-fried white atractylodes) is suitable for fortifying the spleen and drying dampness. *Jiāo bái zhú* (焦白术, scorch-fried white atractylodes) is suitable for aiding digestion, opening the stomach, and dissipating concretions and aggregations. *Tǔ chǎo bái zhú* (土炒白术, earth-fried white atractylodes) is suitable for fortifying the spleen and stomach and for checking diarrhea.[3]

---

[3] There are two common ways to prepare *tǔ chǎo bái zhú* (earth-fried white atractylodes). The first is simply dry-frying the medicinal in fine, red earth until it browns slightly. The second is stir-frying it in mud made by combining fine earth with water, which produces a thin coating of earth. *Chì shí zhī* (halloysite) is sometimes substituted for earth in these methods. (Ed.)

Research

According to the findings of modern research, this medicinal significantly increases gastric and intestinal secretions and accelerates peristalsis. Entering the blood, it accelerates blood circulation. It also lowers blood sugar and has a diuretic action.

Dosage

The dosage is generally 4.5–9 g/1.5–3 qián. In severe cases, use as much as 15–30 g/5 qián–1 liǎng. For example, when *dú shēn tāng* (Pure Ginseng Decoction) is needed to stem vacuity desertion, but *rén shēn* (ginseng) is unavailable, urgently administer a decoction made of 20–45 g/7 qián–1.5 liǎng of *shēng bái zhú* (raw white atractylodes), 30–80 g/1–2.5 liǎng of *dǎng shēn* (codonopsis), and 9–12 g/3–4 qián of *fù piàn* (sliced aconite).

Caution

Use with care in patterns of spleen-stomach yīn vacuity.

---

5. 山药 Shān Yào   Dioscoreae Rhizoma
Dioscorea

Shān yào (dioscorea), sweet in flavor and warm in nature, supplements the spleen and stomach, boosts lung qì, strengthens the kidney and secures essence, and treats vaginal discharge.

1. Supplementing the Spleen and Stomach: *Shān yào* in combination with *bái zhú* (white atractylodes), *dǎng shēn* (codonopsis), *fú líng* (poria), *bái biǎn dòu* (lablab), *lián zǐ* (lotus seed), and *chǎo qiàn shí* (stir-fried euryale) is often used for patterns of spleen-stomach vacuity that result in signs such as persistent vacuity diarrhea, fatigue and lack of strength in the limbs, and a vacuous pulse. This medicinal supplements the spleen and stomach to check diarrhea.

2. Boosting Lung Qì: *Shān yào* supplements the spleen and stomach and boosts lung qì. It is frequently combined with medicinals such as *dǎng shēn* (codonopsis), *wǔ wèi zǐ* (schisandra), *huáng qí* (astragalus), *chén pí* (tangerine peel), and *bái zhú* (white atractylodes) to treat lung qì vacuity that causes shortness of breath, lack of strength, laziness to speak, low voice, a subjective feeling of shortage of qì in the chest, and a vacuous inch pulse on the right side.

3. Strengthening the Kidney and Securing Essence: *Shān yào* strengthens the kidney and secures essence. It is frequently combined with medicinals such as *shēng dì huáng* (dried/fresh rehmannia), *shú dì huáng* (cooked rehmannia), *shān yú ròu* (cornus), *wǔ wèi zǐ* (schisandra), *suǒ yáng* (cynomorium), and *jīn yīng zǐ* (Cherokee rose fruit) to treat seminal efflux and seminal emission from kidney vacuity.

Used raw, *shān yào* supplements the kidney and engenders essence, boosts lung and kidney yīn, and treats dispersion-thirst[546] (消渴 *xiāo kě*). a) For pronounced upper-burner dispersion-thirst (severe thirst, inability to allay thirst, emaciation, copious urine, and spontaneous sweating), *shān yào* is combined with:

tiān huā fěn (天花粉 trichosanthes root, Trichosanthis Radix)

mài dōng (麦冬 ophiopogon, Ophiopogonis Radix)

zhī mǔ (知母 anemarrhena, Anemarrhenae Rhizoma)

huáng qín (黄芩 scutellaria, Scutellariae Radix)

wǔ wèi zǐ (五味子 schisandra, Schisandrae Fructus)

shā shēn (沙参 adenophora/glehnia, Adenophorae seu Glehniae Radix)

shēng shí gāo (生石膏 crude gypsum, Gypsum Fibrosum Crudum)

wū méi (乌梅 mume, Mume Fructus)

b) For pronounced center-burner dispersion-thirst (increased intake of food and drink, rapid hungering, large intake of food and drink, emaciation, and lack of strength in the limbs), it is combined with:

shēng shí gāo (生石膏 crude gypsum, Gypsum Fibrosum Crudum)

zhī mǔ (知母 anemarrhena, Anemarrhenae Rhizoma)

gé gēn (葛根 pueraria, Puerariae Radix)

huáng jīng (黄精 polygonatum, Polygonati Rhizoma)

huáng qín (黄芩 scutellaria, Scutellariae Radix)

tiān huā fěn (天花粉 trichosanthes root, Trichosanthis Radix)

shēng dà huáng (生大黄 raw rhubarb, Rhei Radix et Rhizoma Crudi)

shēng dì huáng (生地黄 dried/fresh rehmannia, Rehmanniae Radix Exsiccata seu Recens)

c) For lower-burner dispersion-thirst (urinary frequency, copious urine, thirst, aching pain in the lumbus, lack of strength in the knees and legs, and impotence), *shān yào* is combined with:

shēng dì huáng (生地黄 dried/fresh rehmannia, Rehmanniae Radix Exsiccata seu Recens)

shú dì huáng (熟地黄 cooked rehmannia, Rehmanniae Radix Praeparata)

shān zhū yú (山茱萸 cornus, Corni Fructus)

wǔ wèi zǐ (五味子 schisandra, Schisandrae Fructus)

zé xiè (泽泻 alisma, Alismatis Rhizoma)

dān pí (丹皮 moutan, Moutan Cortex)

fú líng (茯苓 poria, Poria)

ròu guì (肉桂 cinnamon bark, Cinnamomi Cortex) (small amount)

On the basis of this experience and theory, these formulas have in recent years been varied in accordance with signs to successfully treat diabetes mellitus, diabetes insipidus, and hyperthyroid disorders manifesting in dispersion-thirst patterns.

4. Treating Vaginal Discharge: In dual vacuity of the spleen and kidney, dampness evil pouring into the lower burner can manifest as **vaginal discharge**[566] (带下 *dài xià*). Severe damp-cold generally causes white vaginal discharge, whereas severe damp-heat generally causes yellow vaginal discharge or red vaginal discharge.

Shān yào both supplements the spleen and stomach to transform dampness evil and secures kidney qì to check vaginal discharge. a) White vaginal discharge is commonly treated by combining *shān yào* with:

> *bái zhú* (白术 white atractylodes, Atractylodis Macrocephalae Rhizoma)
>
> *cāng zhú* (苍术 atractylodes, Atractylodis Rhizoma)
>
> *fú líng* (茯苓 poria, Poria)
>
> *lóng gǔ* (龙骨 dragon bone, Mastodi Ossis Fossilia)
>
> *hǎi piāo xiāo* (海螵蛸 cuttlefish bone, Sepiae Endoconcha)
>
> *wú yú* (吴萸 evodia, Evodiae Fructus)
>
> *wū yào* (乌药 lindera, Linderae Radix)
>
> *chē qián zǐ* (车前子 plantago seed, Plantaginis Semen)

b) For yellow vaginal discharge, it is combined with:

> *huáng qín* (黄芩 scutellaria, Scutellariae Radix)
>
> *huáng bǎi* (黄柏 phellodendron, Phellodendri Cortex)
>
> *bái guǒ* (白果 ginkgo, Ginkgo Semen)
>
> *chē qián zǐ* (车前子 plantago seed, Plantaginis Semen)
>
> *qiàn shí* (芡实 euryale, Euryales Semen)
>
> *yǐ mǐ* (苡米 coix, Coicis Semen)

c) For red vaginal discharge, it is combined with:

> *huáng bǎi tàn* (黄柏炭 charred phellodendron, Phellodendri Cortex
>   Carbonisatus)
>
> *qiàn cǎo tàn* (茜草炭 charred madder, Rubiae Radix Carbonisata)
>
> *xù duàn tàn* (续断炭 charred dipsacus, Dipsaci Radix Carbonisata)
>
> *sāng jì shēng* (桑寄生 mistletoe, Taxilli Herba)
>
> *fú líng* (茯苓 poria, Poria)
>
> *dāng guī tàn* (当归炭 charred Chinese angelica, Angelicae Sinensis Radix
>   Carbonisata)
>
> *bái zhú* (白术 white atractylodes, Atractylodis Macrocephalae Rhizoma)
>
> *bái sháo* (白芍 white peony, Paeoniae Radix Alba)

Chǎo shān yào (stir-fried dioscorea)[4] is used to supplement the spleen and stomach, boost lung qì, and treat vaginal discharge; *shēng shān yào* (raw dioscorea) is used to strengthen the kidney and engender essence and to treat dispersion-thirst.

Bái zhú (white atractylodes) dries dampness and fortifies the spleen, and boosts qì and engenders blood more strongly than *shān yào*. *Shān yào* (dioscorea) supplements the kidney and strengthens essence more strongly than *bái zhú*.

Chǎo yǐ mǐ (stir-fried coix) and *chǎo shān yào* (stir-fried dioscorea) both fortify the spleen and check diarrhea; however *yǐ mǐ* (coix) tends to disinhibit dampness to dry the spleen, whereas *shān yào* tends to supplement the spleen and kidney and to secure and astringe.

---

[4] *Chǎo shān yào* (stir-fried dioscorea) is prepared by stir-frying slices of this medicinal with either wheat bran or red earth until it turns pale yellow. (Ed.)

When effulgent yīn vacuity fire gives rise to spleen vacuity diarrhea, if only medicinals such as *bái zhú* (white atractylodes) and *yǐ mǐ* (coix) are used, it is easy to damage kidney yīn. For this type of situation, combining *shān yào* with *lián zǐ* (lotus seed) and *qiàn shí* (euryale) will make the spleen replete and supplement the spleen without damaging the kidney.

Shān yào (dioscorea) occasionally causes side-effects such as qì congestion, distention and oppression in the abdomen, and poor appetite. These can be avoided by adding *chén pí* (tangerine peel).

DOSAGE

The dosage is generally 9–25 g/3–8 qián. When necessary, use up to 30 g/ 1 liǎng or more.[5]

CAUTION

Inappropriate for patients with abdominal distention and for fullness and oppression in the center burner.

---

6. 黄精 Huáng Jīng   Polygonati
Polygonatum   Rhizoma

Huáng jīng (polygonatum) is sweet and neutral, with a nature that is gentle and harmonious. It supplements the center and boosts qì, supplements spleen qì, nourishes stomach yīn, and moistens the lung and heart.

Huáng jīng (polygonatum) combined with *bái zhú* (white atractylodes), *dǎng shēn* (codonopsis), *fú líng* (poria), *gān cǎo* (licorice), *chén pí* (tangerine peel), *mài yá* (barley sprout), and *gǔ yá* (millet sprout) is used for spleen-stomach vacuity with reduced intake of food and drink, lassitude of essence-spirit, laziness of the limbs, and a forceless vacuous soft pulse. Because this medicinal has a gentle and harmonious nature, it is appropriate for use over extended periods and for nourishing and regulating the body after an illness. Physicians of the past learned from experience that "*huáng jīng* can replace *rén shēn* (ginseng) and *huáng qí* (astragalus); *yù zhú* (Solomon's seal) can replace *rén shēn* (ginseng) and *dì huáng* (rehmannia)." This saying is worth bearing in mind in clinical practice.

After a disease with high fever, when stomach yīn has been damaged and there is dry mouth without desire for drink, decreased food intake and dry stool, inability to taste food, and a red tongue with scant fur, use *huáng jīng* combined with *yù zhú* (Solomon's seal), *mài dōng* (ophiopogon), *shā shēn* (adenophora/glehnia), *bīng táng* (rock candy), and *shēng mài yá* (raw barley sprout) to nourish yīn and **open the stomach**[559] (开胃 *kāi wèi*).

---

[5]Large doses (30 g/1 liǎng) of *shān yào* (dioscorea) are usually applied to the treatment of diarrhea. Treatment of dispersion-thirst also calls for large doses. One modern formula for diabetes uses 250 g per day of this medicinal in combination with other medicinals such as *huáng qí* (astragalus), *shēng dì huáng* (dried/fresh rehmannia), and *tiān huā fěn* (trichosanthes root). (Ed.)

For heart-lung yīn vacuity causing cough with scant phlegm, shortness of breath, lack of strength, dry mouth, reduced sleep, and profuse dreaming, *huáng jīng* is combined with the following:

mài dōng (麦冬 ophiopogon, Ophiopogonis Radix)

bèi mǔ (贝母 fritillaria, Fritillariae Bulbus)

shā shēn (沙参 adenophora/glehnia, Adenophorae seu Glehniae Radix)

yuǎn zhì (远志 polygala, Polygalae Radix)

xìng rén (杏仁 apricot kernel, Armeniacae Semen)

fú shén (茯神 root poria, Poria cum Pini Radice)

zǎo rén (枣仁 spiny jujube, Ziziphi Spinosi Semen)

Combined with *màn jīng zǐ* (vitex) and *cǎo jué míng* (fetid cassia), *huáng jīng* supplements the liver and brightens the eyes. Combined with *gǒu qǐ zǐ* (lycium) and *tù sī zǐ* (cuscuta), it supplements the kidney and boosts essence. Combined with *dù zhòng* (eucommia) and *xù duàn* (dipsacus), it assists the sinews and bones. Combined with *qiāng huó* (notopterygium) and *dú huó* (pubescent angelica), it eliminates wind-damp.

DOSAGE

The dosage is generally 6–9 g/2–3 qián.

CAUTION

Contraindicated in patterns with exuberant yīn or qì stagnation.

---

7. 白扁豆 Bái Biǎn Dòu   Lablab
Lablab   Semen Album

Also called *biǎn dòu* 扁豆. Sweet in flavor and slightly warm in nature, *bái biǎn dòu* (lablab) fortifies the spleen and nourishes the stomach, disperses summerheat and eliminates dampness, and is often used in formulas that regulate and supplement the spleen and stomach. This medicinal supplements the spleen without sliminess and transforms dampness without drying. For patterns of spleen-stomach vacuity or after a major illness, when a supplementing formula is first given, *bái biǎn dòu* is the most suitable since it regulates and nourishes right qì without causing a feeling of fullness and oppression.

Bái biǎn dòu combined with *chǎo shān yào* (stir-fried dioscorea), *bái zhú* (white atractylodes), *dǎng shēn* (codonopsis), *fú líng* (poria), and *chǎo qiàn shí* (stir-fried euryale) is used for spleen vacuity diarrhea. Combined with *tiān huā fěn* (trichosanthes root), it treats dispersion-thirst with copious fluid intake.

Bái biǎn dòu resolves summerheat and eliminates dampness. In the summer, for contraction of summerheat-damp evil that results in symptoms such as vomiting, diarrhea, vexation and thirst, cloudy head, and oppression in the chest, *bái biǎn dòu* can be combined with:

huò xiāng (藿香 agastache, Agastaches Herba)

pèi lán (佩兰 eupatorium, Eupatorii Herba)

hé yè (荷叶 lotus leaf, Nelumbinis Folium)

chì xiǎo dòu (赤小豆 rice bean, Phaseoli Semen)

hòu pò (厚朴 officinal magnolia bark, Magnoliae Officinalis Cortex)

bái kòu rén (白蔻仁 cardamom seed, Amomi Cardamomi Semen)

Comparisons

Whereas *shēng bái biǎn dòu* (raw lablab) disperses summerheat and dispels dampness, *chǎo bái biǎn dòu* (stir-fried lablab) fortifies the spleen and nourishes the stomach.

Biǎn dòu huā (lablab flower) resolves and dissipates summerheat evil with greater strength than *bái biǎn dòu*, but *bái biǎn dòu* fortifies the spleen and dispels dampness more powerfully than *biǎn dòu huā*. *Biǎn dòu yī* (lablab seed-coat) clears summerheat-heat and disinhibits summerheat-damp more effectively than *bái biǎn dòu*, but its power to fortify the spleen and support the right does not compare with that of *bái biǎn dòu*.

Lǜ dòu (mung bean) is cool in nature; it disperses summerheat from the heart and stomach and also disinhibits dampness and resolves toxin. *Bái biǎn dòu* is slightly warm in nature; it disperses summerheat from the spleen and stomach and also fortifies the spleen and supports the right.

Hé yè (lotus leaf) upbears clear qì to disperse summerheat, whereas *bái biǎn dòu* downbears damp turbidity to disperse summerheat.

Dosage

The dosage is generally 4.5–12 g/1.5–4 qián. *Biǎn dòu huā* and *biǎn dòu yī* are light so the dosage should be slightly reduced.

---

8. 大枣　Dà Zǎo
Jujube
Jujubae Fructus

Sweet and warm in flavor and nature, *dà zǎo* (jujube) supplements the spleen, harmonizes the stomach, strengthens the spleen and stomach, checks diarrhea, and engenders liquid; it supplements, nourishes, and invigorates. *Dà zǎo* also moderates the nature of medicinals, resolves toxin, and protects the spleen and stomach. For example, the formulas *shí zǎo tāng* (Ten Jujubes Decoction) and *tíng lì dà zǎo xiè fèi tāng* (Lepidium/Descurainia and Jujube Lung-Draining Decoction) both employ *dà zǎo* to moderate the nature of the medicinals, resolve toxin, and safeguard the stomach and spleen.

Dà zǎo combined with *gān cǎo* (licorice) and *xiǎo mài* (wheat), which forms *gān mài dà zǎo tāng* (Licorice, Wheat, and Jujube Decoction), is used for visceral agitation (脏燥 *zàng zào*) in women (with symptoms such as emotional depression, sorrow, and desire to weep). *Dà zǎo* is frequently combined with *xiāng fù* (cyperus), *chái hú* (bupleurum), *shēng lóng gǔ* (crude dragon bone), *shēng mǔ lì* (crude oyster shell), *bái sháo* (white peony), *yù jīn* (curcuma), and *dǎn xīng* (bile arisaema) in formulas varied in accordance with signs.

The kernel of *dà zǎo*, scorch-fried, infused in hot water, and taken as tea, quiets the sleep. For patients with insomnia, this method is used at night in addition to taking a formula. In situations where taking a formula is inconvenient, this medicinal is used alone.

COMPARISONS

Lóng yǎn ròu (longan flesh) and *dà zǎo* both boost the spleen, but *lóng yǎn ròu* (longan flesh) tends to nourish the heart and supplement the blood, thereby treating heart vacuity. *Dà zǎo* tends to supplement the spleen and harmonize the stomach, thereby treating spleen vacuity.

Yí táng (malt sugar), which is sweet in flavor and boosts the spleen, tends to relax tension and harmonize the center, thereby treating pain from center vacuity. *Dà zǎo*, which is also sweet in flavor and boosts the spleen, tends to boost qì, nourish the blood, and also nourish the heart, thereby treating spleen vacuity with flusteredness and anxiety.

DOSAGE

The dosage is generally 3–10 pieces (i.e., 3–10 jujubes).

CAUTION

This medicinal is inappropriate in patterns with gastric distention and fullness or with phlegm-heat.

---

9. 甘草 Gān Cǎo   Glycyrrhizae Radix
Licorice

Sweet and neutral in flavor and nature, *gān cǎo* (licorice) supplements the spleen, clears heat, resolves toxin, relaxes tension, moistens the lung, and harmonizes the nature of medicinals.

1. Supplementing the Spleen: For cases of constitutional vacuity or enduring illness that result in center burner qì vacuity (lack of strength in the limbs, shortness of breath, tendency to speak little, no pleasure in eating, indigestion, and sloppy diarrhea), *gān cǎo* is often combined with medicinals such as *dǎng shēn* (codonopsis), *bái zhú* (white atractylodes), *fú líng* (poria), *bái biǎn dòu* (lablab), and *chén pí* (tangerine peel) to fortify the spleen and boost qì.

2. Clearing Heat and Resolving Toxin: Used raw, *gān cǎo* clears heat and resolves toxin. It is often used for welling- and flat-abscesses and sores. For example, in the treatment of welling-abscesses and sores (fiery redness, swelling, and pain), *gān cǎo* is frequently combined with medicinals such as *jīn yín huā* (lonicera), *lián qiáo* (forsythia), *chì sháo* (red peony), *dān pí* (moutan), *dì dīng* (violet), and *pú gōng yīng* (dandelion). The toxin-resolving action of *gān cǎo* is also used in the treatment of **yīn flat-abscesses**[569] (阴疽 *yīn jū*, characterized by swellings that are hard to the touch and dark in color rather than red), for which *gān căo* is frequently combined with medicinals such as *shú dì huáng* (cooked rehmannia), *má huáng* (ephedra), *ròu guì* (cinnamon bark), *lù jiăo jiāo* (deerhorn glue), *bái jiè zĭ* (white mustard), and *guì zhī* (cinnamon twig). Modern research has shown *gān căo* to have an antidotal effect on *fān mù biē* (nux vomica), chloral hydrate, diphtheria toxin, lockjaw toxin, globefish poison, and snake venom. Physicians of the past also noted that *gān căo* "resolves the hundred toxins."

3. Relaxing Tension: "Tension" means tightness, spasm, and contraction of muscles. A traditional saying based on the experience of past physicians has it that "sweet flavors relax tension," and *gān căo* is a good example. For tense pain in the abdomen, *gān căo* is frequently combined with *bái sháo* (white peony), *yí táng* (malt sugar), *guì zhī* (cinnamon twig), *dà zăo* (jujube), and *shēng jiāng* (fresh ginger). An example of this is *xiăo jiàn zhōng tāng* (Minor Center-Fortifying Decoction), which is suitable for vacuity cold abdominal pain. Modern research has demonstrated that *gān căo* moderates spasms in the smooth muscle of the stomach and intestines. This research has increased our understanding of the tension-relaxing effects of *gān căo*. Combined with *bái sháo* (white peony), a combination known as *sháo yào gān căo tāng* (Peony and Licorice Decoction), it is used for hypertonicity of the feet, inability to stretch, and reverse flow (coolness of the ends of the limbs) that are the result of damage to yīn-blood following inappropriate promotion of sweating.

4. Moistening the Lung: *Shēng gān căo* (raw licorice) also moistens the lung. It is effective for lung heat patterns with sore pharynx and cough. Combined with *xìng rén* (apricot kernel), *bèi mŭ* (fritillaria), *pí pá yè* (loquat leaf), *guā lóu* (trichosanthes), *zhī mŭ* (anemarrhena), and *huáng qín* (scutellaria), it is used for lung heat cough. Combined with *jié gĕng* (platycodon), *shè gān* (belamcanda), *niú bàng zĭ* (arctium), and *xuán shēn* (scrophularia), it is used for sore swollen throat. Modern research has shown that *shēng gān căo* is a moistening expectorant. Taken orally, it reduces irritation of the mucous membrane of the throat, and is suitable for laryngitis. Research has also demonstrated that *gān căo* controls tuberculosis bacteria. Combined with other antiphthisic agents, it is used for pulmonary tuberculosis.

5. Harmonizing the Nature of Medicinals: *Gān căo* is harmonious and moderate in nature. It frees the twelve channels, both upbears and downbears, and harmonizes the natures of supplementing, draining, cold, hot, warm, and cool medicinals. Combined, for example, with supplementing medicinals such as *dāng guī* (Chinese angelica), *bái sháo* (white peony), *dì huáng* (rehmannia), *chuān xiōng* (chuanxiong), *dăng shēn* (codonopsis), *bái zhú* (white atractylodes), and *fú líng* (poria), it makes the supplementing action harmonious and moderate, long-lasting and not abrupt. *Gān căo* combined with precipitating medicinals such as *dà huáng* (rhubarb), *máng xiāo* (mirabilite), and *zhĭ shí* (unripe bitter orange) moderates the draining nature of these medicinals so that they drain without acting too quickly, allowing for their full medicinal strength to come into play without damaging stomach qì. Combined with cold-natured medicinals such as *shēng shí gāo* (crude gypsum) and *zhī mŭ* (anemarrhena), it moderates their cold nature and prevents damage to the stomach. Combined with hot-natured medicinals such as *fù zĭ* (aconite) and *gān jiāng* (dried ginger), it moderates their hot nature to prevent damage to yīn. Combined with warm, acrid, effusing, and dissipating medicinals such as *má huáng* (ephedra), *guì zhī* (cinnamon twig), and *xìng rén* (apricot kernel), it makes them more harmonious and moderate in nature and safeguards the stomach qì, to avoid damaging the fluids through the promotion of sweating. In any formula, *gān cǎo* allows for harmonious interaction between medicinals and prevents struggles between them. This is why physicians of the past said that *gān cǎo* "harmonizes the hundred medicinals."

Gān cǎo combined with *shēng jiāng* (fresh ginger), *guì zhī* (cinnamon twig), *huǒ má rén* (cannabis fruit), *mài dōng* (ophiopogon), *dǎng shēn* (codonopsis), *ē jiāo* (ass hide glue), *shēng dì huáng* (dried/fresh rehmannia), *dà zǎo* (jujube), and *dān pí* (moutan) constitutes a formula called *zhì gān cǎo tāng* (Honey-Fried Licorice Decoction), which is effective for treating yīn-qì vacuity and yáng-qì vacuity that result in bound and intermittent pulses (结代脉 *jié dài mài*) and stirring heart palpitations (心动悸 *xīn dòng jì*). According to modern research, *gān cǎo* has a cardiotonic effect similar to epinephrine.

When mix-fried with honey, it is known as *zhì gān cǎo* (炙甘草, mix-fried licorice). This is suitable for supplementing the center and boosting qì. *Shēng gān cǎo* (生甘草, raw licorice) is suitable for clearing heat and resolving toxin. *Shēng gān cǎo shāo* (生甘草稍, fine licorice root)[6] treats urethral pain and is suitable for strangury. *Shēng cǎo jié* (生草节, raw resinous licorice root) is suitable for dispersing swelling and toxin and for disinhibiting the joints. If *shēng gān cǎo* (raw licorice) is stripped of its bark, it is called *fěn gān cǎo* (粉甘草, shaved licorice), which is suitable for clearing internal heat and draining heart fire.

DOSAGE

The dosage is generally 1–9 g/3 fēn–3 qián.

CAUTION

Contraindicated in patterns of spleen-stomach dampness with center fullness and vomiting. Long-term use at a high dosage causes water swelling and hypertension. This medicinal clashes with *dà jǐ* (euphorbia/knoxia), *gān suì* (kansui), *yuán huā* (genkwa), and *hǎi zǎo* (sargassum).

RESEARCH

Modern research has demonstrated that a liquid extract of *gān cǎo* can control histamine-moderated gastric acid secretion. Thus it is used in the treatment of stomach ulcers. It also has an effect similar to that of the cortical hormones; therefore, it is used for Addison's disease. *Gān cǎo* and cortisone used together have a mutually complementary effect.

---

[6] *Shēng gān cǎo shāo* (生甘草稍, fine licorice root), or *gān cǎo shāo*, is the fine root hairs of licorice. This item is seldom used and is not readily available in the West. *Shēng gān cǎo* (raw licorice) is the usual substitute. (Ed.)

10. 熟地黄 Shú Dì Huáng
Cooked Rehmannia

Rehmanniae
Radix Praeparata

Sweet and slightly bitter in flavor, while slightly warm in nature, *shú dì huáng* (cooked rehmannia)[7] supplements the blood and engenders essence, enriches the kidney and nourishes the liver. It is the most commonly used yīn-enriching, blood-supplementing medicinal.

Shú dì huáng is combined with *dāng guī* (Chinese angelica), *bái sháo* (white peony), and *chuān xiōng* (chuanxiong) to form *sì wù tāng* (Four Agents Decoction), which is a commonly used blood-supplementing formula that treats blood vacuity patterns (withered-yellow facial complexion, pale lips, delayed menstruation and scant flow, dizzy vision, flusteredness, and a fine pulse). In recent times, it has commonly been combined with medicinals such as *dāng guī* (Chinese angelica), *huáng qí* (astragalus), *dǎng shēn* (codonopsis), and *ē jiāo* (ass hide glue), varied in accordance with signs, to treat all forms of anemia.

Shú dì huáng combined with *shān yào* (dioscorea), *shān zhū yú* (cornus), *dān pí* (moutan), *zé xiè* (alisma), and *fú líng* (poria) is called *liù wèi dì huáng wán/tāng* (Six-Ingredient Rehmannia Pill/Decoction). It is used for liver-kidney yīn vacuity patterns (aching lumbus and knees, seminal emission, night sweating, clouded vision, poor vision and hearing, and menstrual irregularities). If yīn vacuity engenders internal heat and results in **steaming bone taxation heat**[564] (骨蒸劳热 *gǔ zhēng láo rè*), dispersion-thirst, tinnitus, deafness, night sweating, emaciation, postmeridian reddening of the cheeks, vexation and agitation at night, dry cough with scant phlegm, and phlegm containing blood, use *shú dì huáng* combined with medicinals such as:

guī bǎn (龟板 tortoise shell, Testudinis Carapax et Plastrum)

zhī mǔ (知母 anemarrhena, Anemarrhenae Rhizoma)

huáng bǎi (黄柏 phellodendron, Phellodendri Cortex)

zhū jǐ suǐ (猪脊髓 pig's spine marrow, Suis Spinae Medulla)

dì gǔ pí (地骨皮 lycium root bark, Lycii Cortex)

qín jiāo (秦艽 large gentian, Gentianae Macrophyllae Radix)

biē jiǎ (鳖甲 turtle shell, Trionycis Carapax)

An example of this use is *dà bǔ yīn wán* (Major Yīn Supplementation Pill).[255]

Shú dì huáng combined with *dāng guī* (Chinese angelica) supplements the blood; with *bái sháo* (white peony), it nourishes the liver; with *bǎi zǐ rén* (arborvitae seed), it nourishes the heart; with *lóng yǎn ròu* (longan flesh), it nourishes the

---

[7]The fresh, unprocessed medicinal is called *xiān dì huáng* (鲜地黄, fresh rehmannia). The shade-dried (or oven-dried) form is called *gān dì huáng* (干地黄, dried rehmannia), or simply 干地 *gān dì*. The wine-steamed form is termed *shú dì huáng* (熟地黄, cooked rehmannia), or simply 熟地 *shú dì*. The Chinese name 生地黄 *shēng dì huáng* (or 生地 *shēng dì*) originally referred to *xiān dì huáng* (鲜地黄, fresh rehmannia), but is now often used to represent *gān dì huáng* (干地黄, dried rehmannia). Only *shú dì huáng* and *gān dì huáng* are generally available in the West. (Ed.)

spleen. When used together with *má huáng* (ephedra), *shú dì huáng* is not sticky or stagnating, and it frees the blood vessels and warms the **interstices**[554] of the flesh. An example of this use is *yáng hé tāng* (Harmonious Yáng Decoction):

Yáng hé tāng 阳和汤   Harmonious Yáng Decoction

---

shú dì huáng (熟地黄 cooked rehmannia, Rehmanniae Radix Praeparata)
má huáng (麻黄 ephedra, Ephedrae Herba)
bái jiè zǐ (白芥子 white mustard, Sinapis Albae Semen)
lù jiǎo jiāo (鹿角胶 deerhorn glue, Cervi Cornus Gelatinum)
ròu guì (肉桂 cinnamon bark, Cinnamomi Cortex)
jiāng tàn (姜炭 blast-charred ginger, Zingiberis Rhizoma Carbonisatum)
gān cǎo (甘草 licorice, Glycyrrhizae Radix)

This formula treats **yīn flat-abscesses**[569] (阴疽 *yīn jū*), bone-clinging flat-abscesses (附骨疽 *fù gǔ jū*), and streaming sores (流注 *liú zhù*), which in Western medicine include cold abscesses, obliterating phlebitis, tuberculosis of the mesenteric lymph nodes, chronic osteomyelitis, and tuberculosis of the joints. It is a commonly used formula for warming yáng and dissipating binds.

COMPARISONS

Ē jiāo (ass hide glue)[115] supplements the blood and also stanches bleeding, while *shú dì huáng* supplements the blood and also replenishes essence and marrow. Whereas *ē jiāo* (ass hide glue) enriches and nourishes the liver and kidney, yet also nourishes lung yīn, *shú dì huáng* enriches and nourishes the liver and kidney, yet also nourishes heart blood.

Sāng shèn (mulberry)[140] supplements the liver and kidney; however, it is cool in nature and its blood-supplementing strength does not compare to that of *shú dì huáng*. *Shú dì huáng* supplements the liver and kidney, but it is warm in nature and enriches yīn and supplements blood far more effectively than *sāng shèn*.

Dāng guī (Chinese angelica)[111] supplements blood and has a moving nature, whereas *shú dì huáng* supplements blood and has a tranquil nature. *Dāng guī* engenders new blood and supplements blood, whereas *shú dì huáng* enriches yīn and essence to nourish blood. The combination of these two medicinals enhances their individual strengths and overcomes their weaknesses.

Hé shǒu wū (flowery knotweed)[118] also supplements the liver and kidney, but its strength to supplement blood is less than *shú dì huáng*. The strength of *shú dì huáng* to blacken the beard and hair, however, is less than that of *hé shǒu wū*.

MISCELLANEOUS

When using *shú dì huáng* for a long period of time, use the type that has been prepared with *shā rén* (amomum) (or else add some *shā rén* (amomum) to the formula) to avoid its sliminess causing blockage that reduces appetite and creates oppression in the chest and stomach duct.

DOSAGE

The dosage is generally 9–25 g/3 qián–8 qián. For severe diseases, as much as 30 g/1 liǎng or more can be used.

CAUTION

Contraindicated in patterns with exuberance of yīn due to yáng vacuity. Its use is inappropriate for patients with copious phlegm, slimy tongue fur, or stagnation and oppression in the chest and diaphragm.

---

11. 当归 Dāng Guī
Chinese angelica

Angelicae
Sinensis Radix

Acrid, sweet, and slightly bitter in flavor and warm in nature, *dāng guī* (Chinese angelica) is the medicinal most commonly used to treat diseases of the blood aspect. Its Chinese name, which literally means "command return," reflects how it makes blood return to the places where it belongs.

1. Supplementing the Blood: The combination of 30 g/10 qián of *huáng qí* (astragalus) and 6–9 g/2–3 qián of *dāng guī* is known as *dāng guī bǔ xuè tāng* (Chinese Angelica Blood-Supplementing Decoction), which is often used after blood loss to treat patterns such as blood vacuity, insufficiency of qì and blood, and excessive postpartum blood loss. *Dāng guī* combined with *shú dì huáng* (cooked rehmannia), *bái sháo* (white peony), and *chuān xiōng* (chuanxiong) is called *sì wù tāng* (Four Agents Decoction), which is the most commonly used blood-supplementing formula. This formula, varied in accordance with signs, is used for various forms of blood vacuity. In recent years variations of *sì wù tāng* have often been used to treat various forms of anemia.

2. Quickening the Blood: *Dāng guī* also quickens the blood and frees the network vessels, dissipates stasis and disperses swelling. *Dāng guī* combined with *hóng huā* (carthamus), *chì sháo* (red peony), *sān qī* (notoginseng), *táo rén* (peach kernel), *rǔ xiāng* (frankincense), and *mò yào* (myrrh) is used for knocks and falls and for pain and swelling from static blood. Combined with *lián qiáo* (forsythia), *jīn yín huā* (lonicera), *chì sháo* (red peony), *hóng huā* (carthamus), *zào jiǎo cì* (gleditsia thorn), and *zhì shān jiǎ* (mix-fried pangolin scales), it is used for the onset of welling-abscesses, sores, swelling, and pain. Combined with *guì zhī* (cinnamon twig), *qiāng huó* (notopterygium), *dú huó* (pubescent angelica), *wēi líng xiān* (clematis), *piàn jiāng huáng* (sliced turmeric), *hóng huā* (carthamus), *yǐ mǐ* (coix), *xù duàn* (dipsacus), and *fù zǐ* (aconite), it is used for wind-cold-damp impediment, and for pain in the arm, lumbus, leg, or foot. Combined with *chuān xiōng* (chuanxiong), *hóng huā* (carthamus), *bàn xià* (pinellia), *fáng fēng* (saposhnikovia), *huáng qí* (astragalus), *guì zhī* (cinnamon twig), *bái sháo* (white peony), *shú dì huáng* (cooked rehmannia), and *zhì shān jiǎ* (mix-fried pangolin scales), it is used for numbness and insensitivity of the skin.

3. Moistening the Intestines and Freeing the Stool: As a result of old age, enduring illness, postpartum blood loss, or insufficiency of the fluids, when blood vacuity intestinal dryness causes bound stool, use *dāng guī* to nourish the blood and moisten the intestines and thereby free the stool. In these cases it is frequently combined with medicinals such as:

huǒ má rén (火麻仁 cannabis fruit, Cannabis Fructus)

shēng dì huáng (生地黄 dried/fresh rehmannia, Rehmanniae Radix Exsiccata seu Recens)

shú dì huáng (熟地黄 cooked rehmannia, Rehmanniae Radix Praeparata)

táo rén (桃仁 peach kernel, Persicae Semen)

ròu cōng róng (肉苁蓉 cistanche, Cistanches Herba)

yù lǐ rén (郁李仁 bush cherry kernel, Pruni Semen)

guā lóu rén (瓜蒌仁 trichosanthes seed, Trichosanthis Semen)

dà huáng (大黄 rhubarb, Rhei Radix et Rhizoma)

4. Regulating Menstruation: *Dāng guī* combined with *shú dì huáng* (cooked rehmannia), *chì sháo* (red peony), *chuān xiōng* (chuanxiong), *hóng huā* (carthamus), *táo rén* (peach kernel), *qiàn cǎo* (madder), and *xiāng fù* (cyperus) is used for menstrual block due to qì and blood stagnation. Combined with *bái sháo* (white peony), *xiāng fù* (cyperus), *yán hú suǒ* (corydalis), and *chǎo chuān liàn zǐ* (stir-fried toosendan), it is used for abdominal pain during menstruation. Combined with *shēng dì huáng* (dried/fresh rehmannia), *bái sháo* (white peony), *bái zhú* (white atractylodes), *ài yè tàn* (charred mugwort), *ē jiāo zhū* (ass hide glue pellets),[8] and *zōng tàn* (charred trachycarpus), it is used for profuse menstruation and for flooding and spotting. In summary, *dāng guī* regulates the thoroughfare (*chōng*), controlling (*rèn*), and girdling (*dài*) vessels. Because *dāng guī* supplements and harmonizes the blood effectively, it is the most commonly used medicinal for regulating the menses. Physicians of the past considered *dāng guī* a "special medicinal for women." For both antepartum and postpartum diseases, *dāng guī* is frequently added to treatments in accordance with the pattern identified.

While *bái sháo* (white peony) also supplements the blood, it tends to nourish yīn; it is tranquil and static in nature. *Dāng guī* also supplements the blood, but tends to warm yáng; it is stirring in nature and is mobile. To treat blood vacuity engendering heat, use *bái sháo* (white peony), whereas to treat blood vacuity with cold, use *dāng guī*.

Dāng guī combined with *huáng qí* (astragalus) and *dǎng shēn* (codonopsis) engenders qì and supplements the blood. Combined with *dà huáng* (rhubarb) and *niú xī* (achyranthes), it breaks static blood in the lower body. Combined with *chuān xiōng* (chuanxiong), *sū mù* (sappan), *hóng huā* (carthamus), and *jié gěng* (platycodon), it quickens static blood in the upper body. Combined with *guì zhī* (cinnamon twig), *sāng zhī* (mulberry twig), *lù lù tōng* (liquidambar fruit), and *sī guā luò* (loofah), it promotes flow in the limbs, quickens the blood, and frees the network vessels.

---

[8]See footnote on page 116.

Dāng guī tóu (Chinese angelica head), i.e., root top, and *dāng guī wěi* (Chinese angelica tail), the root-ends, tend to quicken the blood and break blood. *Dāng guī shēn* (Chinese angelica body), i.e., the main part of the root, tends to supplement the blood and nourish the blood. *Quán dāng guī* (whole Chinese angelica) supplements the blood and quickens the blood. *Dāng guī xū* (Chinese angelica fine root) tends to quicken the blood and free the network vessels.[9]

Jiǔ dāng guī (酒当归, wine-fried Chinese angelica), which is *dāng guī* washed or stir-fried with wine, tends to move and quicken the blood. *Tǔ chǎo dāng guī* (土炒 当归, earth-fried Chinese angelica) is used for blood vacuity patterns and sloppy soft stool. *Dāng guī tàn* (当归炭, charred Chinese angelica) is used to stanch bleeding.

Dosage
The dosage is generally 3–9 g/1 qián–3 qián. In severe or urgent diseases, use up to 15 g/5 qián.

Caution
Inappropriate for use in treating large intestine efflux diarrhea or effulgent fire.

Research
According to modern research, *dāng guī* has both inhibitory and excitatory effects on the uterus. The component that is water-soluble, non-volatile, and crystalline has an excitatory effect on the uterus and increases uterine contractions. The volatile oils present in *dāng guī* inhibit the smooth muscle of the uterus and allow for relaxation of the uterus. *Dāng guī* also fights vitamin E deficiency and has an inhibitory effect on certain types of bacteria, such as *Bacillus dysenteriae*, *Bacillus typhosus*, and hemolytic streptococcus.

---

12. 白芍 Bái Sháo White Peony	Paeoniae Radix Alba

Bái sháo (white peony) is sour and bitter in flavor and slightly cold in nature; it nourishes the blood and enhances the sinews, relaxes tension and relieves pain; it also emolliates the liver and quiets the spleen.

Bái sháo is often used to supplement the blood and nourish yīn. Combined with *dāng guī* (Chinese angelica), *shú dì huáng* (cooked rehmannia), *chuān xiōng* (chuanxiong), *bái zhú* (white atractylodes), and *ē jiāo* (ass hide glue), it supplements blood vacuity. Combined with *mài dōng* (ophiopogon), *wǔ wèi zǐ* (schisandra), and *fú xiǎo*

---

[9]The functions of the various parts of *dāng guī* (Chinese angelica) are subject to some disagreement. This confusion stems from the fact that these medicinals are often mislabeled. *Dāng guī tóu* (Chinese angelica head) is no longer in common use and what is sold for it is generally *dāng guī shēn* (Chinese angelica body). Thus *dāng guī tóu*, which is really *dāng guī shēn*, is said to supplement blood. *Quán dāng guī* (whole Chinese angelica), which is also called *dāng guī piàn* (Chinese angelica slices), both moves blood and supplements blood. There is agreement that *dāng guī wěi* (Chinese angelica tail) quickens and breaks blood. *Dāng guī xū* (Chinese angelica fine root) is not currently found on the market. (Ed.)

mài (light wheat), it is used for yīn vacuity night sweating. Combined with *shēng dì huáng* (dried/fresh rehmannia), *shí hú* (dendrobium), *nǚ zhēn zǐ* (ligustrum), *shēng mǔ lì* (crude oyster shell), and *zhēn zhū mǔ* (mother-of-pearl), it nourishes yīn and subdues yáng. I often use a combination of *bái sháo*, *shēng mǔ lì* (crude oyster shell), *shēng shí jué míng* (crude abalone shell), *shēng dài zhě shí* (crude hematite), *shēng dì huáng* (dried/fresh rehmannia), *huáng qín* (scutellaria), *xiāng fù* (cyperus), *yè jiāo téng* (flowery knotweed stem), *yuǎn zhì* (polygala), *fú shén* (root poria), and *bái jí lí* (tribulus), varied in accordance with signs, for neurasthenia patients manifesting a pattern of yīn vacuity and liver effulgence (headache, dizzy head, dizzy vision, rashness, impatience, irascibility, insomnia, profuse dreaming, **booming heat [effusion]**[543] (轰热 *hōng rè*), forgetfulness, red-tipped tongue, thin yellow tongue fur, and fine rapid stringlike pulse).

For insufficiency of liver blood and loss of luxuriance of the sinews and flesh that manifests in hypertonicity of the limbs, stiffness of the joints, and inhibited bending and stretching, use *bái sháo* combined with *shēn jīn cǎo* (ground pine), *yǐ mǐ* (coix), *jī xuè téng* (spatholobus), *mù guā* (chaenomeles), *gān cǎo jié* (resinous licorice root), and *dāng guī wěi* (Chinese angelica tail). *Bái sháo* combined with *gān cǎo* (licorice), *niú xī* (achyranthes), *mù guā* (chaenomeles), *hóng huā* (carthamus), and *zhì shān jiǎ* (mix-fried pangolin scales) is used for damage to yīn humor causing spasm of the gastrocnemius muscle or contracture and inability to stretch the legs and feet. In severe cases, add *hǔ gǔ* (tiger bone).[10]

Bái sháo combined with *dāng guī* (Chinese angelica), *gān cǎo* (licorice), *guì zhī* (cinnamon twig), and *yí táng* (malt sugar) is used for abdominal pain from blood vacuity and liver exuberance or from spleen vacuity cold. Combined with *mù xiāng* (costusroot), *huáng lián* (coptis), *huáng qín* (scutellaria), *gé gēn* (pueraria), *bīng láng* (areca), and *bái tóu wēng* (pulsatilla), it is used for **dysentery**[547] with abdominal pain. *Bái sháo* relaxes tension and relieves pain and its pain-relieving action is most effective for abdominal pain.

Bái sháo (white peony) supplements the blood, nourishes yīn, and emolliates the liver; thus it also quiets the spleen. When spleen vacuity and liver exuberance result in chronic diarrhea (characteristically exacerbated by anger and associated with abdominal pain prior to, but relieved by, defecation), I often use *bái sháo* with *chǎo fáng fēng* (stir-fried saposhnikovia), *bái zhú* (white atractylodes), and *chén pí* (tangerine peel). This is known as *tòng xiè yào fāng* (Essential Formula for Painful Diarrhea).

Bái sháo is also often used to regulate menstruation. Combined with *dāng guī* (Chinese angelica), *shēng dì huáng* (dried/fresh rehmannia), *huáng qín* (scutellaria), *ài yè tàn* (charred mugwort), and *ē jiāo* (ass hide glue) to form *jiāo ài sì wù tāng* (Ass Hide Glue and Mugwort Four Agents Decoction), it is used for advanced menstruation or profuse menstruation. Combined with *dāng guī* (Chinese angelica), *chuān xiōng* (chuanxiong), *shú dì huáng* (cooked rehmannia), *hóng huā*

---

[10]Because the tiger is an endangered species, the use of tiger bone (and other parts) is no longer considered acceptable. The bones of animals that are not endangered, such as the water buffalo, are recommended as substitutes. (Ed.)

(carthamus), and *táo rén* (peach kernel) to form *táo hóng sì wù tāng* (Peach Kernel and Carthamus Four Agents Decoction) plus *xiāng fù* (cyperus), it is used for delayed menstruation and scant flow. For abdominal pain during menstruation, large quantities of *bái sháo* are often used. Combined with *sāng jì shēng* (mistletoe), *bái zhú* (white atractylodes), and *chǎo huáng qín* (stir-fried scutellaria), it clears heat and quiets the fetus.

To nourish yīn, supplement the blood, and emolliate the liver, use *shēng bái sháo* (raw white peony). To harmonize the center and relax tension, use *jiǔ chǎo bái sháo* (wine-fried white peony). To quiet the spleen and check diarrhea, use *tǔ chǎo bái sháo* (earth-fried white peony).

Comparisons

Chì sháo (red peony)[422] tends to move blood and dissipate stasis, whereas *bái sháo* tends to nourish blood and boost yīn. *Chì sháo* drains liver fire, whereas *bái sháo* nourishes liver yīn. *Chì sháo* dissipates without supplementing, whereas *bái sháo* supplements without dissipating.

Dāng guī (Chinese angelica) enters the liver and moves liver yáng; although *bái sháo* also enters the liver, it constrains liver yáng. *Dāng guī* has a moving nature, whereas *bái sháo* has a tranquil nature. These two medicinals are used together to rectify their respective tendencies and mutually assist the therapeutic effect.

Shú dì huáng (cooked rehmannia) and *bái sháo* both supplement the blood, but *shú dì huáng* supplements blood vis-à-vis entering the kidney to engender essence, whereas *bái sháo* supplements blood vis-à-vis entering the liver to nourish yīn. *Shú dì huáng* is sweet and warm, while *bái sháo* is sour and cold.

Research

According to modern reports, this medicinal inhibits bacteria such as *Bacillus dysenteriae*, *Bacillus typhosus*, and *Bacillus coli*. It also moderates hyperactive peristalsis in the stomach and intestines that causes **mounting pain**[558] (疝痛 *shàn tòng*) in the abdomen.

Dosage

The dosage is generally 4.5–12 g/1.5–4 qián. In severe patterns, use up to 15–30 g/5 qián–1 liǎng.

Caution

Contraindicated in postpartum blood stasis or retention of lochia.

---

13. 阿胶 Ē Jiāo
Ass Hide Glue

Asini
Corii Colla

Ē jiāo (ass hide glue) is sweet and neutral in nature and flavor. It supplements the blood, enriches yīn, moistens the lung, and stanches bleeding. It comes in the form of lumps (*ē jiāo kuài* 阿胶块) that are dissolved in a ready-made decoction.

Ē jiāo supplements the blood and enriches yīn. To treat yīn vacuity, it is combined with *dāng guī* (Chinese angelica), *shú dì huáng* (cooked rehmannia), *bái sháo* (white peony), and *bái zhú* (white atractylodes). In recent years, it has often been used to treat various forms of anemia, depending on the identified patterns. Modern research has demonstrated that *ē jiāo* increases erythrocytes and hemoglobin. For yīn vacuity internal heat and steaming bone consumptive heat, *ē jiāo* is combined with *dì huáng* (rehmannia), *biē jiǎ* (turtle shell), *guī bǎn* (tortoise shell), *qín jiāo* (large gentian), *yín chái hú* (stellaria), and *qīng hāo* (sweet wormwood) to enrich yīn and clear heat.

Ē jiāo zhū (阿胶珠, ass hide glue pellets)[11] are often used to stanch bleeding and to moisten the lung. Combined with *mài dōng* (ophiopogon), *bǎi hé* (lily bulb), *bái jí* (bletilla), *shā shēn* (adenophora/glehnia), *hēi shān zhī* (charred gardenia), and *ǒu jié* (lotus root node), they are used for lung yīn vacuity that results in cough, coughing of blood, and **pulmonary consumption**[560] (肺痨 *fèi láo*). Combined with *bái sháo* (white peony), *dāng guī tàn* (charred Chinese angelica), *ài yè tàn* (charred mugwort), *zōng tàn* (charred trachycarpus), and *bái zhú* (white atractylodes), they are used for profuse menstruation or for flooding and spotting. In recent years, this basic formula has been used with pattern-appropriate additions of spleen-fortifying and kidney-supplementing medicinals such as *shēng dì tàn* (charred dried/fresh rehmannia), *huáng qí* (astragalus), *dǎng shēn* (codonopsis), *shān zhū yú* (cornus), *xù duàn tàn* (charred dipsacus), *tù sī zǐ* (cuscuta), *sāng jì shēng* (mistletoe), and *zǐ hé chē* (placenta) to treat functional metrorrhagia. The combination of *ē jiāo zhū* (ass hide glue pellets) with *chǎo huáng qín* (stir-fried scutellaria), *kǔ shēn* (flavescent sophora), *huái huā tàn* (charred sophora flower), *chǎo dì yú* (stir-fried sanguisorba), *zào xīn tǔ* (oven earth), and *fáng fēng* (saposhnikovia) is used for descent of blood with the stool or bleeding hemorrhoids.

When it is used to moisten the lung and transform phlegm, *ē jiāo* is stir fried with *gé fěn* (clamshell powder). When used to stanch bleeding, it is stir fried with *pú huáng* (typha pollen). When used to enrich yīn and supplement the blood, it is generally used raw (melted into the decoction).

COMPARISONS

Shú dì huáng (cooked rehmannia)[109] and *ē jiāo* both enrich yīn and supplement the blood. However, *shú dì huáng* tends to supplement kidney yīn, replenish essence and marrow, and supplement the blood, whereas *ē jiāo* (ass hide glue) tends to moisten the lung and nourish the liver, supplement the blood and enrich yīn, as well as stanch bleeding.

Huáng míng jiāo (黄明胶, cowhide glue) is very similar to *ē jiāo* in action, so it can be substituted if *ē jiāo* is unavailable. Nonetheless, its supplementing and boosting actions are not so strong as those of *ē jiāo*. Moreover, *huáng míng jiāo* also quickens the blood and resolves toxin.

---

[11] *Ē jiāo zhū* (ass hide glue pellets) are prepared by heating *hǎi gé qiào fěn* (clamshell powder) in a wok and adding small pieces of *ē jiāo* (ass hide glue). After a short time in the heated *hǎi gé qiào fěn*, the *ē jiāo* melts, puffs up, and forms into spherical balls. (Ed.)

Ē jiāo also nourishes the blood, moistens dryness, and lubricates the intestines, and is therefore further used for postpartum constipation, intestinal dryness with constipation in elderly patients, and blood vacuity constipation.

DOSAGE

The dosage is generally 4.5–9 g/1.5–3 qián.

CAUTION

Not suitable when there is a thick slimy tongue fur, poor appetite, or sloppy diarrhea.

---

14. 紫河车 Zǐ Hé Chē   Hominis Placenta
Placenta

Zǐ hé chē (placenta), which literally means "purple river cart," is sometimes referred to in modern literature as *tāi pán* 胎盘. Sweet and salty in flavor and warm in nature, *zǐ hé chē* greatly supplements qì and blood and is an enriching and invigorating medicinal. *Zǐ hé chē*, rich in qì and flavor, is used for all forms of **vacuity detriment**[566] (虚损 *xū sǔn*) and insufficiency of essence-blood. According to traditional experience, "when essence is insufficient, supplement with flavor"; this means use medicinals with rich flavor.

Because *zǐ hé chē* has a fishy smell, it is frequently used in pills, or dried, ground to powder, and taken in capsules, rather than in decoctions. An example is *hé chē dà zào wán* (Placenta Great Creation Pill), which is used for vacuity taxation with marked emaciation, weak health, devitalized essence-spirit, seminal emission, and impotence.

RESEARCH

According to modern research, *zǐ hé chē* promotes development of the mammary glands, female genitals, and ovaries. It also enhances the immune system and strengthens resistance. *Zǐ hé chē* is effective in the treatment of incomplete development of the uterus, uterine atrophy, functional amenorrhea, myometritis, uterine bleeding, scant breast milk, postpartum anterior pituitary hypofunction (Sheehan's syndrome), anemia, pulmonary tuberculosis, and bronchitis.

COMPARISONS

Lù róng (velvet deerhorn) supplements the yáng qì of the kidney and the governing vessel, as well as engendering essence and boosting marrow. *Zǐ hé chē* supplements the yáng qì of the liver and kidney, as well as boosting blood and assisting qì.

DOSAGE

The dosage is generally 2–4.5 g/8 fēn–1.5 qián.

CAUTION

Contraindicated in patterns of vacuity fire.

15. 何首乌 Hé Shǒu Wū
Flowery Knotweed

Polygoni
Multiflori Radix

Hé shǒu wū (flowery knotweed) is slightly warm in nature. When raw, it is bitter and astringent in flavor, but when processed, it takes on an added sweetness. It nourishes the blood and boosts essence, neutrally supplements the liver and kidney, and blackens the beard and hair. It also moistens the stool and lubricates the intestines, disperses scrofula, and treats malaria.

Hé shǒu wū is warm but not drying, and supplementing but not slimy. Being neutral in nature, it can be taken over extended periods and is therefore frequently used in enriching, supplementing, and invigorating pill medicines designed to treat vacuity following an illness, yīn vacuity and blood depletion, and weak sinews and bones. For example, *hé shǒu wū* combined with *shú dì huáng* (cooked rehmannia), *dāng guī* (Chinese angelica), *bái sháo* (white peony), *ē jiāo* (ass hide glue), and *bái zhú* (white atractylodes) is used for insufficiency of liver and kidney, blood and qì vacuity, and various forms of anemia. According to modern research, *hé shǒu wū* promotes development of new blood. Combined with *shān yú ròu* (cornus), *shān yào* (dioscorea), *qiàn shí* (euryale), *wǔ wèi zǐ* (schisandra), *lóng gǔ* (dragon bone), *mǔ lì* (oyster shell), *yuǎn zhì* (polygala), and *fú líng* (poria), it is used for kidney vacuity, seminal efflux or seminal emission, and vaginal discharge.

For insufficiency of liquid and blood that results in lack of fluids in the intestines, stagnation in the intestines, and bound stool, which may be a result of old age, enduring illness, or postpartum loss of blood, use *hé shǒu wū* combined with medicinals such as *dāng guī* (Chinese angelica), *ròu cōng róng* (cistanche), *hēi zhī má* (black sesame), and *huǒ má rén* (cannabis fruit) to nourish the blood, moisten the intestines, and thereby free the stool.

According to modern research, *hé shǒu wū* promotes intestinal peristalsis and is suitable for use in patterns of vacuity-type constipation.

For patterns of liver-kidney depletion, insufficiency of essence blood, and debilitated health in which the hair does not receive sufficient nourishment and becomes dry and white, *hé shǒu wū* is used to make pills in combination with:

bǔ gǔ zhī (补骨脂 psoralea, Psoraleae Fructus)
dāng guī (当归 Chinese angelica, Angelicae Sinensis Radix)
dì huáng (地黄 rehmannia, Rehmanniae Radix)
gǒu qǐ zǐ (枸杞子 lycium, Lycii Fructus)
nǚ zhēn zǐ (女贞子 ligustrum, Ligustri Lucidi Fructus)
tù sī zǐ (菟丝子 cuscuta, Cuscutae Semen)
hēi zhī má (黑芝麻 black sesame, Sesami Semen Nigrum)
hàn lián cǎo (旱莲草 eclipta, Ecliptae Herba)

In the treatment of scrofula or swollen welling-abscesses that arise when the movement of qì and blood stagnates, *shēng hé shǒu wū* (raw flowery knotweed) harmonizes qì and blood and also resolves toxin and disperses swelling. For this type of pattern, *shēng hé shǒu wū* is frequently combined with medicinals such as:

pú gōng yīng (蒲公英 dandelion, Taraxaci Herba)

dì dīng (地丁 violet, Violae Herba)

lián qiáo (连翘 forsythia, Forsythiae Fructus)

xuán shēn (玄参 scrophularia, Scrophulariae Radix)

shēng mǔ lì (生牡蛎 crude oyster shell, Ostreae Concha Cruda)

xià kū cǎo (夏枯草 prunella, Prunellae Spica)

When malarial evil has entered the yīn aspect and persisted without resolution, use *hé shǒu wū* with either *rén shēn* (ginseng) or *dǎng shēn* (codonopsis); this is known as *hé rén yǐn* (Flowery Knotweed and Ginseng Beverage). Alternatively, use 25–30 g/8 qián–1 liǎng of *hé shǒu wū* and 3 g/1 qián of *gān cǎo* (licorice) decocted in water. In the past, I have combined these medicinals with *xiǎo chái hú tāng* (Minor Bupleurum Decoction) and *bái hǔ tāng* (White Tiger Decoction), varied with the signs, to cure several cases of [aversion to] cold and heat [effusion] occurring at set periods for no known cause.

Comparisons

Shú dì huáng (cooked rehmannia)[109] has much greater power to enrich the liver and kidney and to increase essence and boost marrow than *hé shǒu wū*, but its enriching, slimy nature can be excessive and can easily cause clogging and damage to the stomach. Conversely, *hé shǒu wū* is neither cold nor drying, and has no clogging sliminess that harms the stomach. Furthermore, it has a blood-nourishing wind-dispelling action that *shú dì huáng* lacks. When it is necessary to enrich and supplement urgently, *shú dì huáng* is appropriate. When gradual supplementation over an extended period is necessary, *hé shǒu wū* is better. These two medicinals can also be used together.

Huáng jīng (polygonatum) also supplements without being slimy, but tends to supplement the center and boost qì and to moisten and nourish yīn-liquid of the lung and stomach, whereas *hé shǒu wū* tends to enrich the liver and kidney and to nourish the blood and boost essence.

The stem of this medicinal, which is called *shǒu wū téng* (首乌藤, flowery knotweed stem), or more commonly *yè jiāo téng* 夜交藤[162] in Chinese, is decocted with water and taken internally to treat insomnia, dispel wind-damp, soothe the channels and network vessels, and eliminate impediment pain. Decocted with water and used as a topical wash, it resolves toxin, harmonizes the blood, and dispels wind, and is thus used for wind sores and for itching from scabs and lichen.

Shēng hé shǒu wū (raw flowery knotweed) is suitable for dispersing scrofula, resolving sore toxin, and freeing bound stool. *Zhì hé shǒu wū* (processed flowery knotweed) is suitable for supplementing the liver and kidney, strengthening sinew and bone, nourishing the blood, and securing essence.

In the book *Běn Cǎo Gāng Mù* (本草纲目 "The Comprehensive Herbal Foundation"), Lǐ Shí-Zhēn records that this medicinal "relieves heart pain." When I treat hypertensive heart disease, coronary heart disease, or angina pectoris, after considering the nature of the pattern I sometimes add 9–15 g/3–5 qián of *hé shǒu wū*, to good effect. Because in Chinese medicine "heart pain" also includes pain in the stomach duct region, I sometimes use this medicinal when treating vacuity-type stomach duct pain. I usually use equal parts of raw and processed *hé shǒu wū*. According to modern research, *hé shǒu wū* has a pronounced cardiotonic action and is especially effective for fatigue from heart disease. Furthermore, it prevents deposition of cholesterol in the liver and can reduce atherosclerosis. When treating coronary heart disease, I often add this medicinal to pill medicines and have the patient take it over a long period of time.

DOSAGE

The standard dosage is 9–15 g/3–5 qián. In severe patterns, use as much as 20–30 g/7 qián–1 liǎng.

---

16. 龟板 Guī Bǎn
Tortoise Shell
Testudinis
Carapax et Plastrum

Salty and slightly sweet in flavor and cool in nature, *guī bǎn* (tortoise shell) is a yīn-enriching yáng-subduing medicine with the emphasis on enriching yīn. For example, in the treatment of yīn vacuity that manifests in steaming bone consumptive heat, night sweating, pulmonary consumption with cough, or coughing of blood, *guī bǎn* can be used to enrich yīn and nourish the blood in order to clear vacuity heat, and to enrich the liver and kidney in order to invigorate the root. It is frequently combined with medicinals such as the following:

shú dì huáng (熟地黄 cooked rehmannia, Rehmanniae Radix Praeparata)

shēng dì huáng (生地黄 dried/fresh rehmannia, Rehmanniae Radix Exsiccata seu Recens)

zhī mǔ (知母 anemarrhena, Anemarrhenae Rhizoma)

huáng bǎi (黄柏 phellodendron, Phellodendri Cortex)

zhū jǐ suǐ (猪脊髓 pig's spine marrow, Suis Spinae Medulla)

tiān dōng (天冬 asparagus, Asparagi Radix)

mài dōng (麦冬 ophiopogon, Ophiopogonis Radix)

xuán shēn (玄参 scrophularia, Scrophulariae Radix)

shā shēn (沙参 adenophora/glehnia, Adenophorae seu Glehniae Radix)

In warm-heat disease, a prolonged high fever that fails to abate and damages yīn humor leads to yīn vacuity and liquid dryness, and vacuity wind stirring internally, which then results in symptoms such as mild jerking of the limbs, dry tongue without liquid, postmeridian low-grade fever, vexation and agitation at night, and a fine stringlike rapid pulse. For such cases *guī bǎn* can be combined with *mài dōng* (ophiopogon), *bái sháo* (white peony), *ē jiāo* (ass hide glue), *gōu téng* (uncaria), *biē jiǎ* (turtle shell), and *shēng mǔ lì* (crude oyster shell) to enrich yīn and nourish liquid and to subdue yáng and extinguish wind. For this purpose I often use formulas such as *sān jiǎ fù mài tāng* (Triple-Armored Pulse-Restorative Decoction), *dà dìng fēng zhū* (Major Wind Stabilizing Pill), and *xiǎo dìng fēng zhū* (Minor Wind Stabilizing Pill) from *Wēn Bìng Tiáo Biàn* (温病条辨 "Systematized Identification of Warm Diseases").

For patterns of liver-kidney yīn vacuity and ascendant liver yáng that manifest as dizzy head, dizzy vision, tinnitus, vexation, agitation, irascibility, booming heat [effusion] (fever), and **hemilateral headache**[552] (偏头痛 *piān tóu tòng*), *guī bǎn* enriches yīn and subdues yáng and as a result downbears liver heat. For this purpose it is frequently combined with *bái sháo* (white peony), *shēng dì huáng* (dried/fresh rehmannia), *shēng mǔ lì* (crude oyster shell), *shēng shí jué míng* (crude abalone shell), *jú huā* (chrysanthemum), and *huáng qín* (scutellaria), as well as *liù wèi dì huáng wán* (Six-Ingredient Rehmannia Pill).

The liver governs the sinews and the kidney governs the bones. When insufficency of the liver and kidney leads to sinew and bone **wilting**[568] (痿 *wěi*), aching lumbus and limp legs, inability to walk, hunchback and pigeon chest, or nonclosure of the fontanel gate in infants, *guī bǎn* is used to supplement the kidney and strengthen the bones, enrich the liver and enhance the sinews. For this purpose it is frequently combined with:

hǔ gǔ (虎骨 tiger bone, Tigris Os)[12]

niú xī (牛膝 achyranthes, Achyranthis Bidentatae Radix)

shān yào (山药 dioscorea, Dioscoreae Rhizoma)

shān yú ròu (山萸肉 cornus, Corni Fructus)

bǔ gǔ zhī (补骨脂 psoralea, Psoraleae Fructus)

hú táo ròu (胡桃肉 walnut, Juglandis Semen)

dù zhòng (杜仲 eucommia, Eucommiae Cortex)

xù duàn (续断 dipsacus, Dipsaci Radix)

dì huáng (地黄 rehmannia, Rehmanniae Radix)

Guī bǎn also enriches yīn and cools the blood. It is used for effulgent yīn vacuity fire and frenetic movement of hot blood that cause profuse menstruation, incessant flooding and spotting, coughing of blood, or nosebleed. For these cases, it is frequently combined with medicinals such as:

shēng dì huáng (生地黄 dried/fresh rehmannia, Rehmanniae Radix Exsiccata seu Recens)

xuán shēn (玄参 scrophularia, Scrophulariae Radix)

ē jiāo (阿胶 ass hide glue, Asini Corii Colla)

huáng qín (黄芩 scutellaria, Scutellariae Radix)

bái sháo (白芍 white peony, Paeoniae Radix Alba)

huáng bǎi (黄柏 phellodendron, Phellodendri Cortex)

bái máo gēn (白茅根 imperata, Imperatae Rhizoma)

cè bǎi tàn (侧柏炭 charred arborvitae leaf, Platycladi Cacumen Carbonisatum)

zōng tàn (棕炭 charred trachycarpus, Trachycarpi Petiolus Carbonisatus)

---

[12]See note on page 114.

Guī bǎn is salty and softens hardness; it also opens the controlling vessel and harmonizes the blood network vessels. For these reasons, it is used to disperse concretion, conglomeration, and/or aggregation lumps. For blood vacuity and qì stagnation, with evil qì depressed in the channels and network vessels that results in concretion, conglomeration, aggregation lumps in the abdomen, *guī bǎn* is combined with:

> *biē jiǎ* (鳖甲 turtle shell, Trionycis Carapax)
>
> *chì sháo* (赤芍 red peony, Paeoniae Radix Rubra)
>
> *shēng mǔ lì* (生牡蛎 crude oyster shell, Ostreae Concha Cruda)
>
> *hóng huā* (红花 carthamus, Carthami Flos)
>
> *táo rén* (桃仁 peach kernel, Persicae Semen)
>
> *shān zhā hé* (山楂核 crataegus pit, Crataegi Endocarpium et Semen)
>
> *yù jīn* (郁金 curcuma, Curcumae Radix)
>
> *chái hú* (柴胡 bupleurum, Bupleuri Radix)
>
> *xiāng fù* (香附 cyperus, Cyperi Rhizoma)
>
> *é zhú* (莪术 curcuma rhizome, Curcumae Rhizoma)
>
> *sān léng* (三棱 sparganium, Sparganii Rhizoma)

In recent years, this method has frequently been used to treat hepatosplenomegaly.

Comparisons

The glue made from *guī bǎn* (tortoise shell) is called *guī bǎn jiāo* (龟板胶, tortoise shell glue). Sweet in flavor and neutral in nature, *guī bǎn jiāo* possesses a yīn-enriching and blood-supplementing action much stronger than *guī bǎn*, and it also stanches bleeding. Nevertheless, is not as good as *guī bǎn* in freeing the blood vessels and dispersing concretions and conglomerations.

Lù róng (velvet deerhorn)[143] tends to open the governing vessel and supplement kidney yáng, while *guī bǎn* tends to open the controlling vessel and supplement kidney yīn.

Dài mào (hawksbill shell) is effective in calming the liver and settling fright; its strength lies in subduing and downbearing. *Guī bǎn* is effective in supplementing yīn and downbearing fire; its strength lies in enriching and constraining.

Lù jiǎo jiāo (deerhorn glue)[145] supplements the yáng in yīn and frees the blood of the thoroughfare vessel. *Guī bǎn jiāo* (tortoise shell glue) astringes sweating from solitary yáng and quiets yīn that is verging on desertion. *Lù jiǎo jiāo* and *guī bǎn jiāo* are used together; there is a prepared product of this combination called *guī lù èr xiān jiāo* (Tortoise Shell and Deerhorn Two Immortals Glue).

Dosage

The dosage is generally 9–25 g/3–8 qián. When necessary, as much as 30–60 g/ 1–2 liǎng can be used. *Guī bǎn* must be crushed and predecocted.[13]

---

[13] *Zhì guī bǎn* (processed tortoise plastron), usually made by stir-frying with vinegar, is less cold than the unprocessed shell and also is slightly sour. It is less able to nourish yīn than the unprocessed medicinal, but better for softening hardness, stanching bleeding, and strengthening

Caution

Use with care in patients who have slimy tongue fur or poor appetite.

17. 鳖甲 Biē Jiǎ   Trionycis Carapax
Turtle Shell

Biē jiǎ (turtle shell), salty in flavor and cool in nature, is a commonly used yīn-enriching heat-clearing medicine. It also softens hardness and dissipates binds, as well as calming the liver and subduing yáng.

When yīn vacuity internal heat causes steaming bone consumptive heat (骨蒸痨热 *gǔ zhēng láo rè*), night sweating that leaves the hair wet, tidal heat [effusion] (fever), reddening of the cheeks, pulmonary consumption with dry cough, and phlegm containing blood, *biē jiǎ* can be used to enrich yīn and clear heat. For this purpose it is frequently combined with:

yín chái hú (银柴胡 stellaria, Stellariae Radix)

qín jiāo (秦艽 large gentian, Gentianae Macrophyllae Radix)

qīng hāo (青蒿 sweet wormwood, Artemisiae Annuae Herba)

dì gǔ pí (地骨皮 lycium root bark, Lycii Cortex)

zhī mǔ (知母 anemarrhena, Anemarrhenae Rhizoma)

dāng guī (当归 Chinese angelica, Angelicae Sinensis Radix)

wū méi (乌梅 mume, Mume Fructus)

bái sháo (白芍 white peony, Paeoniae Radix Alba)

shēng dì huáng (生地黄 dried/fresh rehmannia, Rehmanniae Radix Exsiccata seu Recens)

xuán shēn (玄参 scrophularia, Scrophulariae Radix)

Biē jiǎ is salty and is used to soften hardness, dissipate binds, and disperse concretions. This action makes it effective for treating chronic malaria in which there is a hard lump under the left rib-side traditionally known as "mother-of-malaria" (疟母 *nüè mǔ*, i.e., splenomegaly). For this purpose, *biē jiǎ* is mix-fried with vinegar,[14] ground to a powder, and taken two or three times a day at a dosage of 30 g/1 qián each time; alternatively, it is combined with:

chái hú (柴胡 bupleurum, Bupleuri Radix)

huáng qín (黄芩 scutellaria, Scutellariae Radix)

dǎng shēn (党参 codonopsis, Codonopsis Radix)

bàn xià (半夏 pinellia, Pinelliae Rhizoma)

táo rén (桃仁 peach kernel, Persicae Semen)

dān pí (丹皮 moutan, Moutan Cortex)

---

the bones. In addition, since the processed medicinal is more friable, it is easier to grind and will not break into potentially dangerous shards when it is broken into pieces before decoction. (Ed.)

[14]Vinegar, according to *Běn Cǎo Bèi Yào* (本草备要 "The Essential Herbal Foundation"), "disperses stasis and resolves toxin, downbears qì, disperses food, opens the stomach, and dissipates water qì." Vinegar enhances the dispersing action of *biē jiǎ* (turtle shell). (Ed.)

shè gān (射干 belamcanda, Belamcandae Rhizoma)

shēng mǔ lì (生牡蛎 crude oyster shell, Ostreae Concha Cruda)

sān léng (三棱 sparganium, Sparganii Rhizoma)

é zhú (莪术 curcuma rhizome, Curcumae Rhizoma)

In *Jīn Guì Yào Lüè* (金匮要略 "Essential Prescriptions of the Golden Coffer") Zhāng Zhòng-Jǐng recorded *biē jiǎ jiān wán* (Turtle Shell Decocted Pill), which is a special formula for mother-of-malaria. In recent years, this pill has been found effective in the treatment of splenomegaly.

For menstrual block, inhibited flow of qì and blood, and stasis accumulation in the abdomen that engenders concretions and lumps, *biē jiǎ* can be used to free the channels and disperse concretions when combined with agents such as the following:

táo rén (桃仁 peach kernel, Persicae Semen)

hóng huā (红花 carthamus, Carthami Flos)

dāng guī wěi (当归尾 Chinese angelica tail, Angelicae Sinensis Radicis Extremitas)

chì sháo (赤芍 red peony, Paeoniae Radix Rubra)

shēng dà huáng (生大黄 raw rhubarb, Rhei Radix et Rhizoma Crudi)

sān léng (三棱 sparganium, Sparganii Rhizoma)

é zhú (莪术 curcuma rhizome, Curcumae Rhizoma)

guì zhī (桂枝 cinnamon twig, Cinnamomi Ramulus)

zhì shān jiǎ (炙山甲 mix-fried pangolin scales, Manis Squama cum Liquido Fricta)

COMPARISONS

Guī bǎn (tortoise shell)[120] tends to enter the kidney and enrich yīn. Its supplementing strength is greater than *biē jiǎ*. *Biē jiǎ* tends to enter the liver and abate heat. Its strength to dissipate binds is greater than *guī bǎn*.

Mǔ lì (oyster shell)[171] tends to transform phlegm binds and disperse scrofula. *Biē jiǎ* tends to eliminate rib-side fullness and dissipate "mother-of-malaria."

DOSAGE

The dosage is generally 9–15 g/3–5 qián. In severe conditions, use up to 30 g/ 1 liǎng. When used in decoction medicines it must be predecocted.

CAUTION

Contraindicated in patterns without yīn vacuity internal heat or with indigestion and intestinal cold diarrhea.

---

18. 山茱萸 **Shān Zhū Yú**   Corni Fructus
Cornus

Also called *shān yú ròu* 山萸肉 and *shān yú* 山萸. Sour, bitter, and astringent in flavor and slightly warm in nature, *shān zhū yú* (cornus) supplements the liver and kidney and strengthens the body. A commonly used enriching and invigorating medicinal, it also astringes essence, checks urinary frequency, constrains sweat, and boosts yīn.

For insufficiency of the liver and kidney that results in aching lumbus and limp legs, dizzy head, tinnitus, seminal emission and premature ejaculation, profuse menstruation, and weak health, *shān zhū yú* is combined with *dì huáng* (rehmannia), *shān yào* (dioscorea), *dān pí* (moutan), *zé xiè* (alisma), and *fú líng* (poria) to form *liù wèi dì huáng wán* (Six-Ingredient Rehmannia Pill). For pronounced seminal emission, add *suŏ yáng* (cynomorium), *jīn yīng zǐ* (Cherokee rose fruit), and *wǔ wèi zǐ* (schisandra). For profuse menstruation, add *huáng bǎi tàn* (charred phellodendron), *ài yè tàn* (charred mugwort), and *ē jiāo zhū* (ass hide glue pellets). For lumbar pain, add *xù duàn* (dipsacus) and *dù zhòng* (eucommia).

For frequent urination from kidney vacuity (aching lumbus and limp legs, frequent urination without pain, normal urine color, and a weak cubit pulse, or for elderly people), *shān zhū yú* is combined with the following:

> *sāng piāo xiāo* (桑螵蛸 mantis egg-case, Mantidis Oötheca)
>
> *yì zhì rén* (益智仁 alpinia, Alpiniae Oxyphyllae Fructus)
>
> *fù pén zǐ* (覆盆子 rubus, Rubi Fructus)
>
> *wū yào* (乌药 lindera, Linderae Radix)
>
> *dì huáng* (地黄 rehmannia, Rehmanniae Radix)
>
> *shān yào* (山药 dioscorea, Dioscoreae Rhizoma)
>
> *wǔ wèi zǐ* (五味子 schisandra, Schisandrae Fructus)

Shān zhū yú is sour, bitter, and astringent in flavor; thus it checks sweating and stems desertion. For patterns of insufficiency of right qì with incessant desertion sweating (dripping cold sweat in shock), use *shān zhū yú* combined with *wǔ wèi zǐ* (schisandra), *mài dōng* (ophiopogon), *huáng qí* (astragalus), *duàn lóng gǔ* (calcined dragon bone), and *duàn mǔ lì* (calcined oyster shell). For severe hypotension, it is combined with *rén shēn* (ginseng) and *fù piàn* (sliced aconite).

COMPARISONS

Wǔ wèi zǐ (schisandra) tends to constrain dissipating lung channel qì that is on the verge of expiration and to astringe the original yáng in the kidney viscus that is dissipating and about to be lost. *Shān zhū yú* enriches liver-kidney yīn and constrains sweating from yīn and yáng on the verge of expiration.

Jīn yīng zǐ (Cherokee rose fruit) and *shān zhū yú* both secure essence and contain qì. However, *jīn yīng zǐ* also astringes lung qì and constrains the large intestine, whereas *shān zhū yú* also reduces urination and astringes yīn sweating (i.e., profuse sweating in the yīn regions).

Note that *shān zhū yú* should be used without the kernel. According to traditional experience, using *shān zhū yú* without removing the kernel can cause seminal efflux. This is why in prescriptions many people write "*shān yú ròu* 山萸肉"[15] to indicate that they want the fleshy fruit without the kernel.

---

[15]The character 肉 *ròu* means flesh and thus implies the flesh of the fruit without the seed. (Ed.)

Dosage

The dosage is generally 3–9 g/1–3 qián. In cases of emergency vacuity desertion, use 20–30 g/7 qián–1 liǎng.

Caution

Inappropriate in patterns with hyperactivity of kidney yáng, heat in the lower burner, and inhibited urination.

---

19. 枸杞子　Gǒu Qǐ Zǐ　　　　　　Lycii Fructus
Lycium

Gǒu qǐ zǐ (lycium) is sweet in flavor and neutral in nature; it enriches the liver and kidney, boosts essence, and brightens the eyes.

For insufficiency of the liver and kidney that manifests in lack of strength in the lumbus and knees, dull pain in the umbilical region, impotence, and sloppy diarrhea, *gǒu qǐ zǐ* is combined with *shú dì huáng* (cooked rehmannia), *shān yào* (dioscorea), *shān zhū yú* (cornus), *ròu guì* (cinnamon bark), *fù piàn* (sliced aconite), *lù jiǎo jiāo* (deerhorn glue), and *tù sī zǐ* (cuscuta) to form *yòu guī wán* (Right-Restoring [Life Gate] Pill).

For insufficiency of the liver and kidney resulting in essence-blood failing to pour into the eyes and leading to clouded vision and blurred vision, *gǒu qǐ zǐ* is combined with medicinals such as *dì huáng* (rehmannia), *shān yào* (dioscorea), *shān zhū yú* (cornus), *fú líng* (poria), *zé xiè* (alisma), and *jú huā* (chrysanthemum), as in *qǐ jú dì huáng wán* (Lycium Berry, Chrysanthemum, and Rehmannia Pill).

This medicinal also engenders liquid and allays thirst; thus it is combined with *tiān dōng* (asparagus), *mài dōng* (ophiopogon), *shān yào* (dioscorea), *yù zhú* (Solomon's seal), *dì huáng* (rehmannia), and *zhī mǔ* (anemarrhena) for dispersion-thirst disease.[16]

Research

According to modern research, *gǒu qǐ zǐ* lowers blood sugar.

In recent years, I have frequently used *gǒu qǐ zǐ* and *wǔ wèi zǐ* (schisandra) together as a substitute for *shān zhū yú* (cornus).[17]

Comparisons

Gǒu qǐ yè (lycium leaf), bitter, sweet, and cool, clears toxic heat from the upper burner. Taken as a tea, it allays dispersion-thirst. The root bark of *gǒu qǐ zǐ*, which is called *dì gǔ pí* (lycium root bark), clears vacuity heat and abates steaming bone heat.

---

[16]Dispersion-thirst disease (消渴 *xiāo kě*) includes, but is not limited to, diabetes mellitus. (Au.)

[17]A substitute for *shān zhū yú* (cornus) is often needed because this medicinal is sometimes very expensive and also because it may become unavailable for long periods of time. (Ed.)

Shān zhū yú (cornus) and *gǒu qǐ zǐ* (lycium) both enrich liver and kidney, but *shān zhū yú* also astringes liver-gallbladder fire, whereas *gǒu qǐ zǐ* also boosts yáng in the kidney.

Sāng shèn (mulberry) enriches yīn and supplements the blood, boosts the brain and moistens dryness. *Gǒu qǐ zǐ* enriches the liver and kidney, boosts essence, and brightens the eyes.

DOSAGE

The dosage is generally 3–9 g/1–3 qián.

CAUTION

Use with care for patterns of externally contracted fever or for indigestion with a tendency to diarrhea.

---

20. 沙参 Shā Shēn
Adenophora/Glehnia

Adenophorae seu Glehniae Radix

Sweet and bitter in flavor and slightly cold in nature, *shā shēn* (adenophora/glehnia) nourishes yīn, moistens the lung, and clears heat.

1. **Nourishing Yīn and Moistening the Lung:** According to a traditional saying, "*Shā shēn* supplements the yīn of the five viscera." Nonetheless, from my clinical experience, this medicinal's effect of nourishing lung and stomach yīn is the most pronounced. For insufficiency of lung yīn that engenders vacuity heat, which results in dry cough with scant phlegm, dry throat, sore pharynx, blood-flecked phlegm, and loss of voice from enduring cough, use *shā shēn* combined with the following:

shēng dì huáng (生地黄 dried/fresh rehmannia, Rehmanniae Radix Exsiccata seu Recens)

zhī mǔ (知母 anemarrhena, Anemarrhenae Rhizoma)

mài dōng (麦冬 ophiopogon, Ophiopogonis Radix)

tiān dōng (天冬 asparagus, Asparagi Radix)

chuān bèi mǔ (川贝母 Sìchuān fritillaria, Fritillariae Cirrhosae Bulbus)

shēng gān cǎo (生甘草 raw licorice, Glycyrrhizae Radix Cruda)

Although the lung is dry in nature, it also has an aversion to dryness, so it easily contracts dryness evil. For lung dryness patterns marked by dry cough with scant phlegm, dry itchy throat, hoarse voice,[18] dry nose and mouth, and a tongue that is red at the tip and margins, use *shā shēn* combined with the following:

sāng yè (桑叶 mulberry leaf, Mori Folium)

mài dōng (麦冬 ophiopogon, Ophiopogonis Radix)

xuán shēn (玄参 scrophularia, Scrophulariae Radix)

---

[18]Hoarse voice (声音嘶哑 *shēng yīn sī yǎ*) is observed in wind-heat invading the lung and damaging fluids, or in patterns of acute or chronic laryngitis, damage to the vocal cords, etc. (Ed.)

shēng shí gāo (生石膏 crude gypsum, Gypsum Fibrosum Crudum)

zhī mǔ (知母 anemarrhena, Anemarrhenae Rhizoma)

shēng dì huáng (生地黄 dried/fresh rehmannia, Rehmanniae Radix Exsiccata seu Recens)

bǎi hé (百合 lily bulb, Lilii Bulbus)

huǒ má rén (火麻仁 cannabis fruit, Cannabis Fructus)

ē jiāo (阿胶 ass hide glue, Asini Corii Colla)

2. Clearing Heat and Engendering Liquid: After high fever with damage to yīn humor or enduring illness that has depleted stomach yīn, with signs such as dry tongue, dry mouth, poor appetite, dry throat and thirst, and peeling tongue fur, use *shā shēn* combined with the following:

mài dōng (麦冬 ophiopogon, Ophiopogonis Radix)

xuán shēn (玄参 scrophularia, Scrophulariae Radix)

shēng dì huáng (生地黄 dried/fresh rehmannia, Rehmanniae Radix Exsiccata seu Recens)

shí hú (石斛 dendrobium, Dendrobii Herba)

yù zhú (玉竹 Solomon's seal, Polygonati Odorati Rhizoma)

tiān huā fěn (天花粉 trichosanthes root, Trichosanthis Radix)

shēng bái sháo (生白芍 raw white peony, Paeoniae Radix Alba Cruda)

This medicinal is used for patterns of yīn vacuity internal heat and pulmonary consumption with damage to yīn because of its capacity to nourish yīn and clear heat. For example, for patterns of pulmonary consumption with cough, **postmeridian tidal heat [effusion]**[559] (下午潮热 *xià wǔ cháo rè*), reddening of the cheeks and night sweating, vexing heat in the five hearts, dry cough with scant phlegm, emaciation, phlegm containing blood, and a fine rapid pulse, use this medicinal combined with the following:

shēng dì huáng (生地黄 dried/fresh rehmannia, Rehmanniae Radix Exsiccata seu Recens)

xuán shēn (玄参 scrophularia, Scrophulariae Radix)

biē jiǎ (鳖甲 turtle shell, Trionycis Carapax)

qín jiāo (秦艽 large gentian, Gentianae Macrophyllae Radix)

dì gǔ pí (地骨皮 lycium root bark, Lycii Cortex)

bèi mǔ (贝母 fritillaria, Fritillariae Bulbus)

bǎi bù (百部 stemona, Stemonae Radix)

bái jí (白及 bletilla, Bletillae Rhizoma)

COMPARISONS

Nán shā shēn (南沙参, adenophora) is lighter and softer in quality; it is cold in nature and bitter in flavor. It clears lung fire and boosts lung yīn, and also is used in wind-heat common cold with lung dryness-heat. *Běi shā shēn* (北沙参, glehnia) is heavier and harder in quality; it is cool in nature and sweet in flavor. It is primarily used to nourish yīn and clear the lung, engender liquid and boost the stomach. It is inappropriate for use in patterns of external contraction. When writing prescriptions, if one only writes *shā shēn* 沙参, pharmacies will generally use *běi shā shēn*. When one wants to use *nán shā shēn*, this should be specified on the prescription.

Dǎng shēn (codonopsis)[92] is sweet and warm, and supplements the lung and stomach qì. *Shā shēn* is sweet and cool, and supplements the lung and stomach yīn.

Rén shēn (ginseng)[89] supplements yáng and engenders yīn, whereas *shā shēn* supplements yīn and restrains yáng.

DOSAGE

The dosage is generally 4.5–12 g/1.5–4 qián.

CAUTION

Inappropriate for use in patterns of wind-cold common cold with cough or lung cold with copious white phlegm.

---

21. 玄参 Xuán Shēn   Scrophulariae Radix
Scrophularia

Also called *yuán shēn* 元参, *xuán shēn* (scrophularia) is bitter and salty in flavor and cold in nature. It mainly enriches yīn and downbears fire, resolves toxin and softens hardness.

When effulgent yīn vacuity fire and fire-heat flaming upward cause sore swollen throat, thirst, and vexation heat, *xuán shēn* can be combined with the following:

shēng gān cǎo (生甘草 raw licorice, Glycyrrhizae Radix Cruda)

jié gěng (桔梗 platycodon, Platycodonis Radix)

mài dōng (麦冬 ophiopogon, Ophiopogonis Radix)

niú bàng zǐ (牛蒡子 arctium, Arctii Fructus)

shēng dì huáng (生地黄 dried/fresh rehmannia, Rehmanniae Radix Exsiccata seu Recens)

huáng qín (黄芩 scutellaria, Scutellariae Radix)

lián qiáo (连翘 forsythia, Forsythiae Fructus)

In warm-heat disease, when a heat evil enters the construction, evil heat damages yīn, causing dry mouth, vexation and agitation, restless sleep, crimson red tongue body, and, in severe patterns, high fever, delirious speech, and dull maculopapular eruptions, *xuán shēn* is combined with medicinals such as *guǎng xī jiǎo* (African rhinoceros horn), *shēng dì huáng* (dried/fresh rehmannia), *huáng lián* (coptis), *lián qiáo* (forsythia), *mài dōng* (ophiopogon), and *dān pí* (moutan), as in *qīng yíng tāng* (Construction-Clearing Decoction). If damage to yīn humor causes bound stool, add *mài dōng* (ophiopogon), *shēng dì huáng* (dried/fresh rehmannia), *yù zhú* (Solomon's seal), *guā lóu* (trichosanthes), and *shēng dà huáng* (raw rhubarb).

Xuán shēn not only enriches yīn and downbears fire, it also cools the blood and resolves toxin. If an exuberant heat toxin gives rise to blood heat macules and vexation and agitation, combine *xuán shēn* with *shēng dì huáng* (dried/fresh rehmannia), *guǎng xī jiǎo* (African rhinoceros horn) (or else *shuǐ niú jiǎo*), *shēng shí gāo* (crude gypsum), *zhī mǔ* (anemarrhena), *gān cǎo* (licorice), *chì sháo* (red peony), and *dān pí* (moutan), as in *huà bān tāng* (Macule-Transforming Decoction).[245]

When depression bind of phlegm heat in the neck engenders scrofula (enlarged lymph nodes in the neck), this medicinal is used to soften hardness and dissipate binds. In such cases, *xuán shēn* is frequently combined with *bèi mǔ* (fritillaria) and *shēng mǔ lì* (crude oyster shell), to form *xiāo luǒ wán* (Scrofula-Dispersing Pill).[437] *Xià kū cǎo* (prunella), *kūn bù* (kelp), and *hǎi zǎo* (sargassum) can also be added. I have applied this empirical combination within a framework of pattern identification as the basis for determining treatment to deal with tuberculosis of the lymph nodes, lymph node granuloma, and thyroid enlargement. To treat tuberculosis of the lymph nodes, judiciously add *bǎi bù* (stemona), *huáng qín* (scutellaria), *xiāng fù* (cyperus), *qīng pí* (unripe tangerine peel), *zhì shān jiǎ* (mix-fried pangolin scales), and *chì bái sháo* (red/white peony). To treat lymph node granuloma, add *lián qiáo* (forsythia), *tiān huā fěn* (trichosanthes root), *pú gōng yīng* (dandelion), *chái hú* (bupleurum), *chì sháo* (red peony), *zào jiǎo cì* (gleditsia thorn), *shān jiǎ* (pangolin scales), and *niú bàng zǐ* (arctium), and take *xiǎo jīn dān* (Minor Golden Elixir) with the decoction. To treat thyroid enlargement, add *huáng qín* (scutellaria), *zhī mǔ* (anemarrhena), *shēng dài zhě shí* (crude hematite), *yù jīn* (curcuma), *bái sháo* (white peony), *zhì shān jiǎ* (mix-fried pangolin scales), *jú hóng* (red tangerine peel), *xuán fù huā* (inula flower), and *huáng yào zǐ* (air potato). This approach is invariably effective.

Shēng dì huáng (dried/fresh rehmannia) and *xuán shēn* (scrophularia) both enrich yīn, but because *shēng dì huáng* is sweet and cold it supplements yīn, and also tends to cool the blood and clear heat; thus it is suitable for fire from blood heat. Because *xuán shēn* is salty and cold, it enriches yīn and also tends to downbear fire; thus it is suitable for yīn vacuity floating fire.

Kǔ shēn (flavescent sophora) is bitter and cold; it drains fire and dries dampness. It is effective in treating skin on the exterior of the body for damp-heat, scab[561] (疥 *jiè*), and lài[556] (癞 *lài*). *Xuán shēn* is salty and cold; it downbears fire and nourishes yīn. It is effective in treating the interior of the body for insufficiency of kidney yīn and steaming bone consumptive heat.

Mài dōng (ophiopogon) nourishes yīn and tends to moisten the lung, whereas *xuán shēn* nourishes yīn and tends to enrich the kidney.

DOSAGE

The dosage is generally 6–12 g/2–4 qián. In severe diseases, use up to 30 g/ 1 liǎng.

CAUTION

Contraindicated in patterns with sloppy diarrhea or exuberant phlegm-damp. This medicinal clashes with *lí lú* (veratrum).

According to modern research, *xuán shēn* is both hypotensive and hypoglycemic (i.e., it lowers both blood pressure and blood sugar). It has a relatively strong inhibitory effect against *Pseudomonas pyocyanea*.

22. 麦冬 Mài Dōng   Ophiopogonis Radix
Ophiopogon

Mài dōng (ophiopogon) is sweet and slightly bitter in flavor and slightly cold in nature.

1. Enriching Yīn and Moistening the Lung: For yīn vacuity internal heat scorching lung liquid and for insufficiency of lung yīn, which are marked by lung heat cough, dry cough with scant phlegm, vexation heat and thirst, or by phlegm containing blood, a red tongue with scant liquid, and a fine rapid pulse, this medicinal is used to enrich yīn and moisten the lung, clear heat and treat cough. For this purpose, *mài dōng* is frequently combined with *sāng yè* (mulberry leaf), *xìng rén* (apricot kernel), *shā shēn* (adenophora/glehnia), *huǒ má rén* (cannabis fruit), *ē jiāo zhū* (ass hide glue pellets), *pí pá yè* (loquat leaf), and *tiān dōng* (asparagus). *Mài dōng* is also appropriate for pulmonary tuberculosis, bronchitis, or whooping cough manifesting with yīn vacuity lung heat cough.

2. Nourishing Yīn and Clearing the Heart: In patterns of heart yīn vacuity with heat vexation in the heart, palpitations, flusteredness, insomnia, red tongue, and a fine rapid pulse, *mài dōng* is frequently combined with medicinals such as the following:

huáng lián (黄连 coptis, Coptidis Rhizoma)

ē jiāo (阿胶 ass hide glue, Asini Corii Colla)

bèi mǔ (贝母 fritillaria, Fritillariae Bulbus)

shēng dì huáng (生地黄 dried/fresh rehmannia, Rehmanniae Radix Exsiccata seu Recens)

xuán shēn (玄参 scrophularia, Scrophulariae Radix)

dān shēn (丹参 salvia, Salviae Miltiorrhizae Radix)

zhēn zhū mǔ (珍珠母 mother-of-pearl, Concha Margaritifera)

yuǎn zhì (远志 polygala, Polygalae Radix)

For dual vacuity of heart qì and yīn that manifests as shortness of breath, fatigue, thirst, sweating, a faint weak pulse verging on expiration, and vacuity desertion, urgently administer *mài dōng* combined with *rén shēn* (ginseng) and *wǔ wèi zǐ* (schisandra). This combination forms *shēng mài sǎn* (Pulse-Engendering Powder), which boosts qì and nourishes yīn, constrains sweat (sweat is the humor of the heart) and stems desertion.

3. Engendering Liquid and Boosting the Stomach: This medicinal nourishes stomach yīn and engenders fluids. After warm-heat disease, damage to fluids can cause an insufficiency of stomach yīn, resulting in dry mouth and throat, poor appetite, and constipation. For this pattern, *mài dōng* is combined with medicinals such as *xuán shēn* (scrophularia), *xì shēng dì* (thin dried rehmannia), *yù zhú* (Solomon's seal), *bīng táng* (rock candy), *guā lóu* (trichosanthes), *shēng dà huáng* (raw rhubarb), *huǒ má rén* (cannabis fruit), and *zhǐ shí* (unripe bitter orange) to form *yì wèi tāng* (Stomach-Boosting Decoction).

4. **Moistening the Lung and Disinhibiting the Throat:** When lung heat damages yīn, resulting in sore dry throat, hoarse voice or loss of voice, dry tongue, and thirst, combine *mài dōng* with *xuán shēn* (scrophularia), *shēng dì huáng* (dried/fresh rehmannia), *jié gěng* (platycodon), *gān cǎo* (licorice), *shān dòu gēn* (bushy sophora), *jīn guǒ lǎn* (tinospora root),[19] and *zhī mǔ* (anemarrhena).

Comparisons

Tiān dōng (asparagus)[133] and *mài dōng* (ophiopogon) both enrich yīn, but *tiān dōng* is sweet, bitter, and very cold and tends to clear heat and downbear fire while also enriching kidney yīn and downbearing kidney fire. In comparison, *mài dōng*, which is sweet and slightly cold, tends to moisten the lung and quiet the heart while also nourishing stomach yīn and relieving vexation and thirst.

Chuān bèi mǔ (Sìchuān fritillaria)[436] and *mài dōng* are both commonly used to moisten the lung and suppress cough, but *chuān bèi mǔ* tends to dissipate lung depression and transform phlegm, while also opening heart depression and clearing heat. In comparison, *mài dōng* tends to enrich lung yīn and clear heat, while also nourishing stomach yīn and allaying thirst.

Mài dōng that has been processed with *zhū shā* (cinnabar) is called *zhū mài dōng* (cinnabar-processed ophiopogon) or *zhū cùn dōng* 朱寸冬, and it is suitable for quieting the heart and quieting the spirit.[20]

Dosage

The dosage is generally 4.5–9 g/1.5–3 qián.[21]

Caution

Inappropriate in patterns with diarrhea, sloppy stool, a slimy white tongue fur, or indigestion.

---

23. 天冬 Tiān Dōng   Asparagi Radix
Asparagus

---

[19] *Jīn guǒ lǎn* (金果榄, tinospora root) is sweet, sour, and cold. It clears heat and resolves toxin. Having the power to disinhibit the throat and disperse welling-abscesses, it is mainly used in the treatment of sore throat (including diphtheria) and lung-heat cough. *Jīn guǒ lǎn* (tinospora root) is also powdered, mixed with vinegar, and applied externally to treat welling-abscesses. The dose in decoction is 3–9 g/1–3 qián. (Ed.)

[20] *Zhū mài dōng* (朱麦冬, cinnabar-processed ophiopogon) is not available in the West and is very infrequently used even in China. (Ed.)

[21] Older books mention that the stringlike fiber in the center of the *mài dōng* (ophiopogon) should be removed before use because that part of the plant can engender heat and heat is antithetical to the function of this medicinal. When the tuber is opened and the center removed this medicinal is referred to as *kāi mài dōng* 开麦冬 or *kāi mén dōng* 开门冬, 开 *kāi* meaning "opened." (Ed.)

Sweet and bitter in flavor and cold in nature, *tiān dōng* (asparagus) is often used to enrich yīn and clear heat.

For effulgent yīn vacuity fire, upward fuming of internal heat, or lung heat that manifest in cough, scant sticky phlegm, dry throat, thirst at night, or with phlegm containing blood and vexing heat in the five hearts, *tiān dōng* is combined with medicinals such as:

mài dōng (麦冬 ophiopogon, Ophiopogonis Radix)

xuán shēn (玄参 scrophularia, Scrophulariae Radix)

shēng dì huáng (生地黄 dried/fresh rehmannia, Rehmanniae Radix Exsiccata seu Recens)

shí hú (石斛 dendrobium, Dendrobii Herba)

bèi mǔ (贝母 fritillaria, Fritillariae Bulbus)

mì pá yè (蜜杷叶 honey-fried loquat leaf, Eriobotryae Folium cum Mele Praeparatum)

xìng rén (杏仁 apricot kernel, Armeniacae Semen)

ǒu jié (藕节 lotus root node, Nelumbinis Rhizomatis Nodus)

bái jí (白及 bletilla, Bletillae Rhizoma)

shēng shí gāo (生石膏 crude gypsum, Gypsum Fibrosum Crudum)

guā lóu (瓜蒌 trichosanthes, Trichosanthis Fructus)

When lung-kidney yīn vacuity gives rise to consumption heat [effusion] (fever), steaming bone, reddening of the cheeks, night sweating, dry cough with scant phlegm, and hoarse voice, this medicinal is combined with:

qín jiāo (秦艽 large gentian, Gentianae Macrophyllae Radix)

bái wēi (白薇 black swallowwort, Cynanchi Atrati Radix)

biē jiǎ (鳖甲 turtle shell, Trionycis Carapax)

dì gǔ pí (地骨皮 lycium root bark, Lycii Cortex)

yín chái hú (银柴胡 stellaria, Stellariae Radix)

shēng dì huáng (生地黄 dried/fresh rehmannia, Rehmanniae Radix Exsiccata seu Recens)

guī bǎn (龟板 tortoise shell, Testudinis Carapax et Plastrum)

huáng bǎi (黄柏 phellodendron, Phellodendri Cortex)

zhī mǔ (知母 anemarrhena, Anemarrhenae Rhizoma)

On the basis of experience, *tiān dōng* is used for diseases such as pulmonary tuberculosis, lung cancer, and pulmonary abscess (final stage).

For lung-kidney yīn vacuity manifesting in thirst with increased fluid intake that fails to resolve the thirst and frequent and copious urination (e.g., diabetes mellitus, diabetes insipidus, and hyperthyroidism), *tiān dōng* is combined with the following:

shēng dì huáng (生地黄 dried/fresh rehmannia, Rehmanniae Radix Exsiccata seu Recens)

shān zhū yú (山茱萸 cornus, Corni Fructus)

tiān huā fěn (天花粉 trichosanthes root, Trichosanthis Radix)

zhī mǔ (知母 anemarrhena, Anemarrhenae Rhizoma)

shā shēn (沙参 adenophora/glehnia, Adenophorae seu Glehniae Radix)

mài dōng (麦冬 ophiopogon, Ophiopogonis Radix)

wǔ wèi zǐ (五味子 schisandra, Schisandrae Fructus)

wū méi (乌梅 mume, Mume Fructus)

gǒu qǐ zǐ (枸杞子 lycium, Lycii Fructus)

COMPARISON

Shí hú (dendrobium)[134] and *tiān dōng* both enrich kidney yīn, but *shí hú* also nourishes the stomach and engenders liquid, whereas *tiān dōng* also clears the lung and moistens dryness.

DOSAGE AND CAUTION

The dosage and cautions are the same as for *mài dōng* (ophiopogon).

---

24. 石斛 Shí Hú   Dendrobii Herba
Dendrobium

Sweet and bland in flavor and cool in nature, *shí hú* (dendrobium) enriches yīn and nourishes the stomach, clears heat and engenders liquid, boosts the kidney, and strengthens sinew and bone.

In the advanced stage of warm-heat disease, when high fever has damaged yīn liquid, resulting in thirst, dry tongue, poor appetite, red tongue body, and yellow or black tongue fur, use *shí hú* to enrich stomach yīn, clear heat and engender liquid, and allay thirst and eliminate vexation. It is important to note that when using this medicinal to treat warm heat disease, it must not be used prematurely, otherwise its enriching and supplementing qualities may constrain the evil.

When yīn vacuity internal heat engenders dry cough, night sweating, low-grade fever, thirst, red tongue, and a fine rapid pulse, use *shí hú* combined with medicinals such as the following:

shēng dì huáng (生地黄 dried/fresh rehmannia, Rehmanniae Radix Exsiccata seu Recens)

mài dōng (麦冬 ophiopogon, Ophiopogonis Radix)

bǎi hé (百合 lily bulb, Lilii Bulbus)

qín jiāo (秦艽 large gentian, Gentianae Macrophyllae Radix)

yín chái hú (银柴胡 stellaria, Stellariae Radix)

dì gǔ pí (地骨皮 lycium root bark, Lycii Cortex)

For insufficiency of kidney essence resulting in clouded vision, dim vision, or loss of visual acuity, *shí hú* is often combined with:

shēng dì huáng (生地黄 dried/fresh rehmannia, Rehmanniae Radix Exsiccata seu Recens)

shú dì huáng (熟地黄 cooked rehmannia, Rehmanniae Radix Praeparata)

shān zhū yú (山茱萸 cornus, Corni Fructus)

cǎo jué míng (草决明 fetid cassia, Cassiae Semen)

tóng jí lí (潼蒺藜 complanate astragalus seed, Astragali Complanati Semen)

dì gǔ pí (地骨皮 lycium root bark, Lycii Cortex)

jú huā (菊花 chrysanthemum, Chrysanthemi Flos)

gǒu qǐ zǐ (枸杞子 lycium, Lycii Fructus)

Chinese medicinal pharmacies have a commonly used ready-prepared pill called *shí hú yè guāng wán* (Dendrobium Night Vision Pill), also called *shí hú míng mù wán* (Dendrobium Eye Brightener Pill), which treats clouded vision, dim vision, and loss of visual acuity. For kidney vacuity causing numbness in the legs and wilting and impediment, use this medicinal combined with the following:

niú xī (牛膝 achyranthes, Achyranthis Bidentatae Radix)

huáng bǎi (黄柏 phellodendron, Phellodendri Cortex)

xù duàn (续断 dipsacus, Dipsaci Radix)

shú dì huáng (熟地黄 cooked rehmannia, Rehmanniae Radix Praeparata)

shān yào (山药 dioscorea, Dioscoreae Rhizoma)

qín jiāo (秦艽 large gentian, Gentianae Macrophyllae Radix)

yǐ mǐ (苡米 coix, Coicis Semen)

mù guā (木瓜 chaenomeles, Chaenomelis Fructus)

hǔ gǔ (虎骨 tiger bone, Tigris Os)

COMPARISONS

Yù zhú (Solomon's seal)[136] and *shí hú* both nourish yīn, but *yù zhú*, which is sweet and neutral, enriching and moistening, nourishes lung and stomach yīn, eliminates dryness-heat, and is supplementing without being slimy. By comparison, *shí hú* clears floating heat from the kidney and contains original qì, eliminates vacuity heat from the stomach, and relieves vexation and thirst; it supplements within clearing and clears within supplementing.

Jīn chāi shí hú (金钗石斛, golden hairpin dendrobium) tends to nourish stomach yīn and supplement the kidney essence. *Huò shí hú* (霍石斛, official dendrobium) is often used for elderly patients or for vacuity patients with insufficiency of yīn humor. *Xiān shí hú* (fresh dendrobium) clears heat and engenders liquid and is stronger for allaying thirst. It is usually used for warm heat disease. In medicinal markets, one mostly finds *gān shí hú* (dried dendrobium) (*chuān shí hú* (Sìchuān dendrobium)), *xiān shí hú* (fresh dendrobium), and *huò shí hú*. Thus, although various forms of *shí hú* are available, their therapeutic effects are quite similar.[22]

DOSAGE

Gān shí hú (dried dendrobium) 6–12 g/2–4 qián; *xiān shí hú* (fresh dendrobium) 15–30 g/5 qián–1 liǎng.

---

[22]Most of what is currently sold for *shí hú* (dendrobium) in the West is 有瓜石斛 *yǒu guā shí hú* (literally, "*shí hú* with a melon"), which is generally classified as a member of the genus *Ephemerantha*, not the genus *Dendrobium*. Its action is considered similar to other forms of *shí hú*. (Ed.)

Caution

Use with care for patients with a thick slimy tongue fur or sloppy stool.

Research

According to research, *jīn chāi shí hú* (golden hairpin dendrobium) has an inhibitory effect on *Staphylococcus*. In acute cholecystitis with high fever, it rapidly abates fever. It also promotes stomach secretions to aid digestion.

| **25. 玉竹 Yù Zhú** | Polygonati Odorati |
| Solomon's Seal | Rhizoma |

Sweet in flavor and neutral in nature, *yù zhú* (Solomon's seal) nourishes qì and blood, neutrally supplements the lung and stomach, and boosts yīn and moistens dryness. It is used as a substitute for *rén shēn* (ginseng) and *dì huáng* (rehmannia).

Yù zhú is often used to treat damage to lung and stomach yīn or damage to the lung by dryness evil that causes cough with scant phlegm, dry throat and tongue, and dryness-heat thirst. It is commonly combined with the following:

shā shēn (沙参 adenophora/glehnia, Adenophorae seu Glehniae Radix)

mài dōng (麦冬 ophiopogon, Ophiopogonis Radix)

sāng yè (桑叶 mulberry leaf, Mori Folium)

xìng rén (杏仁 apricot kernel, Armeniacae Semen)

shí hú (石斛 dendrobium, Dendrobii Herba)

xuán shēn (玄参 scrophularia, Scrophulariae Radix)

In the advanced stage of warm-heat disease, when high fever has damaged stomach yīn and caused thirst with dry tongue, poor appetite, and stomach discomfort, use *yù zhú* combined with the following:

shā shēn (沙参 adenophora/glehnia, Adenophorae seu Glehniae Radix)

shí hú (石斛 dendrobium, Dendrobii Herba)

mài dōng (麦冬 ophiopogon, Ophiopogonis Radix)

bīng táng (冰糖 rock candy, Saccharon Crystallinum)

shēng mài yá (生麦芽 raw barley sprout, Hordei Fructus Germinatus Crudus)

Tiān dōng (asparagus) tends to enrich yīn in the lung and kidney, and its cold nature can cause stagnation in the stomach. *Yù zhú* tends to nourish yīn of the spleen and stomach, and it is neutral in nature so it does not harm the stomach. Although it nourishes stomach yīn, it does not harm spleen yáng.

Dosage

The dosage is generally 6–12 g/2–4 qián. Under special circumstances, use as much as 15–30 g/5 qián–1 liǎng.

Research

According to modern research, *yù zhú* lowers blood sugar.

26. 百合 Bǎi Hé
Lily Bulb
Lilii Bulbus

Sweet in flavor and neutral in nature, *bǎi hé* (lily bulb) is commonly used to constrain yīn and moisten the lung, clear the heart and quiet the spirit. Combined with *shēng dì huáng* (dried/fresh rehmannia), *mài dōng* (ophiopogon), *shā shēn* (adenophora/glehnia), *bèi mǔ* (fritillaria), and *lí pí* (pear peel), it treats cough from yīn vacuity lung dryness. Combined with *shā shēn* (adenophora/glehnia), *wǔ wèi zǐ* (schisandra), *mǎ dōu líng* (aristolochia fruit), *hē zǐ* (chebule), and *mài dōng* (ophiopogon), it treats lung yīn vacuity with lung qì floating and dissipating that manifests in incessant enduring cough, absence of repletion evil, dry throat with scant phlegm, shortness of breath, and slight panting. Combined with *mài dōng* (ophiopogon), *lián zǐ* (lotus seed), *yuǎn zhì* (polygala), *huáng lián* (coptis), *ē jiāo* (ass hide glue), and *xuán shēn* (scrophularia), it is used for spirit-mind abstraction and yīn vacuity vexation and insomnia that result from residual heat from heat disease.

COMPARISONS

Sour and astringent *wǔ wèi zǐ* (schisandra)[193] tends to treat floating and dissipating lung qì. By contrast, sweet, constraining, and lung-moistening *bǎi hé* tends to treat lung yīn vacuity dryness.

Bǎi bù (stemona)[442] warms the lung and transforms phlegm to treat cough and also kills worms.[23] *Bǎi hé*, which is sweet and constraining, moistens the lung to treat cough and also quiets the heart.

Finally, *bǎi hé* boosts qì and regulates the center. For example, 30 g/1 liǎng of *bǎi hé* combined with 9 g/3 qián of *wū yào* (lindera), which forms *bǎi hé tāng* (Lily Bulb Decoction), can be used to treat recalcitrant chronic stomach pain. I often use the following formula to treat chronic stomach pain that results from ulcers and that is ascribed to patterns in which there is concurrent vacuity and repletion, cold-heat complex, and disease of both qì and blood.

    bǎi hé (百合 lily bulb, Lilii Bulbus) 30 g/1 liǎng

    wū yào (乌药 lindera, Linderae Radix) 9 g/3 qián

    dān shēn (丹参 salvia, Salviae Miltiorrhizae Radix) 30 g/1 liǎng

    tán xiāng (檀香 sandalwood, Santali Albi Lignum) 6 g/2 qián (add at end)

    cǎo dòu kòu (草豆蔻 Katsumada's galangal seed, Alpiniae Katsumadai Semen)
        9 g/3 qián

    gāo liáng jiāng (高良姜 lesser galangal, Alpiniae Officinarum Rhizoma)
        9 g/3 qián

    xiāng fù (香附 cyperus, Cyperi Rhizoma) 9 g/3 qián

    chuān liàn zǐ (川楝子 toosendan, Toosendan Fructus) 6 g/2 qián

This formula, which forms a base that can be varied according to signs, invariably yields a satisfactory effect.

---

[23] "Worms" includes many kinds of worms, parasites, and, in some cases, fungi. (Ed.)

Dosage

The dosage is generally 9–12 g/3–4 qián, but when necessary use up to 25–30 g/ 8 qián–1 liǎng.

Caution

Inappropriate for use with externally contracted cough.

---

27. 女贞子 **Nǚ Zhēn Zǐ**   Ligustri
Ligustrum   Lucidi Fructus

Sweet and bitter in flavor and neutral in nature, *nǚ zhēn zǐ* (ligustrum) nourishes yīn and boosts essence, neutrally supplements the liver and kidney, eliminates vacuity heat, blackens the beard and hair, and sharpens hearing and vision.

Nǚ zhēn zǐ combined with *hé shǒu wū* (flowery knotweed), *sāng shèn* (mulberry), *shēng dì huáng* (dried/fresh rehmannia), *dù zhòng* (eucommia), *shān yào* (dioscorea), *hàn lián cǎo* (eclipta), and *gǒu qǐ zǐ* (lycium) is used to treat liver-kidney yīn vacuity that manifests in premature graying of the hair, clouded or flowery vision, tinnitus, deafness, loosening of the teeth, yīn-vacuity heat effusion, and vacuity pain in the lumbus and knees.

Gentle and harmonious in nature, *nǚ zhēn zǐ* supplements yīn without sliminess or stagnation and so is suitable for extended use. While it does not have the same tendency of *shēng dì huáng* (dried/fresh rehmannia) or of *shú dì huáng* (cooked rehmannia) to cause stagnation because of sliminess, it also does not have the same yīn-enriching power as these two.

Combined with *sāng shèn* (mulberry) and *hàn lián cǎo* (eclipta), made into a honey pill, and taken over a long period of time, *nǚ zhēn zǐ* is used for patterns of debilitated health and chronic vacuity detriment.

Comparison

Hé shǒu wū (flowery knotweed) supplements the liver and kidney, blackens the beard and hair, tends to penetrate to the blood aspect, and is slightly warm in nature. *Nǚ zhēn zǐ* also supplements the liver and kidney and blackens the beard and hair, but it clears the qì aspect and has a slightly cool nature.

Dosage

The dosage is generally 6–9 g/2–3 qián.

When using this medicinal for patients with stomach cold or for elderly people, add assistants that supplement the spleen and warm the stomach, such as *bái zhú* (white atractylodes), *chén pí* (tangerine peel), and *cǎo dòu kòu* (Katsumada's galangal seed).

28. 旱莲草 Hàn Lián Cǎo   Ecliptae Herba
Eclipta

Hàn lián cǎo (eclipta) is sweet and sour in flavor and neutral in nature. It is primarily a yīn-enriching medicinal used to supplement the kidney, but it also cools the blood and stanches bleeding.

Hàn lián cǎo combined with *nǔ zhēn zǐ* (ligustrum) to form *èr zhì wán* (Double Supreme Pill) is often used for liver-kidney yīn vacuity with premature graying of the hair or hair loss. The juice of *sāng shèn* (mulberry) can also be added to the pill.

a) *Hàn lián cǎo* combined with *shēng dì huáng* (dried/fresh rehmannia), *xuán shēn* (scrophularia), *bái máo gēn* (imperata), *huáng bǎi tàn* (charred phellodendron), *dà xiǎo jì* (Japanese/field thistle), *qū mài* (dianthus), and *zé xiè* (alisma) is used for bloody urine.

b) Combined with *shēng shí gāo* (crude gypsum), *zhī mǔ* (anemarrhena), *huáng qín* (scutellaria), *bái jí* (bletilla), and *ǒu jié tàn* (charred lotus root node), it is used for blood ejection.

c) Combined with *huái jiǎo* (sophora fruit), *dì yú* (sanguisorba), *huái huā tàn* (charred sophora flower), *huáng bǎi* (phellodendron), and *fáng fēng* (saposhnikovia), it is used for bloody stool.

d) Combined with *sāng jì shēng* (mistletoe), *xù duàn tàn* (charred dipsacus), *bái zhú* (white atractylodes), *zōng tàn* (charred trachycarpus), *ài yè tàn* (charred mugwort), *dāng guī tàn* (charred Chinese angelica), and *ē jiāo* (ass hide glue), it is used for flooding and spotting.

During recent years, *hàn lián cǎo* has often been used in formulas that treat aplastic anemia, functional metrorrhagia, and purpura, according to the identified pattern.

There are two varieties of *hàn lián cǎo*: *mò hàn lián* (墨旱莲, eclipta), which is black, and *hóng hàn lián* (红旱莲, giant hypericum), which is red. *Mò hàn lián* tends to supplement the kidney, enrich yīn, and stanch bleeding. *Hóng hàn lián* tends to cool the blood, quicken stasis, clear heat, and treat sores.[24] When writing a prescription, if one simply writes *hàn lián cǎo* 旱莲草, the pharmacy will generally give *mò hàn lián* 墨旱莲.

DOSAGE

The dosage is generally 9 g/3 qián. In special situations, use up to 15–30 g/ 5 qián–1 liǎng.

---

[24] *Hóng hàn lián* (giant hypericum) is derived from *Hypericum ascyron*. Slightly bitter and cold, it calms the liver and drains fire in the treatment of headache. It also cools blood, stanches bleeding, and disperses swelling in the treatment of vomiting of blood, uterine bleeding, nosebleed, spitting of blood, and bleeding from trauma. The dosage is 4.5–9 g/1.5–3 qián decocted or steeped in wine. (Ed.)

---

29. 桑椹 Sāng Shèn   Mori Fructus
Mulberry

See also

▷ *Sāng piāo xiāo* (桑螵蛸 mantis egg-case, Mantidis Oötheca)[190]

▷ *Sāng bái pí* (桑白皮 mulberry root bark, Mori Cortex)[445]

▷ *Sāng zhī* (桑枝 mulberry twig, Mori Ramulus)[464]

Sweet in flavor and cool in nature, *sāng shèn* (mulberry) enriches yīn and supplements the blood. Markets sell a ready-prepared medicine called *sāng shèn gāo* (Mulberry Paste). This medicine is taken mixed into hot water twice a day in a dosage of 9–15 g/3–5 qián to enrich the liver and kidney and to sharpen the hearing and brighten the eyes.

Sāng shèn combined with *mài dōng* (ophiopogon), *shā shēn* (adenophora/glehnia), and *yù zhú* (Solomon's seal) is used to treat yīn vacuity with scant liquid that results in thirst with dry tongue and dry rough stool.

There are two types of *sāng shèn*: *bái sāng shèn* (white mulberry), the immature fruit of the mulberry, which is mild in action, and *hēi sāng shèn* (black mulberry), the mature fruit, which is the more powerful. *Sāng shèn* is frequently combined with *hé shǒu wū* (flowery knotweed), *hàn lián cǎo* (eclipta), and *nǚ zhēn zǐ* (ligustrum) for premature graying of the hair or hair loss due to yīn-blood vacuity.

DOSAGE

The dosage is generally 6–9 g/2–3 qián.

CAUTION

Contraindicated in patterns with cold in the abdomen or sloppy soft stool.

---

30. 潼蒺藜 Tóng Jí Lí   Astragali
Complanate Astragalus Seed   Complanati Semen

Also called *shā yuàn jí lí* 沙苑蒺藜. Sweet in flavor and warm in nature, *tóng jí lí* (complanate astragalus seed) supplements the kidney and secures essence.

a) *Tóng jí lí* combined with *xù duàn* (dipsacus), *niú xī* (achyranthes), and *dù zhòng* (eucommia) is used to treat kidney vacuity lumbar pain.

b) Combined with *shān zhū yú* (cornus), *wǔ wèi zǐ* (schisandra), *lián xū* (lotus stamen), *lóng gǔ* (dragon bone), *bā jǐ tiān* (morinda), and *xiān máo* (curculigo), it is used for seminal emission and impotence that result from kidney vacuity.

c) Combined with *sāng piāo xiāo* (mantis egg-case), *tù sī zǐ* (cuscuta), *fù pén zǐ* (rubus), *yì zhì rén* (alpinia), and *bǔ gǔ zhī* (psoralea), it is used for elderly people with frequent urination or incontinence that results from kidney vacuity.

d) Combined with *gǒu qǐ zǐ* (lycium), *jú huā* (chrysanthemum), *bái jí lí* (tribulus), *tù sī zǐ* (cuscuta), and *jué míng zǐ* (fetid cassia), it is used for dizzy head and flowery vision that result from kidney vacuity.

Tóng jí lí is best at treating seminal emission and premature ejaculation that result from kidney vacuity. I frequently treat such patterns by adding 9 g/3 qián of *tóng jí lí*, 2 g/6–7 fēn of *lián xū* (lotus stamen), 8 g/2–3 qián of *wǔ wèi zǐ* (schisandra), and 10 g/3 qián of *lóng gǔ* (dragon bone) to a base of *liù wèi dì huáng tāng* (Six-Ingredient Rehmannia Decoction).[347] Taken as a water decoction, it is always effective.

COMPARISONS

Bái jí lí (tribulus)[474] is mainly used to dissipate depression and regulate the liver, whereas *tóng jí lí* is used to supplement the kidney and boost essence.

Tù sī zǐ (cuscuta)[152] and *tóng jí lí* both supplement the kidney and boost essence, but *tù sī zǐ*, which is slightly warm but not drying, tends to engender essence and strengthen the kidney, and is used to treat long-term infertility. *Tóng jí lí* (complanate astragalus seed), which is warm and assists kidney yáng, tends to treat seminal emission and impotence, and it also brightens the eyes.

DOSAGE

The dosage is generally 9–12 g/3–4 qián. When necessary, this dosage can be increased a little.

CAUTION

Contraindicated for patients with excessive sexual desire.

---

31. 黑芝麻 Hēi Zhī Má   Sesami
Black Sesame   Semen Nigrum

Sweet in flavor and neutral in nature, *hēi zhī má* (black sesame) supplements the liver and kidney, supplements essence, moistens dryness, and lubricates the intestines.

a) *Hēi zhī má* combined with *gǒu qǐ zǐ* (lycium), *jú huā* (chrysanthemum), *shú dì huáng* (cooked rehmannia), *shān zhū yú* (cornus), and *bái jí lí* (tribulus) treats dizzy head and flowery vision that result from insufficiency of the liver and kidney.

b) Combined with *hé shǒu wū* (flowery knotweed), *sāng shèn* (mulberry), *hàn lián cǎo* (eclipta), *nǚ zhēn zǐ* (ligustrum), and *shēng dì huáng* (dried/fresh rehmannia), it treats premature graying of the hair resulting from insufficiency of the liver and kidney.

Having a high oil content, *hēi zhī má* moistens dryness and frees the stool. Combined with *dāng guī* (Chinese angelica), *táo rén* (peach kernel), *ròu cōng róng* (cistanche), and *huǒ má rén* (cannabis fruit), it is used for constipation due to liquid dessication and blood dryness.

Comparison

Hé shǒu wū (flowery knotweed)[118] blackens the beard and hair and also nourishes the blood, whereas *hēi zhī má* blackens the beard and hair and also moistens the stool.

Dosage

The dosage is generally 9–12 g/3–4 qián. It is generally used in pill preparations.

Caution

Unsuitable for use in cases of sloppy stool, thirst, or fire toothache.

---

32. 牛膝 Niú Xī Achyranthes	Achyranthis Bidentatae Radix

Also called *huái niú xī* 怀牛膝 to distinguish it from *chuān niú xī* (川牛膝, cyathula) and *tǔ niú xī* (土牛膝, native achyranthes). Bitter and sour in flavor and neutral in nature, *niú xī* (achyranthes) supplements the liver and kidney, strengthens sinew and bone, dissipates static blood, and conducts medicinals downward.

a) *Niú xī* combined with *guī bǎn* (tortoise shell), *huáng bǎi* (phellodendron), *zhī mǔ* (anemarrhena), *shú dì huáng* (cooked rehmannia), *dāng guī* (Chinese angelica), and *hǔ gǔ* (tiger bone) is used for soreness of the lumbus and knees and limp weak legs due to liver-kidney vacuity.

b) *Niú xī* combined with *cāng zhú* (atractylodes) and *huáng bǎi* (phellodendron) to form *sān miào wán* (Mysterious Three Pill) is used for damp-heat pouring downward that results in redness and swelling of the legs, inability to walk, and **damp sores**[545] (湿疮 *shī chuāng*) of the lower extremities.

Niú xī moves blood and dissipates stasis.

a) Combined with *táo rén* (peach kernel), *dāng guī wěi* (Chinese angelica tail), *hóng huā* (carthamus), *chuān xiōng* (chuanxiong), *chì sháo* (red peony), and *dān pí* (moutan), *niú xī* is used for menstrual block or concretions and conglomerations that result from qì and blood stagnation.

b) Combined with *hóng huā* (carthamus), *chuān xiōng* (chuanxiong), *dāng guī* (Chinese angelica), *mù tōng* (trifoliate akebia), *huá shí* (talcum), and *dōng kuí zǐ* (mallow seed), it is used for retention of the placenta.

c) *Niú xī* combined with *zé lán* (lycopus) disinhibits dead blood in the lumbus and knees and is used for lumbus and leg pain resulting from static blood.

Niú xī enters the liver and kidney channels, moves downward, and conducts other medicinals to the legs. It is used as a channel conductor for diseases of the lower body.

For patients with urinary calculi, use a large dosage of *niú xī* combined with *dōng kuí zǐ* (mallow seed), *zé xiè* (alisma), *zé lán* (lycopus), *zhū líng* (polyporus), *fú líng* (poria), *hǎi jīn shā* (lygodium spore), *jīn qián cǎo* (moneywort), *mù tōng* (trifoliate akebia), and *bīng láng* (areca) to promote the downward movement and expulsion of the stone.

COMPARISONS

Shēng niú xī (raw achyranthes) dissipates malign blood, breaks concretions and binds, and quickens the blood and dissipates stasis. *Zhì niú xī* (processed achyranthes), i.e., steeped in wine or steamed with wine, supplements the liver and kidney, strengthens sinew and bone, and strengthens the lumbus and knees.

Huái niú xī (怀牛膝, achyranthes) tends to supplement the liver and kidney, whereas *chuān niú xī* (川牛膝, cyathula) tends to dissipate static blood and also dispel wind to treat impediment.[25]

There is also a medicinal called *tǔ niú xī* (土牛膝, native achyranthes), which is the root of *tiān míng jīng* (天名精, carpesium), whose uses differ from those of *niú xī*. *Tǔ niú xī*, sweet and cold in flavor and nature, breaks blood, stanches bleeding, resolves toxin, and clears heat. It is used for fire-heat toothache, **baby moth**[542] (乳蛾 *rǔ é*), throat impediment (including acute tonsillitis, pharyngitis, and laryngitis), and blood strangury.

When writing a prescription, if one simply writes *niú xī* (achyranthes), pharmacies will generally give *huái niú xī* (achyranthes).

DOSAGE

The dosage is generally 2–9 g/5 fēn–3 qián. When necessary, use as much as 15–30 g/5 qián–1 liǎng.

CAUTION

Because this medicinal moves downward, it should not be used in seminal efflux, sloppy diarrhea, or pregnancy.

RESEARCH

According to modern research, this medicinal temporarily lowers blood pressure. It has a hemolytic effect and can cause protein coagulation. *Niú xī* combined with *jīn yín huā* (lonicera) and *chì sháo* (red peony) can be used for thromboangiitis obliterans (sloughing flat-abscess). It is also effective in treating acute tonsillitis and in preventing diphtheria.

---

33. 鹿茸 **Lù Róng**	Cervi Cornu
Velvet Deerhorn	Pantotrichum

See also
  ▷ *Lù jiǎo* (鹿角 deerhorn, Cervi Cornu)[144]
  ▷ *Lù jiǎo jiāo* (鹿角胶 deerhorn glue, Cervi Cornus Gelatinum)[145]

---

[25] *Chuān niú xī* (cyathula) is more moving than *huái niú xī* (achyranthes) but less able to supplement. Unfortunately most of what is sold for *chuān niú xī* in southern China and in the West is a substitute (most likely *Strobilanthes nemorosus*). (Ed.)

▷ *Lù jiǎo shuāng* (鹿角霜 degelatinated deerhorn, Cervi Cornu Degelatinatum)[146]

Warm in nature and sweet and salty in flavor, *lù róng* (velvet deerhorn) supplements kidney yáng, strengthens sinew and bone, boosts sinew and marrow, and
nourishes the blood. It is used for patterns of vacuity detriment such as kidney
vacuity and cold lumbus, soreness of the limbs, dizzy head and vision, seminal
emission, and impotence. For children with insufficiency of original yáng, slow
development, fear of cold and weakness, wilting and limpness of the legs, and difficulty walking, use a pill preparation comprising the formula for *liù wèi dì huáng
wán* (Six-Ingredient Rehmannia Pill) with the addition of *lù róng* (velvet deerhorn),
nán wǔ jiā pí (acanthopanax), *yín yáng huò* (epimedium), *bǔ gǔ zhī* (psoralea), and
xù duàn (dipsacus).

DOSAGE

The dosage is 0.6–1.5 g/2–5 fēn, once or twice a day. *Lù róng* is not decocted,
but is usually used in powder preparation or taken in capsules. It can be taken
with warm water or with a decoction medicine. It is also frequently added to pills.

---

34. 鹿角 Lù Jiǎo   Cervi Cornu
Deerhorn

See also

▷ *Lù róng* (鹿茸 velvet deerhorn, Cervi Cornu Pantotrichum)[143]

▷ *Lù jiǎo jiāo* (鹿角胶 deerhorn glue, Cervi Cornus Gelatinum)[145]

▷ *Lù jiǎo shuāng* (鹿角霜 degelatinated deerhorn, Cervi Cornu Degelatinatum)[146]

Salty in flavor and warm in nature, *lù jiǎo* (deerhorn) supplements kidney yáng
and boosts essence and blood. It is similar in action to, and can substitute for, *lù
róng* (velvet deerhorn), but it is less effective.

COMPARISON

Lù róng (velvet deerhorn)[143] is commonly used as a drastic liver-kidney supplementing medicinal. It has greater supplementing power than *lù jiǎo*. *Lù jiǎo*,
by contrast, has a moderate liver-kidney supplementing effect, but it quickens the
blood, dissipates stasis, and disperses swelling and toxin with greater strength than
lù róng. For example, *lù jiǎo* combined with *dù zhòng* (eucommia), *xù duàn* (dipsacus), *bǔ gǔ zhī* (psoralea), and *fù piàn* (sliced aconite) is used for lumbar pain
resulting from debilitation of kidney yáng. Combined with *jīn yín huā* (lonicera),
lián qiáo (forsythia), *shān jiǎ* (pangolin scales), *hóng huā* (carthamus), and *chì
sháo* (red peony), it can treat swelling toxin sores.

In prescriptions, *lù jiǎo* (deerhorn) is called *lù jiǎo pǎng* (flaked deerhorn) or *lù
jiǎo piàn* (sliced deerhorn). Used in decoction medicines, it is ground to a powder
and taken drenched, or used in pills. Used raw, it tends to assist yáng and quicken

the blood, dissipate stasis and disperse swelling. Used processed or as glue, it tends to warm and supplement the liver and kidney, enrich and nourish essence-blood.

Dosage

The dosage is generally 3–9 g/1–3 qián. In special situations, use up to 15 g/5 qián. Ground to a powder and taken drenched, it is taken twice or three times a day at a dosage of 0.9–2.5 g/3–8 fēn each time.

---

35. 鹿角胶 Lù Jiǎo Jiāo
Deerhorn Glue

Cervi
Cornus Gelatinum

See also

▷ *Lù róng* (鹿茸 velvet deerhorn, Cervi Cornu Pantotrichum)[143]

▷ *Lù jiǎo* (鹿角 deerhorn, Cervi Cornu)[144]

▷ *Lù jiǎo shuāng* (鹿角霜 degelatinated deerhorn, Cervi Cornu Degelatinatum)[146]

Sweet in flavor and warm in nature, *lù jiǎo jiāo* (deerhorn glue) warms and supplements the lower origin, supplements yáng within yīn, frees the blood of the thoroughfare vessel, engenders essence and blood, and stanches flooding. It is similar in action to *lù róng* (velvet deerhorn), but being slower to supplement it must be taken over a long period of time to be effective. It is mostly used for flooding and spotting, vaginal discharge, vacuity bleeding, and yīn flat-abscesses (lumps that are not red, swollen, hot, or painful).

a) *Lù jiǎo jiāo* (deerhorn glue) combined with *ē jiāo* (ass hide glue), *dāng guī tàn* (charred Chinese angelica), *pú huáng* (typha pollen), and *hǎi piāo xiāo* (cuttlefish bone) is used for vacuity cold flooding and spotting and for vaginal discharge.

b) Combined with *dù zhòng* (eucommia), *ròu cōng róng* (cistanche), and *yín yáng huò* (epimedium), it is used for impotence.

c) Combined with *shú dì huáng* (cooked rehmannia), *shān zhū yú* (cornus), *shān yào* (dioscorea), and *fú líng* (poria), it is used for poor development in children.

d) Combined with *rén shēn* (ginseng), *huáng qí* (astragalus), *dāng guī* (Chinese angelica), and *shú dì huáng* (cooked rehmannia), it is used to warm and supplement qì and blood, enrich and nourish essence-blood, and strengthen the body.

e) Combined with *má huáng* (ephedra), *shú dì huáng* (cooked rehmannia), and *bái jiè zǐ* (white mustard), it is used for yīn flat-abscesses, as in *yáng hé tāng* (Harmonious Yáng Decoction).[364]

Lù jiǎo (deerhorn) quickens the blood and disperses swelling with greater power than *lù jiǎo jiāo* (deerhorn glue). *Lù jiǎo jiāo* enriches and supplements, and it stanches bleeding with greater power than *lù jiǎo*.

Guī bǎn jiāo (tortoise shell glue) is also an enriching and supplementing medicinal, but it tends to be used to enrich yīn. Within supplementing yīn, *lù jiǎo jiāo* also supplements yáng. Used together, this pair of medicinals supplements both yīn and yáng.

Dosage

The dosage is generally 6–9 g/2–3 qián, and it is melted into the decoction.

---

36. 鹿角霜 Lù Jiǎo Shuāng   Cervi Cornu
Degelatinated Deer Antler   Degelatinatum

See also

▷ *Lù róng* (鹿茸 velvet deerhorn, Cervi Cornu Pantotrichum)[143]

▷ *Lù jiǎo* (鹿角 deerhorn, Cervi Cornu)[144]

▷ *Lù jiǎo jiāo* (鹿角胶 deerhorn glue, Cervi Cornus Gelatinum)[145]

Lù jiǎo shuāng (degelatinated deerhorn), which is the dregs left after making *lù jiǎo jiāo* (deerhorn glue), is less warming and supplementing than either *lù jiǎo* (deerhorn) or *lù jiǎo jiāo* (deerhorn glue). *Lù jiǎo shuāng* is used for spleen-stomach vacuity cold, low food intake, and sloppy stool, and it is also used as a substitute for *lù jiǎo* (deerhorn) and *lù jiǎo jiāo* (deerhorn glue), in which case the dosage must be increased.[26]

Dosage

The dosage is generally 6–9 g/2–3 qián. In special cases, use as much as 20–25 g/ 7–8 qián.

---

37. 肉苁蓉 Ròu Cōng Róng   Cistanches Herba
Cistanche

Sour and salty in flavor and warm in nature, *ròu cōng róng* is a kidney-supplementing medicinal that also moistens the intestines and frees the stool.

Being oily and moistening in quality, *ròu cōng róng* supplements kidney yáng without drying.

a) *Ròu cōng róng* combined with *shú dì huáng* (cooked rehmannia), *tù sī zǐ* (cuscuta), *dù zhòng* (eucommia), *shān yào* (dioscorea), *bā jǐ tiān* (morinda), and *yín yáng huò* (epimedium) is used for lumbar pain, limp knees, impotence, reduced sexual function, dizziness, and tinnitus that result from kidney vacuity.

b) Combined with *dāng guī* (Chinese angelica), *chuān xiōng* (chuanxiong), *bái sháo* (white peony), *ài yè* (mugwort), *xiāng fù* (cyperus), and *xù duàn* (dipsacus), it is used for kidney qì vacuity cold, delayed menstruation, uterine cold, and persistent failure to conceive.

c) Combined with *shú dì huáng* (cooked rehmannia), *dāng guī* (Chinese angelica), *táo rén* (peach kernel), *huǒ má rén* (cannabis fruit), and *hēi zhī má* (black

---

[26] *Lù jiǎo shuāng* (degelatinated deerhorn) is also commonly used nowadays to treat flooding and spotting, vaginal discharge, and infertility; it warms the uterus to eliminate uterine cold (胞寒 *bāo hán*). (Ed.)

sesame), it is used for dry stool and constipation that results from qì-blood vacuity and lack of fluids in elderly people or postpartum women.

Comparison

Huǒ má rén (cannabis fruit)[53] frees the stool through enriching the spleen and moistening the intestines, whereas *ròu cōng róng* frees the stool by enriching the kidney and moistening dryness.

Dosage

The dosage is generally 6–12 g/2–4 qián. In special situations, use 15–30 g/ 5 qián–1 liǎng.

Research

According to modern research, this medicinal has a hypotensive action (it lowers blood pressure). It can also be used as a blood-stanching medicinal for cystitis, cystorrhagia (bleeding from the bladder), or renal hemorrhage. In my opinion, when using *ròu cōng róng* to stanch bleeding, it is best to combine it with blood-cooling medicinals, or else confine its use to lower-body vacuity bleeding.

---

38. 巴戟天 Bā Jǐ Tiān
Morinda

Morindae
Officinalis Radix

Acrid and sweet in flavor and slightly warm in nature, *bā jǐ tiān* (morinda) is a kidney-supplementing medicinal that also dispels wind-cold-damp impediment.

In cases where kidney yáng vacuity causes poor sexual function with symptoms such as impotence or premature ejaculation, *bā jǐ tiān* can be combined with *shú dì huáng* (cooked rehmannia), *shān yào* (dioscorea), *yín yáng huò* (epimedium), and *gǒu qǐ zǐ* (lycium). When liver-kidney vacuity cold causes cold pain in the lesser abdomen, cold mounting, or pain in the lumbus, *bā jǐ tiān* can be combined with *wū yào* (lindera), *wú yú* (evodia), *hú lú bā* (fenugreek), *bǔ gǔ zhī* (psoralea), *xiǎo huí xiāng* (fennel), and *xù duàn* (dipsacus). *Bā jǐ tiān* also strengthens sinew and bone and dispels wind-damp. When wind-cold-damp impediment causes lumbar and knee pain, gradual weakening of the lower extremities, and emaciation, use *bā jǐ tiān* with the following:

sāng jì shēng (桑寄生 mistletoe, Taxilli Herba)

dú huó (独活 pubescent angelica, Angelicae Pubescentis Radix)

ròu guì (肉桂 cinnamon bark, Cinnamomi Cortex)

fù zǐ (附子 aconite, Aconiti Radix Lateralis Praeparata)

niú xī (牛膝 achyranthes, Achyranthis Bidentatae Radix)

xù duàn (续断 dipsacus, Dipsaci Radix)

mù guā (木瓜 chaenomeles, Chaenomelis Fructus)

dāng guī (当归 Chinese angelica, Angelicae Sinensis Radix)

dǎng shēn (党参 codonopsis, Codonopsis Radix)

Comparison

Yín yáng huò (epimedium)[148] supplements kidney yáng, tends to enter the qì aspect of the kidney channel, and has a dry nature. *Bā jǐ tiān* supplements kidney yáng, tends to enter the blood aspect of the kidney channel, and is less drying in nature.

Ròu cōng róng (cistanche)[146] supplements kidney yáng and also moistens dryness and frees the stool. *Bā jǐ tiān* supplements kidney yáng and also dispels wind-cold-damp impediment.

Dosage

The dosage is generally 3–9 g / 1–3 qián.

---

39. 淫羊藿 Yín Yáng Huò   Epimedii Herba
Epimedium

Also called *xiān líng pí* 仙灵脾. Sweet and acrid in flavor and warm in nature, *yín yáng huò* (epimedium) is a commonly used kidney-supplementing medicinal that also strengthens sinew and bone and dispels wind-damp.

Drastically supplementing kidney yáng and stimulating sexual function, *yín yáng huò* treats impotence. For this purpose it is frequently combined in pill preparations with:

shú dì huáng (熟地黄 cooked rehmannia, Rehmanniae Radix Praeparata)
xiān máo (仙茅 curculigo, Curculiginis Rhizoma)
ròu cōng róng (肉苁蓉 cistanche, Cistanches Herba)
gǒu qǐ zǐ (枸杞子 lycium, Lycii Fructus)
bā jǐ tiān (巴戟天 morinda, Morindae Officinalis Radix)
tóng jí lí (潼蒺藜 complanate astragalus seed, Astragali Complanati Semen)
shān zhū yú (山茱萸 cornus, Corni Fructus)
suǒ yáng (锁阳 cynomorium, Cynomorii Herba)
yáng qǐ shí (阳起石 actinolite, Actinolitum)
yáng gāo wán (羊睾丸 goat's or sheep's testicle, Caprae seu Ovis Testis)

Yín yáng huò is also used steeped in wine (at a 10% concentration) and taken orally.

Warm in nature and acrid in flavor, *yín yáng huò* dispels wind-cold, supplements the liver and kidney, and strengthens sinew and bone. When wind-cold-damp causes aching pain of the skin and flesh of the limbs, numbness and insensitivity of the limbs, or joint pain and weak legs, combine *yín yáng huò* with:

wēi líng xiān (威灵仙 clematis, Clematidis Radix)
cāng ěr zǐ (苍耳子 xanthium, Xanthii Fructus)
ròu guì (肉桂 cinnamon bark, Cinnamomi Cortex)
fù zǐ (附子 aconite, Aconiti Radix Lateralis Praeparata)
chuān xiōng (川芎 chuanxiong, Chuanxiong Rhizoma)

dú huó (独活 pubescent angelica, Angelicae Pubescentis Radix)

xù duàn (续断 dipsacus, Dipsaci Radix)

These medicinals are taken decocted with water, or ground to a fine powder and taken with warm wine in a dosage of 30 g/1 qián twice a day. I get definite results using *yín yáng huò* combined with *shú dì huáng* (cooked rehmannia), *shān zhū yú* (cornus), *shān yào* (dioscorea), *fú líng* (poria), *fù zǐ* (aconite), *ròu guì* (cinnamon bark), *bā jǐ tiān* (morinda), *ròu cōng róng* (cistanche), *niú xī* (achyranthes), *xù duàn* (dipsacus), and *dù zhòng* (eucommia) to treat myelanalosis or myelitis that result in paraplegia of the legs, lack of strength in the legs, or loss of control of defecation and urination.

Comparisons

Gǒu qǐ zǐ (lycium)[126] supplements the kidney and boosts essence, and it tends to be used for kidney essence vacuity; *yín yáng huò* supplements the kidney and assists yáng, and yet tends to be used for kidney yáng vacuity. *Xiān máo* (curculigo)[151] supplements kidney yáng, enhances the appetite, and assists spleen-stomach movement and transformation, whereas *yín yáng huò* supplements kidney yáng, yet also dispels wind-damp and strengthens sinew and bone to treat wind-cold causing insensitivity in the limbs.

Dosage

The dosage is generally 3–9 g/1–3 qián. In special situations, use 12–15 g/ 4–5 qián.

Caution

Contraindicated for patients with excessive sexual desire.

Research

According to modern research reports, this medicinal promotes secretion of semen.

40. 补骨脂 Bǔ Gǔ Zhī   Psoraleae Fructus
Psoralea

Also called *pò gù zhǐ* 破故纸. Acrid and bitter in flavor and very warm, *bǔ gǔ zhī* mainly supplements kidney yáng, secures the lower origin, warms the stomach and spleen, and checks diarrhea.

When kidney yáng vacuity causes impotence, reduced sexual function, cold pain in the lumbus and knees, cold and damp scrotum, and vacuity cold in the lower abdomen, use *bǔ gǔ zhī* with:

hú táo ròu (胡桃肉 walnut, Juglandis Semen)

dù zhòng (杜仲 eucommia, Eucommiae Cortex)

yáng qǐ shí (阳起石 actinolite, Actinolitum)

xù duàn (续断 dipsacus, Dipsaci Radix)

fù zǐ (附子 aconite, Aconiti Radix Lateralis Praeparata)

shú dì huáng (熟地黃 cooked rehmannia, Rehmanniae Radix Praeparata)

The kidney governs the lower origin, and when kidney yáng vacuity leads to insecurity of the lower origin that manifests in symptoms such as enuresis, frequent urination, or urinary incontinence, *bǔ gǔ zhī* can be used in combination with *sāng piāo xiāo* (mantis egg-case), *tù sī zǐ* (cuscuta), *wū yào* (lindera), and *yì zhì rén* (alpinia). *Bǔ gǔ zhī* can also be stir-fried, ground to a powder, and taken before bed. I have gained satisfactory results using *bǔ gǔ zhī* combined with *sāng piāo xiāo* (mantis egg-case), *fù pén zǐ* (rubus), *wū yào* (lindera), *yì zhì rén* (alpinia), *shú dì huáng* (cooked rehmannia), *shān zhū yú* (cornus), *chǎo jī nèi jīn* (stir-fried gizzard lining), *fú líng* (poria), *lóng gǔ* (dragon bone), *duàn mǔ lì* (calcined oyster shell), *duàn lóng gǔ* (calcined dragon bone), and *sāng jì shēng* (mistletoe) in the treatment of enuresis in young people and adults, as well as stubborn cases in adults.

For spleen-stomach vacuity cold that causes indigestion and chronic diarrhea, combine *bǔ gǔ zhī* with *ròu dòu kòu* (nutmeg), *dà zǎo* (jujube), *shēng jiāng* (fresh ginger) (these ingredients form *èr shén wán* (Two Spirits Pill)), *fú líng* (poria), and *bái zhú* (white atractylodes). *Bǔ gǔ zhī* warms both the kidney and the spleen, so it is most suitable for dual vacuity of the spleen and kidney causing "fifth-watch diarrhea"[549] (五更泄 *wǔ gēng xiè*). For this pattern it is frequently combined with *wú zhū yú* (evodia), *wǔ wèi zǐ* (schisandra), and *ròu dòu kòu* (nutmeg), as in *sì shén wán* (Four Spirits Pill). Using *sì shén wán* (Four Spirits Pill) as a base, I often gain satisfactory results in the treatment of diarrhea in chronic dysentery, chronic enteritis, or intestinal tuberculosis by adding medicinals such as *chǎo shān yào* (stir-fried dioscorea), *hē zǐ* (chebule), *fú líng* (poria), *bái zhú* (white atractylodes), *fù zǐ* (aconite), and *pào jiāng* (blast-fried ginger), depending on the pattern.

COMPARISON

Ròu dòu kòu (nutmeg)[188] and *bǔ gǔ zhī* both check diarrhea, but *ròu dòu kòu* tends to assist spleen yáng and dry spleen dampness, and to astringe the intestines and check diarrhea, whereas *bǔ gǔ zhī* tends to supplement the kidney, warm the spleen, secure the intestines, and check diarrhea.

DOSAGE

The dosage is generally 3–9 g/1–3 qián.

CAUTION

Use with care in patients with bloody urine or constipation, and in pregnant women. Inappropriate for frequent urination due to acute urinary system infection.

---

41. 益智仁 Yì Zhì Rén
Alpinia

Alpiniae
Oxyphyllae Fructus

Acrid in flavor and warm in nature, *yì zhì rén* (alpinia) primarily warms the spleen and kidney, dries spleen dampness, contains drool and spittle, and reduces urination.

When spleen-stomach vacuity cold causes cold pain in the abdomen, vomiting, diarrhea, copious drool, and acid upflow, *yì zhì rén* can be used to supplement spleen yáng and dry spleen dampness. For this purpose, it is frequently combined with:

bái zhú (白术 white atractylodes, Atractylodis Macrocephalae Rhizoma)

huáng qí (黄芪 astragalus, Astragali Radix)

shā rén (砂仁 amomum, Amomi Fructus)

mù xiāng (木香 costusroot, Aucklandiae Radix)

fú líng (茯苓 poria, Poria)

Yì zhì rén is used to contain drool and spittle-humor. I treated a 26-year-old male patient whose primary symptom was severe dribbling. Each night one side of his pillow would be completely wet so that each day he would have to dry the pillow in the sun. This had persisted for 2–3 years and was quite unpleasant. I used *yì zhì rén* combined with *cāng zhú* (atractylodes), *fú líng* (poria), *hē zǐ* (chebule), *bàn xià* (pinellia), and *chén pí* (tangerine peel) and varied the formula as the signs changed. After taking five or six packets, the drooling ceased.

Yì zhì rén is combined with *wū yào* (lindera), ground to a powder, and mixed with flour made from *shān yào* (dioscorea) to form pills. This formula is called *suō quán wán* (Stream-Reducing Pill) and is often used for enuresis, frequent urination, and frequent nocturia. This should be taken with warm water, twice a day, at a dosage of 6 g/2 qián each time. Adding *sāng piāo xiāo* (mantis egg-case), *wǔ wèi zǐ* (schisandra), *shān zhū yú* (cornus), and *bǔ gǔ zhī* (psoralea) makes the effect even better. Combined with *bǔ gǔ zhī* (psoralea) and *ròu dòu kòu* (nutmeg), it is used for spleen-kidney vacuity diarrhea. *Yì zhì rén* combined with *gāo liáng jiāng* (lesser galangal) and *dīng xiāng* (clove) treats stomach cold vomiting (copious water and drool).

Fù pén zǐ (rubus) has greater capacity to supplement the kidney and reduce urine than *yì zhì rén*, but the latter's capacity to dry the spleen and contain drool and spittle is greater than the former's. *Fù pén zǐ* has a strong astringent nature, whereas *yì zhì rén* has a strong drying nature.

DOSAGE

The dosage is generally 3–9 g/1–3 qián.

CAUTION

Should not be used in dryness-heat patterns or urinary frequency with yellow or reddish urine and urethral pain.

---

42. 仙茅 **Xiān Máo**   Curculiginis Rhizoma
Curculigo

Xiān máo (curculigo) is acrid in flavor and warm in nature; it possesses minor toxicity. It is mainly used as a kidney-warming, yáng-invigorating medicinal, and it also warms the stomach. For kidney yáng vacuity that leads to impotence, cold pain in the lumbus and knees, and enuresis in the elderly, *xiān máo* (curculigo) can be combined with *shú dì huáng* (cooked rehmannia), *shān zhū yú* (cornus), *yín yáng huò* (epimedium), *gǒu qǐ zǐ* (lycium), *wǔ wèi zǐ* (schisandra), and *xù duàn* (dipsacus). For cold qì in the stomach duct causing distention and pain, or acid vomiting and poor appetite, use *xiān máo* with:

shā rén (砂仁 amomum, Amomi Fructus)

wú yú (吴萸 evodia, Evodiae Fructus)

mù xiāng (木香 costusroot, Aucklandiae Radix)

gāo liáng jiāng (高良姜 lesser galangal, Alpiniae Officinarum Rhizoma)

RESEARCH

In recent years this medicinal has been used to treat hypertension manifesting as kidney vacuity; it has been found effective when combined with *yín yáng huò* (epimedium), *bā jǐ tiān* (morinda), *huáng bǎi* (phellodendron), *zhī mǔ* (anemarrhena), and *dāng guī* (Chinese angelica) to form *èr xiān tāng* (Two Immortals Decoction).

DOSAGE

The dosage is generally 3–9 g/1–3 qián.

---

43. 菟丝子 **Tù Sī Zǐ**   Cuscutae Semen
Cuscuta

Sweet and acrid in flavor and warm in nature, *tù sī zǐ* (cuscuta) is primarily used as a liver-kidney–supplementing medicinal.

This medicinal is frequently used when insufficiency of the liver and kidney causes lumbus and knee pain, impotence, seminal emission, loss of visual acuity, and dribbling urination. For example, *tù sī zǐ* combined with *wǔ wèi zǐ* (schisandra), *lián zǐ* (lotus seed), *yuǎn zhì* (polygala), and *qiàn shí* (euryale) is used for seminal emission. Combined with *tóng jí lí* (complanate astragalus seed), *yín yáng huò* (epimedium), *gǒu qǐ zǐ* (lycium), and *bā jǐ tiān* (morinda), it is used for impotence. Combined with *cǎo jué míng* (fetid cassia), *gǒu qǐ zǐ* (lycium), *jú huā* (chrysanthcmum), *chē qián zǐ* (plantago seed), *qīng xiāng zǐ* (celosia), *shú dì huáng* (cooked rehmannia), and *shēng dì huáng* (dried/fresh rehmannia), it is used for loss of visual acuity.

On the basis of this medicinal's capacity to supplement the liver and kidney, boost essence-blood, strengthen the lumbus and knees, and secure the lower origin, in recent years it has been used in treatments for functional metrorrhagia, habitual miscarriage, and aplastic anemia. Normally this medicinal is added to formulas within the procedures of pattern identification as the basis for determining treatment.

Shé chuáng zǐ (cnidium seed) supplements the kidney, tends to assist kidney yáng, and is applied topically to dispel dampness and treat pudendal itch. *Tù sī zǐ* supplements the kidney, tends to boost essence, is warm but not drying, and is rarely applied topically.

DOSAGE

The dosage is generally 9–12 g/3–4 qián.

---

44. 杜仲 Dù Zhòng   Eucommiae Cortex
Eucommia

Sweet and slightly acrid in flavor and warm in nature, *dù zhòng* (eucommia) is commonly used to supplement the liver and kidney, strengthen sinew and bone, boost the lumbus and knees, and also to quiet the fetus. The kidney governs the lumbus and knees, the liver governs the sinews, and the kidney governs the bones. When liver-kidney vacuity gives rise to lumbar pain and to limp knees and legs, use this medicinal to supplement the liver and kidney and strengthen sinew and bone in order to boost the lumbus and knees. For such cases, *dù zhòng* (eucommia) is frequently combined with *shú dì huáng* (cooked rehmannia), *xù duàn* (dipsacus), *niú xī* (achyranthes), *shān yào* (dioscorea), *shān zhū yú* (cornus), and *bǔ gǔ zhī* (psoralea). If there is also cold lumbus and legs, liking for warmth, and fear of cold, then add *fù piàn* (sliced aconite), *ròu guì* (cinnamon bark), and *yín yáng huò* (epimedium).

When kidney vacuity in a pregnant woman causes stirring fetus (characterized by the appearance, in the second or third month of pregnancy, of lumbar pain, stirring of the fetus as if about to abort, lack of strength in the lower body, and weak cubit pulse), *dù zhòng* can be used to supplement the kidney and quiet the fetus. For this pattern, *dù zhòng* is frequently combined with:

sāng jì shēng (桑寄生 mistletoe, Taxilli Herba)

xù duàn (续断 dipsacus, Dipsaci Radix)

bái zhú (白术 white atractylodes, Atractylodis Macrocephalae Rhizoma)

shú dì huáng (熟地黄 cooked rehmannia, Rehmanniae Radix Praeparata)

bái sháo (白芍 white peony, Paeoniae Radix Alba)

sū gěng (苏梗 perilla stem, Perillae Caulis)

dāng guī (当归 Chinese angelica, Angelicae Sinensis Radix)

When kidney vacuity gives rise to fetal spotting (uterine bleeding in a pregnant woman), I often use *dù zhòng tàn* (charred eucommia) combined with *xù duàn tàn* (charred dipsacus), *dāng guī* (Chinese angelica), *bái sháo* (white peony), *ē jiāo* (ass hide glue), and *ài yè tàn* (charred mugwort).

In traumatology, *dù zhòng* and *xù duàn* (dipsacus) are frequently used together. It is traditionally believed that *dù zhòng* promotes union of separated sinews and bones, while *xù duàn* (dipsacus) promotes knitting of torn sinews and broken bones. These two medicinals have a mutually complementary therapeutic effect and are also frequently used together in internal medicine to strengthen the effect of supplementing the liver and kidney, strengthening sinew and bone, and invigorating the lumbus and knees.

COMPARISON

Sāng jì shēng (mistletoe) and *dù zhòng* both treat lumbar pain. However, *sāng jì shēng* dispels wind-damp and boosts the blood vessels, and is suitable for lumbar pain that results from kidney channel blood vacuity and wind-damp invasion. By contrast, *dù zhòng* warms qì and dries dampness, and is suitable for lumbar pain due to kidney channel qì vacuity and cold-damp invasion. *Sāng jì shēng* and *dù zhòng* both quiet the fetus. Whereas *sāng jì shēng* quiets the fetus by boosting the liver, kidney, blood, and vessels and by supplementing sinew and bone, *dù zhòng* quiets the fetus by supplementing liver and kidney qì; when liver and kidney qì is sufficient, the fetus is spontaneously quiet. These two medicinals are often used together.

Dù zhòng is warm in nature, dries dampness, and enters the qì aspect of the kidney channel. When using *shú dì huáng* (cooked rehmannia) to supplement the kidney, adding *dù zhòng* as an assistant allows *shú dì huáng* to supplement without causing stagnation.

DOSAGE

The dosage is generally 3–9 g/1–3 qián.

CAUTION

Inappropriate for patterns of insufficiency of kidney yīn with vacuity heat.

RESEARCH

Modern research has demonstrated that *dù zhòng* lowers blood pressure (hypotensive). The hypotensive effect of *chǎo dù zhòng* (stir-fried eucommia) is greater, and this effect is stronger in water decoctions than in tinctures. For heat patterns, *dù zhòng* is combined with *huáng qín* (scutellaria).

---

45. 续断 **Xù Duàn**   Dipsaci Radix
Dipsacus

Also called *chuān xù duàn* 川续断. Bitter and acrid in flavor and slightly warm in nature, *xù duàn* (dipsacus) supplements the liver and kidney, joins sinews and bones, frees the blood vessels, disinhibits the joints, and quiets the fetus.

1. **Kidney Vacuity Lumbar Pain**: For lumbar pain, limp legs, and inhibited walking that result from kidney vacuity, *xù duàn* is frequently combined with *dù zhòng* (eucommia), *gǒu jǐ* (cibotium), *niú xī* (achyranthes), *shēng dì huáng* (dried/fresh rehmannia), *shú dì huáng* (cooked rehmannia), and *zhì fù piàn* (sliced processed aconite). This combination supplements the liver and kidney, disinhibits the joints, strengthens sinew and bone, and relieves pain.

2. **Knocks and Falls**: For knocks and falls, broken sinews and bones, and external injury pain and swelling, *xù duàn* is frequently combined with medicinals such

as *dāng guī* (Chinese angelica), *chuān xiōng* (chuanxiong), *rǔ xiāng* (frankincense), *mò yào* (myrrh), *sān qī* (notoginseng), *dù zhòng* (eucommia), *niú xī* (achyranthes), and *gǔ suì bǔ* (drynaria). This formula disperses swelling and relieves pain, and joins sinew and bones; it is effective in promoting tissue regeneration.

3. Stirring Fetus and Fetal Spotting: In the second or third month of pregnancy, when there is **stirring fetus**[564] (胎动 *tāi dòng*) that may abort, *xù duàn* is frequently used with *sāng jì shēng* (mistletoe), *dù zhòng* (eucommia), *bái zhú* (white atractylodes), and *dāng guī* (Chinese angelica) to secure the kidney and quiet the fetus. For **fetal spotting**[549] (胎漏 *tāi lòu*), which can also give rise to stirring fetus, I frequently combine *xù duàn tàn* (charred dipsacus) with *dāng guī* (Chinese angelica), *bái sháo* (white peony), *shēng dì huáng* (dried/fresh rehmannia), *dù zhòng tàn* (charred eucommia), *ē jiāo* (ass hide glue), and *ài yè tàn* (charred mugwort) to stanch bleeding and quiet the fetus.

COMPARISONS

Dù zhòng (eucommia)[153] enters the qì aspect of the kidney channel and tends to treat aching lumbus and knees. *Xù duàn* enters the blood aspect of the kidney channel and tends to treat inhibition of the joints of the lumbus and knees with difficulty moving. These two medicinals are frequently used together.

Gǒu jǐ (cibotium)[155] enters the governing vessel and tends to treat stiffness and pain of the lumbar spine; it also dispels wind-damp. *Xù duàn* tends to treat pain in the lumbus, knees, legs, and feet; it also quickens the blood.

In recent years, *xù duàn* has frequently been used, where appropriate for the pattern, for lumbar pain due to lumbar muscle strain or sprain, nephritis, or urinary tract infection.

DOSAGE

The dosage is generally 5–10 g/1.5–3 qián. In special situations, use 25–30 g/8 qián–1 liǎng.

---

46. 狗脊 Gǒu Jǐ   Cibotii Rhizoma
Cibotium

Also called *jīn gǒu jǐ* 金狗脊 or *jīn máo gǒu jǐ* 金毛狗脊,[27] *gǒu jǐ* (cibotium) is bitter and sweet in flavor and warm in nature.[28] It supplements the liver and kidney, strengthens the lumbus and knees, and also eliminates wind-damp. For patients with underlying liver-kidney vacuity and insufficiency of qì and blood and who further contract wind-cold-damp evil that results in lumbar spine pain and limp legs with a lack of strength, *gǒu jǐ* can be combined with the following:

---

[27] The names *jīn gǒu jǐ* 金狗脊 and *jīn máo gǒu jǐ* 金毛狗脊 serve to distinguish cibotium from items that are also known as *gǒu jǐ* (cibotium) in Chinese but that are from different botanical sources. (Ed.)

[28] This plant is on the list of endangered species established by the Convention on International Trade in Endangered Species (CITES). (Ed.)

chuān niú xī (川牛膝 cyathula, Cyathulae Radix)

hǎi fēng téng (海风藤 kadsura pepper stem, Piperis Kadsurae Caulis)

mù guā (木瓜 chaenomeles, Chaenomelis Fructus)

xù duàn (续断 dipsacus, Dipsaci Radix)

qín jiāo (秦艽 large gentian, Gentianae Macrophyllae Radix)

dú huó (独活 pubescent angelica, Angelicae Pubescentis Radix)

Gǒu jǐ is a gentle and harmonious liver- and kidney-supplementing medicinal. Besides the symptoms described above, it is also used when insufficiency of the liver and kidney causes profuse menstruation, white vaginal discharge, or frequent urination.

Profuse Menstruation

gǒu jǐ (狗脊 cibotium, Cibotii Rhizoma)

dāng guī tàn (当归炭 charred Chinese angelica, Angelicae Sinensis Radix Carbonisata)

bái sháo (白芍 white peony, Paeoniae Radix Alba)

ài yè tàn (艾叶炭 charred mugwort, Artemisiae Argyi Folium Carbonisatum)

shēng dì huáng (生地黄 dried/fresh rehmannia, Rehmanniae Radix Exsiccata seu Recens)

huáng qín (黄芩 scutellaria, Scutellariae Radix)

White Vaginal Discharge

gǒu jǐ (狗脊 cibotium, Cibotii Rhizoma)

bái zhú (白术 white atractylodes, Atractylodis Macrocephalae Rhizoma)

bái liǎn (白蔹 ampelopsis, Ampelopsis Radix)

cāng zhú (苍术 atractylodes, Atractylodis Rhizoma)

fú líng (茯苓 poria, Poria)

bái jī guān huā (白鸡冠花 white cockscomb, Celosiae Cristatae Flos Albus)

Frequent Urination

gǒu jǐ (狗脊 cibotium, Cibotii Rhizoma)

tù sī zǐ (菟丝子 cuscuta, Cuscutae Semen)

wǔ wèi zǐ (五味子 schisandra, Schisandrae Fructus)

sāng piāo xiāo (桑螵蛸 mantis egg-case, Mantidis Oötheca)

These formulas should be varied in accordance with signs. *Gǒu jǐ* is even more suitable for elderly people with signs such as aching pain of the lumbar spine and limp legs and weak feet.

In recent years, I have added 12–25 g/4–8 qián of *gǒu jǐ* to appropriate formulas that supplement the liver and kidney, free the blood vessels, and dispel wind-cold in the treatment of spondylarthritis, myelopathy, and sequelae of spinal compression fractures. For example, I have used the following formula, varied in accordance with signs, to treat compression fracture of the thoracic vertebrae with satisfactory results:

shēng shú dì (生熟地 raw/cooked rehmannia, Rehmanniae Radix Praeparata seu Cruda) *shān yào* (山药 dioscorea, Dioscoreae Rhizoma)

shān zhū yú (山茱萸 cornus, Corni Fructus)

gǔ suì bǔ (骨碎补 drynaria, Drynariae Rhizoma)

bǔ gǔ zhī (补骨脂 psoralea, Psoraleae Fructus)

nán hóng huā (南红花 carthamus, Carthami Flos)

xù duàn (续断 dipsacus, Dipsaci Radix)

dù zhòng (杜仲 eucommia, Eucommiae Cortex)

dú huó (独活 pubescent angelica, Angelicae Pubescentis Radix)

zhì fù piàn (制附片 sliced processed aconite, Aconiti Radix Lateralis Praeparata Secta)

yín yáng huò (淫羊藿 epimedium, Epimedii Herba)

jīn gǒu jǐ (金狗脊 cibotium, Cibotii Rhizoma)

niú xī (牛膝 achyranthes, Achyranthis Bidentatae Radix)

zhì hǔ gǔ (炙虎骨 mix-fried tiger bone, Tigris Os cum Liquido Frictum)

ròu guì (肉桂 cinnamon bark, Cinnamomi Cortex)

Char-fried *gǒu jǐ* stanches bleeding, and it is primarily used to stanch bleeding in external injury.

DOSAGE

The dosage is generally 6–9 g/2–3 qián. When necessary, use 12–30 g/4 qián–1 liǎng.

---

47. 蛇床子 Shé Chuáng Zǐ   Cnidii Fructus
Cnidium Seed

Acrid and bitter in flavor and warm in nature, *shé chuáng zǐ* (cnidium seed) warms the kidney yáng and warms the uterus. *Shé chuáng zǐ* (cnidium seed) is used for male impotence, reduced sexual function, and infertility from uterine cold. It is frequently combined with *shú dì huáng* (cooked rehmannia), *shān zhū yú* (cornus), *fú líng* (poria), *tù sī zǐ* (cuscuta), *tóng jí lí* (complanate astragalus seed), *dāng guī* (Chinese angelica), *ròu guì* (cinnamon bark), and *yín yáng huò* (epimedium). Applied topically, *shé chuáng zǐ* dries dampness, kills worms, and relieves itching. For trichomonas that causes white vaginal discharge (trichomonas vaginitis), use this medicinal as a wash, a sitz bath, or an ointment, to dry dampness, kill worms, and relieve itching. *Shé chuáng zǐ* is combined with *kǔ shēn* (flavescent sophora), *huáng bǎi* (phellodendron), and *mì tuó sēng* (litharge), ground to a powder, mixed with oil, and applied topically to treat stubborn lichen and damp sores.

Decocted alone and used as an external wash, *shé chuáng zǐ* is used for damp, watery itching of the scrotum.

DOSAGE

When taken internally, the dosage is generally 3–9 g/1–3 qián. It is frequently used in pill preparations. When decocted as an external wash, the dosage is 9–30 g/ 3 qián–1 liǎng.

CAUTION

Contraindicated for patterns with fire in the kidney channel or for excessive sexual desire.

48. 阳起石 Yáng Qǐ Shí   Actinolitum
Actinolite

Salty in flavor and slightly warm in nature, *yáng qǐ shí* (actinolite) is primarily used as a kidney-yáng-supplementing medicinal. It is combined with *shú dì huáng* (cooked rehmannia), *shān yào* (dioscorea), *shān zhū yú* (cornus), *fú líng* (poria), *zé xiè* (alisma), *yín yáng huò* (epimedium), *bā jǐ tiān* (morinda), and *fù zǐ* (aconite) for kidney yáng vacuity that causes impotence and cold sweating in the genitals in men, and uterine cold, abdominal pain, and persistent failure to conceive in women. For impotence, use *yáng qǐ shí* 30 g/1 liǎng and *shú dì huáng* (cooked rehmannia) 30 g/ 1 liǎng, taken decocted with water.

DOSAGE

The dosage is generally 9–30 g/3 qián–1 liǎng.

CAUTION

Inappropriate for patterns of hyperactive kidney yáng.

49. 韭菜子 Jiǔ Cài Zǐ   Allii
Chinese Leek Seed   Tuberosi Semen

Acrid and sweet in flavor and warm in nature, *jiǔ cài zǐ* (Chinese leek seed) warms and supplements the liver and kidney. Combined with *lóng gǔ* (dragon bone), ground to a powder, and taken with warm water or wine, 1 qián per dose, twice a day, it can be used to treat seminal emission. Combined with *sāng piāo xiāo* (mantis egg-case), it can be used to treat vacuity cold of the lower origin and urinary incontinence. *Jiǔ cài zǐ* combined with *qiàn shí* (euryale) and *bái zhú* (white atractylodes) is used for white vaginal discharge.

DOSAGE

The dosage is generally 3–9 g/1–3 qián.

CAUTION

Contraindicated in patterns of kidney channel heat.

---

50. 酸枣仁 Suān Zǎo Rén   Ziziphi
Spiny Jujube   Spinosi Semen

Sweet and sour in flavor and neutral in nature, *suān zǎo rén* (spiny jujube) nourishes the liver, quiets the heart, quiets the spirit, and constrains sweat. By supplementing heart and liver blood, it quiets the spirit and stabilizes the mind. It is most commonly used for vacuous blood of the liver-gallbladder that is unable to nourish the heart, which results in vexation and sleeplessness, profuse dreaming, and susceptibility to fright. For patients who tend to heart-spleen insufficiency and dual vacuity of qì and blood, it is frequently combined with medicinals such as *huáng qí* (astragalus), *bái zhú* (white atractylodes), *dāng guī* (Chinese angelica), and *bái sháo* (white peony). An example of this use is *guī pí tāng* (Spleen-Returning Decoction):

Guī pí tāng 归脾汤   Spleen-Returning Decoction

---

huáng qí (黄芪 astragalus, Astragali Radix)

bái zhú (白术 white atractylodes, Atractylodis Macrocephalae Rhizoma)

dāng guī (当归 Chinese angelica, Angelicae Sinensis Radix)

lóng yǎn ròu (龙眼肉 longan flesh, Longan Arillus)

suān zǎo rén (酸枣仁 spiny jujube, Ziziphi Spinosi Semen)

dǎng shēn (党参 codonopsis, Codonopsis Radix)

fú líng (茯苓 poria, Poria)

yuǎn zhì (远志 polygala, Polygalae Radix)

mù xiāng (木香 costusroot, Aucklandiae Radix)

gān cǎo (甘草 licorice, Glycyrrhizae Radix)

For patients with a tendency toward liver-gallbladder vacuity heat, *suān zǎo rén* is frequently combined with medicinals such as *zhī mǔ* (anemarrhena), *fú líng* (poria), and *huáng qín* (scutellaria). An example of this use is *jīn guì suān zǎo rén tāng* (Golden Coffer Spiny Jujube Decoction):

Jīn guì suān zǎo rén tāng 金匮酸枣仁汤   Golden Coffer Spiny Jujube Decoction

---

suān zǎo rén (酸枣仁 spiny jujube, Ziziphi Spinosi Semen)

zhī mǔ (知母 anemarrhena, Anemarrhenae Rhizoma)

fú líng (茯苓 poria, Poria)

chuān xiōng (川芎 chuanxiong, Chuanxiong Rhizoma)

gān cǎo (甘草 licorice, Glycyrrhizae Radix)

For patients with a tendency toward yīn vacuity and liver exuberance, *suān zǎo rén* is frequently combined with *bái sháo* (white peony), *shēng shí jué míng* (crude abalone shell), *shēng dì huáng* (dried/fresh rehmannia), *lóng chǐ* (dragon tooth), *fú líng* (poria), and *shēng mǔ lì* (crude oyster shell).

RESEARCH

According to modern research, *suān zǎo rén* inhibits the central nervous system and has a sedative and soporific effect. Use raw or lightly stir-fried; if stir-fried until dry, it loses its sedative action.

Sweet and sour, *suān zǎo rén* both constrains vacuity sweating and engenders liquid. For enduring illness with blood loss, or for anxiety and thought causing taxation damage of the heart and spleen, which manifest in fatigue, sweating, vexation and thirst, and palpitations, *suān zǎo rén* is combined with:

shēng dì huáng (生地黄 dried/fresh rehmannia, Rehmanniae Radix Exsiccata seu Recens)

bái sháo (白芍 white peony, Paeoniae Radix Alba)

shān zhū yú (山茱萸 cornus, Corni Fructus),

wǔ wèi zǐ (五味子 schisandra, Schisandrae Fructus)

mǔ lì (牡蛎 oyster shell, Ostreae Concha)

Comparisons

Huáng lián (coptis)[246] treats hyperactive heart fire and vexation heat in the heart causing inability to sleep. *Suān zǎo rén* treats vacuity vexation, timidity, and inability to sleep due to insufficiency of the liver and gallbladder.

Raw, *suān zǎo rén* is sweet, sour, and moistening; it tends to be used for liver-gallbladder vacuity heat patterns. Stir fried, it is sour, warm, and fragrant; it arouses the spleen and tends to be used for reduced sleep due to blood vacuity of the liver, gallbladder, heart, and spleen.

Physicians of the past have claimed that *shēng zǎo rén* (raw spiny jujube) treats hypersomnia, whereas *chǎo zǎo rén* (stir-fried spiny jujube) treats insomnia. Modern pharmacological laboratory animal studies, however, have failed to show evidence of these opposite effects. Other physicians of the past believed that the two forms of *suān zǎo rén* had been confused with *suān zǎo ròu* (spiny jujube) and *suān zǎo rén*, suggesting that *suān zǎo ròu* (spiny jujube) treats hypersomnia, while *suān zǎo rén* treats insomnia, just as *má huáng* (ephedra) promotes sweating and *má huáng jié* (ephedra node) checks sweating. I personally use *chǎo zǎo rén* (stir-fried spiny jujube) when treating insomnia. I find that it is more effective if freshly stir-fried than if stored a time after stir-frying.

Dosage

The dosage is generally 3–9 g/1–3 qián. In special situations, use as much as 15–30 g/5 qián–1 liǎng.

Caution

Inappropriate for patterns of liver, gallbladder, heart, or spleen repletion heat, for summerheat-damp collecting in the interior, or for initial-stage externally contracted wind-cold.

---

51. 柏子仁 Bǎi Zǐ Rén   Platycladi Semen
Arborvitae Seed

Sweet in flavor and neutral in nature, *bǎi zǐ rén* (arborvitae seed) nourishes the heart and quiets the spirit, moistens dryness and frees the stool.

Bǎi zǐ rén supplements heart qì, nourishes heart blood, and quiets the spirit. For spleen and heart that have been harmed because of excessive thought and preoccupation, causing flusteredness, fright palpitations, insomnia, and night sweating, *bǎi zǐ rén* is combined with medicinals such as the following:

dì huáng (地黄 rehmannia, Rehmanniae Radix)

suān zǎo rén (酸枣仁 spiny jujube, Ziziphi Spinosi Semen)

dāng guī (当归 Chinese angelica, Angelicae Sinensis Radix)

dǎng shēn (党参 codonopsis, Codonopsis Radix)

fú líng (茯苓 poria, Poria)

mài dōng (麦冬 ophiopogon, Ophiopogonis Radix)

wǔ wèi zǐ (五味子 schisandra, Schisandrae Fructus)

yuǎn zhì (远志 polygala, Polygalae Radix)

Bǎi zǐ rén also nourishes the blood and moistens the intestines. For patients with bound stool due to dessication of liquid-blood, whether from old age, enduring illness, or debilitated health, *bǎi zǐ rén* can be combined with:

táo rén (桃仁 peach kernel, Persicae Semen)

xìng rén (杏仁 apricot kernel, Armeniacae Semen)

dāng guī (当归 Chinese angelica, Angelicae Sinensis Radix)

huǒ má rén (火麻仁 cannabis fruit, Cannabis Fructus)

guā lóu (瓜蒌 trichosanthes, Trichosanthis Fructus)

sōng zǐ rén (松子仁 pine nut, Pini Semen)

COMPARISONS

Hé huān huā (silk tree flower) treats insomnia from liver depression; *yè jiāo téng* (flowery knotweed stem)[162] treats insomnia from noninteraction of yīn and yáng; *bǎi zǐ rén* treats insomnia from heart vacuity.

Yù lǐ rén (bush cherry kernel)[54] tends to treat constipation due to qì bind in the pylorus, whereas *bǎi zǐ rén* tends to treat constipation due to blood vacuity and intestinal dryness.

DOSAGE

The dosage is generally 3–9 g/1–3 qián.

CAUTION

Contraindicated for copious phlegm in the diaphragm or for diarrhea.

52. 远志 Yuǎn Zhì
Polygala

Polygalae Radix

Bitter in flavor and warm in nature, *yuǎn zhì* (polygala) quiets the spirit and boosts the mind, dispels phlegm and opens the orifices.

This medicinal promotes heart-kidney interaction and quiets the spirit. In normal physiology, the heart yáng reaches down to interact with the kidney, and the kidney yīn ascends to interact with the heart, so that there is a regulating interaction between the two organs. For noninteraction of the heart and kidney that results in insomnia and fright palpitations, combine *yuǎn zhì* with:

fú líng (茯苓 poria, Poria)

suān zǎo rén (酸枣仁 spiny jujube, Ziziphi Spinosi Semen)

dì huáng (地黄 rehmannia, Rehmanniae Radix)

dǎng shēn (党参 codonopsis, Codonopsis Radix)

yè jiāo téng (夜交藤 flowery knotweed stem, Polygoni Multiflori Caulis)

wǔ wèi zǐ (五味子 schisandra, Schisandrae Fructus)

Yuǎn zhì boosts the memory. It is used for deteriorating memory, forgetfulness, and lack of concentration that are caused by heart-kidney insufficiency. For this purpose, *yuǎn zhì* is frequently combined with *chāng pú* (acorus), *lóng gǔ* (dragon bone), *guī bǎn* (tortoise shell), *mài dōng* (ophiopogon), *wǔ wèi zǐ* (schisandra), and *bǎi zǐ rén* (arborvitae seed).

For patterns of phlegm obstructing the orifices of the heart that gives rise to unclear spirit-mind, **fright epilepsy**[550] (惊痫 *jīng xián*), and poor hearing and vision, use *yuǎn zhì* to transform phlegm and open the orifices. For this purpose it is frequently combined with medicinals such as *tiān zhú huáng* (bamboo sugar), *yù jīn* (curcuma), *chāng pú* (acorus), and *dǎn xīng* (bile arisaema). According to modern research, *yuǎn zhì* increases bronchial secretions, makes the contents of the bronchi easier to expectorate, and has an expectorant action. It can therefore be used for bronchitis and is frequently combined with medicinals such as *xìng rén* (apricot kernel), *zǐ wǎn* (aster), *qián hú* (peucedanum), and *gān cǎo* (licorice) to dispel phlegm and suppress cough.

Dosage

The dosage is generally 3–9 g/1–3 qián.

53. 夜交藤 Yè Jiāo Téng
Flowery Knotweed Stem

Polygoni
Multiflori Caulis

Yè jiāo téng (flowery knotweed stem), also called *shǒu wū téng* 首乌藤, is the stem of *hé shǒu wū* (flowery knotweed). Sweet in flavor and neutral in nature, it is commonly used as a spirit-quieting medicinal, but it also frees the channels and network vessels and eliminates impediment pain.

Yè jiāo téng regulates the yīn and yáng of the body. It is suitable for liver-kidney yīn vacuity with exuberant yáng that results in vacuity vexation, insomnia, and profuse dreaming. For this pattern, it is combined with medicinals such as *shēng dì huáng* (dried/fresh rehmannia), *bái sháo* (white peony), *lóng gǔ* (dragon bone), *mǔ lì* (oyster shell), *yuǎn zhì* (polygala), and *xuán shēn* (scrophularia).

In addition, *yè jiāo téng* frees the channels and quickens the network vessels. Thus it is used for wind-cold-damp impediment and scurrying pain of the whole body. For this pattern it is frequently combined with medicinals such as:

sāng jì shēng (桑寄生 mistletoe, Taxilli Herba)

sāng zhī (桑枝 mulberry twig, Mori Ramulus)

dú huó (独活 pubescent angelica, Angelicae Pubescentis Radix)

qiāng huó (羌活 notopterygium, Notopterygii Rhizoma et Radix)

guì zhī (桂枝 cinnamon twig, Cinnamomi Ramulus)

dāng guī (当归 Chinese angelica, Angelicae Sinensis Radix)

hóng huā (红花 carthamus, Carthami Flos)

fù zǐ (附子 aconite, Aconiti Radix Lateralis Praeparata)

DOSAGE

The dosage for internal use is generally 9–30 g/3 qián–1 liǎng.

---

54. 珍珠母 **Zhēn Zhū Mǔ**   Concha Margaritifera
Mother-of-Pearl

Also called *zhēn zhū mǔ* 真珠母. *Zhēn zhū mǔ* (mother-of-pearl) is salty in flavor and cool in nature.

1. Downbearing Heart Fire and Clearing Liver Heat: For febrile disease in which exuberant internal phlegm-heat, heat entering the pericardium, or extreme heat engendering wind causes clouded spirit and delirious speech, fright epilepsy, and convulsions, *zhēn zhū mǔ* is combined with the following:

yù jīn (郁金 curcuma, Curcumae Radix)

huáng lián (黄连 coptis, Coptidis Rhizoma)

tiān zhú huáng (天竹黄 bamboo sugar, Bambusae Concretio Silicea)

dǎn xīng (胆星 bile arisaema, Arisaema cum Bile)

chāng pú (菖蒲 acorus, Acori Tatarinowii Rhizoma)

yuǎn zhì (远志 polygala, Polygalae Radix)

guǎng xī jiǎo (广犀角 African rhinoceros horn, Rhinocerotis Cornu Africanum)

zhū shā (朱砂 cinnabar, Cinnabaris)

gōu téng (钩藤 uncaria, Uncariae Ramulus cum Uncis)

quán xiē (全蝎 scorpion, Scorpio)

2. Subduing Liver Yáng and Quieting the Heart Spirit: For patterns of heart-liver yīn vacuity with agitation of liver yáng, and unquiet heart spirit causing dizziness, tinnitus, palpitations, insomnia, vacuity vexation, and profuse dreaming, *zhēn zhū mǔ* is combined with the following:

shēng bái sháo (生白芍 raw white peony, Paeoniae Radix Alba Cruda)

shēng dì huáng (生地黄 dried/fresh rehmannia, Rehmanniae Radix Exsiccata seu Recens)

bái jí lí (白蒺藜 tribulus, Tribuli Fructus)

yuǎn zhì (远志 polygala, Polygalae Radix)

huáng qín (黄芩 scutellaria, Scutellariae Radix)

xiāng fù (香附 cyperus, Cyperi Rhizoma)

gōu téng (钩藤 uncaria, Uncariae Ramulus cum Uncis)

shēng dài zhě shí (生代赭石 crude hematite, Haematitum Crudum)

I often have satisfactory results from using medicinals of this kind to treat neurasthenia that is ascribed to yīn vacuity and exuberant yáng.

Comparisons

Zhēn zhū mǔ, yuǎn zhì (polygala), *yè jiāo téng* (flowery knotweed stem), *suān zǎo rén* (spiny jujube), and *bǎi zǐ rén* (arborvitae seed) all quiet the spirit and treat insomnia. However, *zhēn zhū mǔ* tends to be used for insomnia from heart-liver yīn vacuity with heart channel heat; *yuǎn zhì* (polygala) tends to be used for insomnia from noninteraction of the heart and kidney, or phlegm obstructing the orifices of the heart; *yè jiāo téng* (flowery knotweed stem) tends to be used for insomnia from liver-kidney insufficiency and yīn-yáng disharmony; *suān zǎo rén* (spiny jujube) tends to be used for insomnia from liver-gallbladder blood vacuity; and *bǎi zǐ rén* (arborvitae seed) tends to be used for insomnia from insufficiency of heart blood.

Zhēn zhū mǔ and *shí jué míng* (abalone shell) both subdue yáng. Nevertheless, *zhēn zhū mǔ* tends to downbear heart fire, whereas *shí jué míng* (abalone shell) tends to downbear liver fire. I often use *zhēn zhū mǔ* for heart channel spirit-mind diseases and *shí jué míng* (abalone shell) for liver channel yáng hyperactivity diseases.

Lóng chǐ (dragon tooth) effectively tranquilizes and quiets the spirit, while *zhēn zhū mǔ* is effective in nourishing the heart and quieting the spirit.

Dosage

The dosage is generally 9–30 g/3 qián–1 liǎng and it must be predecocted.

Caution

Inappropriate for patterns with cold in the heart channel or for water-rheum intimidating the heart.

55. 朱砂 Zhū Shā   Cinnabaris
Cinnabar

Also called *chén shā* (cinnabar). Sweet in flavor and slightly cold in nature, *zhū shā* (cinnabar)[29] is a heavy settling spirit-quieting medicinal that also resolves toxin.

Cold in nature and heavy in substance, *zhū shā* enters the heart channel, clears heat, settles fright, and quiets the spirit. For fright palpitations, **mania and withdrawal**[557] (癫狂 *diān kuáng*), or insomnia that result from excessively exuberant heart heat or heart channel phlegm-heat, it is combined with medicinals such as *huáng lián* (coptis), *shēng dì huáng* (dried/fresh rehmannia), *dāng guī* (Chinese angelica), and *gān cǎo* (licorice), as in *zhū shā ān shén wán* (Cinnabar Spirit-Quieting Pill); or it is combined with *cí shí* (loadstone) and *shén qū* (medicated leaven), as in *cí zhū wán* (Loadstone and Cinnabar Pill). *Zhū shā* is not used in decoction medicines, but is frequently used in pill medicines (as, for example, in the formula above), or else ground into a fine powder and taken drenched. For the pattern described above, for example, one can decoct *huáng lián* (coptis), *shēng dì huáng* (dried/fresh rehmannia), *yuǎn zhì* (polygala), *tiān zhú huáng* (bamboo sugar), *yù jīn* (curcuma), and *shēng tiě luò* (iron flakes), and give 0.6–0.9 g/ 2–3 fēn of *zhū shā fěn* (cinnabar powder) to be taken drenched with the decoction. *Zhū shā* is also sometimes used as an outside coating for medicinal pills. I have had definite results treating manically agitated schizophrenic patients using medicinals such as the following, varied according to presenting signs:

xiāng fù (香附 cyperus, Cyperi Rhizoma)
bái sháo (白芍 white peony, Paeoniae Radix Alba)
huáng qín (黄芩 scutellaria, Scutellariae Radix)
huáng lián (黄连 coptis, Coptidis Rhizoma)
tiān zhú huáng (天竹黄 bamboo sugar, Bambusae Concretio Silicea)
chāng pú (昌浦 acorus, Acori Tatarinowii Rhizoma)
yuǎn zhì (远志 polygala, Polygalae Radix)
yù jīn (郁金 curcuma, Curcumae Radix)
shēng dài zhě shí (生代赭石 crude hematite, Haematitum Crudum)
shēng mǔ lì (生牡蛎 crude oyster shell, Ostreae Concha Cruda)
shēng tiě luò (生铁落 iron flakes, Ferri Frusta)
zhū shā (朱砂 cinnabar, Cinnabaris) 0.6–0.9 g/2–3 fēn (taken drenched)

Cold in nature, *zhū shā* clears heat and quiets the spirit; thus it often figures in formulas designed to clear summerheat-heat and quiet the heart spirit. An example of this use is *yì yuán sǎn* (Origin-Boosting Powder), which contains *huá shí* (talcum), *gān cǎo* (licorice), and *zhū shā*. *Rén dān* (Human Elixir) and *bì wēn sǎn* (Scourge-Repelling Powder) are two summerheat-dispelling formulas that often contain *zhū shā*.

---

[29]Owing to its toxic nature, this medicinal is not readily available in the West. (Ed.)

Physicians of the past noted that "all painful, itchy sores belong to the heart" (诸痛痒疮皆属于心 *zhū tòng yǎng chuāng jiē shǔ yú xīn*). They believed that fire-heat in the blood could engender toxic sores and swollen welling-abscesses. *Zhū shā*, which clears heart heat, is also a commonly used heat-clearing toxin-resolving medicinal in external medicine and laryngology. For example, *zhū shā* combined with *bái jiāng cán* (silkworm) and *péng shā* (borax), ground to a fine powder, and used as a laryngeal insufflation, treats acute tonsillitis and sore swollen throat. *Yù yào shí sǎn* (Jade Key Powder), an ancient formula for sore throat comprised of *xī guā shuāng* (watermelon frost), *xī yuè shí* (borax), *fēi zhū shā* (water-ground cinnabar), *bái jiāng cán* (silkworm), and *bīng piàn* (borneol), is an effective laryngeal insufflation.

COMPARISONS

Zhēn zhū mǔ (mother-of-pearl)[163] quiets the spirit primarily through nourishing the heart yīn and downbearing heart fire, whereas *zhū shā* quiets the spirit primarily through settling fright and clearing heat.

Shēng tiě luò (iron flakes), a heavy settler that acts on the heart and liver, expels phlegm and precipitates qì, and treats mania and withdrawal irascibility. *Zhū shā*, a heart-settling and fire-downbearing medicinal, tends to treat evil heat in the heart channel with clouded spirit and delirious raving.

DOSAGE

The dosage is generally 0.3–0.9 g/1–3 fēn taken drenched with a decoction medicine. In severe patterns, use as much as 1.5–2.5 g/5–8 fēn.

RESEARCH

According to modern research, this medicinal reduces excitation in the central nervous system; thus it has a sedative effect.

CAUTION

Zhū shā must not be directly exposed to heat, otherwise it decomposes into metallic mercury, which causes poisoning. It must not be used in excessive dosages or for prolonged periods since this may also cause poisoning.

---

56. 琥珀 Hǔ Pò   Succinum
Amber

Hǔ pò (amber) is sweet in flavor and neutral in nature and has three main actions.

1. **Tranquilizing and Quieting the Spirit:** *Hǔ pò* is primarily used to treat epilepsy. When a severe sudden fright causes clouded spirit, ejection of white foam, hoisted eyes[552] (吊眼 *diào yǎn*, i.e., upturned eyes), and convulsions, this is called "fright epilepsy" (惊痫 *jīng xián*). In children this disease can be caused by seeing a strange sight or hearing a strange sound. *Hǔ pò* settles fright, quiets the spirit, and frees the orifices of the heart. It is frequently combined with medicinals such as *zhū shā* (cinnabar), *dǎn xīng* (bile arisaema), *niú huáng* (bovine bezoar), *quán*

xiē (scorpion), and *tiān zhú huáng* (bamboo sugar). An example of this use is *hŭ pò zhèn jīng wán* (Amber Fright-Settling Pill).

2. Disinhibiting Water and Freeing Strangury: *Hŭ pò* disinhibits urine through bland percolation. For bladder heat bind with bloody urine, painful urination, and urinary difficulty, it is combined with medicinals such as *mù tōng* (trifoliate akebia), *biăn xù* (knotgrass), *huá shí* (talcum), *fú líng* (poria), *zé xiè* (alisma), and *qū mài* (dianthus).

3. Dissipating Static Blood: When a woman has lochia that fails to clear and gradually develops pain in the lower abdomen that refuses pressure, and a hard, painful lump, this is the result of static blood. In such cases, *hŭ pò* is used to dissipate stasis and quicken the blood, frequently in combination with medicinals such as:

dāng guī (当归 Chinese angelica, Angelicae Sinensis Radix)

chuān xiōng (川芎 chuanxiong, Chuanxiong Rhizoma)

biē jiă (鳖甲 turtle shell, Trionycis Carapax)

sān léng (三棱 sparganium, Sparganii Rhizoma)

yán hú suŏ (延胡索 corydalis, Corydalis Rhizoma)

mò yào (没药 myrrh, Myrrha)

hóng huā (红花 carthamus, Carthami Flos)

táo rén (桃仁 peach kernel, Persicae Semen)

wŭ líng zhī (五灵脂 squirrel's droppings, Trogopteri Faeces)

COMPARISONS

Zhū shā (cinnabar)[165] settles with heaviness, clears heat, and quiets the spirit. *Hŭ pò* settles fright, frees the orifices, and quiets the spirit.

Zhēn zhū mŭ (mother-of-pearl)[163] settles the heart, calms the liver, and quiets the spirit, and it also removes **eye screens**[549] (目翳 *mù yì*) and closes sores. *Hŭ pò* settles the heart, frees the orifices, and quiets the spirit, and it also disinhibits water and frees strangury.

DOSAGE

The dosage is generally 0.3–2.5 g/1–8 fēn, taken drenched with a decoction medicine.

CAUTION

Contraindicated for scant urine or inhibited urination that result from yīn vacuity internal heat or insufficiency of the fluids.

---

57. 磁石 Cí Shí   Magnetitum
Loadstone

Acrid and salty in flavor and cold in nature, *cí shí* (loadstone) is a heavy-settling medicinal that supplements the kidney to promote qì absorption, settles the liver and subdues yáng, and stabilizes the mind and quiets the spirit.

1. Supplementing the Kidney to Promote Qì Absorption: For patterns of kidney vacuity with dilation of the pupils and unclear vision, or for dual vacuity of liver and kidney with visual clouding and darkness, black flowery spots in the vision (眼生黑花 yǎn shēng hēi huā), and cataracts, cí shí is often combined with medicinals such as:

> shú dì huáng (熟地黄 cooked rehmannia, Rehmanniae Radix Praeparata)
>
> shēng dì huáng (生地黄 dried/fresh rehmannia, Rehmanniae Radix Exsiccata seu Recens)
>
> gǒu qǐ zǐ (枸杞子 lycium, Lycii Fructus)
>
> jú huā (菊花 chrysanthemum, Chrysanthemi Flos)
>
> shí hú (石斛 dendrobium, Dendrobii Herba)
>
> bái sháo (白芍 white peony, Paeoniae Radix Alba)
>
> dāng guī (当归 Chinese angelica, Angelicae Sinensis Radix)
>
> tù sī zǐ (菟丝子 cuscuta, Cuscutae Semen)
>
> yè míng shā (夜明砂 bat's droppings, Verspertilionis Faeces)
>
> qīng xiāng zǐ (青葙子 celosia, Celosiae Semen)
>
> yáng gān (羊肝 goat's or sheep's liver, Caprae seu Ovis Iecur)
>
> zhū shā (朱砂 cinnabar, Cinnabaris)

Alternatively, it can be combined with zhū shā (cinnabar) and shén qū (medicated leaven) and made into pills. (Cí shí checks outward emission of essence and water, and zhū shā (cinnabar) does not allow fire-evil to invade upward.) This pill, which is called cí zhū wán (Loadstone and Cinnabar Pill), is commonly used to treat cataracts and is available in Chinese medicinal pharmacies. Enduring illness with enduring cough or weak constitution lead to kidney qì depletion or failure of the kidney to absorb qì. This gives rise to vacuity panting with signs such as shortness of breath and panting exacerbated by fatigue, inhalation more difficult than exhalation, a feeling that inhaled qì fails to reach the cinnabar field (the region below the umbilicus), or limp aching lumbus and knees, black face, and a weak cubit pulse. This pattern is known as vacuity panting caused by kidney failing to absorb qì. Cí shí, which conducts lung qì to the kidney, is used for this purpose in combination with medicines such as:

> shú dì huáng (熟地黄 cooked rehmannia, Rehmanniae Radix Praeparata)
>
> shān zhū yú (山茱萸 cornus, Corni Fructus)
>
> shān yào (山药 dioscorea, Dioscoreae Rhizoma)
>
> dān pí (丹皮 moutan, Moutan Cortex)
>
> fú líng (茯苓 poria, Poria)
>
> zé xiè (泽泻 alisma, Alismatis Rhizoma)
>
> ròu guì (肉桂 cinnamon bark, Cinnamomi Cortex)
>
> wǔ wèi zǐ (五味子 schisandra, Schisandrae Fructus)
>
> fù piàn (附片 sliced aconite, Aconiti Radix Lateralis Praeparata Secta)
>
> chén xiāng (沉香 aquilaria, Aquilariae Lignum Resinatum)
>
> sū zǐ (苏子 perilla fruit, Perillae Fructus)
>
> xìng rén (杏仁 apricot kernel, Armeniacae Semen)

This formula promotes absorption of qì by the kidney to calm panting.

2. Settling the Liver and Subduing Yáng: When in liver-kidney yīn vacuity, the vacuous liver and kidney allow yáng to harass the upper body, causing tinnitus, deafness, dizziness, flowery vision, and headache, *cí shí* is frequently combined with medicinals such as:

shēng dì huáng (生地黄 dried/fresh rehmannia, Rehmanniae Radix Exsiccata seu Recens)

bái sháo (白芍 white peony, Paeoniae Radix Alba)

shēng dài zhě shí (生代赭石 crude hematite, Haematitum Crudum)

shēng shí jué míng (生石决明 crude abalone shell, Haliotidis Concha Cruda)

chán tuì (蝉蜕 cicada molting, Cicadae Periostracum)

jú huā (菊花 chrysanthemum, Chrysanthemi Flos)

huáng qín (黄芩 scutellaria, Scutellariae Radix)

sāng jì shēng (桑寄生 mistletoe, Taxilli Herba)

3. Stabilizing the Mind and Quieting the Spirit: For disquieted heart spirit[546] (心神不安 *xīn shén bù ān*), fright, fear, insomnia, flusteredness, vacuity timidity, and epilepsy, *cí shí* is combined with:

yuǎn zhì (远志 polygala, Polygalae Radix)

zhū shā (朱砂 cinnabar, Cinnabaris)

zhēn zhū mǔ (珍珠母 mother-of-pearl, Concha Margaritifera)

dāng guī (当归 Chinese angelica, Angelicae Sinensis Radix)

bái sháo (白芍 white peony, Paeoniae Radix Alba)

bǎi zǐ rén (柏子仁 arborvitae seed, Platycladi Semen)

lóng chǐ (龙齿 dragon tooth, Mastodi Dentis Fossilia)

fú shén (茯神 root poria, Poria cum Pini Radice)

COMPARISONS

Shēng dài zhě shí (crude hematite)[332] settles qì in the reverting yīn (pericardium), eliminates heat from the blood vessels, nourishes the blood and settles counterflow, and also settles and downbears liver yáng. *Cí shí* settles and absorbs upward floating lesser yīn (*shào yīn*) fire, promotes interaction of the heart and kidney, and stabilizes the mind and quiets the spirit. *Zhě shí* (hematite) tends to enter the heart and liver, whereas *cí shí* tends to enter the liver and kidney.

Zǐ shí yīng (fluorite) is a heavy settling medicinal that supplements the blood aspect of the heart and liver and also warms the uterus. *Cí shí* is a heavy settling medicinal that supplements the kidney and nourishes the liver, as well as promotes qì absorption in the kidney.

Hēi qiān (minium) promotes absorption of qì by the kidney; working from the upper body downward, it settles and downbears counterflow ascent of kidney qì. *Cí shí* also promotes absorption of qì by the kidney; working from the lower body upward, it conducts lung fire downward and promotes qì absorption in the kidney.

Líng cí shí (magnetic loadstone), i.e., *cí shí* (loadstone) that is magnetized, is even more effective.

Miscellaneous

Because *cí shí* (loadstone) is a ferrous ore, it is best combined with medicinals such as *shén qū* (medicated leaven) and *jī nèi jīn* (gizzard lining) that aid digestion by promoting absorption of iron and preventing damage to the stomach.

Dosage

The dosage is generally 9–30 g/3 qián–1 liǎng. It should be crushed and predecocted.

---

58. 龙骨 Lóng Gǔ
Dragon Bone

Mastodi
Ossis Fossilia

Lóng gǔ (dragon bone) is sweet and astringent in flavor and neutral in nature. It is used raw (crude) or calcined. *Shēng lóng gǔ* (crude dragon bone) calms the liver and subdues yáng, and tranquilizes and quiets the spirit; *duàn lóng gǔ* (calcined dragon bone) secures and astringes.

For vexation and agitation, insomnia, and dizzy head and vision that are a result of yīn vacuity and yáng hyperactivity, *shēng lóng gǔ* is used to calm the liver and subdue yáng. It is frequently combined with medicinals such as *shēng dì huáng* (dried/fresh rehmannia), *bái sháo* (white peony), *xuán shēn* (scrophularia), *bái jí lí* (tribulus), *huáng qín* (scutellaria), *yuǎn zhì* (polygala), and *shēng mǔ lì* (crude oyster shell). When receiving a fright causes disquieted heart spirit, or when heart vacuity causes susceptibility to fright, palpitations, insomnia, and susceptibility to being awoken from sleep by fright, *shēng lóng gǔ* can be used to settle fright and quiet the spirit. For this pattern it is frequently combined with medicinals such as:

yuǎn zhì (远志 polygala, Polygalae Radix)

fú shén (茯神 root poria, Poria cum Pini Radice)

hǔ pò (琥珀 amber, Succinum)

lóng chǐ (龙齿 dragon tooth, Mastodi Dentis Fossilia)

dāng guī (当归 Chinese angelica, Angelicae Sinensis Radix)

shú dì huáng (熟地黄 cooked rehmannia, Rehmanniae Radix Praeparata)

zhēn zhū mǔ (珍珠母 mother-of-pearl, Concha Margaritifera)

When appropriate according to pattern identification, *shēng lóng gǔ* is used in formulas that treat insomnia, headache, or vexation and agitation.

Duàn lóng gǔ astringes, secures, and astringes more effectively than *shēng lóng gǔ*, and hence is often used to treat profuse sweating, seminal emission, flooding and spotting, excessive white vaginal discharge, enuresis, and enduring dysentery. For example, to treat spontaneous sweating, *duàn lóng gǔ* is combined with medicinals such as *má huáng gēn* (ephedra root), *fú xiǎo mài* (light wheat), *shēng huáng qí* (raw astragalus), and *bái zhú* (white atractylodes); to treat night sweating, it is combined with *mài dōng* (ophiopogon), *wǔ wèi zǐ* (schisandra), *shēng dì huáng* (dried/fresh rehmannia), and *mǔ lì* (oyster shell); to treat seminal emission, it is combined with *jīn yīng zǐ* (Cherokee rose fruit), *suǒ yáng* (cynomorium), *huáng bǎi* (phellodendron), *yuǎn zhì* (polygala), and *lián zǐ xīn* (lotus plumule); to treat flooding and spotting, it is combined with *sāng jì shēng* (mistletoe), *xù duàn tàn* (charred dipsacus), *duàn mǔ lì* (calcined oyster shell), *zōng tàn* (charred trachycarpus), and *ē jiāo* (ass hide glue); to treat white vaginal discharge, it is combined with *shū gēn bái pí* (ailanthus root bark), *cāng zhú* (atractylodes), *yǐ mǐ* (coix), and *fú líng* (poria); to treat enuresis, it is combined with *sāng piāo xiāo* (mantis egg-case), *fù pén zǐ* (rubus), *yì zhì rén* (alpinia), *wū yào* (lindera), and *shān zhū yú* (cornus); and, finally, to treat enduring dysentery, it is combined with *chì shí zhī* (halloysite), *mù xiāng* (costusroot), and *wū méi* (mume).

COMPARISONS

Lóng chǐ (dragon tooth) and *lóng gǔ* are broadly similar in their effects, but *lóng chǐ* quiets the spirit and tranquilizes more effectively, while *lóng gǔ* secures and astringes essential qì in the lower burner more effectively.

Although both *mǔ lì* (oyster shell)[171] and *lóng gǔ* calm the liver and subdue yáng, *mǔ lì* (oyster shell) also softens hardness and dissipate binds, downbears phlegm and eliminates concretions, whereas *lóng gǔ* also stanches bleeding and checks dysentery.

In external medicine, *duàn lóng gǔ* is commonly used in topically-applied medicinal preparations to engender flesh and close sores.

DOSAGE

The dosage is generally 9–15 g/3–5 qián. *Shēng lóng gǔ* (生龙骨, crude dragon bone) dosages can be as much as 20–30 g/7 qián–1 liǎng, but it is inappropiate to use *duàn lóng gǔ* in very large doses.[30]

CAUTION

Contraindicated for patterns with exuberant fire and seminal emission. Mistaken use can result in painful, inhibited voidings of reddish urine.

---

59. 牡蛎 Mǔ Lì   Ostreae Concha
Oyster Shell

Mǔ lì (oyster shell) is salty in flavor and cold in nature. *Shēng mǔ lì* boosts yīn and subdues yáng, clears heat and resolves thirst, softens hardness and dissipates binds. *Duàn mǔ lì* (煅牡蛎, Calcined oyster shell) reduces urination and checks vaginal discharge.[31]

For vexation and agitation, insomnia, and night sweating that are the result of yīn vacuity and yáng hyperactivity, *mǔ lì* boosts yīn and subdues yáng. For this purpose it is frequently combined with:

---

[30] The restriction on the dosage of *duàn lóng gǔ* (calcined dragon bone) is primarily attributable to its strongly astringent nature. (Ed.)

[31] Modern practitioners also use *mǔ lì* (oyster shell) to neutralize excess stomach acid in the treatment of gastric or duodenal ulcers. (Ed.)

shēng lóng gǔ (生龙骨 crude dragon bone, Mastodi Ossis Fossilia Cruda)

shēng dì huáng (生地黄 dried/fresh rehmannia, Rehmanniae Radix Exsiccata seu Recens)

bái sháo (白芍 white peony, Paeoniae Radix Alba)

huáng qín (黄芩 scutellaria, Scutellariae Radix)

xiāng fù (香附 cyperus, Cyperi Rhizoma)

yuǎn zhì (远志 polygala, Polygalae Radix)

yè jiāo téng (夜交藤 flowery knotweed stem, Polygoni Multiflori Caulis)

Shēng mǔ lì boosts the kidney, nourishes yīn, clears heat, allays thirst, and eliminates vexation. For nighttime thirst and vacuity heat vexation and agitation that result from yīn vacuity, *shēng mǔ lì* is combined with:

xuán shēn (玄参 scrophularia, Scrophulariae Radix)

shēng dì huáng (生地黄 dried/fresh rehmannia, Rehmanniae Radix Exsiccata seu Recens)

tiān huā fěn (天花粉 trichosanthes root, Trichosanthis Radix)

bái sháo (白芍 white peony, Paeoniae Radix Alba)

shí hú (石斛 dendrobium, Dendrobii Herba)

Shēng mǔ lì transforms phlegm and dissipates binds. For example, *shēng mǔ lì*, *xuán shēn* (scrophularia), and *chuān bèi mǔ* (Sìchuān fritillaria), ground to a powder, formed into a honey pill, and taken twice a day at a dosage of 9 g/ 3 qián each time, are used to disperse scrofula or phlegm nodes (as in tuberculosis of the cervical lymph nodes, thyroma, and granuloma of the cervical lymph nodes).

For concretions and aggregations in the abdomen, and mother-of-malaria (hepatosplenomegaly and hard swellings in the abdomen), *shēng mǔ lì* softens hardness, dissipates binds, and disperses swellings. I often use *shēng mǔ lì* (crude oyster shell) combined with the following medicinals:

biē jiǎ (鳖甲 turtle shell, Trionycis Carapax)

hóng huā (红花 carthamus, Carthami Flos)

táo rén (桃仁 peach kernel, Persicae Semen)

sān léng (三棱 sparganium, Sparganii Rhizoma)

é zhú (莪术 curcuma rhizome, Curcumae Rhizoma)

yù jīn (郁金 curcuma, Curcumae Radix)

chái hú (柴胡 bupleurum, Bupleuri Radix)

shén qū (神曲 medicated leaven, Massa Medicata Fermentata)

shān zhā hé (山楂核 crataegus pit, Crataegi Endocarpium et Semen)

shè gān (射干 belamcanda, Belamcandae Rhizoma)

bái zhú (白术 white atractylodes, Atractylodis Macrocephalae Rhizoma)

This can also be prepared in pill form for long-term use.

Duàn mǔ lì has a stronger securing and astringing action. It is often used for white vaginal discharge, flooding and spotting, seminal emission, and enuresis. For these patterns it is combined with medicinals such as:

bái zhú (白术 white atractylodes, Atractylodis Macrocephalae Rhizoma)

cāng zhú (苍术 atractylodes, Atractylodis Rhizoma)

shān zhū yú (山茱萸 cornus, Corni Fructus)

shān yào (山药 dioscorea, Dioscoreae Rhizoma)

lián zǐ xīn (莲子心 lotus plumule, Nelumbinis Plumula)

sāng piāo xiāo (桑螵蛸 mantis egg-case, Mantidis Oötheca)

yì zhì rén (益智仁 alpinia, Alpiniae Oxyphyllae Fructus)

fù pén zǐ (覆盆子 rubus, Rubi Fructus)

Mǔ lì contains calcium; in combination with medicinals such as *cāng zhú* (atractylodes) it treats rickets due to calcium deficiency in children.

COMPARISON

Hǎi gé fěn (clamshell powder), which is salty and transforms phlegm, tends to be used for cough with sticky phlegm that is not easily expectorated. *Mǔ lì*, which likewise is salty and transforms phlegm, tends to be used to soften hardness and dissipate binds, such as in the treatment of scrofula, phlegm nodes, and concretions and conglomerations.

DOSAGE

The dosage is generally 9–30 g/3 qián–1 liǎng. The dosage of *duàn mǔ lì* should be slightly less.

---

60. 浮小麦 Fú Xiǎo Mài
Light Wheat
Tritici
Fructus Levis

Including

  ▷ *Xiǎo mài* (小麦 wheat, Tritici Fructus)
  ▷ *Mài miáo* (麦苗 wheat sprouts, Tritici Fructus Germinatus)

Sweet in flavor and cool in nature, *fú xiǎo mài* (light wheat) is a commonly used sweat-checking medicinal.

"Sweat is the humor of the heart." *Fú xiǎo mài* enters the heart channel and checks sweating with sweetness and coolness. To treat yáng vacuity spontaneous sweating, it is combined with *shēng huáng qí* (raw astragalus), *má huáng gēn* (ephedra root), and *mǔ lì* (oyster shell). To treat yīn vacuity night sweating, it is combined with:

bǎi zǐ rén (柏子仁 arborvitae seed, Platycladi Semen)

mài dōng (麦冬 ophiopogon, Ophiopogonis Radix)

wǔ wèi zǐ (五味子 schisandra, Schisandrae Fructus)

bái sháo (白芍 white peony, Paeoniae Radix Alba)

shēng dì huáng (生地黄 dried/fresh rehmannia, Rehmanniae Radix Exsiccata seu Recens)

Fú xiǎo mài is also used during enduring illness or after a major illness when consumption of fluids and essence-blood results in yīn vacuity that manifests in vexation, night sweating, postmeridian tidal heat [effusion] (fever), emaciation, dry tender red tongue, and fine rapid pulse. For this purpose, *fú xiǎo mài* is frequently combined with medicinals such as:

shā shēn (沙参 adenophora/glehnia, Adenophorae seu Glehniae Radix)

mài dōng (麦冬 ophiopogon, Ophiopogonis Radix)

wǔ wèi zǐ (五味子 schisandra, Schisandrae Fructus)

bái sháo (白芍 white peony, Paeoniae Radix Alba)

shēng dì huáng (生地黄 dried/fresh rehmannia, Rehmanniae Radix Exsiccata seu Recens)

dì gǔ pí (地骨皮 lycium root bark, Lycii Cortex)

xuán shēn (玄参 scrophularia, Scrophulariae Radix)

qín jiāo (秦艽 large gentian, Gentianae Macrophyllae Radix)

biē jiǎ (鳖甲 turtle shell, Trionycis Carapax)

Fú xiǎo mài is selected from *xiǎo mài* (wheat) that is placed in a container of water. The lighter grains that are dry and shrivelled or that still bear their husk float to the surface of the water and are separated out for use as *fú xiǎo mài*.[32] *Fú xiǎo mài* is a commonly used medicinal substance. *Xiǎo mài* (wheat), i.e., the part that does not float to the surface of the water, can also be used as medicine. Neutral and sweet, it nourishes the heart and eliminates vexation, and is used for signs such as sorrow, frequent crying, and depression in visceral agitation (脏躁 *zàng zào*, recognized in modern medicine as hysteria). An example of this use is *gān mài dà zǎo tāng* (Licorice, Wheat, and Jujube Decoction) (*gān cǎo* (licorice), *xiǎo mài* (wheat), and *dà zǎo* (jujube)) from *Jīn Guì Yào Lüè* (金匮要略 "Essential Prescriptions of the Golden Coffer"). When the symptoms are appropriate, *xiǎo mài* (wheat) is used in combination with medicinals that course the liver, resolve depression, nourish the heart, and quiet the spirit. For example, it is combined with medicinals such as the following:

xiāng fù (香附 cyperus, Cyperi Rhizoma)

bái sháo (白芍 white peony, Paeoniae Radix Alba)

chái hú (柴胡 bupleurum, Bupleuri Radix)

yuǎn zhì (远志 polygala, Polygalae Radix)

fú shén (茯神 root poria, Poria cum Pini Radice)

zhēn zhū mǔ (珍珠母 mother-of-pearl, Concha Margaritifera)

lóng chǐ (龙齿 dragon tooth, Mastodi Dentis Fossilia)

Because *xiǎo mài* (wheat) and *fú xiǎo mài* (light wheat) are not the same, when writing a prescription, *xiǎo mài* (wheat) is usually written as *huái xiǎo mài* 淮小麦 or *jìng xiǎo mài* 净小麦.

Mài miào (wheat sprouts) are acrid and cold; they eliminate heat vexation and abate jaundice.

Comparison

Má huáng gēn (ephedra root)[175] secures the interstices to check sweating. *Fú*

---

[32]The selection process is reflected in the Chinese name of the medicinal, *fú xiǎo mài* 浮小麦, which literally means "floating wheat." (Ed.)

xiǎo mài eliminates vacuity heat in the heart channel to check sweating. *Xiǎo mài* nourishes the heart and eliminates vexation, but does not check sweating.

DOSAGE

The dosage is generally 9–30 g/3 qián–1 liǎng. The dosage of *xiǎo mài* (wheat) is the same.

---

61. 麻黄根 Má Huáng Gēn   Ephedrae Radix
Ephedra Root

Sweet in flavor and neutral in nature, *má huáng gēn* (ephedra root) is a commonly used sweat-checking medicinal. It conducts qì-supplementing medicinals to the defense aspect and secures the interstices to check sweating. Combined with *shēng huáng qí* (raw astragalus), *duàn mǔ lì* (calcined oyster shell), *fú xiǎo mài* (light wheat), *dǎng shēn* (codonopsis), and *bái zhú* (white atractylodes), it is often used for spontaneous sweating that results from yáng vacuity and insecurity of defense qì. Combined with *dì huáng* (rehmannia), *shān zhū yú* (cornus), *wǔ wèi zǐ* (schisandra), *bǎi zǐ rén* (arborvitae seed), *mài dōng* (ophiopogon), and *shēng mǔ lì* (crude oyster shell), it is used for yīn vacuity internal heat, vacuity vexation, insomnia, tidal heat, and night sweating. *Má huáng gēn* combined with blood-nourishing and exterior-securing medicinals such as *dāng guī* (Chinese angelica) and *huáng qí* (astragalus) treats postpartum vacuity sweating.

DOSAGE

The dosage is generally 6–9 g/2-3 qián.

---

62. 金樱子 Jīn Yīng Zǐ   Rosae
Cherokee Rose Fruit   Laevigatae Fructus

Sour and astringent in flavor and neutral in nature, *jīn yīng zǐ* (Cherokee rose fruit) supplements the kidney and secures qì, astringes essence and secures the intestines.

For seminal efflux[562] (滑精 *huá jīng*) and seminal emission[562] (遺精 *yí jīng*) due to kidney vacuity, *jīn yīng zǐ* is combined with *qiàn shí* (euryale), *lóng gǔ* (dragon bone), *mǔ lì* (oyster shell), and *suǒ yáng* (cynomorium). For enuresis, it is combined with *sāng piāo xiāo* (mantis egg-case), *fù pén zǐ* (rubus), *shān yào* (dioscorea), and *lián xū* (lotus stamen). For excessive vaginal discharge, it is combined with *shān yào* (dioscorea), *qiàn shí* (euryale), *lián zǐ* (lotus seed), *cāng zhú* (atractylodes), and *fú líng* (poria).

"The kidney controls urine and stool." *Jīn yīng zǐ* not only supplements the kidney and secures qì, secures the essence gate, checks vaginal discharge, and constrains urine, it also secures and astringes the large intestine and checks diarrhea. It is frequently used to treat chronic diarrhea in combination with medicinals such as:

> *bǔ gǔ zhī* (补骨脂 psoralea, Psoraleae Fructus)
> *shān yào* (山药 dioscorea, Dioscoreae Rhizoma)
> *qiàn shí* (芡实 euryale, Euryales Semen)
> *fú líng* (茯苓 poria, Poria)
> *wǔ wèi zǐ* (五味子 schisandra, Schisandrae Fructus)
> *ròu dòu kòu* (肉豆蔻 nutmeg, Myristicae Semen)
> *dǎng shēn* (党参 codonopsis, Codonopsis Radix)
> *bái zhú* (白术 white atractylodes, Atractylodis Macrocephalae Rhizoma)

I often treat chronic dysentery and intractable chronic enteritis with satisfactory effect by using *sì shén wán* (Four Spirits Pill) combined with *fù zǐ lǐ zhōng tāng* (Aconite Center-Rectifying Decoction) (both formulas are given below) as well as *jīn yīng zǐ* (Cherokee rose fruit), *hē zǐ* (chebule), and *fú líng* (poria), varying the formula according to the pattern.

Sì shén wán 四神丸   Four Spirits Pill

> *bǔ gǔ zhī* (补骨脂 psoralea, Psoraleae Fructus)
> *wú zhū yú* (吴茱萸 evodia, Evodiae Fructus)
> *wǔ wèi zǐ* (五味子 schisandra, Schisandrae Fructus)
> *ròu dòu kòu* (肉豆蔻 nutmeg, Myristicae Semen)

Fù zǐ lǐ zhōng tāng 附子理中汤   Aconite Center-Rectifying Decoction

---

> *fù zǐ* (附子 aconite, Aconiti Radix Lateralis Praeparata)
> *bái zhú* (白术 white atractylodes, Atractylodis Macrocephalae Rhizoma)
> *dǎng shēn* (党参 codonopsis, Codonopsis Radix)
> *gān jiāng* (干姜 dried ginger, Zingiberis Rhizoma)
> *zhì gān cǎo* (炙甘草 mix-fried licorice, Glycyrrhizae Radix cum Liquido Fricta)

COMPARISON

Lián xū (lotus stamen) treats seminal emission by clearing the heart and securing essence. *Jīn yīng zǐ* (Cherokee rose fruit) treats seminal emission by tightening kidney qì and securing essence. Use *lián xū* for seminal emission with dreams; use *jīn yīng zǐ* for seminal efflux or seminal emission without dreaming.

Jīn yīng zǐ is made into a liquid paste that is commercially available as *jīn yīng zǐ gāo* (Cherokee Rose Fruit Paste). This is used for seminal emission, enuresis, vaginal discharge, and enduring diarrhea and is convenient to take.

RESEARCH

According to modern research, *jīn yīng zǐ* causes contraction of the intestinal mucosa, reduces secretions, and therefore has an antidiarrheal action. It is also used for chronic enteritis.

DOSAGE

The dosage is generally 4.5–9 g/1.5–3 qián.

Caution

Contraindicated for seminal emission, painful urination, or frequent urination that are the result of repletion fire and evil heat in the heart and kidney.

---

63. 莲子 Lián Zǐ
Lotus Seed
Nelumbinis Semen

Including

> ▷ *Lián zǐ xīn* (莲子心 lotus plumule, Nelumbinis Plumula)

Sweet and astringent in flavor and neutral in nature, *lián zǐ* (lotus seed) nourishes the heart, fortifies the spleen, supplements the kidney, and secures and astringes. When *lián zǐ* is used as medicine, the skin and embryo (heart) are removed; thus it is also called *lián ròu* 莲肉 or *lián zǐ ròu* 莲子肉.[33]

Lián zǐ (lotus seed) enters the heart channel. For patterns of heart vacuity or noninteraction of the heart and kidney with disquieted heart spirit, insomnia, and profuse dreaming, it is frequently combined with medicinals such as *fú shén* (root poria), *yuǎn zhì* (polygala), *bǎi zǐ rén* (arborvitae seed), *zhēn zhū mǔ* (mother-of-pearl), and *lóng chǐ* (dragon tooth).

Lián zǐ fortifies the spleen, and thickens the stomach and intestines (厚肠胃 *hòu cháng wèi*).[34] For this purpose it is frequently combined with *bái zhú* (white atractylodes), *shān yào* (dioscorea), *bái biǎn dòu* (lablab), *fú líng* (poria), *dǎng shēn* (codonopsis), *qiàn shí* (euryale), and *mù xiāng* (costusroot); this combination is used to treat spleen vacuity diarrhea, indigestion, sloppy stool, reduced eating, yellow-white face, emaciation, and other signs of spleen vacuity.

For seminal emission that results from heart-kidney vacuity, *lián zǐ* is frequently combined with *shēng dì huáng* (dried/fresh rehmannia), *shān zhū yú* (cornus), *wǔ wèi zǐ* (schisandra), *yuǎn zhì* (polygala), *jīn yīng zǐ* (Cherokee rose fruit), and *suǒ yáng* (cynomorium).

For dual vacuity of the spleen and kidney with dampness evil pouring downward and causing enduring diarrhea, excessive vaginal discharge, and **white turbidity**[567] (白浊 *bái zhuó*), *lián zǐ* is used to secure the lower burner. For this purpose it is frequently combined with medicinals such as the following:

ròu dòu kòu (肉豆蔻 nutmeg, Myristicae Semen)

qiàn shí (芡实 euryale, Euryales Semen)

bái jī guān huā (白鸡冠花 white cockscomb, Celosiae Cristatae Flos Albus)

chǎo shān yào (炒山药 stir-fried dioscorea, Dioscoreae Rhizoma Frictum)

chǎo yǐ mǐ (炒苡米 stir-fried coix, Coicis Semen Frictum)

hē zǐ (诃子 chebule, Chebulae Fructus)

---

[33] The 肉 *ròu* in the name of this medicinal means "flesh" in reference to the edible substance of the lotus seed. (Ed.)

[34] Thicken the stomach and intestines, 厚肠胃 *hòu cháng wèi*: To improve stomach and intestinal function. (Ed.)

bái zhú (白术 white atractylodes, Atractylodis Macrocephalae Rhizoma)

fú líng (茯苓 poria, Poria)

bái shí zhī (白石脂 kaolin, Kaolin)

Lián zǐ (lotus seed) nourishes the heart and fortifies the spleen. *Lián zǐ xīn* (lotus plumule) clears and discharges heart heat. *Lián fáng tàn* (charred lotus receptacle) stanches bleeding. *Lián xū* (lotus stamen) astringes essence and secures the kidney.

Qiàn shí (euryale) and *lián zǐ* are both sweet and neutral securing and astringing medicinals. However, *qiàn shí* is used to secure the kidney and astringe essence, whereas *lián zǐ* is used to nourish the heart and fortify the spleen.

DOSAGE

The dosage is generally 2–10 g/7 fēn–3 qián.

---

64. 海螵蛸 Hǎi Piāo Xiāo   Sepiae Endoconcha
Cuttlefish Bone

Also called *wū zéi gǔ* 乌贼骨. Salty and astringent in flavor and slightly warm in nature, *hǎi piāo xiāo* (cuttlefish bone) enters the blood aspect of the liver and kidney, frees the blood vessels, quickens the channels and network vessels, supplements liver blood, and dispels cold-damp. It also stanches bleeding, checks vaginal discharge, secures essence, and has an antacid effect.

Physicians of the past used *hǎi piāo xiāo* and *qiàn cǎo* (madder), ground to a powder, mixed with sparrow's egg, and made into pills that were swallowed with abalone soup, to treat menstrual block in women with liver damage or blood dessication. I often use this formula in combination with an appropriate decoction medicine to treat menstrual block in young women for which laboratory testing, fluoroscopy, and physical examination have not revealed any cause, and that is accompanied by steaming bone tidal heat [effusion] (fever), emaciation, and night sweating. This treatment usually produces satisfactory results.

Hǎi piāo xiāo frees the blood vessels, quickens the channels and network vessels, and dispels cold-damp. Physicians of the past often used this medicinal to treat periumbilical abdominal pain, stomach duct pain, and vomiting of acid and water. It frees the network vessels, quickens the blood, relieves pain, and controls acid. In accordance with pattern indentification, it is frequently combined with medicinals such as:

gāo liáng jiāng (高良姜 lesser galangal, Alpiniae Officinarum Rhizoma)

xiāng fù (香附 cyperus, Cyperi Rhizoma)

wǔ líng zhī (五灵脂 squirrel's droppings, Trogopteri Faeces)

dān shēn (丹参 salvia, Salviae Miltiorrhizae Radix)

bái sháo (白芍 white peony, Paeoniae Radix Alba)

dāng guī (当归 Chinese angelica, Angelicae Sinensis Radix)

wū yào (乌药 lindera, Linderae Radix)

In recent years there have been reports of using *hǎi piāo xiāo* combined with *bái jí* (bletilla), *bèi mǔ* (fritillaria), and *gān cǎo* (licorice), ground to a powder, and taken drenched, to treat bleeding from ulcers. This method has achieved excellent effects.

Hǎi piāo xiāo astringes and stanches bleeding, and so it is used to treat various forms of bleeding. Because it enters the blood aspect of the liver and kidney, and because the liver and kidney govern the lower burner, it is often used for flooding (major bleeding from the womb). For this purpose it is combined with:

bái zhú (白术 white atractylodes, Atractylodis Macrocephalae Rhizoma)

huáng qí (黄芪 astragalus, Astragali Radix)

duàn lóng gǔ (煅龙骨 calcined dragon bone, Mastodi Ossis Fossilia Calcinata)

duàn mǔ lì (煅牡蛎 calcined oyster shell, Ostreae Concha Calcinata)

shān yú ròu (山萸肉 cornus, Corni Fructus)

wǔ wèi zǐ (五味子 schisandra, Schisandrae Fructus)

tù sī zǐ (菟丝子 cuscuta, Cuscutae Semen)

xù duàn tàn (续断炭 charred dipsacus, Dipsaci Radix Carbonisata)

lián fáng tàn (莲房炭 charred lotus receptacle, Nelumbinis Receptaculum Carbonisatum)

zōng lǘ tàn (棕榈炭 charred trachycarpus, Trachycarpi Petiolus Carbonisatus)

Gǔ chōng tāng (Thoroughfare-Securing Decoction) from *Zhōng Zhōng Cān Xī Lù* (衷中参西录 "Chinese Medicine with Reference to Western Medicine") contains this medicinal, because it has an excellent capacity to treat flooding[550] (血崩 *xuè bēng*).

Hǎi piāo xiāo is often used to treat red and white vaginal discharge[566] (带下 *dài xià*). For this purpose it is commonly combined with *shān yào* (dioscorea), *lóng gǔ* (dragon bone), and *mǔ lì* (oyster shell).

RESEARCH

According to modern research, *hǎi piāo xiāo* contains calcium and colloids and is a good antacid and hemostatic agent. It is taken internally or applied topically. When taken internally, a powder preparation is more effective than a decoction preparation.

Lóng gǔ (dragon bone)[170] and *hǎi piāo xiāo* are both astringent, but the astringent quality of *lóng gǔ* can cause stagnation, whereas within the astringent quality of *hǎi piāo xiāo* there is strength to quicken stasis.

Sāng piāo xiāo (mantis egg-case)[190] supplements the kidney qì and is often used to secure kidney essence and reduce urination. *Hǎi piāo xiāo* supplements liver blood and is often used to check flooding and vaginal discharge and to treat abdominal pain.

DOSAGE

The dosage is generally 3–9 g/1–3 qián. In powder preparations that are swallowed, 0.3–2 g/1–7 fēn can be used.

CAUTION

Inappropriate when there is evil heat in the inner body or for exterior patterns.

---

65. 瓦楞子 Wǎ Léng Zǐ   Arcae Concha
Ark Shell

Wǎ léng zǐ (ark shell) is salty in flavor and neutral in nature. *Shēng wǎ léng zǐ* (crude ark shell) softens hardness and dissipates binds, disperses phlegm and dispels stasis, whereas *duàn wǎ léng zǐ* (calcined ark shell) checks hyperchlorhydria (excessive stomach acid).

For concretions, conglomerations, aggregations, and glomus in the abdomen, old phlegm accumulations and lumps, and undefined swellings, *wǎ léng zǐ* softens hardness and dissipates binds, disperses accumulation lumps, and dispels blood stasis. It can be combined with medicinals such as those given below, care being taken to vary the formula according to the pattern identified.

zhǐ shí (枳实 unripe bitter orange, Aurantii Fructus Immaturus)

bái zhú (白术 white atractylodes, Atractylodis Macrocephalae Rhizoma)

shēng mǔ lì (生牡蛎 crude oyster shell, Ostreae Concha Cruda)

shān zhā hé (山楂核 crataegus pit, Crataegi Endocarpium et Semen)

lái fú zǐ (莱菔子 radish seed, Raphani Semen)

hóng huā (红花 carthamus, Carthami Flos)

chì sháo (赤芍 red peony, Paeoniae Radix Rubra)

dāng guī (当归 Chinese angelica, Angelicae Sinensis Radix)

guì zhī (桂枝 cinnamon twig, Cinnamomi Ramulus)

chuān shān jiǎ (穿山甲 pangolin scales, Manis Squama)

é zhú (莪术 curcuma rhizome, Curcumae Rhizoma)

For stomach duct pain, acid upflow, acid vomiting, and hyperchlorhydria, *duàn wǎ léng zǐ* (calcined ark shell) is used to control acid and relieve pain. For this purpose it is frequently combined with:

gāo liáng jiāng (高良姜 lesser galangal, Alpiniae Officinarum Rhizoma)

xiāng fù (香附 cyperus, Cyperi Rhizoma)

wú zhū yú (吴茱萸 evodia, Evodiae Fructus)

huáng lián (黄连 coptis, Coptidis Rhizoma)

cǎo dòu kòu (草豆蔻 Katsumada's galangal seed, Alpiniae Katsumadai Semen)

mù xiāng (木香 costusroot, Aucklandiae Radix)

bàn xià (半夏 pinellia, Pinelliae Rhizoma)

fú líng (茯苓 poria, Poria)

yán hú suǒ (延胡索 corydalis, Corydalis Rhizoma)

In recent years a combination of *duàn wǎ léng zǐ* (calcined ark shell) and *gān cǎo* (licorice) (in equal proportions), ground to a fine powder and taken at a dosage of 2–4 g/7 fēn–1.3 qián, three times a day with warm water, has been effective in the treatment of stomach and duodenal ulcers and hyperchlorhydria (excessive stomach acid). For dry stool, add *shēng dà huáng* (raw rhubarb); for liking of warmth in the stomach region, add *gāo liáng jiāng* (lesser galangal); for pronounced stomach pain with a fixed location, add *yán hú suŏ* (corydalis) and *wŭ líng zhī* (squirrel's droppings).

The use of *duàn wă léng zĭ* can cause dry stool. Thus, for patterns of stomach duct pain and acid vomiting in which there is also dry stool, *duàn wă léng zĭ* should be combined with *shēng dà huáng* (raw rhubarb) and *fān xiè yè* (senna).

Comparisons

Hăi piāo xiāo[178] frees the blood vessels, dispels cold-damp, and treats abdominal pain. *Wă léng zĭ* softens hardness and dissipates binds, disperses phlegm accumulations, and treats stomach pain.

Yán hú suŏ (corydalis)[382] treats stomach pain because it quickens the blood and moves qì, whereas *wă léng zĭ* treats stomach pain because it controls acid and dispels stasis.

Dosage

The dosage is generally 6–9 g/2–3 qián. When necessary, use 12–18 g/4–6 qián. When used raw, *wă léng zĭ* should be crushed and predecocted.

Caution

Inappropriate for patients who normally have dry bound stool.

---

66. 赤石脂 Chì Shí Zhī   Halloysitum Rubrum
Halloysite

Including

> ▷ *bái shí zhī* (白石脂 kaolin, Kaolin)

Chì shí zhī (halloysite) is a naturally occurring, red-colored, *gāo lĭng tŭ* (kaolin) with high water content; it is primarily produced in Shānxī, Hénán, and Jiāngsū provinces. Once the impurities are removed, it is ground into a fine powder and used as a medicinal substance. Sweet, sour, and astringent in flavor and warm in nature, *chì shí zhī* secures and astringes, contracts dampness, constrains desertion and checks diarrhea, stanches bleeding, and checks vaginal discharge. It also is applied topically for sores and flat-abscesses that fail to close.[35]

Chì shí zhī is sweet, sour, and astringent in flavor, warm in nature, and heavy in substance. It astringes and secures the intestines, and hence is most commonly used for enduring diarrhea or dystentery and for large intestinal vacuity cold efflux desertion that in prolonged cases can lead to prolapse of the rectum. For enduring patterns of gastrointestinal vacuity cold, cold pain in the abdomen, or dysentery with pus and blood, combine *chì shí zhī* with *gān jiāng* (dried ginger) and *gēng mĭ* (non-glutinous rice). The *chì shí zhī* is first ground to a fine powder and half is set aside. The other half is decocted with the *gān jiāng* and *gēng mĭ*. After the rice is cooked, the dregs are removed and the remaining *chì shí zhī* is then

---

[35]It is important to insure that the sore is not infected before applying any method of closing the wound. (Ed.)

added to the decoction, which is then divided into two doses and taken warm. (This is *táo huā tāng* (Peach Blossom Decoction) from *Shāng Hán Lùn* (伤寒论 "On Cold Damage").) For **incontinent intestinal efflux**[552] (肠滑不禁 *cháng huá bù jìn*) or incessant diarrhea, *chì shí zhī* can be combined with *yǔ yú liáng* (limonite), as in *chì shí zhī yǔ yú liáng tāng* (Halloysite and Limonite Decoction), adding, if necessary, medicinals such as *chē qián zǐ* (plantago seed) and *fú líng* (poria) in order to disinhibit urine. In summary, *chì shí zhī* is used to treat insecurity of the lower burner.

For flooding (heavy uterine bleeding) or incessant spotting (frequent light uterine bleeding), *chì shí zhī* is used as a securing astringent to stanch bleeding. It is frequently combined with medicinals such as:

> *shēng dì huáng* (生地黄 dried/fresh rehmannia, Rehmanniae Radix Exsiccata seu Recens)
>
> *dāng guī* (当归 Chinese angelica, Angelicae Sinensis Radix)
>
> *bái sháo* (白芍 white peony, Paeoniae Radix Alba)
>
> *bái zhú* (白术 white atractylodes, Atractylodis Macrocephalae Rhizoma)
>
> *jiǔ chǎo huáng qín* (酒炒黄芩 wine-fried scutellaria, Scutellariae Radix cum Vino Fricta)
>
> *xù duàn tàn* (续断炭 charred dipsacus, Dipsaci Radix Carbonisata)
>
> *zōng lǘ tàn* (棕榈炭 charred trachycarpus, Trachycarpi Petiolus Carbonisatus)
>
> *ài yè tàn* (艾叶炭 charred mugwort, Artemisiae Argyi Folium Carbonisatum)
>
> *ē jiāo* (阿胶 ass hide glue, Asini Corii Colla)
>
> *sāng jì shēng* (桑寄生 mistletoe, Taxilli Herba)
>
> *zhì huáng qí* (炙黄芪 mix-fried astragalus, Astragali Radix cum Liquido Fricta)

For chronic dysentery, chronic enteritis, ulcerative colitis, or intestinal tuberculosis, *chì shí zhī* reduces the frequency of bowel movements when used in an appropriate formula chosen on the basis of pattern identification. For functional metrorrhagia or enduring bloody stool, the addition of this medicinal helps to stanch bleeding.

Research

According to modern research reports, this medicinal safeguards against inflammation of the intestinal mucosa. On the one hand, it reduces irritation caused by foreign matter, and on the other it absorbs the inflammatory exudate and thus reduces inflammation. It acts as a hemostat in gastrointestinal hemorrhage. It also absorbs toxic matter in the digestive tract, and hence can be used to treat mercury or phosphorous poisoning and prevent the absorption of these toxins.

Comparisons

Both *yǔ yú liáng* (limonite) and *chì shí zhī* astringe the intestines, check dysentery, and stanch bleeding. Yet *yǔ yú liáng*[183] is sweet and salty with a cold nature, whereas *chì shí zhī* is sweet and sour with a warm nature.

Both *huā ruǐ shí* (ophicalcite) and *chì shí zhī* are sour and astringent and stanch bleeding. Nevertheless, *huā ruǐ shí* tends to treat coughing of blood and blood ejection, whereas *chì shí zhī* tends to treat flooding and spotting as well as bloody stool.

The indications for *Bái shí zhī* (kaolin)[36] and *chì shí zhī* are essentially the same, but *chì shí zhī* tends to enter the blood aspect.

Chì shí zhī is frequently used calcined to increase its astringent nature.

DOSAGE

The dosage is generally 9–15 g/3–5 qián. In severe patterns, use up to 30 g/ 1 liǎng.

CAUTION

Contraindicated when there is repletion evil in the large intestine. Because *chì shí zhī* has a heavy nature, it should be used with care for pregnant women. Continual use can cause a severe decrease in appetite.

---

67. 禹馀粮 Yǔ Yú Liáng   Limonitum
Limonite

Sweet, salty, and astringent in flavor and slightly cold in nature, *yǔ yú liáng* (limonite) is almost the same in its effect as *chì shí zhī* (halloysite). It is an astringent and securing medicinal for the lower origin, and it is used for enduring dysentery, enduring diarrhea, red and white vaginal discharge, uterine bleeding, or descent of blood with the stool. Nevertheless, *yǔ yú liáng* is slightly cold in nature, so it also clears heat.

DOSAGE AND CAUTION

The dosage and cautions are the same as those for *chì shí zhī* (halloysite).

---

68. 乌梅 Wū Méi   Mume Fructus
Mume

Wū méi (mume) is sour and astringent in flavor and warm in nature.

1. **Sourness and Astringency:** *Wū méi* is often used to check diarrhea, stanch bleeding, and check dysentery, as well as to constrain the lung and suppress cough. For enduring diarrhea in spleen vacuity and incessant large intestine efflux diarrhea, which in severe cases can lead to unretractable prolapse of the rectum, *wū méi* secures the intestines with sour and astringent flavor to check diarrhea. For this purpose it is frequently combined with medicinals such as:

dǎng shēn (党参 codonopsis, Codonopsis Radix)

cāng zhú (苍术 atractylodes, Atractylodis Rhizoma)

---

[36] *bái shí zhī* 白石脂 is the name by which *gāo lǐng tǔ* (高岭土, kaolin) is usually referred in medical Chinese. (Ed.)

bái zhú (白术 white atractylodes, Atractylodis Macrocephalae Rhizoma)

fú líng (茯苓 poria, Poria)

shān yào (山药 dioscorea, Dioscoreae Rhizoma)

mù xiāng (木香 costusroot, Aucklandiae Radix)

hē zǐ (诃子 chebule, Chebulae Fructus)

ròu dòu kòu (肉豆蔻 nutmeg, Myristicae Semen)

wǔ wèi zǐ (五味子 schisandra, Schisandrae Fructus)

For descent of blood with the stool or profuse menstruation, the sour, astringent flavor of *wū méi* stanches bleeding. For this purpose it is frequently combined with medicinals such as:

dì yú tàn (地榆炭 charred sanguisorba, Sanguisorbae Radix Carbonisata)

huái huā tàn (槐花炭 charred sophora flower, Sophorae Flos Carbonisatus)

huáng qín tàn (黄芩炭 charred scutellaria, Scutellariae Radix Carbonisata)

ài yè tàn (艾叶炭 charred mugwort, Artemisiae Argyi Folium Carbonisatum)

ē jiāo (阿胶 ass hide glue, Asini Corii Colla)

For incessant dysentery, *wū méi* is frequently combined with medicinals such as:

huáng lián (黄连 coptis, Coptidis Rhizoma)

mù xiāng (木香 costusroot, Aucklandiae Radix)

chì shí zhī (赤石脂 halloysite, Halloysitum Rubrum)

yǔ yú liáng (禹馀粮 limonite, Limonitum)

bái sháo (白芍 white peony, Paeoniae Radix Alba)

wēi gé gēn (煨葛根 roasted pueraria, Puerariae Radix Tostum)

hē zǐ (诃子 chebule, Chebulae Fructus)

pào jiāng (炮姜 blast-fried ginger, Zingiberis Rhizoma Praeparatum)

In the treatment of enduring cough causing lung damage, in which lung qì floats and dissipates and the cough is dry and persistent, *wū méi* constrains lung qì; it is frequently combined with medicinals such as:

bǎi hé (百合 lily bulb, Lilii Bulbus)

wǔ wèi zǐ (五味子 schisandra, Schisandrae Fructus)

zǐ wǎn (紫菀 aster, Asteris Radix)

hē zǐ (诃子 chebule, Chebulae Fructus)

2. Engendering Liquid and Allaying Thirst: For dispersion-thirst with heat vexation and thirst, *wū méi* is frequently combined with:

mài dōng (麦冬 ophiopogon, Ophiopogonis Radix)

shí hú (石斛 dendrobium, Dendrobii Herba)

shā shēn (沙参 adenophora/glehnia, Adenophorae seu Glehniae Radix)

yù zhú (玉竹 Solomon's seal, Polygonati Odorati Rhizoma)

tiān huā fěn (天花粉 trichosanthes root, Trichosanthis Radix)

It is also decocted and taken singly. In recent years, *liù wèi dì huáng tāng* (Six-Ingredient Rehmannia Decoction), which contains *shēng dì huáng* (dried/fresh rehmannia), *shān zhū yú* (cornus), *shān yào* (dioscorea), *fú líng* (poria), *dān pí* (moutan), and *zé xiè* (alisma), with the addition of *wū méi*, *wŭ wèi zĭ* (schisandra), and a small amount of *ròu guì* (cinnamon bark), has achieved excellent results in the treatment of diabetes mellitus, diabetes insipidus, and hyperthyroidism that manifests in severe thirst.

3. Expelling Roundworm and Relieving Pain: *Wū méi* expels roundworms. When treating roundworm, physicians traditionally used sour, bitter, acrid, and hot medicinals together. They believed that roundworms soften with sourness, descend with bitterness, subside with acridity, and quiet with heat. For this purpose *wū méi* is generally combined with medicinals such as:

chuān jiāo (川椒 zanthoxylum, Zanthoxyli Pericarpium)

wú zhū yú (吴茱萸 evodia, Evodiae Fructus)

gān jiāng (干姜 dried ginger, Zingiberis Rhizoma)

shĭ jūn zĭ (使君子 quisqualis, Quisqualis Fructus)

shēng dà huáng (生大黄 raw rhubarb, Rhei Radix et Rhizoma Crudi)

huáng lián (黄连 coptis, Coptidis Rhizoma)

Two commonly used formulas for this pattern are *wū méi wán* (Mume Pill) and *ān huí tāng* (Roundworm-Quieting Decoction).

Wū méi wán 乌梅丸   Mume Pill

---

wū méi (乌梅 mume, Mume Fructus)

xì xīn (细辛 asarum, Asari Herba)

guì zhī (桂枝 cinnamon twig, Cinnamomi Ramulus)

dăng shēn (党参 codonopsis, Codonopsis Radix)

fù zĭ (附子 aconite, Aconiti Radix Lateralis Praeparata)

huáng băi (黄柏 phellodendron, Phellodendri Cortex)

huáng lián (黄连 coptis, Coptidis Rhizoma)

gān jiāng (干姜 dried ginger, Zingiberis Rhizoma)

chuān jiāo (川椒 zanthoxylum, Zanthoxyli Pericarpium)

dāng guī (当归 Chinese angelica, Angelicae Sinensis Radix)

Ān huí tāng 安蛔汤   Roundworm-Quieting Decoction

---

dăng shēn (党参 codonopsis, Codonopsis Radix)

bái zhú (白术 white atractylodes, Atractylodis Macrocephalae Rhizoma)

fú líng (茯苓 poria, Poria)

pào jiāng (炮姜 blast-fried ginger, Zingiberis Rhizoma Praeparatum)

chuān jiāo (川椒 zanthoxylum, Zanthoxyli Pericarpium)

wū méi (乌梅 mume, Mume Fructus)

Wū méi also relieves pain from worms. Traditionally, when worms are suspected as the cause of stomach or abdominal pain, 6–9 g/2–3 qián of *wū méi* is decocted and the patient drinks a large cupful. If the pain is significantly relieved, then one can diagnose and treat for worm pain. If the pain is unrelieved after drinking the decoction, it may not be due to worms, and further investigation should be made to gain a more accurate diagnosis. This method is easy and convenient, so readers may wish to try it. In rural areas, if one cannot find *wū méi*, having the patient drink a half bowl of vinegar (about 60 ml/2 liǎng) will also work.

When using *wū méi* to engender liquid and allay thirst, to astringe the intestines, or to constrain the lung, it should be used raw without the pit. To stanch bleeding, it should be used char-fried (*wū méi tàn* (charred mume)).

Finally, *wū méi* also softens hardness and disperses excrescences to treat corns[545] (鸡眼 *jī yǎn*). After steeping 30 g/1 liǎng of *wū méi* in brine for twenty-four hours, remove the pits, add an appropriate amount of vinegar, and grind into an ointment. Apply to the corn or callus, cover with *xiàng pí gāo* (Elephant Hide Plaster), and remove after several days.

In the summer, *wū méi tāng* (Mume Decoction) is taken to engender liquid, clear heat, disperse summerheat, and allay thirst.

COMPARISON

Shān zhā (crataegus)[504] and *wū méi* are both sour, but *shān zhā* is neither astringent nor contracting, and it disperses accumulations and breaks qì. On the other hand, *wū méi*, which is sour and astringent, constrains the lung and astringes the intestines.

DOSAGE

The dosage is generally 1–4.5 g/3 fēn–1.5 qián. When necessary, one can use 6–9 g/2–3 qián.

CAUTION

Contraindicated in patterns in which a repletion evil is still present or in which effusing and dissipating treatment is required.

RESEARCH

According to modern research, *wū méi* has an antibacterial effect against *Staphylococcus aureus*, *Pseudomonas pyocyanea*, various types of intestinal disease-causing bacteria, tuberculosis bacteria, and cutaneous fungus. It is effective in the treatment of enteritis and bacterial dysentery. *Wū méi* also causes contractions of the gallbladder and stimulates bile secretion; it is effective in the treatment of biliary ascariasis, malaria, and hookworm.

---

69. 诃子 Hē Zǐ   Chebulae Fructus
Chebule

Including
  ▷ *Hē zǐ pí* (诃子皮 chebule husk, Chebulae Pericarpium)

Also called *hē lí lè* 诃黎勒 and *hē zǐ ròu* 诃子肉. Bitter, sour, and astringent in flavor and warm in nature, *hē zǐ* (chebule) astringes the intestines, constrains the lung, precipitates qì, regulates the center, transforms phlegm, and opens the voice.

Hé zǐ (chebule) astringes the large intestines and is used to treat enduring diarrhea and enduring dysentery. For this purpose it is combined with the following:

ròu dòu kòu (肉豆蔻 nutmeg, Myristicae Semen)

wú zhū yú (吴茱萸 evodia, Evodiae Fructus)

qiàn shí (芡实 euryale, Euryales Semen)

mù xiāng (木香 costusroot, Aucklandiae Radix)

ròu guì (肉桂 cinnamon bark, Cinnamomi Cortex)

wǔ wèi zǐ (五味子 schisandra, Schisandrae Fructus)

bǔ gǔ zhī (补骨脂 psoralea, Psoraleae Fructus)

fú líng (茯苓 poria, Poria)

bái zhú (白术 white atractylodes, Atractylodis Macrocephalae Rhizoma)

chì shí zhī (赤石脂 halloysite, Halloysitum Rubrum)

For descent of blood with the stool, it is combined with the following:

fáng fēng (防风 saposhnikovia, Saposhnikoviae Radix)

huái huā tàn (槐花炭 charred sophora flower, Sophorae Flos Carbonisatus)

dì yú tàn (地榆炭 charred sanguisorba, Sanguisorbae Radix Carbonisata)

huáng bǎi tàn (黄柏炭 charred phellodendron, Phellodendri Cortex Carbonisatus)

bái zhú (白术 white atractylodes, Atractylodis Macrocephalae Rhizoma)

xù duàn tàn (续断炭 charred dipsacus, Dipsaci Radix Carbonisata)

I have had satisfactory results treating chronic dysentery using *sì shén wán* (Four Spirits Pill)[176] and *bā wèi dì huáng wán* (Eight-Ingredient Rehmannia Pill)[341] with the addition of *hé zǐ*, *chì shí zhī* (halloysite), and *wū méi* (mume).

For women with flooding and spotting, vaginal discharge, fetal spotting, or stirring fetus that may abort, *hé zǐ* promotes astriction, stanches bleeding, and secures the fetus when combined with medicinals such as:

bái zhú (白术 white atractylodes, Atractylodis Macrocephalae Rhizoma)

shān yào (山药 dioscorea, Dioscoreae Rhizoma)

xù duàn tàn (续断炭 charred dipsacus, Dipsaci Radix Carbonisata)

huáng qín tàn (黄芩炭 charred scutellaria, Scutellariae Radix Carbonisata)

sāng jì shēng (桑寄生 mistletoe, Taxilli Herba)

bǔ gǔ zhī (补骨脂 psoralea, Psoraleae Fructus)

ài yè tàn (艾叶炭 charred mugwort, Artemisiae Argyi Folium Carbonisatum)

zhù má gēn (苎麻根 ramie, Boehmeriae Radix)

Hé zǐ astringes lung qì. For unresolved enduring cough that causes the lung qì to float and dissipate, producing symptoms such as enduring cough without phlegm, shortness of breath, and hoarse voice, it is combined with *bǎi hé* (lily bulb), *wū méi* (mume), *wǔ wèi zǐ* (schisandra), *mài dōng* (ophiopogon), and *mǎ dōu líng* (aristolochia fruit); this combination constrains lung qì to suppress cough. Nonetheless, one must be aware that treating cough with the above lung-qì–restraining medicinals must be performed in the final stage of an illness when there is absolutely no repletion evil. Otherwise, it is possible to constrain the evil and make its departure difficult, resulting in an enduring cough that is very difficult to treat.

For chronic laryngitis, chronic pharyngitis, and hoarse voice, *hē zǐ* is combined with *wū méi* (mume), *xuán fù huā* (inula flower), *jīn guǒ lǎn* (tinospora root), *wǔ bèi zǐ* (sumac gallnut), *shè gān* (belamcanda), and *chán tuì* (cicada molting); when properly varied in accordance with pattern identification this formula is quite effective.

Comparison

Wǔ bèi zǐ (sumac gallnut) and *hē zǐ* both promote constraining and astriction and stanch bleeding, but *wǔ bèi zǐ* is cold in nature, while *hē zǐ* is warm in nature.

Jīn yīng zǐ (Cherokee rose fruit), which is sour and astringent, is primarily used to secure the essence gate. *Hē zǐ* is primarily used to astringe the intestines and check diarrhea and dysentery.

Ròu dòu kòu (nutmeg) warms the spleen and dries dampness to check diarrhea. *Hē zǐ* astringes the intestines and stems desertion to check diarrhea, while *wū méi* (mume) checks enduring dysentery and precipitation of blood; it also engenders liquid and allays thirst, and it kills worms. *Hē zǐ* checks enduring dysentery and descent of blood; however, it is more bitter than sour, and so is able to precipitate qì and downbear lung fire.

Hē zǐ is used raw (*shēng hē zǐ* 生诃子) to move qì, disperse distention, protect the lung, and clear phlegm. It is used roasted (*wēi hē zǐ* 煨诃子) to warm the stomach and secure the intestines. *Hē zǐ pí* (诃子皮, chebule husk) is used for enduring cough, panting counterflow, and enduring diarrhea, because it is more strongly astringent.

Dosage

The dosage is generally 3–9 g/1–3 qián.

Caution

Contraindicated for patterns of cough, early-stage dysentery, repletion heat in the lung, damp-heat dysentery, and panting from fire surging into the upper burner.

Research

According to modern research, *hē zǐ* has an inhibitory effect on *Bacillus diphtheriae*, *Bacillus dysenteriae*, *Diplococcus pneumoniae*, *Pseudomonas pyocyanea*, *Staphylococcus aureus*, *Staphylococcus albus*, *Bacillus proteus*, and hemolytic streptococcus. In the lower region of the intestines, it has astringent and antidysenteric effects. When sucked in the mouth, it treats laryngitis.

---

70. 肉豆蔻 Ròu Dòu Kòu   Myristicae Semen
Nutmeg

Acrid in flavor and warm in nature, *ròu dòu kòu* (nutmeg) dries the spleen, warms the stomach, and astringes the intestines.

1. Warming the Spleen and Checking Diarrhea: For enduring diarrhea and enduring dysentery that result from spleen-stomach vacuity cold, *ròu dòu kòu* warms the spleen and dries dampness, astringes the intestines and checks diarrhea. For this purpose it is frequently combined with medicinals such as:

dǎng shēn (党参 codonopsis, Codonopsis Radix)

bái zhú (白术 white atractylodes, Atractylodis Macrocephalae Rhizoma)

fú líng (茯苓 poria, Poria)

hē zǐ (诃子 chebule, Chebulae Fructus)

mù xiāng (木香 costusroot, Aucklandiae Radix)

qiàn shí (芡实 euryale, Euryales Semen)

shā rén (砂仁 amomum, Amomi Fructus)

Ròu dòu kòu is even more effective for **fifth-watch diarrhea**[549] (五更泄 *wǔ gēng xiè*), daily occurrences of early morning diarrhea that are attributable to spleen-kidney vacuity cold. *Ròu dòu kòu* warms the spleen and dries dampness, and it astringes the intestines. For fifth-watch diarrhea, it is frequently combined with *wú zhū yú* (evodia), *wǔ wèi zǐ* (schisandra), and *bǔ gǔ zhī* (psoralea), to form *sì shén wán* (Four Spirits Pill),[176] which is the most commonly used prescription for this condition. I often get excellent results in the treatment of chronic enteritis, chronic dysentery, and chaotic intestinal function (manifesting as chronic diarrhea) using *sì shén wán* (Four Spirits Pill) with the addition of medicinals such as the following, in accordance with signs:

dǎng shēn (党参 codonopsis, Codonopsis Radix)

bái zhú (白术 white atractylodes, Atractylodis Macrocephalae Rhizoma)

fú líng (茯苓 poria, Poria)

hē zǐ (诃子 chebule, Chebulae Fructus)

shān yào (山药 dioscorea, Dioscoreae Rhizoma)

shān zhū yú (山茱萸 cornus, Corni Fructus)

ròu guì (肉桂 cinnamon bark, Cinnamomi Cortex)

fù piàn (附片 sliced aconite, Aconiti Radix Lateralis Praeparata Secta)

gān jiāng (干姜 dried ginger, Zingiberis Rhizoma)

wū yào (乌药 lindera, Linderae Radix)

zào xīn tǔ (灶心土 oven earth, Terra Flava Usta)

This formula should be adjusted on the basis of the identified pattern.

2. Warming the Stomach and Moving Qì: *Ròu dòu kòu* warms the stomach and aids digestion, precipitates qì and disperses distention. For non-transformation of food, poor appetite, and distending pain in the stomach duct that result from center burner vacuity cold, it is frequently combined with medicinals such as:

mù xiāng (木香 costusroot, Aucklandiae Radix)

gāo liáng jiāng (高良姜 lesser galangal, Alpiniae Officinarum Rhizoma)

shā rén (砂仁 amomum, Amomi Fructus)

xiāng fù (香附 cyperus, Cyperi Rhizoma)

bàn xià (半夏 pinellia, Pinelliae Rhizoma)

hòu pò (厚朴 officinal magnolia bark, Magnoliae Officinalis Cortex)

zhǐ qiào (枳壳 bitter orange, Aurantii Fructus)

Modern research has shown *ròu dòu kòu* to contain volatile oils that stimulate stomach secretions, increase peristalsis, enhance the appetite, and relieve pain and distention. Nevertheless, in large doses, it has an inhibitory effect on both peristalsis and stomach secretions. Thus, when it is used to warm the stomach and move qì, and to open the stomach and increase food intake, it is appropriate to use a light dosage, 1.5–4.5 g/5 fēn–1.5 qián. When it is used to warm the spleen and check diarrhea, it is appropriate to use a heavier dosage, such as 9–12 g/ 3–4 qián.

Comparisons

Yì zhì rén (alpinia)[150] and *ròu dòu kòu* both dry the spleen, but *yì zhì rén* tends to be used for spleen dampness with copious drool and also for supplementing the kidney and reducing urine to treat enuresis. *Ròu dòu kòu* tends to be used for spleen vacuity diarrhea and also for warming the stomach and moving qì.

Bǔ gǔ zhī (psoralea)[149] and *ròu dòu kòu* both treat diarrhea, but *bǔ gǔ zhī* warms and supplements kidney yáng to treat sloppy diarrhea that results from kidney vacuity-cold, whereas *ròu dòu kòu* warms the spleen and dries dampness to treat intestinal efflux diarrhea that results from spleen vacuity-cold.

Dosage

The dosage is generally 1.5–9 g/5 fēn–3 qián.

Caution

Contraindicated when repletion heat or fire evil is present.

---

71. 桑螵蛸 Sāng Piāo Xiāo   Mantidis Oötheca
Mantis Egg-Case

Sweet and salty in flavor and neutral in nature, *sāng piāo xiāo* (mantis egg-case) supplements the kidney, secures essence, and reduces urination.

For seminal emission and premature ejaculation that result from kidney vacuity with insecurity of the essence gate, *sāng piāo xiāo* is combined with medicinals such as *lóng gǔ* (dragon bone), *lián xū* (lotus stamen), *shān yào* (dioscorea), *dì huáng* (rehmannia), and *jīn yīng zǐ* (Cherokee rose fruit).

Sāng piāo xiāo is most commonly used to treat kidney vacuity with a failure to perform its office (contracting and containing), which results in enuresis or frequent urination (with absence of urethral pain). For this pattern, it is combined with medicinals such as *yì zhì rén* (alpinia), *wū yào* (lindera), *shān zhū yú* (cornus), *shān yào* (dioscorea), *lóng gǔ* (dragon bone), and *dǎng shēn* (codonopsis). I frequently treat enuresis with satisfactory results using a pattern-appropriate combination of *sāng piāo xiāo* with medicinals such as the following:

shú dì huáng (熟地黄 cooked rehmannia, Rehmanniae Radix Praeparata)

shān zhū yú (山茱萸 cornus, Corni Fructus)

shān yào (山药 dioscorea, Dioscoreae Rhizoma)

wŭ wèi zĭ (五味子 schisandra, Schisandrae Fructus)

yì zhì rén (益智仁 alpinia, Alpiniae Oxyphyllae Fructus)

fù pén zĭ (覆盆子 rubus, Rubi Fructus)

chăo jī nèi jīn (炒鸡内金 stir-fried gizzard lining, Galli Gigeriae Endothelium Corneum Frictum)

xù duàn (续断 dipsacus, Dipsaci Radix).

This formula must be varied in accordance with pattern identification. For example, I treated a patient who had had enuresis with involuntary loss of urine once or twice a night for more than twenty years. The patient frequently slept on a wooden board, not daring to use bedclothes, thereby incurring considerable suffering. On the basis of the pulse and signs, the diagnosis was a kidney vacuity-cold pattern, which I treated with the following formula:

sāng piāo xiāo (桑螵蛸 mantis egg-case, Mantidis Oötheca) 12 g/4 qián

yì zhì rén (益智仁 alpinia, Alpiniae Oxyphyllae Fructus) 9 g/3 qián

wū yào (乌药 lindera, Linderae Radix) 12 g/4 qián

fù pén zĭ (覆盆子 rubus, Rubi Fructus) 12 g/4 qián

xù duàn (续断 dipsacus, Dipsaci Radix) 15 g/5 qián

yín yáng huò (淫羊藿 epimedium, Epimedii Herba) 12 g/4 qián

ròu guì (肉桂 cinnamon bark, Cinnamomi Cortex) 4 g/1.5 qián

zhì fù piàn (制附片 sliced processed aconite, Aconiti Radix Lateralis Praeparata Secta) 6 g/2 qián

suŏ yáng (锁阳 cynomorium, Cynomorii Herba) 12 g/4 qián

jī nèi jīn (鸡内金 gizzard lining, Galli Gigeriae Endothelium Corneum) 12 g/4 qián

shú dì huáng (熟地黄 cooked rehmannia, Rehmanniae Radix Praeparata) 24 g/8 qián

sāng jì shēng (桑寄生 mistletoe, Taxilli Herba) 30 g/1 liăng

After slightly more than 40 packets of this formula, his condition resolved.

Comparisons

Yì zhì rén (alpinia), *fù pén zĭ* (rubus), *tái wū yào* (lindera), and *sāng piāo xiāo* all reduce urination. Nevertheless, they differ in action: a) *yì zhì rén* (alpinia)[150] supplements the spleen and kidney, astringes essence, reduces urination, and also contains drool and spittle; b) *fù pén zĭ* (rubus)[192] supplements the liver and kidney, secures essential qì, is sour and astringent in flavor, and reduces urination; c) *tái wū yào* (lindera)[234] warms cold qì in the bladder and kidney and normalizes bladder and kidney counterflow qì to treat frequent urination; d) *sāng piāo xiāo* secures the kidney to reduce urination.

Hăi piāo xiāo (cuttlefish bone) frees the channels, quickens the blood, relieves abdominal pain, and controls stomach acid. *Sāng piāo xiāo* supplements the kidney, secures essence, treats seminal emission, and reduces urination.

DOSAGE

The dosage is generally 4.5–9 g/1.5–3 qián.

CAUTION

Contraindicated in patterns of effulgent yīn vacuity fire and heat in the bladder. Inappropriate for urinary frequency due to acute urinary infection (which generally is ascribed to damp-heat).

---

72. 覆盆子 Fù Pén Zǐ   Rubi Fructus
Rubus

Sweet and sour in flavor and warm in nature, *fù pén zǐ* (rubus) supplements the liver and kidney, secures essence, and reduces urination.

1. Clouded Vision: When insufficiency of liver and kidney causes clouded and flowery vision and decreased and weakened visual acuity, *fù pén zǐ* is combined with medicinals such as *gǒu qǐ zǐ* (lycium), *chē qián zǐ* (plantago seed), *tù sī zǐ* (cuscuta), *wǔ wèi zǐ* (schisandra), *dì huáng* (rehmannia), *chén xiāng* (aquilaria), *cí shí* (loadstone), and *yè míng shā* (bat's droppings).

2. Enuresis: The kidney controls urine and stool. When a vacuous kidney fails to contain and secure urine, causing enuresis, dribble after voiding, and frequent urination, *fù pén zǐ* is used to supplement the kidney, reduce urination, and check enuresis. It is frequently combined with medicinals such as *sāng piāo xiāo* (mantis egg-case), *wǔ wèi zǐ* (schisandra), *shān zhū yú* (cornus), *wū yào* (lindera), and *yì zhì rén* (alpinia). It is effective for treating diabetes insipidus.

3. Seminal Emission: For seminal emission, seminal efflux, and premature ejaculation due to kidney vacuity and insecurity of the essence gate, *fù pén zǐ* is used to supplement the kidney and secure essence. For this purpose it is combined with:

shēng dì huáng (生地黄 dried/fresh rehmannia, Rehmanniae Radix Exsiccata seu Recens)

shú dì huáng (熟地黄 cooked rehmannia, Rehmanniae Radix Praeparata)

shān zhū yú (山茱萸 cornus, Corni Fructus)

wǔ wèi zǐ (五味子 schisandra, Schisandrae Fructus)

suǒ yáng (锁阳 cynomorium, Cynomorii Herba)

jīn yīng zǐ (金樱子 Cherokee rose fruit, Rosae Laevigatae Fructus)

Jīn yīng zǐ (Cherokee rose fruit) and *fù pén zǐ* both treat seminal emission and seminal efflux; however, *jīn yīng zǐ* also treats diarrhea, enduring dysentery, and frequent defecation, whereas *fù pén zǐ* also treats enuresis and frequent urination.

DOSAGE

The dosage is generally 4.5–9 g/1.5–3 qián.

Caution

Contraindicated for patterns with inhibited urination, roughness and pain in the urethra, and hyperactive sexual function.

---

73. 五味子 Wǔ Wèi Zǐ   Schisandrae Fructus
Schisandra

Wǔ wèi zǐ (schisandra) is sour and salty in flavor, its skin is sweet, and its kernel is acrid and bitter; hence it contains all five flavors.[37] It is warm in nature.

1. **Constraining the Lung:** Wǔ wèi zǐ constrains lung qì and also boosts the kidney to make it absorb qì. For enduring cough when the lung qì floats and dissipates, causing dry cough, loss of voice, shortness of breath and panting, fatigue and lack of strength, and facial complexion without luster, wǔ wèi zǐ is combined with bǎi hé (lily bulb), shēng dì huáng (dried/fresh rehmannia), shān zhū yú (cornus), zǐ wǎn (aster), mǎ dōu líng (aristolochia fruit), and pí pá yè (loquat leaf). Nonetheless, it is important to pay attention to the fact that when there is still a repletion evil in the lung and cough, one should not use lung-contracting medicinals.

2. **Supplementing the Kidney:** For seminal emission, seminal efflux, and enuresis that result from kidney vacuity, wǔ wèi zǐ supplements the kidney and secures essence, and promotes absorption of kidney qì. For this purpose it is frequently combined with:

dì huáng (地黄 rehmannia, Rehmanniae Radix)

shān zhū yú (山茱萸 cornus, Corni Fructus)

lóng gǔ (龙骨 dragon bone, Mastodi Ossis Fossilia)

mǔ lì (牡蛎 oyster shell, Ostreae Concha)

jīn yīng zǐ (金樱子 Cherokee rose fruit, Rosae Laevigatae Fructus)

dān pí (丹皮 moutan, Moutan Cortex)

zé xiè (泽泻 alisma, Alismatis Rhizoma)

fú líng (茯苓 poria, Poria)

yuǎn zhì (远志 polygala, Polygalae Radix)

"The kidney controls urine and stool." For kidney vacuity that results in enduring diarrhea or dysentery, wǔ wèi zǐ is frequently combined with medicinals such as the following to supplement both the spleen and kidney:

bǔ gǔ zhī (补骨脂 psoralea, Psoraleae Fructus)

wú zhū yú (吴茱萸 evodia, Evodiae Fructus)

ròu dòu kòu (肉豆蔻 nutmeg, Myristicae Semen)

chǎo bái zhú (炒白术 stir-fried white atractylodes, Atractylodis Macrocephalae Rhizoma Frictum)

---

[37]The Chinese wǔ wèi zǐ 五味子, which literally means "five-flavored seed," reflects this understanding. (Ed.)

chǎo shān yào (炒山药 stir-fried dioscorea, Dioscoreae Rhizoma Frictum)

fú líng (茯苓 poria, Poria)

pào jiāng (炮姜 blast-fried ginger, Zingiberis Rhizoma Praeparatum)

dǎng shēn (党参 codonopsis, Codonopsis Radix)

mù xiāng (木香 costusroot, Aucklandiae Radix)

3. **Nourishing the Heart and Constraining Sweat:** For insomnia, palpitations, susceptibility to fright, and profuse dreaming that result from insufficiency of heart qì, *wǔ wèi zǐ* is used to contract and nourish heart qì and quiet the spirit. For this purpose it is frequently combined with medicinals such as:

bǎi zǐ rén (柏子仁 arborvitae seed, Platycladi Semen)

yuǎn zhì (远志 polygala, Polygalae Radix)

fú shén (茯神 root poria, Poria cum Pini Radice)

lóng chǐ (龙齿 dragon tooth, Mastodi Dentis Fossilia)

zhēn zhū mǔ (珍珠母 mother-of-pearl, Concha Margaritifera)

lóng yǎn ròu (龙眼肉 longan flesh, Longan Arillus)

dǎng shēn (党参 codonopsis, Codonopsis Radix)

According to modern research, *wǔ wèi zǐ* has been demonstrated to elevate work capacity of the cerebral cortex, stimulate the respiratory center, regulate physiological function in the cardiovascular system, and improve blood circulation. In the vasomotor center, the effect is especially pronounced. Made into a 90% *wǔ wèi zǐ* tincture, and taken over a long period of time, it treats neurasthenia and forgetfulness (take 1–2 ml three times a day). Alternatively, steep *wǔ wèi zǐ* 30 g/ 1 liáng, in 300 ml. of *bái jiǔ* (white liquor) for seven days. A small cup (about 8–10 ml) of this is then taken two or three times a day. In traditional practice, *wǔ wèi zǐ* is often used in combinations varied according to signs.

"The heart governs sweating" and "the kidney governs the five humors." *Wǔ wèi zǐ* nourishes the heart and enriches the kidney. Being sour and contracting, it checks sweating. For yáng vacuity spontaneous sweating, it is frequently combined with medicinals such as:

fú xiǎo mài (浮小麦 light wheat, Tritici Fructus Levis)

shēng huáng qí (生黄芪 raw astragalus, Astragali Radix Cruda)

má huáng gēn (麻黄根 ephedra root, Ephedrae Radix)

suān zǎo rén (酸枣仁 spiny jujube, Ziziphi Spinosi Semen)

For yīn vacuity night sweating, it is frequently combined with:

mài dōng (麦冬 ophiopogon, Ophiopogonis Radix)

shēng dì huáng (生地黄 dried/fresh rehmannia, Rehmanniae Radix Exsiccata seu Recens)

xuán shēn (玄参 scrophularia, Scrophulariae Radix)

shān zhū yú (山茱萸 cornus, Corni Fructus)

lóng gǔ (龙骨 dragon bone, Mastodi Ossis Fossilia)

duàn mǔ lì (煅牡蛎 calcined oyster shell, Ostreae Concha Calcinata)

huáng bǎi (黄柏 phellodendron, Phellodendri Cortex)

wū méi (乌梅 mume, Mume Fructus)

4. Engendering Liquid and Allaying Thirst: *Wǔ wèi zǐ* enriches the yīn of the liver and kidney, engenders spleen-stomach liquid, and contracts the dissipated qì of the lung and kidney; therefore, it is effective in engendering liquid and allaying thirst. For thirst with taking of fluids that results from insufficiency of yīn liquid, *wǔ wèi zǐ* is used in combination with medicinals such as *mài dōng* (ophiopogon), *shēng dì huáng* (dried/fresh rehmannia), *xuán shēn* (scrophularia), and *wū méi* (mume). For diabetes mellitus that belongs to a pattern of kidney vacuity dispersion-thirst, use *liù wèi dì huáng wán* (Six-Ingredient Rehmannia Pill) with the addition of 9–12 g/3–4 qián of *wǔ wèi zǐ* and 0.5–1.5 g/2–5 fēn of *ròu guì* (cinnamon bark). Taken decocted with water, this formula has a definite effect.

COMPARISON

Shān zhū yú (cornus) and *wǔ wèi zǐ* both check sweating, but *shān zhū yú*[124] tends to enrich liver and kidney yīn, whereas *wǔ wèi zǐ* contracts and nourishes heart and lung qì, as well as kidney qì that is dissipating and verging on desertion.

Jīn yīng zǐ (Cherokee rose fruit)[175] is sour and astringent in flavor, and it enters the kidney. It secures essence and also astringes the intestines and checks diarrhea. *Wǔ wèi zǐ* is sour and contracting, and also enters the kidney and secures essence, but it also constrains the lung and suppresses cough.

When used to supplement and boost, *wǔ wèi zǐ* should be stir fried. When used to treat cough, it should be raw.

RESEARCH

According to modern research reports, *wǔ wèi zǐ* has an inhibitory effect against *Staphylococcus aureus*, *Staphylococcus albus*, *Pneumococcus*, *Bacillus typhosus*, *Vibrio cholerae*, and *Pseudomonas pyocyanea*. It excites the smooth muscle of the uterus; thus it strengthens contractions during delivery. During recovery from hepatitis, *wǔ wèi zǐ* is effective in lowering transaminase levels that have been elevated for a long period. (It is generally used as a powder for this purpose.) One can integrate this measure with treatment designed to address each patient's specific condition.

DOSAGE

The dosage is generally 1.5–9 g/5 fēn–3 qián.

CAUTION

Contraindicated in patterns with hyperactivity of kidney yáng, repletion heat in the lung, amassed phlegm and collecting rheum, liver fire stirring frenetically, or in the initial stage of sand papules.

---

74. 白果 Bái Guǒ   Ginkgo Semen
Ginkgo

Also called *yín xìng* 银杏. Sweet, bitter, and astringent in flavor and neutral in nature, *bái guǒ* (ginkgo)[38] possesses minor toxicity. It constrains the lung and boosts qì, stabilizes panting and treats cough. It also reduces urination and checks white vaginal discharge.

a) For wheezing and panting and phlegm cough, *bái guǒ* is frequently combined with medicinals such as *má huáng* (ephedra), *sū zǐ* (perilla fruit), *kuǎn dōng huā* (coltsfoot), *bàn xià* (pinellia), *sāng pí* (mulberry root bark), *xìng rén* (apricot kernel), *huáng qín* (scutellaria), and *gān cǎo* (licorice), as in *bái guǒ dìng chuǎn tāng* (Ginkgo Panting-Stabilizing Decoction).

b) For enduring cough and loss of voice, *bái guǒ* is combined with medicinals such as *sāng pí* (mulberry root bark), *fú líng* (poria), *mài dōng* (ophiopogon), and *chán tuì* (cicada molting). Because *bái guǒ* is astringent, it is more appropriate for enduring cough in which repletion evil is absent from the lung or combined with medicinals that diffuse lung qì, such as *jié gěng* (platycodon), *má huáng* (ephedra), and *xì xīn* (asarum), to avoid constraining the evil.

For frequent urination and enuresis, *bái guǒ* is combined with medicinals such as *wū yào* (lindera), *yì zhì rén* (alpinia), *fù pén zǐ* (rubus), *jī nèi jīn* (gizzard lining), *shú dì huáng* (cooked rehmannia), *shān yào* (dioscorea), and *shān zhū yú* (cornus). For white vaginal discharge, it is combined with:

bái zhú (白术 white atractylodes, Atractylodis Macrocephalae Rhizoma)

fú líng (茯苓 poria, Poria)

chǎo yǐ mǐ (炒苡米 stir-fried coix, Coicis Semen Frictum)

bái jī guān huā (白鸡冠花 white cockscomb, Celosiae Cristatae Flos Albus)

chūn gēn bái pí (椿根白皮 toona root bark, Toonae Radicis Cortex)

Wǔ wèi zǐ (schisandra)[193] warms and contracts lung qì and promotes the absorption of qì by the kidney; it tends to be used for enduring cough with panting. *Bái guǒ* contracts the lung and boosts qì; it tends to be used for phlegm panting with cough.

Used stir-fried, *bái guǒ* boosts the lung and stabilizes panting. Used raw, it downbears phlegm.

DOSAGE

The dosage is generally 1.5–9 g/5 fēn–3 qián. The dosage should not be too high if distention and oppression or poisoning is to be avoided. Poisoning manifests in signs such as headache, vomiting, difficulty breathing, and cramps. If poisoning

---

[38]This medicinal is not readily available because it is frequently infested with insects and also easily becomes moldy. The shelled flesh of the seed can sometimes be purchased in vacuum sealed packaging, but it must be refrigerated once it is opened. The seed (shell included) can often be purchased at Oriental markets because it is used as an ingredient in some Chinese dishes. (Ed.)

occurs, use 30–60 g/1–2 liǎng of *shēng gān cǎo* (raw licorice) decocted in water, or use 30 g/1 liǎng of *bái guǒ qiào* (ginkgo nut shell) decocted in water.

CAUTION

Inappropriate during the onset of an external contraction cough.

Lecture Five
Qì-Rectifying Medicinals
理气药 *Lǐ Qì Yào*

In this lecture, I discuss medicines that move qì, downbear qì, and break qì. The notion of "rectifying qì" also includes "supplementing qì." Nevertheless, I will not discuss qì-supplementing medicinals in this lecture since they have already been discussed in Lecture Four.

---

1. 陈皮 Chén Pí
Tangerine Peel

Citri Reticulatae
Pericarpium

Including
- ▷ *Jú hóng* (橘红 red tangerine peel, Citri Reticulatae Exocarpium Rubrum)
- ▷ *Jú luò* (橘络 tangerine pith, Citri Fructus Fasciculus Vascularis)
- ▷ *Jú hé* (橘核 tangerine pip, Citri Reticulatae Semen)
- ▷ *Jú yè* (橘叶 tangerine leaf, Citri Reticulatae Folium)

Chén pí (tangerine peel)[1] is acrid and bitter in flavor and warm in nature. It is a commonly used qì-rectifying medicinal and has an additional effect of drying dampness and transforming phlegm.

1. **Dispersing Distention and Checking Retching:** For lung-stomach qì stagnation that manifests in signs such as oppression in the chest, epigastric distention and fullness, nausea, vomiting, and distention and pain in the chest and abdomen, *chén pí* is combined with medicinals such as *zhǐ qiào* (bitter orange), *bàn xià* (pinellia), *sū gěng* (perilla stem), and *sū zǐ* (perilla fruit). a) For concurrent presence of stomach heat (yellow tongue fur, liking for cold foods and drinks, rapid

---

[1] *Chén pí* (tangerine peel) is derived from *Citrus reticulata* BLANCO. The same item grown in Guǎngdōng Province is termed *guǎng chén pí* (southern tangerine peel) and is considered to be the best. *Huà jú hóng* (red Huàzhōu pomelo peel) is *Citrus grandis* (L.) OSBECK. The various forms of *jú hóng* (red tangerine peel) generally come wrapped in packets with string and often are cut in a flower petal pattern. *Jú hóng* (red tangerine peel) is about twice as thick as *chén pí*. *Chén pí* is usually orange or red whereas *jú hóng* usually has a green or brown tinge. (Ed.)

pulse), one can add *huáng qín* (scutellaria) and *chuān liàn zǐ* (toosendan). b) For concurrent presence of stomach cold (white tongue fur, liking for hot compresses and hot food and drink, slow or moderate pulse), one can add *wū yào* (lindera) and *gāo liáng jiāng* (lesser galangal). c) For the concurrent presence of exuberant dampness in the center burner (thick slimy white tongue fur, no desire to drink water, slippery pulse), one can add *fú líng* (poria) and *cāng zhú* (atractylodes).

2. Dispelling Phlegm and Suppressing Cough: a) For center burner damp phlegm invading the upper body or externally contracted wind-cold that cause inhibition of lung qì and give rise to signs such as cough, copious phlegm, oppression in the chest, no thought of food, slimy white tongue fur, and slippery pulse, *chén pí* is frequently combined with medicinals such as *bàn xià* (pinellia), *fú líng* (poria), *sū zǐ* (perilla fruit), *xìng rén* (apricot kernel), *chǎo lái fú zǐ* (stir-fried radish seed), *jīn fèi cǎo* (inula),[2] and *qián hú* (peucedanum). b) When external contraction signs are pronounced, *jīng jiè* (schizonepeta), *jié gěng* (platycodon), and *má huáng* (ephedra) may be further added.

3. Rectifying Qì and Opening the Stomach: For center burner qì stagnation with poor appetite, this medicinal is combined with *mài yá* (barley sprout), *gǔ yá* (millet sprout), *bái dòu kòu qiào* (cardamom husk), *shén qū* (medicated leaven), and *shān zhā* (crataegus). This combination increases the appetite.

4. Enhancing Medicinals that Supplement: When supplementing medicinals such as *dǎng shēn* (codonopsis), *huáng qí* (astragalus), *bái zhú* (white atractylodes), *shān yào* (dioscorea), *shú dì huáng* (cooked rehmannia), and *shēng dì huáng* (dried/fresh rehmannia) are being used, the inclusion of *chén pí* prevents oppression in the chest, center fullness, poor appetite, and other side-effects and thus enhances their supplementing action.

Běn Cǎo Bèi Yào (本草备要 "The Essential Herbal Foundation") succinctly summarizes the actions of *chén pí* in the following statement:

> [*Chén pí*] is acrid and can dissipate, is bitter and can dry and drain, is warm and can supplement and harmonize. It supplements when combined with supplementing medicinals, and drains when combined with draining medicinals; it upbears when combined with upbearing medicinals, downbears when combined with downbearing medicinals. It is a medicinal for the qì aspect of the spleen and lung. It regulates the center and disinhibits the diaphragm, abducts stagnation and disperses phlegm, disinhibits water and breaks concretions, and frees the five viscera.

Chén pí (tangerine peel) is the skin of the tangerine that has been kept for a long period of time. It is best when matured, so that in Chinese it is called "matured peel" (陈皮 *chén pí*). High quality *chén pí* comes from Guǎngzhōu in the south of China, and so it is often called *guǎng chén pí* (southern tangerine peel). When the white inner pithy layer is removed, it is called *guǎng jú hóng* (southern red tangerine

---

[2] *Xuán fù huā* (inula flower) in former times was called *jīn fèi cǎo* 金沸草. Nowadays, the name *jīn fèi cǎo* 金沸草 is reserved for the whole herb. See page 211 for more about the flower. (Ed.)

peel). A similar product is *huà jú hóng* (red Huàzhōu pomelo peel), which is the red part of the peel of the pomelo[3] that traditionally comes from Huàzhōu.

COMPARISONS

Huà jú hóng (red Huàzhōu pomelo peel), *guǎng jú hóng* (southern red tangerine peel), and *chén pí* (tangerine peel) all have the effect of transforming phlegm, but *huà jú hóng* (red Huàzhōu pomelo peel) has the strongest phlegm-transforming action and is used for copious phlegm, thick phlegm, and white sticky phlegm. *Guǎng jú hóng* tends to be light and clearing and to enter the lung, and it is suitable for external contractions with cough, copious phlegm, and oppression in the chest. *Chén pí* compared to *jú hóng* has a more powerful ability to rectify qì, disperse distention, and open the stomach, but *jú hóng* is better at transforming phlegm.

There are other products from the tangerine: a) *Jú luò* (tangerine pith) transforms phlegm and frees the network vessels and is often used for cough, oppression and pain in the chest and rib-side, and numbness and tingling of the fingers. b) *Jú hé* (tangerine pip) dissipates binds and relieves pain and is often used to treat mounting qì[558] (疝气 *shàn qì*) pain. c) *Jú yè* (tangerine leaf) soothes the liver and resolves depression and is often used for oppression and pain in the chest and rib-side, and for distention of the breasts.

Qīng pí (unripe tangerine peel)[201] tends to enter the liver and gallbladder; it breaks qì and dissipates stagnation, and also treats mounting. *Chén pí* (tangerine peel) tends to enter the spleen and lung; it rectifies qì and harmonizes the stomach and can also transform phlegm. *Huà jú hóng* has a stronger phlegm-transforming action than *jú hóng* (red tangerine peel).

DOSAGE

The dosage is generally 3–9 g/1–3 qián.

CAUTION

This medicinal is aromatic in flavor and dry in nature. Used to excess, it can dissipate right qì. It should not be used in the absence of qì stagnation.

---

2. 青皮 **Qīng Pí** Unripe Tangerine Peel	Citri Reticulatae Pericarpium Viride

---

Bitter and acrid in flavor and warm in nature, *qīng pí* (unripe tangerine peel) breaks qì, disperses stagnation, soothes depression, and downbears counterflow. In particular, it treats mounting qì (疝气 *shàn qì*) pain.

In binding depression of liver qì that causes signs such as distention and oppression in the chest and diaphragm, qì counterflow with inability to eat, rib-side pain and distention, irascibility, and qì stagnation stomach pain, use *qīng pí* to break

---

[3]The pomelo is a large, coarse-grained, pear-shaped citrus fruit resembling the grapefruit. (Ed.)

qì binds and soothe liver depression. For this purpose it is often combined with medicinals such as:

zhǐ qiào (枳壳 bitter orange, Aurantii Fructus)

sū gěng (苏梗 perilla stem, Perillae Caulis)

xiāng fù (香附 cyperus, Cyperi Rhizoma)

bīng láng (槟榔 areca, Arecae Semen)

hòu pò (厚朴 official magnolia bark, Magnoliae Officinalis Cortex)

chén pí (陈皮 tangerine peel, Citri Reticulatae Pericarpium)

Qīng pí breaks qì and calms the liver, and it conducts all medicinals into the liver channel. *Qīng pí* combined with medicinals such as *wū yào* (lindera), *chuān liàn zǐ* (toosendan), *wú zhū yú* (evodia), *xiǎo huí xiāng* (fennel), and *jú hé* (tangerine pip) treats mounting pain (疝痛 *shàn tòng*). For example, in *tiān tái wū yào sǎn* (Tiāntái Lindera Powder), which is given below, *qīng pí* is used to break qì and calm the liver.

Tiān tái wū yào sǎn 天台乌药散   Tiāntái Lindera Powder

---

wū yào (乌药 lindera, Linderae Radix)

chuān liàn zǐ (川楝子 toosendan, Toosendan Fructus)

mù xiāng (木香 costusroot, Aucklandiae Radix)

xiǎo huí xiāng (小茴香 fennel, Foeniculi Fructus)

gāo liáng jiāng (高良姜 lesser galangal, Alpiniae Officinarum Rhizoma)

qīng pí (青皮 unripe tangerine peel, Citri Reticulatae Pericarpium Viride)

bīng láng (槟榔 areca, Arecae Semen)

This is a commonly used formula for small intestinal mounting qì (小肠疝气 *xiǎo cháng shàn qì*) with pain stretching into the umbilical region. I often apply this traditional experience in the treatment of diseases such tuberculosis of the testis, chronic orchitis, or prostatitis, which are marked by signs such as painful sagging of the testicles with smaller abdomen pain, sagging distention in the perineum, and liking for warmth and fear of cold. For such conditions I use the following combination:

chǎo chuān liàn zǐ (炒川楝子 stir-fried toosendan, Toosendan Fructus Frictus)
9–12 g/3–4 qián

chǎo jú hé (炒橘核 stir-fried tangerine pip, Citri Reticulatae Semen Frictum)
9 g/3 qián

qīng pí (青皮 unripe tangerine peel, Citri Reticulatae Pericarpium Viride)
6–9 g/2–3 qián

chǎo xiǎo huí xiāng (炒小茴香 stir-fried fennel, Foeniculi Fructus Frictus)
6–9 g/2–3 qián

wū yào (乌药 lindera, Linderae Radix) 9 g/3 qián

wú yú (吴萸 evodia, Evodiae Fructus) 3–6 g/1–2 qián

lì zhī hé (荔枝核 litchee pit, Litchi Semen) 9 g/3 qián

bái sháo (白芍 white peony, Paeoniae Radix Alba) 12–15 g/4–5 qián *ròu guì* (肉桂 cinnamon bark, Cinnamomi Cortex) 0.9–3 g/3 fēn–1 qián

This formula, varied in accordance with signs, usually produces satisfactory results.

Comparisons

Xiāng fù (cyperus)[225] frees the qì aspect of the twelve channels, moves qì and opens depression, and also regulates menstruation and rectifies the blood. *Qīng pí* (unripe tangerine peel) mainly enters the liver channel; it breaks qì and opens depression, and also treats mounting pain.

Zhǐ shí[203] breaks qì and is cold, bitter, and downbearing. It tends to be used to disinhibit the chest and diaphragm, and to disperse and abduct gastrointestinal accumulation and stagnation. *Qīng pí* also breaks qì, but it a) dissipates with warmth and acridity and b) downbears with warmth and bitterness. It tends to be used to treat rib-side pain and to break liver channel qì bind.[4]

Dosage

The dosage is generally 3–9 g/1–3 qián.

Caution

Use with care in qì vacuity. Do not use in the absence of qì stagnation or in profuse sweating. This medicinal should not be used to excess or taken over extended periods because it can damage right qì.

---

3. 枳实 Zhǐ Shí   Aurantii Fructus
Unripe Bitter Orange   Immaturus

Zhǐ shí (unripe bitter orange) is bitter in flavor and slightly cold in nature.[5] Its main actions are breaking qì, dispersing accumulations, abducting stagnation, and eliminating glomus.

Zhǐ shí is good for breaking and discharging **gastrointestinal qì bind**[551] (肠胃结气 *cháng wèi jié qì*). It is effective for signs such as glomus and pain below the heart, hard distention in the stomach duct, food stagnation with abdominal distention, abdominal pain, and gastrointestinal qì bind with inhibited defecation. For this purpose it is often combined with medicinals such as *zhǐ qiào* (bitter orange), *mù xiāng* (costusroot), *bīng láng* (areca), *shén qū* (medicated leaven), *mài yá* (barley sprout), *shān zhā* (crataegus), and *dà huáng* (rhubarb). For fullness and distention in the stomach duct and abdomen, retching counterflow, inability to get food down, and distention in both rib-sides due to infection of the biliary tract or cholecystitis, one can use *xiǎo chái hú tāng* (Minor Bupleurum Decoction) with variations: remove the *dǎng shēn* (codonopsis) and *gān cǎo* (licorice) and add *zhǐ shí* (unripe

---

[4]Note that *qīng pí* (unripe tangerine peel) is said to enter the liver, gallbladder, and spleen, while *zhǐ shí* (unripe bitter orange) enters the spleen and stomach. This can be a convenient way to remember the differences in use. (Ed.)

[5]Many sources also say that *zhǐ shí* (unripe bitter orange) is acrid. This designation partially explains its dispersing nature. (Ed.)

bitter orange), *bīng láng* (areca), *dà huáng* (rhubarb), and *yuán míng fěn* (refined mirabilite). This often produces good results. However, it is important to vary the formula in accordance with signs.

Xiǎo chái hú tāng 小柴胡汤   Minor Bupleurum Decoction

chái hú (柴胡 bupleurum, Bupleuri Radix)
huáng qín (黄芩 scutellaria, Scutellariae Radix)
bàn xià (半夏 pinellia, Pinelliae Rhizoma)
dǎng shēn (党参 codonopsis, Codonopsis Radix)
gān cǎo (甘草 licorice, Glycyrrhizae Radix)
shēng jiāng (生姜 fresh ginger, Zingiberis Rhizoma Recens)
dà zǎo (大枣 jujube, Jujubae Fructus)

Zhǐ shí precipitates qì, abducts stagnation, and frees the stool. It is often used for accumulation and stagnation in the stomach and intestines with bound stool and constipation. It is combined with medicinals such as *dà huáng* (rhubarb), *hòu pò* (officinal magnolia bark), *máng xiāo* (mirabilite), *yuán míng fěn* (refined mirabilite), *guā lóu* (trichosanthes), *bīng láng* (areca), and *huǒ má rén* (cannabis fruit). Here are some examples of formulas:

Dà chéng qì tāng 大承气汤   Major Qì-Coordinating Decoction

zhǐ shí (枳实 unripe bitter orange, Aurantii Fructus Immaturus)
hòu pò (厚朴 officinal magnolia bark, Magnoliae Officinalis Cortex)
shēng dà huáng (生大黄 raw rhubarb, Rhei Radix et Rhizoma Crudi)
máng xiāo (芒硝 mirabilite, Natrii Sulfas)

Xiǎo chéng qì tāng 小承气汤   Minor Qì-Coordinating Decoction

zhǐ shí (枳实 unripe bitter orange, Aurantii Fructus Immaturus)
hòu pò (厚朴 officinal magnolia bark, Magnoliae Officinalis Cortex)
shēng dà huáng (生大黄 raw rhubarb, Rhei Radix et Rhizoma Crudi)

Zhǐ shí dǎo zhì wán 枳实导滞丸   Unripe Bitter Orange Stagnation-Abducting Pill

zhǐ shí (枳实 unripe bitter orange, Aurantii Fructus Immaturus)
dà huáng (大黄 rhubarb, Rhei Radix et Rhizoma)
huáng qín (黄芩 scutellaria, Scutellariae Radix)
huáng lián (黄连 coptis, Coptidis Rhizoma)
shén qū (神曲 medicated leaven, Massa Medicata Fermentata)
bái zhú (白术 white atractylodes, Atractylodis Macrocephalae Rhizoma)
fú líng (茯苓 poria, Poria)
zé xiè (泽泻 alisma, Alismatis Rhizoma)

Zhǐ shí is powerful in breaking qì binds. In hard accumulations due to qì bind, it breaks the qì bind; when the qì moves, the accumulation disperses. In phlegm obstruction due to qì bind, *zhǐ shí* breaks the qì bind; when qì moves, the phlegm moves. In glomus and oppression in the chest and stomach duct and chest pain due to qì bind, *zhǐ shí* breaks the qì bind, and so the glomus and oppression spontaneously disappear.

Zhǐ shí combined with *bái zhú* (white atractylodes) eliminates accumulations and gatherings in the abdomen as well as glomus and fullness that is hard and painful under pressure. For example, *zhǐ zhú tāng* (Unripe Bitter Orange and White Atractylodes Decoction) from *Jīn Guì Yào Lüè* (金匮要略 "Essential Prescriptions of the Golden Coffer"), which contains *zhǐ shí* and *bái zhú* (white atractylodes), is designed to treat hardness below the heart as large as a plate, as well as glomus and fullness. *Sháo yào zhǐ shí wán* (Peony and Unripe Bitter Orange Pill), which is given below, treats food accumulation glomus and fullness in children or abdominal enlargement, distention, and fullness with constant pain in children. Combined with *hòu pò* (officinal magnolia bark), it eliminates center fullness. Combined with *dà huáng* (rhubarb) and *máng xiāo* (mirabilite), it breaks and drains repletion binds in the intestines.

Sháo yào zhǐ shí wán 芍药枳实丸   Peony and Unripe Bitter Orange Pill

---

chì sháo (赤芍 red peony, Paeoniae Radix Rubra)

zhǐ shí (枳实 unripe bitter orange, Aurantii Fructus Immaturus)

bái zhú (白术 white atractylodes, Atractylodis Macrocephalae Rhizoma)

chén pí (陈皮 tangerine peel, Citri Reticulatae Pericarpium)

COMPARISONS

Qīng pí (unripe tangerine peel)[201] breaks liver channel qì binds. *Zhǐ shí* breaks gastrointestinal qì bind.

Mù xiāng (costusroot)[225] moves gastrointestinal qì stagnation and tends to rectify qì and disperse distention. *Zhǐ shí* breaks gastrointestinal qì binds, and tends to eliminate glomus and disperse accumulation.

DOSAGE

The dosage is generally 1.5–9 g/5 fēn–3 qián.

CAUTION

Use with care in pregnancy. Contraindicated in qì vacuity center fullness, qì fall with sloppy stool, and stomach vacuity with no thought of food.

---

4. 枳壳 Zhǐ Qiào   Aurantii Fructus
Bitter Orange

Bitter and sour in flavor, and slightly cold in nature, *zhǐ qiào* (bitter orange) is similar in action to *zhǐ shí* (unripe bitter orange). However, *zhǐ shí* mainly enters the spleen and stomach, while *zhǐ qiào* mainly enters the spleen and lung. *Zhǐ qiào* is moderate in strength and tends to rectify qì and disperse distention. *Zhǐ shí* is a powerful medicinal; it breaks qì and disperses accumulation. *Zhǐ shí* is powerful in breaking and downbearing, while *zhǐ qiào* has a greater power to open the chest and loosen the intestines.[6]

COMBINATIONS

a) *Zhǐ qiào* combined with *jié gěng* (platycodon) loosens the chest and disperses distention. b) With *bīng láng* (areca), it causes bound counterflow qì in the chest to move downward. c) With *jīng jiè* (schizonepeta), *fáng fēng* (saposhnikovia), *hóng huā* (carthamus), and *chì sháo* (red peony), it treats generalized numbness and itching of the skin.

DOSAGE

The dosage is generally 3–9 g/1–3 qián.

CAUTION

Use with care in spleen-stomach vacuity and qì vacuity.

RESEARCH

According to modern research reports, the decocted combination of *zhǐ shí* (unripe bitter orange) and *zhǐ qiào* (bitter orange) strengthens excitation of the smooth muscle of the stomach, intestines, and uterus and enhances the regularity of gastrointestinal peristalsis. It is effective for gastrectasia, gastroptosis, indigestion, prolapse of the rectum, hernia, and prolapse of the uterus.

| 5. 沉香 Chén Xiāng | Aquilariae Lignum |
| Aquilaria | Resinatum |

Acrid and bitter in flavor and slightly warm in nature, *chén xiāng* (aquilaria)[7] is chiefly a qì-downbearing medicinal, but it also warms the kidney and calms panting.

1. **Warming the Center and Downbearing Qì:** *Chén xiāng* (aquilaria) treats qì counterflow due to impaired center qì harmony and downbearing, which manifests as oppression and distention in the chest, stomach duct, and rib-side, pain in the heart [region] and abdomen, as well as vomiting and diarrhea, stomach cold, and hiccup. Use this medicinal to downbear qì, warm the stomach, and regulate the center. For oppression and distention in the chest, stomach duct, and rib-side,

---

[6]On the basis of research, some modern books ascribe yáng-uplifting actions to *zhǐ qiào* (bitter orange). (Ed.)

[7]*Aquilaria agallocha* ROXB. is a CITES II plant, but most of what is used for *chén xiāng* (aquilaria) in China is *Aquilaria sinensis* (LOUR.) GILG, whose use need not be prohibited. Because of confusion around this issue, it is often difficult to import *chén xiāng*. Note that China imports some very expensive *chén xiāng* (which is *Aquilaria agallocha*) from Indonesia, Malaysia, and Thailand. *Aquilaria agallocha* is more red and dense than *Aquilaria sinensis*, which is grey and fibrous. As with all expensive medicinals, it is important to purchase *chén xiāng* from a trusted supplier. A common practice is to paint various woods black and sell them as *chén xiāng*. (Ed.)

combine it with medicinals such as *xiāng fù* (cyperus), *zhǐ qiào* (bitter orange), *chǎo chuān liàn zǐ* (stir-fried toosendan), and *qīng pí* (unripe tangerine peel). For pain in the heart [region] and abdomen, combine it with medicinals such as *gāo liáng jiāng* (lesser galangal), *wú yú* (evodia), *yán hú suǒ* (corydalis), and *pú huáng* (typha pollen). For vomiting and diarrhea, combine it with medicinals such as:

bàn xià (半夏 pinellia, Pinelliae Rhizoma)

huò xiāng (藿香 agastache, Agastaches Herba)

zhú rú (竹茹 bamboo shavings, Bambusae Caulis in Taenia)

fú líng (茯苓 poria, Poria)

mù xiāng (木香 costusroot, Aucklandiae Radix)

bái zhú (白术 white atractylodes, Atractylodis Macrocephalae Rhizoma)

For stomach cold hiccup, combine it with medicinals such as

zǐ sū (紫苏 perilla, Perillae Folium, Caulis et Calyx)

dòu kòu (豆蔻 Katsumada's galangal seed, Alpiniae Katsumadai Semen)

dīng xiāng (丁香 clove, Caryophylli Flos)

shì dì (柿蒂 persimmon calyx, Kaki Calyx)

2. Warming the Kidney and Calming Panting: *Chén xiāng* is warm and downbearing in nature. It conducts qì to the kidney, warms and supplements kidney yáng, and is used for panting due to kidney vacuity cold. This pattern is characterized by inhalation more difficult than exhalation and inability for inhaled breath to reach the cinnabar field (region below the umbilicus), cold pain in the lumbus and knees, impotence, seminal efflux, limp legs, and a cubit pulse that is moderate and weak. For this purpose *chén xiāng* is often combined with medicinals such as:

bǔ gǔ zhī (补骨脂 psoralea, Psoraleae Fructus)

hú lú bā (胡芦巴 fenugreek, Trigonellae Semen)

yáng qǐ shí (阳起石 actinolite, Actinolitum)

hēi xí (黑锡 galenite, Galenitum)

liú huáng (硫黄 sulfur, Sulphur)[8]

fù zǐ (附子 aconite, Aconiti Radix Lateralis Praeparata)

xiǎo huí xiāng (小茴香 fennel, Foeniculi Fructus)

ròu dòu kòu (肉豆蔻 nutmeg, Myristicae Semen)

jīn líng zǐ (金铃子 toosendan, Toosendan Fructus)

mù xiāng (木香 costusroot, Aucklandiae Radix)

ròu guì (肉桂 cinnamon bark, Cinnamomi Cortex)

For example, *jú fāng hēi xí dān* (Bureau Formula Galenite Elixir) is composed of the above medicinals. The dosage for this formula is 1.5–2.5 g/5–8 fēn, not exceeding 3 g/1 qián, once or twice a day. *Chén xiāng* can sometimes also be used for repletion panting and cough due to lung qì failing to downbear, and congesting phlegm turbidity, for which it is often combined with *sū zǐ* (perilla fruit), *qián hú* (peucedanum), *bàn xià* (pinellia), *hòu pò* (officinal magnolia bark), and *chén pí*

---

[8] *Hēi xí* (galenite) and *liú huáng* (sulfur) are not included in decoction medicine; they are only in pill formulas. (Au.)

(tangerine peel). For example, *jú fāng sū zǐ jiàng qì tāng* (Bureau Formula Perilla Fruit Qì-Downbearing Decoction), given below, makes use of the qì-downbearing strength of *chén xiāng* to disperse phlegm and calm panting.

Jú fāng sū zǐ jiàng qì tāng 局方苏子降气汤	Bureau Formula Perilla Fruit Qì-Downbearing Decoction

> *sū zǐ* (苏子 perilla fruit, Perillae Fructus)
> *bàn xià* (半夏 pinellia, Pinelliae Rhizoma)
> *qián hú* (前胡 peucedanum, Peucedani Radix)
> *hòu pò* (厚朴 officinal magnolia bark, Magnoliae Officinalis Cortex)
> *chén pí* (陈皮 tangerine peel, Citri Reticulatae Pericarpium)
> *gān cǎo* (甘草 licorice, Glycyrrhizae Radix)
> *dāng guī* (当归 Chinese angelica, Angelicae Sinensis Radix)
> *chén xiāng* (沉香 aquilaria, Aquilariae Lignum Resinatum)

COMPARISONS

Xuán fù huā (inula flower)[211] downbears lung-spleen phlegm qì, while *chén xiāng* downbears spleen and kidney counterflow qì.

Bīng láng (areca)[237] downbears qì, but it tends to be used to break, drain, and downbear, and hence is contraindicated in vacuity of right qì. *Chén xiāng* likewise downbears qì, but having no breaking and draining effect, it does not damage right qì. According to traditional experience, *chén xiāng* "moves qì but does not damage qì, and warms the center without assisting fire [evil]." This is worth bearing in mind.

Jiàng xiāng (dalbergia) downbears the qì in blood and stanches bleeding. *Chén xiāng* downbears the qì that a vacuous kidney fails to absorb and thereby calms panting.

PREPARATION

Chén xiāng is usually ground to a fine powder and taken with decoction medicine. This method is economical, and the effect is reliable. It is generally not boiled in a decoction medicine.

DOSAGE

The dosage is generally 0.6–2.5 g/2–8 fēn, taken with decoction medicine.

CAUTION

Contraindicated in qì vacuity fall.

---

6. 檀香 Tán Xiāng   Santali Albi Lignum
Sandalwood

Acrid in flavor and warm in nature, *tán xiāng* (sandalwood) is a qì-rectifying and depression-opening medicinal that mainly regulates the spleen and lung and disinhibits the chest and diaphragm.

Tán xiāng conducts the qì of the spleen and stomach upward and enhances intake of food and drink. It opens and effuses qì depression in the chest and lung, and thereby loosens and disinhibits the chest and diaphragm. It is therefore used for impaired regulation of spleen and lung qì in conditions such as oppression and distention in the chest and diaphragm, pain in the heart [region] and abdomen, decreased intake of food and drink, and **dysphagia-occlusion**[548] (噎膈 *yē gé*) with vomiting of food. For this purpose, *tán xiāng* is often combined with *sū gěng* (perilla stem), *guā lóu pí* (trichosanthes rind), and *zhǐ qiào* (bitter orange) for oppression and distention in the chest and diaphragm; with *dān shēn* (salvia), *shā rén* (amomum), *wū yào* (lindera), *bǎi hé* (lily bulb), and *gāo liáng jiāng* (lesser galangal) for pain in the heart [region] and abdomen; with *chén pí* (tangerine peel), *shēng mài yá* (raw barley sprout), *shā shēn* (adenophora/glehnia), and *mài dōng* (ophiopogon) for decreased intake of food and drink.

COMBINATIONS

For coronary heart disease and angina pectoris, I often combine *tán xiāng* with the following:

guā lóu (瓜蒌 trichosanthes, Trichosanthis Fructus)

xiè bái (薤白 Chinese chive, Allii Macrostemonis Bulbus)

guì zhī (桂枝 cinnamon twig, Cinnamomi Ramulus)

hóng huā (红花 carthamus, Carthami Flos)

chì sháo (赤芍 red peony, Paeoniae Radix Rubra)

yuǎn zhì (远志 polygala, Polygalae Radix)

wǔ líng zhī (五灵脂 squirrel's droppings, Trogopteri Faeces)

pú huáng (蒲黄 typha pollen, Typhae Pollen)

bīng láng (槟榔 areca, Arecae Semen)

I find it produces satisfactory results for oppression and pain of fixed location in the chest. Also, I often combine this medicinal with *dān shēn* (salvia), *shā rén* (amomum), *gāo liáng jiāng* (lesser galangal), *xiāng fù* (cyperus), *bǎi hé* (lily bulb), and *wū yào* (lindera) to treat persistent stomach duct pain (including pain from ulcers). The two formulas above should be varied in accordance with signs. Note that for both formulas I recommend 31 g/1 liǎng of *dān shēn* (salvia) and *bǎi hé* (lily bulb), and only 6–9 g/2–3 qián of the other medicinals.

COMPARISONS

In Chinese we speak of two different kinds of 檀香 *tán xiāng*, purple (紫檀 *zǐ tán xiāng*) and white (白檀 *bái tán*). The purple kind is not a true sandalwood.[9] It is cold in nature, salty in flavor, and tends to enter the blood aspect. It is applied topically to **incised wounds**[552] (金创 *jīn chuāng*) to disperse swelling and settle pain. If one writes *tán xiāng* 檀香 on a prescription, the pharmacist will give 白檀 *bái tán*, the white kind. If one wants *zǐ tán*, one has to specify it explicitly.

Chén xiāng (aquilaria)[206] downbears qì. Within its downbearing there is also upbearing, but it tends to be used to downbear qì. *Tán xiāng* rectifies qì. Within its upbearing there is downbearing, but it tends to be used to diffuse qì depression.

---

[9] *Zǐ tán* (紫檀 Burmese rosewood, Pterocarpi Lignum). (Ed.)

Jiàng xiāng (dalbergia), which rectifies qì and also enters the blood aspect, tends to be used to treat fractures, to stanch bleeding, to quicken the blood, and to disperse swelling and settle pain. *Tán xiāng* (sandalwood) tends to rectify qì and open depression, and it can treat any pain in the heart [region] and abdomen.

Dosage

The dosage is generally 1.5–9 g/5 fēn–3 qián. When used in decoction medicines, it should be added at the end.

---

7. 柿蒂 Shì Dì   Kaki Calyx
Persimmon Calyx

Bitter and astringent in flavor and neutral in nature, *shì dì* (persimmon calyx) downbears counterflow qì and stops hiccup.

Combinations

When used to treat retching, *shì dì* is often combined with medicinals such as *bàn xià* (pinellia), *zhú rú* (bamboo shavings), *shēng jiāng* (fresh ginger), *huò xiāng* (agastache), and *dài zhě shí* (hematite). To treat hiccup, it is often combined with medicinals such as *dīng xiāng* (clove), *chén xiāng* (aquilaria), and *xuán fù huā* (inula flower). For vacuity-pattern hiccup (as observed in severe illness, enduring illness, or in the elderly and weak), *dǎng shēn* (codonopsis), *rén shēn* (ginseng), *fù zǐ* (aconite), *bái zhú* (white atractylodes), and *chén pí* (tangerine peel) can also be added. For hiccup due to cerebrovascular accident or other diseases of the brain and nervous system, I have found that the formula given below produces results. It should be varied in accordance with signs and taken decocted with water.

shì dì (柿蒂 persimmon calyx, Kaki Calyx) 7–10 pieces

gōng dīng xiāng (公丁香 clove, Caryophylli Flos) 2.5–4.5 g/8 fēn–1.5 qián (add at end)

shēng dài zhě shí (生代赭石 crude hematite, Haematitum Crudum) 30–40 g/1–1.5 liǎng (predecoct)

xuán fù huā (旋覆花 inula flower, Inulae Flos) 9 g/3 qián (wrapped in cloth)

dǎng shēn (党参 codonopsis, Codonopsis Radix) 9–12 g/3–4 qián

bàn xià (半夏 pinellia, Pinelliae Rhizoma) 9 g/3 qián

dāo dòu zǐ (刀豆子 sword bean, Canavaliae Semen) 9 g/3 qián[10]

sū zǐ (苏子 perilla fruit, Perillae Fructus) 6–9 g/2–3 qián

Dosage

The dosage is generally 3–9 g/1–3 qián, or 3–7 calyxes.

---

[10]*Dāo dòu zǐ* (sword bean) is sweet and warm; it downbears qì and relieves belching. It is principally employed in the treatment of vacuity-cold counterflow characterized by belching, nausea, and vomiting. The dosage in decoctions is typically 10–15 grams. (Ed.)

8. 旋覆花 Xuán Fù Huā   Inulae Flos
Inula Flower

Including

> *jīn fèi cǎo* (金沸草 inula, Inulae Herba)

Xuán fù huā (inula flower) is bitter, acrid, and salty in flavor and warm in nature. Its main actions are downbearing qì, transforming phlegm, and moving water.

1. **Belching and Retching Counterflow:** *Xuán fù huā* is used to treat counterflow ascent of lung and stomach qì that occurs a) when great sweating or draining precipitation has caused damage to stomach qì or b) when damp phlegm becomes obstructed and fails to bear downward, which manifests in frequent belching, glomus and oppression in the stomach duct, painful distention in the chest and rib-side, and immediate vomiting of ingested food with vomitus composed of food mixed with phlegm-water. *Xuán fù huā* is often combined with medicinals such as *dài zhě shí* (hematite), *bàn xià* (pinellia), *shēng jiāng* (fresh ginger), *dǎng shēn* (codonopsis), *zhú rú* (bamboo shavings), *sū zǐ* (perilla fruit), and *fú líng* (poria). For exuberant phlegm-damp, one can add *chén pí* (tangerine peel) and *chǎo lái fú zǐ* (stir-fried radish seed).

2. **Cough and Panting with Copious Phlegm:** This medicinal downbears qì and transforms phlegm, causing qì to downbear and phlegm to disperse, thereby calming cough and panting. When impaired downbearing of lung qì causes phlegm turbidity, amassment of water-rheum, or stagnation and blockage in the chest and diaphragm that further inhibit qì dynamic, signs that arise include cough with copious thick sticky phlegm and qì counterflow with panting. For this purpose, *xuán fù huā* is often combined with medicinals such as:

chén pí (陈皮 tangerine peel, Citri Reticulatae Pericarpium)
bàn xià (半夏 pinellia, Pinelliae Rhizoma)
sāng pí (桑皮 mulberry root bark, Mori Cortex)
xìng rén (杏仁 apricot kernel, Armeniacae Semen)
zǐ wǎn (紫菀 aster, Asteris Radix)
sū zǐ (苏子 perilla fruit, Perillae Fructus)
bīng láng (槟榔 areca, Arecae Semen)
chǎo lái fú zǐ (炒莱菔子 stir-fried radish seed, Raphani Semen Frictum)[11]

The whole herb, including flowers, stalks, and leaves, is called *jīn fèi cǎo* (金沸草, inula). Besides downbearing qì and transforming phlegm, *jīn fèi cǎo* is also used to treat wind-cold. It is therefore used for externally contracted wind-cold that causes cough with copious phlegm. For this, it is often used in combination with:

jīng jiè (荆芥 schizonepeta, Schizonepetae Herba)

---

[11] *Jīn fèi cǎo sǎn* (Inula Powder) is an example of this type of combination. Nowadays, *xuán fù huā* (inula flower) is often substituted for *jīn fèi cǎo* (inula). (Ed.)

qián hú (前胡 peucedanum, Peucedani Radix)

bàn xià (半夏 pinellia, Pinelliae Rhizoma)

xì xīn (细辛 asarum, Asari Herba)

fú líng (茯苓 poria, Poria)

sū yè (苏叶 perilla leaf, Perillae Folium)

jié gěng (桔梗 platycodon, Platycodonis Radix)

chén pí (陈皮 tangerine peel, Citri Reticulatae Pericarpium)

COMPARISONS

Sū zǐ (perilla fruit)[216] downbears qì and also opens depression and warms the center. *Xuán fù huā* downbears qì and also disperses phlegm and moves water.

Hǎi fú shí (costazia bone/pumice) treats phlegm-bind manifesting as hard lumps. *Xuán fù huā* treats spittle and sticky phlegm that is like glue or lacquer.

MISCELLANEOUS

This medicinal is downbearing in nature, hence the traditional saying "All flowers bear upward; only *xuán fù huā* (inula flower) bears downward."[12] On the basis of traditional experience, I have found that *xuán fù huā* combined with *sū gěng* (perilla stem), *hòu pò* (officinal magnolia bark), *bàn xià* (pinellia), *shēng mǔ lì* (crude oyster shell), *fú líng* (poria), *xiāng fù* (cyperus), *huáng qín* (scutellaria), *jīn guǒ lǎn* (tinospora root), and *wū méi tàn* (charred mume), when varied in accordance with signs, is effective in the treatment of **plum-pit qì**[559] (梅核气 *méi hé qì*). Plum-pit qì is caused by phlegm qì congealing and stagnating, and so medicinals that downbear qì and disperse phlegm are invariably effective in treating it.

DOSAGE

Dosage is generally 3–9 g/1–3 qián. This medicinal is covered with hairs and so is wrapped in gauze for decoction.

CAUTION

Contraindicated in qì vacuity and large intestine cold diarrhea.

---

9. 莱菔子 Lái Fú Zǐ   Raphani Semen
Radish Seed

Lái fú zǐ (radish seed) is acrid and sweet in flavor and neutral in nature. Its main actions are to downbear qì and calm panting, transform phlegm and disperse accumulations, as well as rectify qì and eliminate distention.

1. **Phlegm Panting and Cough:** For panting, cough, copious phlegm, and oppression in the chest due to phlegm turbidity obstructing the lung and impaired depurative downbearing of the lung, one can use this medicinal combined with *sū zǐ* (perilla fruit) and *bái jiè zǐ* (white mustard). This combination is traditionally called *sān zǐ yǎng qīn tāng* (Three-Seed Filial Devotion Decoction). Depending

---

[12]This, like many sayings in Chinese, is a generalization intended as a mnemonic device. Other flowers, such as *kuǎn dōng huā* (coltsfoot),[440] also have downbearing actions. (Ed.)

on signs, it is combined with medicinals such as *chén pí* (tangerine peel), *bàn xià* (pinellia), *fú líng* (poria), and *zhì gān cǎo* (mix-fried licorice). In clinical practice, I often find that *lái fú zǐ* is effective for cough and panting with copious phlegm due to chronic bronchitis in the elderly. For this purpose, I combine *lái fú zǐ* with *má huáng* (ephedra), *xìng rén* (apricot kernel), *chǎo lái fú zǐ* (stir-fried radish seed), *chǎo sū zǐ* (stir-fried perilla fruit), *chǎo bái jiè zǐ* (stir-fried white mustard), *bàn xià* (pinellia), *chén pí* (tangerine peel), *fú líng* (poria), and *zhì gān cǎo* (mix-fried licorice) according to the signs. As a way of remembering this formula, I call it *má xìng èr sān tāng* (Ephedra and Apricot Kernel Two-Three Decoction), "Two" standing for *èr chén tāng* (Two Matured Ingredients Decoction),[13] and "Three" standing for *sān zǐ yǎng qīn tāng* (Three-Seed Filial Devotion Decoction).[14] If the tongue fur is thick and slimy and the stool is dry, add *shú dà huáng* (cooked rhubarb), *bīng láng* (areca), and *guā lóu* (trichosanthes). If exhaling is more difficult than inhaling, add *zhǐ qiào* (bitter orange), *jié gěng* (platycodon), and *qián hú* (peucedanum). If inhaling is more difficult, add *cí shí* (loadstone) and *chén xiāng* (aquilaria). For pronounced cough, add *zǐ wǎn* (aster), *pí pá yè* (loquat leaf), and *bèi mǔ* (fritillaria). For coughing of clear phlegm, add *gān jiāng* (dried ginger), *xì xīn* (asarum), and *wǔ wèi zǐ* (schisandra).

2. Food Accumulation and Abdominal Distention: For blockage and oppression in the stomach duct, belching and acid swallowing, and abdominal fullness and distention that occurs when food and drink accumulates and stagnates, this medicinal is used in combination with *jiāo sān xiān* (scorch-fried three immortals),[555] *bīng láng* (areca), *zhǐ shí* (unripe bitter orange), and *mù xiāng* (costusroot).

Used raw, *lái fú zǐ* tends to upbear, and when taken in large quantities, it can cause nausea and vomiting. (In clinical practice, therefore, it is not commonly used raw, except for in food stagnation patterns, when the treatment involves making the patient vomit.) When stir-fried,[15] it is downbearing in nature and is used to downbear qì and transform phlegm and to disperse distention and calm panting.

COMPARISON

Shān zhā hé (crataegus pit) tends to aid digestion and disintegrate accumulation lumps. *Lái fú zǐ* tends to disperse phlegm and transform stagnation and to downbear qì and eliminate phlegm.

DOSAGE

The dosage is generally 4.5–9 g/1.5–3 qián.

CAUTION

Contraindicated in qì vacuity without phlegm accumulation.

---

[13]The translation of *èr chén tāng* 二陈汤 as "Two Matured Ingredients Decoction" reflects the use of two ingredients that are aged before use. These are *chén pí* (tangerine peel) and *bàn xià* (pinellia). (Ed.)

[14]In the original text, *sān zǐ yǎng qīn tāng* (Three-Seed Filial Devotion Decoction) is called *sān zǐ tāng* (Three-Seed Decoction). See footnote on page 3 on term changes in the People's Republic of China. (Ed.)

[15]Stir-fried *lái fú zǐ* is typically dry-fried in a wok over a medium flame. The medicinal is stirred and fried until it puffs up and gives off its characteristic aroma. (Ed.)

10. 薤白 Xiè Bái
Chinese Chive

Allii Macrostemonis
Bulbus

Acrid and bitter in flavor and warm in nature, *xiè bái* (Chinese chive) mainly assists chest yáng, opens the orifices of the heart, and dissipates qì stagnation in the chest and large intestine. It also quickens the blood.

For chest impediment with stabbing pain, heart pain and blood stagnation, and rapid panting that result from devitalized yáng qì in the chest, *xiè bái* is often combined with medicinals such as:

guā lóu (瓜蒌 trichosanthes, Trichosanthis Fructus)

bái jiǔ (白酒 white liquor, Granorum Spiritus Incolor)

guì zhī (桂枝 cinnamon twig, Cinnamomi Ramulus)

zhǐ qiào (枳壳 bitter orange, Aurantii Fructus)

wǔ líng zhī (五灵脂 squirrel's droppings, Trogopteri Faeces)

pú huáng (蒲黄 typha pollen, Typhae Pollen)

tán xiāng (檀香 sandalwood, Santali Albi Lignum)

hóng huā (红花 carthamus, Carthami Flos)

sū gěng (苏梗 perilla stem, Perillae Caulis)

sū zǐ (苏子 perilla fruit, Perillae Fructus)

bīng láng (槟榔 areca, Arecae Semen)

chuān xiōng (川芎 chuanxiong, Chuanxiong Rhizoma)

On the basis of clinical experience, it is used to treat what modern medicine calls angina pectoris.

For dysentery with rectal heaviness and rough stagnant stool due to large intestine qì stagnation, *xiè bái* is often combined with medicinals such as:

bái sháo (白芍 white peony, Paeoniae Radix Alba)

mù xiāng (木香 costusroot, Aucklandiae Radix)

huáng lián (黄连 coptis, Coptidis Rhizoma)

bīng láng (槟榔 areca, Arecae Semen)

zhǐ shí (枳实 unripe bitter orange, Aurantii Fructus Immaturus)

zhǐ qiào (枳壳 bitter orange, Aurantii Fructus)

Xiè bái also dissipates blood, quickens stasis, and engenders the new. For chronic illness with qì stagnation and blood stasis, and pain in the limbs, it is combined with medicinals such as:

guì zhī (桂枝 cinnamon twig, Cinnamomi Ramulus)

dāng guī (当归 Chinese angelica, Angelicae Sinensis Radix)

hóng huā (红花 carthamus, Carthami Flos)

qiāng huó (羌活 notopterygium, Notopterygii Rhizoma et Radix)

piàn jiāng huáng (片姜黄 sliced turmeric, Curcumae Longae Rhizoma Sectum)

sōng jié (松节 knotty pine wood, Pini Nodi Lignum)

An example of such a formula is *chèn tòng sàn* (Pain-Chasing Powder).[16]

Chèn tòng sàn 趁痛散   Pain-Chasing Powder

---

niú xī (牛膝 achyranthes, Achyranthis Bidentatae Radix) 15 g/5 qián

dāng guī (当归 Chinese angelica, Angelicae Sinensis Radix) 15 g/5 qián

guì zhī (桂枝 cinnamon twig, Cinnamomi Ramulus) 15 g/5 qián

bái zhú (白术 white atractylodes, Atractylodis Macrocephalae Rhizoma)
   15 g/5 qián

huáng qí (黄芪 astragalus, Astragali Radix) 15 g/5 qián

dú huó (独活 pubescent angelica, Angelicae Pubescentis Radix) 15 g/5 qián

shēng jiāng (生姜 fresh ginger, Zingiberis Rhizoma Recens) 15 g/5 qián

xiè bái (薤白 Chinese chive, Allii Macrostemonis Bulbus) 7.5 g/2.5 qián

zhì gān cǎo (炙甘草 mix-fried licorice, Glycyrrhizae Radix cum Liquido Fricta)
   7.5 g/2.5 qián

Grind to a rough powder, and take 15 g/5 qián at a time, decocted with water. This is a commonly used formula for treating generalized pain in women with postpartum weak qì and blood stagnation who contract wind and catch cold.

Comparisons

Gān jiāng (dried ginger)[348] warms the lung and assists chest yáng. It tends to be used to dispel cold evil in the heart and lung. *Xiè bái* enters the heart and diffuses the orifices, moves qì, quickens the blood, and assists chest yáng. It tends to be used for stabbing pain due to chest impediment (胸痹 *xiōng bì*, i.e., heart and chest pain).

Xì xīn (asarum) enters the heart and assists yáng, but it mainly enters the liver and kidney. Thus for cough and panting and ejection of drool and foam due to water collecting below the heart, one can use *xì xīn*. *Xiè bái* dissipates large intestine qì stagnation and mainly enters the heart and assists chest yáng. Thus it is often used to treat chest impediment (胸痹 *xiōng bì*) due to devitalized heart yáng.

Dosage

The dosage is generally 3–9 g/1–3 qián. For especially severe conditions, up to 15 g/5 qián or more may be used.

Caution

Inappropriate in the absence of qì and blood stagnation.

---

[16]This version of *chèn tòng sàn* (Pain-Chasing Powder) is from *Fù Rén Liáng Fāng* (妇人良方 "Good Remedies for Women"). (Ed.)

11. 苏子 Sū Zǐ   Perillae Fructus
Perilla Fruit

Acrid in flavor and warm in nature, *sū zǐ* (perilla fruit) mainly precipitates qì and calms panting, disperses phlegm and suppresses cough, and disinhibits the diaphragm and opens depression.

Sū zǐ moistens the lung and heart, downbears qì, and disperses phlegm. For impaired depurative downbearing of the lung with copious phlegm and qì counterflow, which manifests in signs such as cough and panting, and oppression in the chest, it is often combined with:

xìng rén (杏仁 apricot kernel, Armeniacae Semen)

chǎo lái fú zǐ (炒莱菔子 stir-fried radish seed, Raphani Semen Frictum)

chǎo bái jiè zǐ (炒白芥子 stir-fried white mustard, Sinapis Albae Semen Frictum)

chén pí (陈皮 tangerine peel, Citri Reticulatae Pericarpium)

zǐ wǎn (紫菀 aster, Asteris Radix)

qián hú (前胡 peucedanum, Peucedani Radix)

hòu pò (厚朴 official magnolia bark, Magnoliae Officinalis Cortex)

dāng guī (当归 Chinese angelica, Angelicae Sinensis Radix)

chén xiāng (沉香 aquilaria, Aquilariae Lignum Resinatum)

Commonly used formulas for this pattern include:

Sān zǐ tāng 三子汤   Three-Seed Decoction

---

chǎo sū zǐ (炒苏子 stir-fried perilla fruit, Perillae Fructus Frictus)

chǎo lái fú zǐ (炒莱菔子 stir-fried radish seed, Raphani Semen Frictum)

chǎo bái jiè zǐ (炒白芥子 stir-fried white mustard, Sinapis Albae Semen Frictum)

Sū zǐ jiàng qì tāng 苏子降气汤   Perilla Fruit Qì-Downbearing Decoction

---

chǎo sū zǐ (炒苏子 stir-fried perilla fruit, Perillae Fructus Frictus)

bàn xià (半夏 pinellia, Pinelliae Rhizoma)

chén pí (陈皮 tangerine peel, Citri Reticulatae Pericarpium)

qián hú (前胡 peucedanum, Peucedani Radix)

hòu pò (厚朴 official magnolia bark, Magnoliae Officinalis Cortex)

gān cǎo (甘草 licorice, Glycyrrhizae Radix)

dāng guī (当归 Chinese angelica, Angelicae Sinensis Radix)

chén xiāng (沉香 aquilaria, Aquilariae Lignum Resinatum)

Sū zǐ has the further action of warming the center and downbearing counterflow. For stomach qì ascending counterflow and phlegm turbidity flooding upward causing nausea and vomiting, it is often combined with medicinals such as *bàn xià* (pinellia), *huò xiāng* (agastache), *fú líng* (poria), *chén pí* (tangerine peel), *dīng xiāng* (clove), *jiāo sān xiān* (scorch-fried three immortals),[555] and *zhǐ shí* (unripe bitter orange).

Sū gěng (perilla stem) is also commonly used to regulate qì. See "*zǐ sū* (perilla)," page 18.

Comparisons

Lái fú zǐ (radish seed)[212] is like *sū zǐ* in that it is effective for downbearing qì and calming panting, but it has greater power to disperse phlegm and break accumulations, while *sū zǐ* has greater power to precipitate qì and open depression. *Lái fú zǐ* (radish seed) tends to be used to disperse abdominal distention, while *sū zǐ* tends to be used to disinhibit the chest and diaphragm. The two medicinals are often used together to treat distention and oppression in the chest and abdomen.

Dosage

The dosage is generally 3–9 g/1–3 qián. It is stir-fried and crushed for use.

Caution

Contraindicated in qì vacuity fall.

---

12. 草豆蔻 Căo Dòu Kòu — Alpiniae Katsumadai
Katsumada's Galangal Seed — Semen

Acrid in flavor and warm in nature, *căo dòu kòu* (Katsumada's galangal seed) principally dries dampness, warms the center, breaks qì, and opens depression.

1. Center Burner Cold-Damp Failing to Transform: This medicinal is warm, acrid, and aromatic. Its dry harsh qì transforms damp turbidity. It is often used when due to cold-damp the center burner fails to transform and gives rise to signs such as vomiting, **stomach reflux**[564] (反胃 *fǎn wèi*), dysphagia-occlusion (噎膈 *yē gé*), glomus and oppression, diarrhea, abdominal distention, thick slimy white tongue fur, and oppression in the stomach duct with reduced food intake. For this, *căo dòu kòu* is combined with medicinals such as the following:

huò xiāng (藿香 agastache, Agastaches Herba)

chén pí (陈皮 tangerine peel, Citri Reticulatae Pericarpium)

mù xiāng (木香 costusroot, Aucklandiae Radix)

shā rén (砂仁 amomum, Amomi Fructus)

hòu pò (厚朴 officinal magnolia bark, Magnoliae Officinalis Cortex)

sū gěng (苏梗 perilla stem, Perillae Caulis)

fú líng (茯苓 poria, Poria)

xuán fù huā (旋覆花 inula flower, Inulae Flos)

2. Stomach Duct Pain: *Căo dòu kòu* dissipates stagnant qì with acridity and warms and transforms cold-damp. When cold-damp settles in the center burner, which results in stomach qì stagnation with signs such as stomach duct pain, thick white tongue fur, blockage and oppression in the chest and stomach duct, and epigastric fullness and distention, *căo dòu kòu* is combined with medicinals such as:

gāo liáng jiāng (高良姜 lesser galangal, Alpiniae Officinarum Rhizoma)

xiāng fù (香附 cyperus, Cyperi Rhizoma)

tán xiāng (檀香 sandalwood, Santali Albi Lignum)

shā rén (砂仁 amomum, Amomi Fructus)

sū gěng (苏梗 perilla stem, Perillae Caulis)

bīng láng (槟榔 areca, Arecae Semen)

wū yào (乌药 lindera, Linderae Radix)

dān shēn (丹参 salvia, Salviae Miltiorrhizae Radix)

bǎi hé (百合 lily bulb, Lilii Bulbus)

See *sān hé tāng* (Three-Combination Decoction) under *"xiāng fù* (cyperus)," page 227. In that formula, I often use *cǎo dòu kòu* instead of *shā rén* (amomum).

In clinical practice, whenever I observe aversion to cold and heat effusion (fever) occurring at set periods and mealy white tongue fur attributable to depressed cold-damp depression (whether or not a blood test shows the presence of plasmodium), to transform damp turbidity with aroma, I often add *cǎo dòu kòu* to suitable formulas containing medicinals such as:

chái hú (柴胡 bupleurum, Bupleuri Radix)

hòu pò (厚朴 officinal magnolia bark, Magnoliae Officinalis Cortex)

zhī mǔ (知母 anemarrhena, Anemarrhenae Rhizoma)

huáng qín (黄芩 scutellaria, Scutellariae Radix)

bīng láng (槟榔 areca, Arecae Semen)

cháng shān (常山 dichroa, Dichroae Radix)

huò xiāng (藿香 agastache, Agastaches Herba)

cāng zhú (苍术 atractylodes, Atractylodis Rhizoma)

Traditional literature states that this medicinal can "eliminate miasma and interrupt malaria" (除瘴截疟 *chú zhàng jié nüè*), so this is worth bearing in mind.

Comparisons

Bái dòu kòu (cardamom)[221] has functions broadly similar to those of *cǎo dòu kòu*. However, *bái dòu kòu* often tends to be used to move qì and loosen the diaphragm, and its power to dry dampness with aroma is not as strong as that of *cǎo dòu kòu*. On the other hand, *cǎo dòu kòu* tends to be used to break qì and open depression and to warm the center and dry dampness. *Bái dòu kòu* tends to enter the lung, while *cǎo dòu kòu* tends to enter the spleen.

Hóng dòu kòu (galangal fruit) is the seed of a closely related plant (*Alipinia galanga*). It is hot in nature and tends to be used to warm the lung and dissipate cold and to arouse the spleen and dry dampness. It is not an aromatic qì-moving medicinal.

Ròu dòu kòu (nutmeg)[188] astringes the large intestine and checks diarrhea. *Cǎo dòu kòu* dries dampness, breaks qì, and opens depression.

Cǎo guǒ (tsaoko)[508] has an acrid, aromatic, dry, harsh qì that is even more powerful than that of *cǎo dòu kòu*. It interrupts malaria and disperses phlegm.

Cǎo dòu kòu is effective in transforming dampness by warming the center and regulating qì.

DOSAGE

The dosage is generally 3–9 g/1–3 qián.

CAUTION

Taken over a long period of time or in excess, this medicinal can assist spleen heat and dissipate right qì.

---

13. 砂仁 **Shā Rén**   Amomi Fructus
Amomum

Acrid in flavor and warm in nature, *shā rén* (amomum) mainly moves qì and regulates the center, arouses the spleen and opens the stomach, and aids digestion. It also conducts qì to the kidney and further has the effect of warming the kidney and transforming dampness.

1. Fullness and Distention in the Stomach Duct and Abdomen: For fullness and distention in the stomach duct and abdomen, phlegm-damp accumulation and stagnation, vomiting, diarrhea, abdominal pain, and indigestion that are due to qì stagnation and spleen-stomach damp cold, *shā rén* (amomum) is used to move qì and dissipate cold, to transform dampness and harmonize the stomach, and to aid digestion. For this purpose it is often combined with medicinals such as:

zhǐ shí (枳实 unripe bitter orange, Aurantii Fructus Immaturus)

bái zhú (白术 white atractylodes, Atractylodis Macrocephalae Rhizoma)

mù xiāng (木香 costusroot, Aucklandiae Radix)

bàn xià (半夏 pinellia, Pinelliae Rhizoma)

chén pí (陈皮 tangerine peel, Citri Reticulatae Pericarpium)

fú líng (茯苓 poria, Poria)

huò xiāng (藿香 agastache, Agastaches Herba)

jiāo shén qū (焦神曲 scorch-fried medicated leaven, Massa Medicata Fermentata Usta)

2. Diarrhea: For diarrhea due to spleen-stomach vacuity cold (cold pain in the abdomen with a liking for pressure and warmth, absence of thirst, and clear thin stool), *shā rén* is used to warm the spleen, dissipate cold, and dry dampness. For this purpose, it is often combined with medicinals such as:

dǎng shēn (党参 codonopsis, Codonopsis Radix)

bái zhú (白术 white atractylodes, Atractylodis Macrocephalae Rhizoma)

mù xiāng (木香 costusroot, Aucklandiae Radix)

pào jiāng (炮姜 blast-fried ginger, Zingiberis Rhizoma Praeparatum)

fú líng (茯苓 poria, Poria)

3. Cold Dysentery: For cold dysentery due to spleen-stomach vacuity cold (cold pain in the abdomen, tenesmus, and stool containing white mucus, which are exacerbated by exposure to cold), *shā rén* can be used to warm the spleen, move qì, and transform dampness. It is often combined with medicinals such as:

mù xiāng (木香 costusroot, Aucklandiae Radix)

cǎo dòu kòu (草豆蔻 Katsumada's galangal seed, Alpiniae Katsumadai Semen)

wú yú (吴萸 evodia, Evodiae Fructus)

bīng láng (槟榔 areca, Arecae Semen)

dāng guī (当归 Chinese angelica, Angelicae Sinensis Radix)

tǔ chǎo bái sháo (土炒白芍 earth-fried white peony, Paeoniae Radix Alba cum Terra Fricta)

Because *shā rén* moves qì, promoting the free movement of stool, it is also sometimes used for ungratifying defecation and in cases of damp-heat dysentery. However, for this it needs to be combined with cold-natured medicinals such as *huáng lián* (coptis), *huáng qín* (scutellaria), *mǎ chǐ xiàn* (purslane), and *bái tóu wēng* (pulsatilla) in order to counteract its warm nature.

4. Stirring Fetus: For stirring fetus[564] (胎动不安 *tāi dòng bù ān*) due to stomach qì ascending counterflow manifesting in oppression in the chest, retching, and vomiting, use *shā rén* combined with medicinals such as *sū yè* (perilla leaf), *huò xiāng* (agastache), *huáng qín* (scutellaria), *bái zhú* (white atractylodes), *mù xiāng* (costusroot), and *dāng guī* (Chinese angelica). This quiets the fetus and harmonizes the center.

5. Preventing Side-Effects of Slimy Supplementing Medicinals: When using large quantities of slimy, clogging, supplementing medicinals such as *shú dì huáng* (cooked rehmannia), a little *shā rén* is included to prevent the side-effects of impairing digestion and reducing appetite.[17] Traditional literature often suggests the use of "*shú dì huáng* mixed with *shā rén*" (so that it sticks to the *shú dì huáng*). This method not only prevents *shú dì huáng* from damaging the stomach, but also helps it to reach the kidney. Thus it accomplishes two tasks at the same time.

COMPARISONS

Bái dòu kòu (cardamom)[221] is like *shā rén* in that it moves qì and regulates the center. But *bái dòu kòu* (cardamom) harmonizes the stomach and checks vomiting much better than *shā rén*, while *shā rén* warms the stomach and dries dampness much more effectively than *bái dòu kòu*.

Ròu guì (cinnamon bark)[343] is like *shā rén* in that it also enters the kidney. When conducting fire to the origin (the kidney), *ròu guì* is used; when conducting qì to the origin (the kidney), *shā rén* is used.

Shā qiào (amomum husk) also rectifies qì and arouses the stomach, but it lacks the power of *shā rén* to warm the center and dissipate cold. *Shā qiào* is weak in qì and flavor and has minor dryness, so it is appropriate for effulgent liver and weak stomach.

---

[17] Preparing this form of *shú dì huáng* (cooked rehmannia) involves pounding *shā rén* (amomum) powder into freshly steamed *shú dì huáng*. (Ed.)

RESEARCH

According to modern pharmacological research, *shā rén* has an aromatic stomach-fortifying effect, enhances stomach function, stimulates the secretion of gastric juices, and expels accumulated gas in the digestive tract.

DOSAGE

The dosage is generally 1.5–4.5 g/5 fēn–1.5 qián. Under special circumstances, one can use up to 6–9 g/2–3 qián. When *shā rén* is used in decoctions, it should be crushed and added at the end since its medicinal power diminishes with long boiling. *Shā qiào* (amomum husk) is light in substance and is generally used in doses of 0.9–1.5 g/3–5 fēn or 2–2.5 g/7–8 fēn.

CAUTION

This medicinal is aromatic, warm, and dry in nature. It should be used with caution in yīn vacuity with repletion heat.

---

14. 白豆蔻 Bái Dòu Kòu — Amomi Fructus
Cardamom — Rotundus

Acrid in flavor and warm in nature, *bái dòu kòu* (cardamom) is commonly used to move qì, transform dampness, fortify the stomach, and check retching. It diffuses stagnant qì in the lung, warms and moves cold qì in the stomach, and dries and transforms damp qì in the spleen channel.

1. Indigestion, Vomiting, and Stomach Reflux: This medicinal is suitable for pathoconditions such as indigestion, vomiting, stomach reflux, fullness and oppression in the chest and stomach duct, and abdominal distention and pain that are due to spleen-stomach vacuity cold, damp depression, or qì stagnation. For this purpose it is often combined with medicinals such as *huò xiāng* (agastache), *bàn xià* (pinellia), *chén pí* (tangerine peel), *shēng jiāng* (fresh ginger), and *dīng xiāng* (clove).

2. Damp Warm Disease: *Bái dòu kòu* is an especially effective aromatic, qì-moving, dryness-warming, and dampness-transforming medicinal. It is used to treat **damp warm disease**[545] (湿温病 *shī wēn bìng*) at the turn of season between summer and autumn, which manifests in **unsurfaced heat**[566] (身热不扬 *shēn rè bù yáng*), sweating that brings no abatement of heat [effusion], headache, generalized heaviness, blockage and oppression in the chest and stomach duct, poor appetite, absence of thirst sometimes with a sweet taste in the mouth, inhibited urination, thick glossy slimy white tongue fur, and soggy, slippery, and moderate pulse. For this purpose it is often combined with *xìng rén* (apricot kernel), *yǐ rén* (coix), *hòu pò* (officinal magnolia bark), *bàn xià* (pinellia), *huá shí* (talcum), *tōng cǎo* (rice-paper plant pith), and *zhú yè* (lophatherum) to bring about acrid opening, bitter downbearing, and bland percolation. This combination is *sān rén tāng* (Three Kernels Decoction), which is commonly used in the treatment of damp warmth.

Combinations

Bái dòu kòu combined with medicinals such as *chén pí* (tangerine peel), *shēng mài yá* (raw barley sprout), and *xiāng dào yá* (rice sprout) treats poor appetite. Combined with medicinals such as *gāo liáng jiāng* (lesser galangal), *xiāng fù* (cyperus), *gān jiāng* (dried ginger), and *wú yú* (evodia), it treats stomach cold pain.

Comparisons

Bái kòu yī (cardamom husk), also called *bái kòu pí* 白蔻皮, is effective in rectifying qì, loosening the chest, and dispersing distention; it has a less pronounced warm nature than *bái dòu kòu*, and is used accordingly.

Dosage

The dosage is generally 1.5–6 g/5 fēn–2 qián. If used without the husk it is called *bái kòu rén* (cardamom seed), which when used in decoctions is added at the end of cooking to preserve its medicinal strength.

Caution

Contraindicated in exuberant lung-stomach fire and qì vacuity.

Note

If one merely writes "蔻仁 *kòu rén*" on a prescription, the pharmacy will provide *zǐ kòu rén* (purple nutmeg), which is the highest quality of this medicinal. It is large, its flavor is concentrated, and its medicinal strength is full. *Zǐ kòu rén* (purple nutmeg) mainly moves qì with aroma, warms the center, and regulates the stomach. Its therapeutic action is between that of *shā rén* (amomum) and *bái dòu kòu* (cardamom). Its aromatic, warm, and dry nature is less than that of *shā rén*, but more than that of *bái dòu kòu*. Thus, in terms of stomach-regulating medicinals, *zǐ kòu rén* (purple nutmeg) can sometimes be substituted for *shā rén* (amomum).

---

15. 荔枝核 Lì Zhī Hé   Litchi Semen
Litchee Pit

Sweet in flavor and warm in nature, *lì zhī hé* (litchee pit) moves and dissipates stagnant qì and is suitable for various forms of qì stagnation with pain.

    1. Mounting Qì Pain: This medicinal enters the liver channel and is most commonly used to treat mounting qì pain (疝气痛 *shàn qì tòng*) and sagging, distention, and pain in the testicles. For this purpose it is often combined with medicinals such as *xiǎo huí xiāng* (fennel), *jú hé* (tangerine pip), *qīng pí* (unripe tangerine peel), *wū yào* (lindera), and *chuān liàn zǐ* (toosendan).

    2. Abdominal Pain: *Lì zhī hé* that is subjected to **nature-preservative burning**[558] (炒存性 *chǎo cún xìng*) is combined with *chǎo xiāng fù* (stir-fried cyperus) to treat women with stabbing abdominal pain from congealing blood and stagnant qì. Combined with *gāo liáng jiāng* (lesser galangal), *xiāng fù* (cyperus), and *wǔ líng zhī* (squirrel's droppings), it is used for stomach duct pain.

3. Running Piglet Qì: *Lì zhī hé* is also used to treat running piglet qì (奔豚 气 *bēn tún qì*, a subjective sensation of qì surging up from the smaller abdomen to below the heart or epigastric region that gives rise to pain). For this it is often combined with medicinals such as *xiǎo huí xiāng* (fennel), *mù xiāng* (costusroot), *wú yú* (evodia), and *ròu guì* (cinnamon bark). An example of such a combination is *bēn tún wán* (Running Piglet Pill) from *Yī Xué Xīn Wù* (医学心悟 "Medical Insights").

Bēn tún wán 奔豚丸   Running Piglet Pill

> *lì zhī hé* (荔枝核 litchee pit, Litchi Semen) 24 g/8 qián
>
> *xiǎo huí xiāng* (小茴香 fennel, Foeniculi Fructus) 21 g/7 qián
>
> *mù xiāng* (木香 costusroot, Aucklandiae Radix) 21 g/7 qián
>
> *ròu guì* (肉桂 cinnamon bark, Cinnamomi Cortex) 9 g/3 qián
>
> *fù zǐ* (附子 aconite, Aconiti Radix Lateralis Praeparata) 15 g/5 qián
>
> *wú yú* (吴萸 evodia, Evodiae Fructus) 15 g/5 qián
>
> *fú líng* (茯苓 poria, Poria) 45 g/1.5 liǎng
>
> *jú hé* (橘核 tangerine pip, Citri Reticulatae Semen) 45 g/1.5 liǎng
>
> *chuān liàn zǐ* (川楝子 toosendan, Toosendan Fructus) 30 g/1 liǎng

The above medicinals are ground together to a fine powder that is mixed with *chǎo shā táng* (stir-fried granulated sugar) and formed into pills. The dosage is 6 g/ 2 qián at a time, to be swallowed with weak brine. In heat patterns, *ròu guì* (cinnamon bark) and *fù zǐ* (aconite) are removed.

I often use *bēn tún wán* (Running Piglet Pill) combined with *guì zhī jiā guì tāng* (Cinnamon Twig Decoction with Extra Cinnamon) and *xuán fù dài zhě tāng* (Inula and Hematite Decoction).

Guì zhī jiā guì tāng 桂枝加桂汤   Cinnamon Twig Decoction with Extra Cinnamon

> *guì zhī* (桂枝 cinnamon twig, Cinnamomi Ramulus)
>
> *bái sháo* (白芍 white peony, Paeoniae Radix Alba)
>
> *zhì gān cǎo* (炙甘草 mix-fried licorice, Glycyrrhizae Radix cum Liquido Fricta)
>
> *shēng jiāng* (生姜 fresh ginger, Zingiberis Rhizoma Recens)
>
> *dà zǎo* (大枣 jujube, Jujubae Fructus)
>
> *ròu guì* (肉桂 cinnamon bark, Cinnamomi Cortex)

Ròu guì can be replaced with a larger dosage of *guì zhī*.

Xuán fù dài zhě tāng 旋覆代赭汤   Inula and Hematite Decoction

> *xuán fù huā* (旋覆花 inula flower, Inulae Flos)
>
> *shēng dài zhě shí* (生代赭石 crude hematite, Haematitum Crudum)
>
> *bàn xià* (半夏 pinellia, Pinelliae Rhizoma)
>
> *dǎng shēn* (党参 codonopsis, Codonopsis Radix)
>
> *shēng jiāng* (生姜 fresh ginger, Zingiberis Rhizoma Recens)

gān cǎo (甘草 licorice, Glycyrrhizae Radix)

dà zǎo (大枣 jujube, Jujubae Fructus)

When the main ingredients of these three formulas are combined, the resulting formula, varied in accordance with signs and prepared as a decoction medicine, is always effective in the treatment of running piglet qì disease, which in Western medicine is usually diagnosed as neurosis.

Dosage

The dosage is generally 6–12 g/2–4 qián.

Caution

Use with care in the absence of cold-damp qì stagnation.

---

16. 川楝子 **Chuān Lián Zǐ**   Toosendan Fructus
Toosendan

Also called *jīn líng zǐ* 金铃子. *Chuān lián zǐ* (toosendan) is bitter in flavor, cold in nature, and slightly toxic.

1. Liver Qì Pain: This medicinal enters the liver channel and soothes liver qì. It is therefore often used to treat liver qì pain, liver qì distention, rib-side pain, mounting pain, fullness and oppression in the chest, and stomach duct pain. For such purposes *chuān lián zǐ* is often combined with medicinals such as:

yán hú suǒ (延胡索 corydalis, Corydalis Rhizoma)

mù xiāng (木香 costusroot, Aucklandiae Radix)

qīng pí (青皮 unripe tangerine peel, Citri Reticulatae Pericarpium Viride)

hòu pò (厚朴 officinal magnolia bark, Magnoliae Officinalis Cortex)

xiāng fù (香附 cyperus, Cyperi Rhizoma)

Chuān lián zǐ can also conduct pericardium channel fire-heat downward, and abducts small intestine and bladder damp-heat; thus it is used to clear heat and disinhibit dampness. For this purpose it is used in combination with medicinals such as *mù tōng* (trifoliate akebia), *zhú yè* (lophatherum), *shēng dì huáng* (dried/fresh rehmannia), and *zé xiè* (alisma).

2. Mounting Qì: On the basis of their experience, physicians of the past considered *chuān lián zǐ* to be "an important medicinal for mounting qì (疝气 *shàn qì*)."[558] Nevertheless, it is cold or cool in nature; therefore, when treating cold patterns it needs to be combined with medicinals such as:

xiǎo huí xiāng (小茴香 fennel, Foeniculi Fructus)

lì zhī hé (荔枝核 litchee pit, Litchi Semen)

wú yú (吴萸 evodia, Evodiae Fructus)

ròu guì (肉桂 cinnamon bark, Cinnamomi Cortex)

wū yào (乌药 lindera, Linderae Radix)

bǔ gǔ zhī (补骨脂 psoralea, Psoraleae Fructus)

It can also be stir-fried to reduce its cold nature.

COMBINATIONS

Chuān liàn zǐ combined with *yán hú suǒ* (corydalis) is used to treat heat-type stomach pain. Combined with *zhǐ qiào* (bitter orange) and *xiāng fù* (cyperus), it is used to treat liver heat rib-side pain. Combined with *wū méi* (mume) and *chuān jiāo* (zanthoxylum), it treats roundworm abdominal pain.

COMPARISONS

Lì zhī hé (litchee pit)²²² treats mounting and is warm in nature. *Chuān liàn zǐ* (toosendan) also treats mounting, but is cold in nature.

Kǔ liàn zǐ (chinaberry seed), or more usually *kǔ liàn gēn pí* (chinaberry root bark),⁵¹¹ tends to be used to kill worms. *Chuān liàn zǐ* (toosendan) tends to be used to soothe the liver and rectify qì and to treat mounting. *Chuān liàn pí* (toosendan bark) is also used to kill worms.¹⁸

PROCESSING

Use stir-fried to treat mounting and course the liver; use raw to clear heat.

DOSAGE

The dosage is generally 3–12 g/1–4 qián.

CAUTION

Contraindicated in spleen-stomach vacuity cold.

---

17. 香附 **Xiāng Fù**   Cyperi Rhizoma
Cyperus

Acrid and slightly bitter in flavor and neutral in nature,¹⁹ *xiāng fù* (cyperus) is the most commonly used qì-rectifying and depression-opening medicinal. It is diffusing in nature and is able to free the qì aspect of the twelve channels and eight vessels. In older literature, it was said to "govern all qì," resolve the six depressions (qì depression, blood depression, phlegm depression, food depression, damp depression, and fire depression), and regulate menstruation.

1. Soothing the Liver and Resolving Depression: *Xiāng fù* is aromatic, acrid, and dissipating. It regulates qì, soothes the liver, and resolves depression. It treats liver qì depression due to inhibited emotions, which manifests in abdominal fullness and distention, rib-side distention and pain, no pleasure in eating, and oppression in the chest with a liking for long exhalation. For this purpose it is often combined with medicinals such as:

---

¹⁸Technically, *kǔ liàn pí* (chinaberry bark) is tree bark (or the root bark) of *Melia azedarach* L., whereas the recognized source of *chuān liàn pí* (toosendan bark) is *Melia toosendan* SIEB. ET ZUCC. In practice the two species are used interchangeably, and *Melia toosendan* is also considered to be *kǔ liàn pí* (chinaberry bark). (Ed.)

¹⁹Many sources, including the *Běn Cǎo Gāng Mù* (本草纲目 "The Comprehensive Herbal Foundation"), include sweet among the flavors of *xiāng fù* (cyperus). (Ed.)

chái hú (柴胡 bupleurum, Bupleuri Radix)

bái sháo (白芍 white peony, Paeoniae Radix Alba)

yù jīn (郁金 curcuma, Curcumae Radix)

qīng pí (青皮 unripe tangerine peel, Citri Reticulatae Pericarpium Viride)

chén pí (陈皮 tangerine peel, Citri Reticulatae Pericarpium)

mù xiāng (木香 costusroot, Aucklandiae Radix)

hòu pò (厚朴 officinal magnolia bark, Magnoliae Officinalis Cortex)

sū gěng (苏梗 perilla stem, Perillae Caulis)

For different forms of depression, other medicinals may be judiciously added: a) For liver qì depression with concurrent blood depression (dark purple tongue, absence of menstruation, lusterless facial complexion, etc.), add *chuān xiōng* (chuanxiong) and *hóng huā* (carthamus). b) For concurrent phlegm depression (slimy white tongue fur, retching and nausea, copious phlegm, obesity, no desire to drink water, etc.), add *bàn xià* (pinellia), *jú hóng* (red tangerine peel), and *fú líng* (poria). c) For concurrent food depression (poor appetite, putrid belching and acid swallowing, thick tongue fur, glomus and oppression in the stomach duct, etc.), add *chǎo bīng láng* (stir-fried areca), *jiāo shén qū* (scorch-fried medicated leaven), and *chǎo mài yá* (stir-fried barley sprout). d) For concurrent damp depression (with signs such as watery glossy tongue fur, oppression in the chest, no desire to drink water, in some cases slight puffy swelling, sloppy stool, etc.), add *cāng zhú* (atractylodes), *bái zhú* (white atractylodes), *qiāng huó* (notopterygium), *zhū líng* (polyporus), and *zé xiè* (alisma). e) For fire depression (symptoms such as bitter taste in the mouth, vexation, yellow urine, red-tipped tongue, etc.), add *zhī zǐ* (gardenia), *huáng qín* (scutellaria), and *chuān liàn zǐ* (toosendan).

2. Moving Qì and Settling Pain: *Xiāng fù* (cyperus) moves qì and frees stagnation; when there is free flow, there is no pain. *Xiāng fù* is most commonly used for qì stagnation stomach pain (stomach pain caused by anger, or stomach pain exacerbated by bad moods, with rib-side distention and pain, and stringlike pulse, etc.). For this it is often combined with medicinals such as *gāo liáng jiāng* (lesser galangal), *mù xiāng* (costusroot), *bái dòu kòu* (cardamom), *chuān liàn zǐ* (toosendan), *yán hú suǒ* (corydalis), *bái sháo* (white peony), and *sū gěng* (perilla stem). It is often used in prescriptions such as *liáng fù sǎn* (Lesser Galangal and Cyperus Powder): Take 60–90 g/2–3 liǎng of *xiāng fù*, grind to a fine powder, pour into a jar, and secure the lid tightly. Then take 60–90 g/2–3 liǎng *gāo liáng jiāng* (lesser galangal), grind to a fine powder, pour into another jar, and secure the lid tightly. When stomach duct pain due to qì stagnation cold depression occurs, if the qì stagnation is more pronounced than the cold depression (pain exacerbated by anger or attacking the rib-side, with rashness and irascibility, and stringlike pulse), take 2.1 g/7 fēn of the powdered *xiāng fù* and 0.9 g/3 fēn of the powdered *gāo liáng jiāng*, mix them in a small packet, and swallow with warm water. If the cold depression is more pronounced than the qì stagnation (stomach duct liking warmth, liking for hot foods and drinks, pain exacerbated by exposure to cold, and a slow or moderate stringlike pulse), take 2.1 g/7 fēn of the powdered *gāo liáng jiāng* and 0.9 g/3 fēn of the powdered *xiāng fù*, mix them in a small packet, and swallow with warm water. If qì stagnation and cold depression are equally pronounced, take 1.5 g/ 5 fēn of each of the powdered *xiāng fù* and *gāo liáng jiāng*, mix them together, and swallow with warm water. Note that the two powders are more effective when mixed just before they are taken. I also often combine *liáng fù sǎn* (Lesser Galangal and Cyperus Powder), *bǎi hé tāng* (Lily Bulb Decoction), and *dān shēn yǐn* (Salvia Beverage) to form what I call *sān hé tāng* (Three-Combination Decoction), which I use to treat stomach duct pain that has persisted over a long period or that takes the form of vacuity, repletion, cold, and heat complex patterns (including ulcers, chronic gastritis, antral gastritis, etc.), invariably getting satisfactory results. Such a combination can take the following form:

Sān hé tāng 三合汤   Three-Combination Decoction

> *gāo liáng jiāng* (高良姜 lesser galangal, Alpiniae Officinarum Rhizoma)
>   9 g/3 qián
>
> *xiāng fù* (香附 cyperus, Cyperi Rhizoma) 9 g/3 qián
>
> *bǎi hé* (百合 lily bulb, Lilii Bulbus) 30 g/1 liǎng
>
> *wū yào* (乌药 lindera, Linderae Radix) 9 g/3 qián
>
> *dān shēn* (丹参 salvia, Salviae Miltiorrhizae Radix) 30 g/1 liǎng
>
> *tán xiāng* (檀香 sandalwood, Santali Albi Lignum) 6 g/2 qián (add at end)
>
> *shā rén* (砂仁 amomum, Amomi Fructus) 2.5 g/8 fēn or *cǎo dòu kòu* (草豆蔻
>   Katsumada's galangal seed, Alpiniae Katsumadai Semen) 9 g/3 qián

If the location of the pain remains markedly fixed and the tongue body is dark or has stasis macules on it, one can add *shī xiào sǎn* (Sudden Smile Powder), which contains *wǔ líng zhī* (squirrel's droppings) and *pú huáng* (typha pollen). For vomiting of acid water, add *duàn wǎ léng zǐ* (calcined ark shell). For dry stool, add *shēng dà huáng* (raw rhubarb) and *bīng láng* (areca). Further additions can be made as necessary.

3. Rectifying Qì and Regulating Menstruation: Because *xiāng fù* is a qì-moving medicinal that can also enter the blood aspect, it is traditionally called a "qì-in-blood medicinal" (that is, a qì-moving medicinal that enters the blood aspect). It rectifies qì and regulates menstruation (adjusts the menstrual cycle), and it is effective for signs such as menstrual irregularities, overdue periods, and abdominal pain during menstruation that are due to liver qì depression in emotionally inhibited women. For this purpose it is combined with medicinals such as:

> *dāng guī* (当归 Chinese angelica, Angelicae Sinensis Radix)
>
> *bái sháo* (白芍 white peony, Paeoniae Radix Alba)
>
> *shú dì huáng* (熟地黄 cooked rehmannia, Rehmanniae Radix Praeparata)
>
> *hóng huā* (红花 carthamus, Carthami Flos)
>
> *wǔ líng zhī* (五灵脂 squirrel's droppings, Trogopteri Faeces)
>
> *chuān liàn zǐ* (川楝子 toosendan, Toosendan Fructus)
>
> *xiǎo huí xiāng* (小茴香 fennel, Foeniculi Fructus)
>
> *wū yào* (乌药 lindera, Linderae Radix)
>
> *táo rén* (桃仁 peach kernel, Persicae Semen)

Xiāng fù (cyperus) also conducts blood-supplementing medicinals to the qì aspect in order to engender blood. It is used in combination with other medicinals to treat any antepartum or postpartum pathocondition, and for this reason it is traditionally said to be "an important women's medicinal."

Processing

a) Used raw, *xiāng fù* (cyperus) tends to ascend to the chest and diaphragm, and to reach outward to the skin. b) Used processed, it tends to enter the liver and kidney and to disinhibit the lumbus and feet. c) When used to free the channels and network vessels, it is processed by steeping in wine and then stir-frying. d) When used to disperse accumulations and gatherings, it should be steeped in vinegar and stir-fried. e) When it is used to disperse and transform phlegm-rheum, it should be soaked in *jiāng zhī* (ginger juice) and then stir-fried. f) When used for flooding and spotting or for profuse menstruation, it should be stir-fried until black. This last form is called *hēi xiāng fù* (charred cyperus) and has the additional action of stanching bleeding.

Combinations

a) Combining *xiāng fù* with *dǎng shēn* (codonopsis) and *bái zhú* (white atractylodes) helps them boost qì. b) Combining it with *shú dì huáng* (cooked rehmannia) and *dāng guī* (Chinese angelica) helps them supplement the blood. c) Combined with *mù xiāng* (costusroot), it courses stagnation and harmonizes the center, and moves gastrointestinal qì stagnation. d) Combined with *tán xiāng* (sandalwood), it rectifies qì and loosens the chest, disperses distention and arouses the spleen. e) Combined with *chén xiāng* (aquilaria) and *chái hú* (bupleurum), it restores normal upbearing and downbearing of all qì. f) Combined with *chuān xiōng* (chuanxiong) and *cāng zhú* (atractylodes), it resolves all depression. g) Combined with *zhī zǐ* (gardenia) and *huáng lián* (coptis), it downbears fire and clears heat. h) Combined with *fú líng* (poria) and *yuǎn zhì* (polygala), it promotes the interaction of heart and kidney qì. i) Combined with *xiǎo huí xiāng* (fennel) and *bǔ gǔ zhī* (psoralea), it moves stagnant qì in the kidney channel. j) Combined with *hòu pò* (official magnolia bark) and *bàn xià* (pinellia), it downbears phlegm and disperses distention. k) Combined with *sān léng* (sparganium) and *é zhú* (curcuma rhizome), it disperses accumulation lumps. l) Combined with *cōng bái* (scallion white) and *zǐ sū* (perilla), it diffuses and resolves exterior evil. m) Combined with *ài yè* (mugwort), it warms the uterus and quickens qì and blood.

Comparisons

Mù xiāng (costusroot)[229] is acrid and warm and tends to move gastrointestinal qì stagnation; it enters the qì aspect. *Xiāng fù* is neutral and acrid and tends to perfuse the qì aspect of the twelve channels, as well as to enter the blood aspect.

Qīng pí (unripe tangerine peel) enters the liver; it breaks qì and dissipates bind, and also treats mounting (疝 *shàn*).[558] *Xiāng fù* also enters the liver; it rectifies qì, opens depression, and furthermore regulates menstruation.

Hòu pò (official magnolia bark) moves qì and tends to disperse distention and eliminate fullness. *Xiāng fù* moves qì, but tends to soothe the liver and resolve depression.

DOSAGE

The dosage is generally 3–9 g/1–3 qián.

CAUTION

Use with care in qì vacuity and blood dryness.

RESEARCH

According to modern research reports, *xiāng fù* inhibits contractions of the uterine muscles and relaxes muscular tension.

---

18. 木香 Mù Xiāng   Aucklandiae Radix
Costusroot

Acrid and bitter in flavor and warm in nature, *mù xiāng* (costusroot)[20] moves gastrointestinal qì stagnation, courses the liver and opens depression, as well as harmonizing the stomach and fortifying the spleen. By the principle, "when qì is moved, pain is settled," *mù xiāng* is a frequently used qì-moving medicinal that is applicable for any type of cold qì stagnation pain.

Mù xiāng tends to move stagnant qì in the stomach and intestines. It is often used to treat signs such as stomach duct pain, distention and oppression in the stomach duct, distention and oppression between the diaphragm and stomach duct, frequent belching, abdominal distention, and abdominal pain that result from gastrointestinal qì stagnation. For this purpose it is combined with medicinals such as:

huò xiāng (藿香 agastache, Agastaches Herba)

xiāng fù (香附 cyperus, Cyperi Rhizoma)

gāo liáng jiāng (高良姜 lesser galangal, Alpiniae Officinarum Rhizoma)

bīng láng (槟榔 areca, Arecae Semen)

shā rén (砂仁 amomum, Amomi Fructus)

cǎo dòu kòu (草豆蔻 Katsumada's galangal seed, Alpiniae Katsumadai Semen)

dīng xiāng (丁香 clove, Caryophylli Flos)

If there is concurrent rib-side pain, add *chǎo chuān liàn zǐ* (stir-fried toosendan), *zhǐ qiào* (bitter orange), and *qīng pí* (unripe tangerine peel).

Mù xiāng is also an aromatic dampness-transforming medicinal. For vomiting, abdominal pain, and diarrhea due to qì stagnation in the stomach and intestines and due to collected dampness failing to transform, it is often combined with medicinals such as:

huò xiāng (藿香 agastache, Agastaches Herba)

pèi lán (佩兰 eupatorium, Eupatorii Herba)

---

[20] *Aucklandia lappa* CLARKE (also called *Aucklandia lappa* DECNE), is considered an endangered species according to CITES. According to this international convention, *mù xiāng* that is marketed should be accompanied by a valid Certificate of Cultivation. *Chuān mù xiāng* (common vladimiria) is not on the endangered species list. (Ed.)

zhú rú (竹茹 bamboo shavings, Bambusae Caulis in Taenia)

bàn xià (半夏 pinellia, Pinelliae Rhizoma)

fú líng (茯苓 poria, Poria)

zào xīn tǔ (灶心土 oven earth, Terra Flava Usta)

mù guā (木瓜 chaenomeles, Chaenomelis Fructus)

huáng bǎi (黄柏 phellodendron, Phellodendri Cortex)

huáng lián (黄连 coptis, Coptidis Rhizoma)

COMBINATIONS

Mù xiāng combined with *huáng lián* (coptis)[246] makes a formula called *xiāng lián wán* (Costusroot and Coptis Pill), which is commonly used in the treatment of dysentery. In this formula, *mù xiāng* moves gastrointestinal qì stagnation, eliminates tenesmus, and furthermore transforms dampness with aroma. *Huáng lián* dries dampness and clears heat, cools the blood and resolves toxin, and furthermore eliminates pus and blood from the stool. This combination is very effective for dysentery due to accumulation and stagnation of damp-heat in the stomach and intestines. In clinical practice, *xiāng lián wán* (Costusroot and Coptis Pill) is varied in accordance with signs to treat various forms of dysentery. For example: a) For pronounced dampness, add *fú líng* (poria), *yǐ mǐ* (coix), *cāng zhú* (atractylodes), and *chē qián zǐ* (plantago seed). b) For pronounced heat, add *huáng qín* (scutellaria), *huáng bǎi* (phellodendron), *bái tóu wēng* (pulsatilla), and *mǎ chǐ xiàn* (purslane). c) For food stagnation, add *jiāo sān xiān* (scorch-fried three immortals),[555] *bīng láng* (areca), and *chǎo jī nèi jīn* (stir-fried gizzard lining). d) If there are exterior heat signs, add *gé gēn* (pueraria) and *jīng jiè* (schizonepeta). e) For the presence of cold, add *wú yú* (evodia), *ròu guì* (cinnamon bark), and *gān jiāng* (dried ginger). f) For pronounced abdominal pain or stool containing copious pus and blood, add *bái sháo* (white peony) (in large amounts) and *dāng guī* (Chinese angelica). These formulas are used to treat bacterial dysentery and ulcerative colitis.

There are other notable ways of combining *mù xiāng*. a) Combined with *shā rén* (amomum), it treats stomach duct and abdominal glomus and fullness. b) Combined with *bīng láng* (areca), it eliminates tenesmus. c) Combined with *lái fú zǐ* (radish seed), it treats abdominal distention. d) Combined with *xiǎo huí xiāng* (fennel), it treats **mounting pain**[558] (疝痛 *shàn tòng*). e) Combined with *wū yào* (lindera), it treats pain due to qì counterflow in the smaller abdomen.

COMPARISONS

Shā rén (amomum)[219] moves qì and tends to be used to harmonize the center, disperse food, and eliminate glomus and oppression. It also conducts qì to the kidney. *Mù xiāng* moves qì, but it tends to be used to move stagnant gastrointestinal qì and disperse abdominal distention. It also dries dampness, treats diarrhea, and strengthens the large intestine.

Bīng láng (areca) breaks qì, eliminates stagnation, and disperses food; it is downbearing in nature and also treats **leg qì**[556] (脚气 *jiǎo qì*). *Mù xiāng* moves qì, disperses distention, and harmonizes the stomach and intestines; it is dry in nature and also treats dysentery.

Wū yào (lindera) tends to be used to normalize bladder and kidney counterflow qì (marked by smaller abdominal qì distention and qì pain), while *mù xiāng* is used to treat thoroughfare vessel counterflow qì with abdominal urgency (counterflow qì surging from the two sides of the smaller abdomen to the bladder and causing pain).

Processing

When using *mù xiāng* with qì-moving medicinals, one should use *shēng mù xiāng* (raw costusroot). When using it with medicinals to treat diarrhea and strengthen the large intestine, one should use *wēi mù xiāng* (roasted costusroot).[21]

When using supplementing medicinals, a small quantity of *mù xiāng* as an assistant prevents their enriching slimy natures from causing stagnation, thereby strengthening the therapeutic effect. *Xiāng shā liù jūn zǐ tāng* (Costusroot and Amomum Six Gentlemen Decoction) and *guī pí tāng* (Spleen-Returning Decoction) are examples of formulas that use a small amount of *mù xiāng* for this purpose.

Dosage

The dosage is generally 0.9–9 g/3 fēn–3 qián. Under special circumstances, up to 12 g/4 qián can be used.

Caution

Contraindicated in lung vacuity with heat, blood-aspect dryness heat, and vacuity fire surging upward.

Research

According to modern research reports, *mù xiāng* has an inhibitory effect on paratyphoid and a number of pathological fungi. It is effective for distention and pain in the stomach duct and abdomen and for counterflow qì attacking pain that occurs with gallbladder colic.

---

19. 厚朴 Hòu Pò
Official Magnolia Bark

Magnoliae Officinalis Cortex

Hòu pò (official magnolia bark) is bitter and acrid in flavor and warm in nature. Its main actions are to precipitate qì, eliminate fullness, dry dampness, and disperse distention.

Hòu pò is used to treat fullness and oppression in the chest and abdomen, vomiting, and abdominal distention and fullness that arise when poor movement and transformation of the spleen and stomach is exacerbated by contraction of cold-damp that further impairs movement and transformation in the center burner

---

[21] *Wēi mù xiāng* (roasted costusroot) is prepared by placing slices of *mù xiāng* on boards that are covered with absorbent paper and then covering the medicinal with another layer of absorbent paper. Several layers are placed on top of each other. The setup is then tightly wrapped with string so as to squeeze the boards together and force the oil into the paper. The wrapped, layered press is then placed into a drying oven or other warm place until the oil from the medicinal is completely absorbed into the paper. (Ed.)

and encourages the collection and stagnation of dampness. For this purpose it is combined with medicinals such as:

mù xiāng (木香 costusroot, Aucklandiae Radix)

gān jiāng (干姜 dried ginger, Zingiberis Rhizoma)

cǎo dòu kòu (草豆蔻 Katsumada's galangal seed, Alpiniae Katsumadai Semen)

chén pí (陈皮 tangerine peel, Citri Reticulatae Pericarpium)

fú líng (茯苓 poria, Poria)

bàn xià (半夏 pinellia, Pinelliae Rhizoma)

huò xiāng (藿香 agastache, Agastaches Herba)

If there is pronounced dampness evil (oppression in the chest, reduced eating, thick slimy white tongue fur, and a soggy, slippery, moderate pulse), add medicinals such as *cāng zhú* (atractylodes), *chǎo yǐ mǐ* (stir-fried coix), and *shā qiào* (amomum husk). If cold evil enters the interior and transforms into heat, which then binds in the intestines and stomach and results in abdominal distention and fullness, glomus and hardness that does not like pressure, bound stool, postmeridian generalized heat [effusion], and delirious speech, combine *hòu pò* with *zhǐ shí* (unripe bitter orange), *shēng dà huáng* (raw rhubarb), and *máng xiāo* (mirabilite). Examples of this are seen in the following formulas from the *Shāng Hán Lùn* (伤寒论 "On Cold Damage"):

Dà chéng qì tāng 大承气汤   Major Qì-Coordinating Decoction

---

hòu pò (厚朴 officinal magnolia bark, Magnoliae Officinalis Cortex)

zhǐ shí (枳实 unripe bitter orange, Aurantii Fructus Immaturus)

shēng dà huáng (生大黄 raw rhubarb, Rhei Radix et Rhizoma Crudi)

máng xiāo (芒硝 mirabilite, Natrii Sulfas)

Xiǎo chéng qì tāng 小承气汤   Minor Qì-Coordinating Decoction

---

hòu pò (厚朴 officinal magnolia bark, Magnoliae Officinalis Cortex)

zhǐ shí (枳实 unripe bitter orange, Aurantii Fructus Immaturus)

shēng dà huáng (生大黄 raw rhubarb, Rhei Radix et Rhizoma Crudi)

Because *hòu pò* can downbear qì, it is often included in formulas to treat fullness and distention in the chest and abdomen, counterflow qì ascent, and panting and cough. Examples include: *guì zhī jiā hòu pò xìng rén tāng* (Cinnamon Twig Decoction Plus Officinal Magnolia Bark and Apricot Kernel) for cough and panting in externally contracted wind-cold with spontaneous sweating; and *sū zǐ jiàng qì tāng* (Perilla Fruit Qì-Downbearing Decoction) for copious phlegm and qì counterflow, fullness in the chest, and cough and panting.

Guì zhī jiā hòu pò xìng rén tāng 桂枝加厚朴杏仁汤   Cinnamon Twig Decoction
Plus Officinal Magnolia Bark and Apricot Kernel

---

guì zhī (桂枝 cinnamon twig, Cinnamomi Ramulus)

bái sháo (白芍 white peony, Paeoniae Radix Alba)

zhì gān cǎo (炙甘草 mix-fried licorice, Glycyrrhizae Radix cum Liquido Fricta)

shēng jiāng (生姜 fresh ginger, Zingiberis Rhizoma Recens)

dà zǎo (大枣 jujube, Jujubae Fructus)

hòu pò (厚朴 officinal magnolia bark, Magnoliae Officinalis Cortex)

xìng rén (杏仁 apricot kernel, Armeniacae Semen)

Sū zǐ jiàng qì tāng 苏子降气汤   Perilla Fruit Qì-Downbearing Decoction

---

sū zǐ (苏子 perilla fruit, Perillae Fructus)

bàn xià (半夏 pinellia, Pinelliae Rhizoma)

zhì gān cǎo (炙甘草 mix-fried licorice, Glycyrrhizae Radix cum Liquido Fricta)

qián hú (前胡 peucedanum, Peucedani Radix)

hòu pò (厚朴 officinal magnolia bark, Magnoliae Officinalis Cortex)

chén pí (陈皮 tangerine peel, Citri Reticulatae Pericarpium)

dāng guī (当归 Chinese angelica, Angelicae Sinensis Radix)

shēng jiāng (生姜 fresh ginger, Zingiberis Rhizoma Recens)

ròu guì (肉桂 cinnamon bark, Cinnamomi Cortex)

COMPARISONS

Zhǐ shí (unripe bitter orange)[203] breaks qì and tends to be used to disperse accumulation and stagnation, and to eliminate glomus and hardness; it also drains fire. *Hòu pò* precipitates qì, and tends to be used to disperse abdominal distention and eliminate gastric fullness; it also dries dampness.

Dà fù pí (areca husk) precipitates qì and disperses distention; it also disinhibits water, and tends to be used to treat ascites. *Hòu pò* likewise precipitates qì and disperses distention; in addition, it dries dampness and eliminates fullness, and tends to be used to treat abdominal distention and bound stool. *Dà fù pí* has a much greater power to disinhibit water than *hòu pò*; but the latter has a much greater power to precipitate qì.

Cāng zhú (atractylodes) dries dampness, eliminates spleen dampness, and up-bears clear yáng. *Hòu pò* dries dampness, eliminates stomach fullness, and down-bears accumulation and stagnation. Although both dry dampness, they differ in that one is upbearing while the other is downbearing.

Qīng pí (unripe tangerine peel) breaks binding depression of liver qì and treats rib-side pain due to anger. *Hòu pò* precipitates accumulated qì in the stomach and intestines, and treats abdominal distention, fullness, and pain.

Hòu pò huā (official magnolia flower) is broadly similar to *hòu pò* in nature, flavor, and function, but its medicinal strength is not as great. Its special feature is that it also rectifies liver qì and treats liver-stomach qì stagnation with oppression and pain in the stomach duct. *Hòu pò huā* (official magnolia flower) tends to be used for the upper and center burners, while *hòu pò* tends to be used for the center and lower burners.

When used raw, *hòu pò* tends to precipitate qì; used stir-fried with ginger juice, it checks retching. Combined with medicinals such as *dǎng shēn* (codonopsis), *bái zhú* (white atractylodes), *fú líng* (poria), *ròu dòu kòu* (nutmeg), and *wǔ wèi zǐ* (schisandra), it treats diarrhea. Combined with *qīng pí* (unripe tangerine peel) and *chuān liàn zǐ* (toosendan), it is used for pain from liver-stomach qì stagnation.

Dosage

The dosage is generally 2–6 g/7 fēn–2 qián. In acute and severe conditions, one can use as much as 9–12 g/3–4 qián or more.

Caution

This is a warming, drying, qì-precipitating medicinal; it should be used with care in vacuity and in pregnancy.

Research

Modern research reports suggest that this medicinal has a stong inhibitory effect on *Staphylococcus aureus* in vitro.

---

20. 乌药 Wū Yào   Linderae Radix
Lindera

Also called *tái wū yào* 台乌药. *Wū yào* (lindera) is acrid in flavor and warm in nature. Its main actions are to move qì and loosen distention, to normalize counterflow and relieve pain, to warm and dissipate liver-kidney cold qì, and to course counterflow qì in the abdomen. It is a commonly used warm-natured qì-moving medicinal that has the additional effect of warming the kidney and reducing urine.

This medicinal is effective in treating cold-type qì pain in the lower burner. In clinical practice, *wū yào* is most commonly used to warm the kidney and treat mounting. For attacks of lesser abdominal pain and **mounting qì pain**[558] (疝气痛 *shàn qì tòng*), and cold pain, sagging, and distention of the testes caused by cold qì in the kidney affecting the liver channel, *wū yào* is combined with medicinals such as *wú yú* (evodia), *mù xiāng* (costusroot), *qīng pí* (unripe tangerine peel), *chǎo xiǎo huí xiāng* (stir-fried fennel), *chǎo jú hé* (stir-fried tangerine pip), *lì zhī hé* (litchee pit), *ròu guì* (cinnamon bark), and *chuān liàn zǐ* (toosendan). A commonly used prescription is *tiān tái wū yào sǎn* (Tiāntái Lindera Powder).

Tiān tái wū yào sǎn 天台乌药散   Tiāntái Lindera Powder

---

wū yào (乌药 lindera, Linderae Radix)

mù xiāng (木香 costusroot, Aucklandiae Radix)

xiǎo huí xiāng (小茴香 fennel, Foeniculi Fructus)

gāo liáng jiāng (高良姜 lesser galangal, Alpiniae Officinarum Rhizoma) *qīng pí* (青皮 unripe tangerine peel, Citri Reticulatae Pericarpium Viride)

bīng láng (槟榔 areca, Arecae Semen)

chuān liàn zǐ (川楝子 toosendan, Toosendan Fructus) (stir-fried with *bā dòu* (croton) and *xiǎo mài fū* (wheat bran), which are then discarded)

When cold evil invading the spleen and stomach results in center burner cold that inhibits the movement of qì and causes signs such as indigestion, continuous distention and pain in the chest and abdomen (in severe cases with vomiting), and liking for warmth in the region of the stomach, all of which are exacerbated by taking even small quantities of cold food, *wū yào* warms and dissipates spleen cold, moves qì and loosens distention, and normalizes counterflow and relieves pain. For this purpose it is often combined with medicinals such as:

xiāng fù (香附 cyperus, Cyperi Rhizoma)

gāo liáng jiāng (高良姜 lesser galangal, Alpiniae Officinarum Rhizoma)

chén pí (陈皮 tangerine peel, Citri Reticulatae Pericarpium)

bàn xià (半夏 pinellia, Pinelliae Rhizoma)

shén qū (神曲 medicated leaven, Massa Medicata Fermentata)

shēng jiāng (生姜 fresh ginger, Zingiberis Rhizoma Recens)

wú yú (吴萸 evodia, Evodiae Fructus)

For women suffering from abdominal pain during menstruation due to contractions of cold, it is combined with medicinals such as:

dāng guī (当归 Chinese angelica, Angelicae Sinensis Radix)

wú yú (吴萸 evodia, Evodiae Fructus)

xiāng fù (香附 cyperus, Cyperi Rhizoma)

chǎo xiǎo huí xiāng (炒小茴香 stir-fried fennel, Foeniculi Fructus Frictus)

chuān xiōng (川芎 chuanxiong, Chuanxiong Rhizoma)

chǎo bái sháo (炒白芍 stir-fried white peony, Paeoniae Radix Alba Fricta)

ròu guì (肉桂 cinnamon bark, Cinnamomi Cortex)

pào jiāng (炮姜 blast-fried ginger, Zingiberis Rhizoma Praeparatum)

For frequent urination due to kidney channel vacuity cold (pale-colored urine, absence of pain in the urethra, and symptoms exacerbated by exposure to cold), *wū yào* is often combined with *sāng piāo xiāo* (mantis egg-case), *yì zhì rén* (alpinia), *shān yào* (dioscorea), and *wǔ wèi zǐ* (schisandra). On the basis of this traditional experience, I once treated a woman who suffered from postpartum urinary incontinence for ten years, and who was diagnosed in Western medicine as having cystoparalysis. The many treatments she had received in different places were ineffective and she usually had to line her underwear with cotton, which she found most troublesome. After performing the four examinations (inspection, inquiry, listening-smelling, and palpation) and correlating the findings gained through them, I diagnosed her as having loss of control over urination due to kidney channel vacuity cold. I treated this by warming the kidney and securing and containing. I prescribed *bā wèi dì huáng wán* (Eight-Ingredient Rehmannia Pill) plus medicinals such as *wū yào* (lindera) and *sāng piāo xiāo* (mantis egg-case). After taking ten packets of the formula, her symptoms were reduced by more than half. After ten more packets of an adjusted formula, she had completely recovered. The main ingredients of the prescriptions were:

shú dì huáng (熟地黄 cooked rehmannia, Rehmanniae Radix Praeparata)

shān yào (山药 dioscorea, Dioscoreae Rhizoma)

shān zhū yú (山茱萸 cornus, Corni Fructus)

fú líng (茯苓 poria, Poria)

zé xiè (泽泻 alisma, Alismatis Rhizoma)

dān pí (丹皮 moutan, Moutan Cortex)

fù zǐ (附子 aconite, Aconiti Radix Lateralis Praeparata)

ròu guì (肉桂 cinnamon bark, Cinnamomi Cortex)

wū yào (乌药 lindera, Linderae Radix)

sāng piāo xiāo (桑螵蛸 mantis egg-case, Mantidis Oötheca)

yì zhì rén (益智仁 alpinia, Alpiniae Oxyphyllae Fructus)

fù pén zǐ (覆盆子 rubus, Rubi Fructus)

wǔ wèi zǐ (五味子 schisandra, Schisandrae Fructus)

duàn lóng gǔ (煅龙骨 calcined dragon bone, Mastodi Ossis Fossilia Calcinata)

duàn mǔ lì (煅牡蛎 calcined oyster shell, Ostreae Concha Calcinata)

yín yáng huò (淫羊藿 epimedium, Epimedii Herba)

These medicinals should be varied in accordance with signs. Readers might like to try this remedy.

COMPARISONS

Xiǎo huí xiāng (fennel)[353] and *wū yào* both relieve **mounting pain**[558] (疝痛 *shàn tòng*). However, *xiǎo huí xiāng* warms the lower burner and dissipates cold evil, whereas *wū yào* warms the liver and kidney, dissipates cold qì, and normalizes counterflow qì.

Xiāng fù (cyperus)[225] moves stagnant qì in the twelve channels, opens depression and dissipates binds, and tends to enter the liver and gallbladder. It is effective in treating lesser abdomen qì stagnation. *Wū yào* normalizes bladder and kidney counterflow qì, treats mounting, and reduces urine; it tends to enter the kidney channel and is effective in treating smaller-abdominal qì counterflow.

DOSAGE

The dosage is generally 4.5–9 g/1.5–3 qián.

CAUTION

Use carefully in qì vacuity with internal heat.

21. 槟榔 Bīng Láng
Areca

Arecae Semen

Including

▷ *Dà fù pí* (大腹皮 areca husk, Arecae Pericarpium)

Bīng láng (areca) is acrid in flavor and warm in nature. Its forte is downbearing qì and breaking stagnation. It also moves phlegm and precipitates water, disperses accumulations, and kills worms.

This medicinal is effective in downbearing the qì. There is a traditional saying that "its nature is downbearing like that of *tiě shí* (loadstone)," which is able to downbear qì stagnation from the highest part of the body to the lowest. Thus, it is used to treat distention and oppression in the chest and abdomen, belching and retching counterflow, abdominal fullness and difficult defecation, dysentery[547] (痢疾 *lì jí*) with rectal heaviness, and leg qì[556] (脚气 *jiǎo qì*) with water swelling due to qì counterflow and qì stagnation. For example, for distention and oppression in the chest and abdomen, it is often combined with medicinals such as *zhǐ qiào* (bitter orange), *sū gěng* (perilla stem), *huò xiāng gěng* (agastache stem), and *hòu pò huā* (official magnolia flower). For belching and retching counterflow, it is often combined with medicinals such as *shēng dài zhě shí* (crude hematite) (predecocted), *xuán fù huā* (inula flower) (cloth-wrapped), *sū zǐ* (perilla fruit), *dīng xiāng* (clove), *bàn xià* (pinellia), and *zhú rú* (bamboo shavings). For abdominal fullness and difficult defecation, it is often combined with *hòu pò* (official magnolia bark), *zhǐ shí* (unripe bitter orange), and *shēng dà huáng* (raw rhubarb). For dysentery with rectal heaviness (in former times, physicians believed that rectal heaviness[561] (后重 *hòu zhòng*, tenesmus) could be eliminated by regulating qì), it is often combined with *mù xiāng* (costusroot) and *hòu pò* (official magnolia bark). For leg qì with water swelling, it is often combined with:

zǐ sū (紫苏 perilla, Perillae Folium, Caulis et Calyx)

chén pí (陈皮 tangerine peel, Citri Reticulatae Pericarpium)

mù guā (木瓜 chaenomeles, Chaenomelis Fructus)

fáng jǐ (防己 fangji, Stephaniae Tetrandrae Radix)

For phlegm-food accumulations and gatherings, strings and aggregrations[565] (痃癖 *xián pǐ*), concretions and conglomerations[544] (癥瘕 *zhēng jiǎ*, including hepatosplenomegaly and benign lumps, cysts, and tensing of particular muscles), worm and gān accumulations, distention and fullness due to ascites, etc., all of which are due to qì stagnation, *bīng láng* downbears qì and breaks stagnation, moves phlegm and precipitates water, and kills worms and disperses accumulation. It is often combined with medicinals that disperse food, transform phlegm, quicken the blood and dispel stasis, disinhibit urine, and disperse accumulations, with the formula varied in accordance with signs. For example, for phlegm-food accumulations and gatherings, strings and aggregations,[22] concretions and conglomerations, it is combined with medicinals such as:

jiāo sān xiān (焦三仙 scorch-fried three immortals, Tres Immortales Usti)[555]

lái fú zǐ (莱菔子 radish seed, Raphani Semen)

hēi bái chǒu (黑白丑 morning glory, Pharbitidis Semen)

táo rén (桃仁 peach kernel, Persicae Semen)

hóng huā (红花 carthamus, Carthami Flos)

sān léng (三棱 sparganium, Sparganii Rhizoma)

é zhú (莪术 curcuma rhizome, Curcumae Rhizoma)

shēng mǔ lì (生牡蛎 crude oyster shell, Ostreae Concha Cruda)

xiāng fù (香附 cyperus, Cyperi Rhizoma)

yù jīn (郁金 curcuma, Curcumae Radix)

zào jiǎo zǐ (皂角子 gleditsia seed, Gleditsiae Semen)

shān zhā hé (山楂核 crataegus pit, Crataegi Endocarpium et Semen)

cāng zhú (苍术 atractylodes, Atractylodis Rhizoma)

bái zhú (白术 white atractylodes, Atractylodis Macrocephalae Rhizoma)

zhǐ shí (枳实 unripe bitter orange, Aurantii Fructus Immaturus)

For worms and gān accumulation, it is combined with medicinals such as:

shǐ jūn zǐ (使君子 quisqualis, Quisqualis Fructus)

wū méi (乌梅 mume, Mume Fructus)

fěi zǐ (榧子 torreya, Torreyae Semen)

léi wán (雷丸 omphalia, Omphalia)

nán guā zǐ (南瓜子 pumpkin seed, Cucurbitae Semen)

hú huáng lián (胡黄连 picrorhiza, Picrorhizae Rhizoma)

chuān jiāo (川椒 zanthoxylum, Zanthoxyli Pericarpium)

xì xīn (细辛 asarum, Asari Herba)

jiāo sān xiān (焦三仙 scorch-fried three immortals, Tres Immortales Usti)[555]

chǎo jī nèi jīn (炒鸡内金 stir-fried gizzard lining, Galli Gigeriae Endothelium Corneum Frictum)

For abdominal distention and fullness due to ascites, it is combined with medicinals such as:

fú líng (茯苓 poria, Poria)

zhū líng (猪苓 polyporus, Polyporus)

zé xiè (泽泻 alisma, Alismatis Rhizoma)

dà fù pí (大腹皮 areca husk, Arecae Pericarpium)

guì zhī (桂枝 cinnamon twig, Cinnamomi Ramulus)

chén pí (陈皮 tangerine peel, Citri Reticulatae Pericarpium)

---

[22]Strings, 痃 *xián*, and aggregations, 癖 *pì*, are two different types of symptoms, but they are sometimes mixed together. Strings are raised sinews or lumps on the sides of the umbilicus that are like bowstrings in form, can vary in size, and which may or may not be painful. Aggregations are lumps that are hidden within the rib-sides. They are usually only felt when the patient feels pain and then palpates the area. See **strings and aggregations**[565] (痃癖 *xián pì*) (Au.).

dōng guā pí (冬瓜皮 wax gourd rind, Benincasae Exocarpium)

Combined with *tíng lì zǐ* (lepidium/descurainia), it downbears phlegm and treats panting. Combined with *shān zhā hé* (crataegus pit) and *é zhú* (curcuma rhizome), it disperses accumulations and transforms stagnation.

Comparisons

Zhǐ shí (unripe bitter orange)[203] has greater power than *bīng láng* to abduct and disperse accumulation and stagnation and to eliminate glomus and fullness. *Bīng láng* has greater power than *zhǐ shí* to downbear qì and in addition it kills worms.

Dà fù pí (areca husk) dissipates formless qì stagnation, disperses distention, and disinhibits water. *Bīng láng* disperses hard accumulations, downbears qì, and moves phlegm.

Shǐ jūn zǐ (quisqualis)[510] kills roundworm and fortifies movement and transformation. *Bīng láng* (areca) expels tapeworm and disperses gān accumulation.

Dosage

The dosage is generally 4.5–9 g/1.5–3 qián. To expel tapeworm, use as much as 60–90 g/2–3 liǎng or more.

Caution

This medicinal is inappropriate for qì vacuity and sloppy diarrhea.

---

22. 香櫞 Xiāng Yuán   Citri Fructus
Citron

Acrid, sour, and bitter in flavor and warm in nature, *xiāng yuán* (citron)[23] regulates qì, loosens the chest, and transforms phlegm.

Xiāng yuán is suitable for liver qì depression that causes rib-side pain, stomach duct pain, fullness and oppression in the stomach duct and abdomen, belching, and vomiting. It is often combined with medicinals such as:

bàn xià (半夏 pinellia, Pinelliae Rhizoma)

shēng jiāng (生姜 fresh ginger, Zingiberis Rhizoma Recens)

mù xiāng (木香 costusroot, Aucklandiae Radix)

shā rén (砂仁 amomum, Amomi Fructus)

kòu rén (蔻仁 nutmeg, Myristicae Semen)

xiāng fù (香附 cyperus, Cyperi Rhizoma)

sū gěng (苏梗 perilla stem, Perillae Caulis)

---

[23]This medicinal is difficult to import into the United States owing to the concerns of the Department of Agriculture. There is a fear that *xiāng yuán* (citron) will bring with it diseases or pests that will infect citrus plants. The US Department of Agriculture often requires medicinals like this to be heated to a given temperature before importation to prevent the spread of pests and disease. This is also true of other citrus products, such as *chén pí* (tangerine peel), *qīng pí* (unripe tangerine peel), and *fó shǒu* (Buddha's hand). (Ed.)

hòu pò huā (厚朴花 officinal magnolia flower, Magnoliae Officinalis Flos)

For phlegm qì counterflow fullness that causes cough and oppression in the chest, and copious phlegm and panting, *xiāng yuán* is combined with medicinals such as *sū zǐ* (perilla fruit), *xìng rén* (apricot kernel), *guā lóu* (trichosanthes), *zǐ sū* (perilla), and *lái fú zǐ* (radish seed).

COMPARISONS

Méi guī huā (rose) soothes the liver and harmonizes the stomach, and also quickens the blood and frees the network vessels. *Xiāng yuán*[239] arouses the spleen and disinhibits the lung, and also transforms phlegm.

This medicinal enhances the appetite during the initial stage of pregnancy.

DOSAGE

The dosage is generally 4.5–9 g/1.5–3 qián.

---

23. 佛手 Fó Shǒu
Buddha's Hand

Citri Sarcodactylis
Fructus

Acrid, bitter, and sour in flavor and warm in nature, *fó shǒu* (Buddha's hand) rectifies qì and harmonizes the center, and soothes the liver and resolves depression.

This medicinal is suitable for liver-stomach disharmony, qì stagnation stomach pain, oppression in the chest, rib-side distention, poor appetite, and vomiting. For this purpose it is combined with medicinals such as:

xiāng yuán (香橼 citron, Citri Fructus)

xiāng fù (香附 cyperus, Cyperi Rhizoma)

sū gěng (苏梗 perilla stem, Perillae Caulis)

hòu pò (厚朴 officinal magnolia bark, Magnoliae Officinalis Cortex)

bàn xià (半夏 pinellia, Pinelliae Rhizoma)

chén pí (陈皮 tangerine peel, Citri Reticulatae Pericarpium)

huò xiāng (藿香 agastache, Agastaches Herba)

Fó shǒu is used in various other combinations. Combined with *qīng pí* (unripe tangerine peel) and *chuān liàn zǐ* (toosendan), it treats stomach duct pain due to binding depression of liver qì. Combined with *zhú rú* (bamboo shavings) and *huáng qín* (scutellaria), it treats vomiting in pregnancy. Combining it with *jiàng xiāng* (dalbergia) and *chén xiāng qū* (aquilaria leaven) strengthens its ability to downbear counterflow and check vomiting.

COMPARISONS

Xiāng yuán (citron)[239] has a stronger phlegm-transforming effect than *fó shǒu*, but the latter is more effective in checking retching.[24]

---

[24]Some practitioners consider *xiāng yuán* (citron) to be an inexpensive substitute for *fó shǒu* (Buddha's hand). (Ed.)

Fó shǒu huā (Buddha's hand flower) tends to be used for pain from chest and rib-side qì stagnation. It also opens the stomach and arouses the spleen. *Fó shǒu* tends to be used for center burner qì stagnation with stomach pain and retching.

Chén pí (tangerine peel) has a greater phlegm-transforming and dampness-drying effect than *fó shǒu*, but the latter has a more powerful effect for soothing the liver and resolving depression than *chén pí*.

DOSAGE

The dosage is generally 4.5–9 g/1.5–3 qián.

Although both *xiāng yuán* (citron) and *fó shǒu* are qì-rectifying medicinals, their medicinal strength is moderate, and their nature is gentle and neutral. They are suitable for mild conditions. In severe cases of qì depression and qì stagnation, they need to be combined with other qì-rectifying medicinals.

Lecture Six
Cold & Cool Medicinals
寒凉药 *Hán Liáng Yào*

In this lecture, I discuss medicinals with the following natures and flavors that are commonly used to clear heat: acrid and cold, sweet and cold, bitter and cold, salty and cold, sour and cold, as well as acrid and cool, and sweet and cool. This group includes medicinals that clear heat and drain fire, clear heat and resolve toxin, clear heat and resolve summerheat, clear heat and dry dampness, clear heat and transform phlegm, and clear heat and cool the blood.

1. 石膏 Shí Gāo
Gypsum
Gypsum Fibrosum

Shí gāo (gypsum) is acrid and sweet in flavor and cold in nature. When used raw, it clears lung and stomach fire, clears fire, allays thirst, eliminates vexation, and abates heat. When used in its calcined form, it is called *shú shí gāo* (cooked gypsum) or *duàn shí gāo* (calcined gypsum).[1] Calcining greatly reduces its heat-clearing action and gives it an astringent effect; thus it is often used in external applications to close sores, dispel dampness, and relieve itching.[2] It is also used with bandages to make casts. *Shí gāo* is often used internally in the following situations:

1. **Cold Damage Yáng Brightness Channel Pattern:** *Shēng shí gāo* (crude gypsum) is used for externally contracted wind-cold that has shifted and transformed into heat, manifesting as a fever so hot that it is burning to the touch, profuse sweating over the entire body with a high fever that fails to abate, great thirst, desire for cold drinks, vexation and agitation (possibly with unconsciousness

---

[1] *Duàn shí gāo* (calcined gypsum) is traditionally used in external medicine. It is often a component in powders that are sprinkled in open sores to generate flesh and close the sore. Bear in mind that the powder must be sterilized before this method is applied and the powder ground to a fine powder. The powder should be able to pass through a 120-mesh screen or finer. In addition, it is necessary that there be no infection present before this method is applied. (Ed.)

[2] *Shí gāo* (gypsum) medicinal plasters are used in modern China to aid in the treatment of severe burns. (Ed.)

and mania in severe cases), and a surging large and rapid pulse. It clears and resolves yáng brightness channel fire-heat; and, for this purpose, it is used as the chief medicinal in combination with medicinals such as *zhī mǔ* (anemarrhena), *gān cǎo* (licorice), *gēng mǐ* (non-glutinous rice), *tiān huā fěn* (trichosanthes root), and *lú gēn* (phragmites), as in the formula *bái hǔ tāng* (White Tiger Decoction). If there has been high fever, great sweating, and thirst for several days, and if one observes a dry tongue without liquid and a large vacuous pulse, add *dǎng shēn* (codonopsis).

2. Seasonal Heat Epidemic: Epidemic febrile infectious diseases manifest as aversion to cold with heat effusion (fever), headache and eye pain (this pattern is similar to cold damage but differs in that it includes a splitting headache and clouded and painful eyes), high fever with manic agitation, vexation, dry mouth, and manic activity with reduced sleep. In severe cases, there is vomiting of blood, nosebleed, macular eruptions, a red prickly tongue, dry parched lips, either great sweating and thirst or scant sweating, and a pulse that is either deep or floating but that is rapid. These symptoms indicate exuberant toxic heat in both qì and blood. In this case use *shēng shí gāo* (crude gypsum) combined with medicinals such as:

shēng dì huáng (生地黄 dried/fresh rehmannia, Rehmanniae Radix Exsiccata seu Recens)

xī jiǎo (犀角 rhinoceros horn, Rhinocerotis Cornu)

huáng lián (黄连 coptis, Coptidis Rhizoma)

zhī zǐ (栀子 gardenia, Gardeniae Fructus)

huáng qín (黄芩 scutellaria, Scutellariae Radix)

zhī mǔ (知母 anemarrhena, Anemarrhenae Rhizoma)

chì sháo (赤芍 red peony, Paeoniae Radix Rubra)

xuán shēn (玄参 scrophularia, Scrophulariae Radix)

lián qiáo (连翘 forsythia, Forsythiae Fructus)

dān pí (丹皮 moutan, Moutan Cortex)

zhú yè (竹叶 lophatherum, Lophatheri Herba)

dà qīng yè (大青叶 isatis leaf, Isatidis Folium)

This combination of medicinals is similar to *qīng wēn bài dú yǐn* (Scourge-Clearing Toxin-Vanquishing Beverage), a formula that appears in Yú Shī-Yú's book of 1794, *Yì Zhěn Yī Dé* (疫疹一得 "Revelations on Epidemic Papules"). (See Lecture One, page 4, for a discussion of medicinal dosages and modifications of formulas.) I have achieved definite results using *qīng wēn bài dú yǐn* varied in accordance with signs to treat epidemic cerebrospinal meningitis, infectious encephalitis B (Japanese encephalitis), and other epidemic, infectious febrile diseases. Some hospitals use a modified version of this formula and have made it into an injection fluid that is convenient and quick to administer. Readers may reference reports from each area.

3. Warm Disease with Papules: When warm disease heat toxin enters the blood aspect, it causes high fever and outbreaks of papules on the skin, red papules under the skin that resemble the markings of brocade, or papules that form patches. There is also mania, a tongue that is dark, dry, crimson, and prickly and that has a yellow fur with scant liquid, and a fine, rapid pulse. In such cases, use the following formula.

Huà bān tāng 化斑汤   Macule-Transforming Decoction

---

shēng shí gāo (生石膏 crude gypsum, Gypsum Fibrosum Crudum)

xuán shēn (玄参 scrophularia, Scrophulariae Radix)

zhī mǔ (知母 anemarrhena, Anemarrhenae Rhizoma)

shēng gān cǎo (生甘草 raw licorice, Glycyrrhizae Radix Cruda)

gēng mǐ (粳米 non-glutinous rice, Oryzae Semen)

xī jiǎo (犀角 rhinoceros horn, Rhinocerotis Cornu)

4. Stomach Fire Toothache: When stomach channel fire-heat causes toothache, red swollen gums, thirst, and dry stool or constipation, *shēng shí gāo* may be combined with medicinals such as:

dì gǔ pí (地骨皮 lycium root bark, Lycii Cortex)

shēng dì huáng (生地黄 dried/fresh rehmannia, Rehmanniae Radix Exsiccata seu Recens)

shēng dà huáng (生大黄 raw rhubarb, Rhei Radix et Rhizoma Crudi)

dān pí (丹皮 moutan, Moutan Cortex)

shēng má (升麻 cimicifuga, Cimicifugae Rhizoma)

bò hé (薄荷 mint, Menthae Herba)

If there is also wind damage, one can add *jīng jiè* (schizonepeta) and *fáng fēng* (saposhnikovia).

5. Lung-Heat Cough and Panting: In patients with preexisting lung heat, when externally contracted wind-cold fetters the skin and [body] hair, causing non-diffusion of lung qì so that the evil heat is depressed internally, the result is symptoms such as cough, panting, thirst, yellow phlegm, red facial complexion, hot breath from the nose and mouth, and a rapid floating pulse. Treat this pattern with the following modified formula:

Má xìng shí gān tāng 麻杏石甘汤   Ephedra, Apricot Kernel, Gypsum, and
                                          Licorice Decoction

---

shēng shí gāo (生石膏 crude gypsum, Gypsum Fibrosum Crudum)

má huáng (麻黄 ephedra, Ephedrae Herba)

xìng rén (杏仁 apricot kernel, Armeniacae Semen)

gān cǎo (甘草 licorice, Glycyrrhizae Radix)

This is modified by the addition of:

jīng jiè (荆芥 schizonepeta, Schizonepetae Herba)

bò hé (薄荷 mint, Menthae Herba)

qián hú (前胡 peucedanum, Peucedani Radix)

huáng qín (黄芩 scutellaria, Scutellariae Radix)

I often use *má xìng shí gān tāng* (Ephedra, Apricot Kernel, Gypsum, and Licorice Decoction) with the following additions: *jīn yín huā* (lonicera), *lián qiáo* (forsythia), *bò hé* (mint), *jīng jiè* (schizonepeta), *lú gēn* (phragmites), *huáng qín* (scutellaria), and *jié gěng* (platycodon) for lobar pneumonia and acute bronchitis that present as lung-heat cough and panting. If there is also phlegm containing blood, eliminate *má huáng* and add *bái máo gēn* (imperata) and *chǎo zhī zǐ* (stir-fried gardenia).

COMPARISONS

Hán shuǐ shí (glauberite) and *shēng shí gāo* both clear heat and drain fire. Nevertheless, *hán shuǐ shí* clears lung and stomach repletion fire and enters the blood aspect; it has no ability to resolve the flesh and outthrust the exterior. *Shēng shí gāo* clears lung and stomach fire-heat and enters the qì aspect; it also resolves the flesh and outthrusts the exterior, and can outthrust evils through the exterior.

Dà qīng yè (isatis leaf)[264] and *shēng shí gāo* are both commonly used for seasonal heat epidemic. Nevertheless, *dà qīng yè* is bitter, salty, and very cold. It tends to be used for toxic heat in the stomach and heart, manic heat with vexation and derangement, red macules due to blood heat, and heat toxin red dysentery. *Shēng shí gāo* is acrid, sweet, and cold. It tends to be used for intense epidemic heat in the lung and stomach, scorching heat in the flesh, splitting headache, great sweating, and vexation thirst.

DOSAGE

The dosage for *shēng shí gāo* is generally 9–45 g/3 qián–1.5 liǎng; in special cases one can use up to 90–120 g/3–4 liǎng. For decoctions it should be crushed and predecocted. Note that when treating severe conditions, the dosage must not be too small. *Duàn shí gāo* (calcined gypsum) is primarily used topically and is not commonly used internally.

CAUTION

Shí gāo should not be used in blood vacuity heat effusion (fever), weakness of the stomach, lung vacuity, or in the absence of repletion heat.

RESEARCH

According to modern research reports, decocted *shí gāo* has a pronounced antipyretic effect when given to rabbits with artificially-induced fevers. Nevertheless, the pharmacology of *shí gāo* has not yet been fully explored.

---

2. 黄连 Huáng Lián   Coptidis Rhizoma
Coptis

Huáng lián (coptis) is also called *chuān huáng lián* 川黄连 because the variety produced in Sìchuān Province has the strongest medicinal effect.[3] It is bitter in

---

[3] *Huáng lián* (coptis) comes in two basic varieties: 1) the multi-branched root known as *wèi lián* 味连 (*Coptis chinensis*) and 2) the single-branched root that is either *yǎ lián* 雅连 (*Coptis deltoidea* C.Y. CHENG ET HSIAO) or *yún lián* 云连 (*Coptis teetoides* C.Y. CHENG). *Wèi lián*, which is also known as *chuān lián* 川连, is preferred by most practitioners. (Ed.)

flavor and cold in nature. It mainly clears and drains fire-heat from the heart and stomach, cools the liver and gallbladder, and resolves heat toxins. It also has the effect of drying dampness.

In treating heart and stomach fire-heat that manifests as mouth and tongue sores, red eyes, toothache, reddish urine, and constipation, *huáng lián* is combined with medicinals such as *shēng dì huáng* (dried/fresh rehmannia), *mù tōng* (trifoliate akebia), *zhú yè* (lophatherum), *huáng qín* (scutellaria), and *shēng dà huáng* (raw rhubarb). If there is depressed and accumulated blood-aspect heat toxin with sores, boils, and swellings, it is combined with medicinals such as:

huáng qín (黄芩 scutellaria, Scutellariae Radix)

zhī zǐ (栀子 gardenia, Gardeniae Fructus)

huáng bǎi (黄柏 phellodendron, Phellodendri Cortex)

chì sháo (赤芍 red peony, Paeoniae Radix Rubra)

dì dīng (地丁 violet, Violae Herba)

jīn yín huā (金银花 lonicera, Lonicerae Flos)

lián qiáo (连翘 forsythia, Forsythiae Fructus)

For warm disease heat evil entering the heart and causing clouded spirit and delirious speech, vexation and agitation, sweating and thirst, generalized heat (fever), and a red tongue, *huáng lián* is combined with medicinals such as:

tiān zhú huáng (天竹黄 bamboo sugar, Bambusae Concretio Silicea)

yù jīn (郁金 curcuma, Curcumae Radix)

chāng pú (菖蒲 acorus, Acori Tatarinowii Rhizoma)

yuǎn zhì (远志 polygala, Polygalae Radix)

lián qiáo (连翘 forsythia, Forsythiae Fructus)

xī jiǎo (犀角 rhinoceros horn, Rhinocerotis Cornu)

shēng dì huáng (生地黄 dried/fresh rehmannia, Rehmanniae Radix Exsiccata seu Recens)

xuán shēn (玄参 scrophularia, Scrophulariae Radix)

In treating exuberant heart heat that causes signs such as vexation and insomnia, dry mouth, red tongue, yellow urine, and a rapid pulse, it is combined with medicinals such as:

zhī zǐ (栀子 gardenia, Gardeniae Fructus)

shēng dì huáng (生地黄 dried/fresh rehmannia, Rehmanniae Radix Exsiccata seu Recens)

dāng guī (当归 Chinese angelica, Angelicae Sinensis Radix)

gān cǎo (甘草 licorice, Glycyrrhizae Radix)

zhū shā (朱砂 cinnabar, Cinnabaris)

dòu chǐ (豆豉 fermented soybean, Sojae Semen Praeparatum)

For heat evil stagnating and binding in the stomach duct that causes glomus below the heart together with heat and pain in the stomach and abdomen, *huáng lián* is combined with medicinals such as *hòu pò* (officinal magnolia bark), *zhǐ shí* (unripe bitter orange), *bàn xià* (pinellia), *guā lóu* (trichosanthes), *chén pí* (tangerine peel), *fú líng* (poria), and *shēng dà huáng* (raw rhubarb). *Huáng lián* and *zhǐ shí* (unripe bitter orange) is a commonly used medicinal pair that treats "glomus below the heart" (a feeling of blockage in the stomach duct).

This medicinal also has the effect of clearing the liver and brightening the eyes. *Huáng lián yáng gān wán* (Coptis and Goat's Liver Pill) is a commonly used formula with this effect.

Huáng lián yáng gān wán 黄连羊肝丸   Coptis and Goat's Liver Pill

> *huáng lián* (黄连 coptis, Coptidis Rhizoma)
>
> *lóng dǎn cǎo* (龙胆草 gentian, Gentianae Radix)
>
> *cǎo jué míng* (草决明 fetid cassia, Cassiae Semen)
>
> *shí jué míng* (石决明 abalone shell, Haliotidis Concha)
>
> *mì méng huā* (密蒙花 buddleia, Buddleja Flos)
>
> *yè míng shā* (夜明砂 bat's droppings, Verspertilionis Faeces)
>
> *chōng wèi zǐ* (茺蔚子 leonurus fruit, Leonuri Fructus)
>
> *huáng qín* (黄芩 scutellaria, Scutellariae Radix)
>
> *chái hú* (柴胡 bupleurum, Bupleuri Radix)
>
> *mù zéi cǎo* (木贼草 equisetum, Equiseti Hiemalis Herba)
>
> *qīng pí* (青皮 unripe tangerine peel, Citri Reticulatae Pericarpium Viride)
>
> *huáng bǎi* (黄柏 phellodendron, Phellodendri Cortex)
>
> *yáng gān* (羊肝 goat's or sheep's liver, Caprae seu Ovis Iecur)
>
> *fēng mì* (蜂蜜 honey, Mel)

This formula is indicated for exuberant liver channel fire and vacuous blood failing to nourish the eyes producing symptoms such as dark and clouded vision, unclear vision, aversion to light and sun, **sparrow-vision night blindness**[564] (雀目夜盲 *què mù yè máng*), and **excrescence creeping over the eyes**[548] (胬肉攀睛 *nǔ ròu pān jīng*). For such conditions, *huáng lián* is decocted with water and used externally as an eye wash. This wash also treats symptoms such as red eyes and eye pain, or fulminant fire eye (including acute conjunctivitis).

Huáng lián can also dry dampness to treat damp-heat accumulation and stagnation causing dysentery with symptoms of abdominal pain, frequent ungratifying defecation with stool containing pus and blood, tenesmus, a slimy yellow tongue fur, dry mouth with no desire to drink large quantities, and a slippery rapid pulse. For this purpose it is commonly used with medicinals such as:

> *mù xiāng* (木香 costusroot, Aucklandiae Radix)
>
> *bái sháo* (白芍 white peony, Paeoniae Radix Alba)
>
> *dāng guī* (当归 Chinese angelica, Angelicae Sinensis Radix)
>
> *bīng láng* (槟榔 areca, Arecae Semen)
>
> *huáng qín* (黄芩 scutellaria, Scutellariae Radix)
>
> *bái tóu wēng* (白头翁 pulsatilla, Pulsatillae Radix)
>
> *fú líng* (茯苓 poria, Poria)
>
> *hòu pò* (厚朴 officinal magnolia bark, Magnoliae Officinalis Cortex)

zhǐ shí (枳实 unripe bitter orange, Aurantii Fructus Immaturus)

Huáng lián combined with *wú yú* (evodia) is used for effulgent liver fire or liver-stomach disharmony causing stomach pain or **clamoring stomach**[544] (嘈杂 *cáo zá*), and upwelling and vomiting of sour water. Combined with *xì xīn* (asarum), it is used to treat mouth sores. Combined with *ròu guì* (cinnamon bark), it is used to treat noninteraction of the heart and kidney. Combined with *mù xiāng* (costusroot), it is used for dysentery. Combined with *gān jiāng* (dried ginger), it is used to treat cold abdominal pain and dysentery. Combined with *dà suàn* (garlic), it is used for descent of blood with the stool. The combinations above, which were used by physicians of the past, achieve their effects by using one cold and one hot medicinal or one yīn and one yáng medicinal, thereby creating mutually benefitting and mutually balancing formulas. When devising prescriptions today, we can learn from their experience.

COMPARISONS

Huáng bǎi (phellodendron)[254] primarily clears lower burner damp-heat and also consolidates the kidney. *Huáng lián* primarily clears center burner damp-heat and also drains heart fire.

Hú huáng lián (picrorhiza)[285] is used for steaming bone taxation heat and vexing heat in the five hearts. It also treats gān disease and fright epilepsy in children. *Huáng lián*, by contrast, is used for center burner damp-heat and various types of sores and toxin swellings.

DOSAGE

The dosage is generally 0.9–6 g/3 fēn–2 qián or 9 g/3 qián.

CAUTION

Do not use in cases of yīn vacuity with heat vexation, spleen-kidney vacuity diarrhea, qì vacuity with diarrhea, or similar patterns.

RESEARCH

According to modern research reports, *huáng lián* has a general antibacterial effect, with its effect on *Bacillus dysenteriae* being the strongest. The active ingredient is berberine.

---

3. 黄芩 Huáng Qín
Scutellaria   Scutellariae Radix

Cold in nature and bitter in flavor, *huáng qín* (scutellaria) is a commonly used heat-clearing dampness-drying and heat-clearing toxin-resolving medicinal. It drains center burner repletion fire, dries gastrointestinal damp-heat, and clears lesser yáng evil heat. In addition, it cools the blood and quiets the fetus.

1. **Draining Center Burner Repletion Fire:** For stomach fire congesting in the upper body and causing sore pharynx, toothache, mouth ulcers, sore swollen tonsils, oppression and heat in the diaphragm, dry bound stool, and lung heat

cough, one can use this medicinal to clear heat and drain fire. For this purpose it is often combined with medicinals such as:

shēng dì huáng (生地黄 dried/fresh rehmannia, Rehmanniae Radix Exsiccata seu Recens)

xuán shēn (玄参 scrophularia, Scrophulariae Radix)

lián qiáo (连翘 forsythia, Forsythiae Fructus)

huáng lián (黄连 coptis, Coptidis Rhizoma)

shēng dà huáng (生大黄 raw rhubarb, Rhei Radix et Rhizoma Crudi)

For patients who also have an exterior pattern, add *jīng jiè* (schizonepeta) and *bò hé* (mint). If there is severe cough, add *jié gěng* (platycodon), *guā lóu* (trichosanthes), *xìng rén* (apricot kernel), and *pí pá yè* (loquat leaf).

2. Drying Gastrointestinal Damp-Heat: For damp-heat in the stomach and intestines and damp-heat pouring downwards that cause diarrhea, dysentery[547] (痢疾 *lì jí*), and heat strangury, use *huáng qín* to clear heat and dry dampness in combination with medicinals such as *huáng bǎi* (phellodendron), *fú líng* (poria), *zhū líng* (polyporus), *chǎo bái biǎn dòu* (stir-fried lablab), and *chǎo yǐ mǐ* (stir-fried coix) (for damp-heat diarrhea); *huáng lián* (coptis), *gé gēn* (pueraria), *mù xiāng* (costusroot), and *bīng láng* (areca) (for damp-heat dysentery); *mù tōng* (trifoliate akebia), *biǎn xù* (knotgrass), *huá shí* (talcum), *zhū líng* (polyporus), and *zé xiè* (alisma) (for damp-heat strangury). For center burner damp-heat causing jaundice (yáng jaundice), this medicinal is often combined with medicinals such as *huáng bǎi* (phellodendron), *zhī zǐ* (gardenia), *yīn chén* (virgate wormwood), *zhū líng* (polyporus), *zé xiè* (alisma), and *chē qián zǐ* (plantago seed).

3. Clearing Lesser Yáng Evil Heat: For disease evil harbored in the lesser yáng and causing alternating heat and cold, bitter mouth and dry pharynx, fullness in the chest and rib-side, poor appetite, nausea, and desire to retch, *huáng qín* is combined with medicinals such as *chái hú* (bupleurum), *bàn xià* (pinellia), *shēng jiāng* (fresh ginger), *gān cǎo* (licorice), and *dǎng shēn* (codonopsis), as in *xiǎo chái hú tāng* (Minor Bupleurum Decoction). I often modify *xiǎo chái hú tāng* (Minor Bupleurum Decoction) by removing *dǎng shēn* (codonopsis) and *gān cǎo* (licorice) and by adding *yīn chén* (virgate wormwood), *huáng bǎi* (phellodendron), *zhī zǐ* (gardenia), *shēng dà huáng* (raw rhubarb), *chē qián zǐ* (plantago seed), *jiāo sān xiān* (scorch-fried three immortals), and *chǎo bīng láng* (stir-fried areca) to treat infectious icteric hepatitis because it is effective in both abating heat and abating jaundice. Another effective modification for treating infectious icteric hepatitis also eliminates *dǎng shēn* and *gān cǎo*, but adds *chǎo chuān liàn zǐ* (stir-fried toosendan), *cǎo dòu kòu* (Katsumada's galangal seed), *chǎo lái fú zǐ* (stir-fried radish seed), *hóng huā* (carthamus), *qiàn cǎo* (madder), *bái jí lí* (tribulus), *zào jiǎo cì* (gleditsia thorn), *jiāo sān xiān* (scorch-fried three immortals), and *bīng láng* (areca); this second modification of *xiǎo chái hú tāng* (Minor Bupleurum Decoction) is also varied according to the signs.

4. Cooling the Blood and Quieting the Fetus: For pregnant women who experience fetal heat and restlessness that cause nausea and vomiting, heat vexation in the heart, vomiting of water, abdominal discomfort, and hunger without desire for food, *huáng qín* is combined with medicinals such as:

zhú rú (竹茹 bamboo shavings, Bambusae Caulis in Taenia)

jú pí (橘皮 tangerine peel, Citri Reticulatae Pericarpium)

shēng jiāng (生姜 fresh ginger, Zingiberis Rhizoma Recens)

huáng lián (黄连 coptis, Coptidis Rhizoma)

sū gěng (苏梗 perilla stem, Perillae Caulis)

fú líng (茯苓 poria, Poria)

Huáng qín stir-fried with wine is best for draining lung fire and treating upper burner damp-heat. *Huáng qín tàn* (黄芩炭, charred scutellaria) is used for any form of hot-natured bleeding. *Kū qín* (枯芩, old scutellaria), also called *piàn qín* 片芩 in Chinese, is hollow in the center and black in color; it tends to drain the lung and clear heat from the fleshy exterior. *Zǐ qín* (子芩, young scutellaria), also called *tiáo qín* 条芩 in Chinese, is hard and solid on both the inside and the outside and is greenish yellow in color; it tends to drain gastrointestinal fire and is often used to clear heat and quiet the fetus.[4]

COMPARISONS

Sāng pí (mulberry root bark)[445] and *dì gǔ pí* (lycium root bark)[306] drain heat in the qì aspect of the lung channel. *Huáng qín* and *zhī zǐ* (gardenia) drain heat in the blood aspect of the lung channel.

Chái hú (bupleurum)[37] clears heat because it can "diffuse with bitterness" (苦以发之 *kǔ yǐ fā zhī*). "Diffuse" refers to diffusing and dissipating fire and heat; *chái hú* dissipates the tip of fire and heat. *Huáng qín* clears heat because it can "overcome with cold" (寒以胜之 *hán yǐ shèng zhī*). Coldness and bitterness attack directly and cold overcomes heat; thus *huáng qín* directly attacks the root of fire and heat. Although both of these medicinals clear heat, their uses are quite different. Used together, they are a special formula for treating heat-evil in the lesser yáng (*shào yáng*).

RESEARCH

According to modern research reports, *huáng qín* has antipyretic, diuretic, and hypotensive effects. It also has an antibacterial effect against the following: *Bacillus dysenteriae*, *Bacillus typhosus*, *Bacillus coli*, *Bordatella pertussis*, *Staphylococcus*, *hemolytic streptococcus* and *Diplococcus pneumoniae*. In addition, it has been shown to have an inhibitory effect on contagious viruses.

DOSAGE

The dosage is generally 3–9 g/1–3 qián.

CAUTION

Do not use in cases of spleen-stomach vacuity cold.

---

[4]These various forms of *huáng qín* (scutellaria) are all *Scutellaria baicalensis* GEORGI, but *kū qín* (枯芩, old scutellaria) is older roots and *zǐ qín* (子芩, young scutellaria) is younger roots. (Ed.)

4. 栀子 Zhī Zǐ   Gardeniae Fructus
Gardenia

Also called *shān zhī* 山栀 and *shān zhī zǐ* 山栀子. Cold in nature and bitter in flavor, *zhī zǐ* (gardenia) is commonly used to clear heat and drain fire. It clears and drains triple burner fire-heat, and dispels dampness and resolves toxin.

1. **All Forms of Febrile Disease:** *Zhī zǐ* is used to clear heat and drain fire for any condition caused by fire-heat that manifests with symptoms such as headache, red eyes, toothache, sore throat, mouth and tongue sores, fire toxin and swollen boils, heat [effusion] (fever) with agitation and vexation, dry bound stool, and yellow or reddish urine. For these conditions it is often combined with medicinals such as:

> *huáng lián* (黄连 coptis, Coptidis Rhizoma)
>
> *xuán shēn* (玄参 scrophularia, Scrophulariae Radix)
>
> *huáng qín* (黄芩 scutellaria, Scutellariae Radix)
>
> *chì sháo* (赤芍 red peony, Paeoniae Radix Rubra)
>
> *shēng shí gāo* (生石膏 crude gypsum, Gypsum Fibrosum Crudum)
>
> *shēng dà huáng* (生大黄 raw rhubarb, Rhei Radix et Rhizoma Crudi)

2. **Frenetic Movement of Hot Blood:** For blood heat causing nosebleed, blood ejection, coughing of blood, or bloody urine, *zhī zǐ* is combined with medicinals such as *shēng dì huáng* (dried/fresh rehmannia), *dān pí* (moutan), *cè bǎi yè* (arborvitae leaf), *bái máo gēn* (imperata), *shēng ǒu jié* (raw lotus root node), and *bái jí* (bletilla). I have used *zhī zǐ tàn* (charred gardenia) in combination with the following medicinals to successfully treat a stubborn case of coughing of blood.

> *shēng shí gāo* (生石膏 crude gypsum, Gypsum Fibrosum Crudum)
>
> *shēng dì tàn* (生地炭 charred dried/fresh rehmannia, Rehmanniae Radix Exsiccata seu Recens Carbonisata)
>
> *huáng qín tàn* (黄芩炭 charred scutellaria, Scutellariae Radix Carbonisata)
>
> *ǒu jié tàn* (藕节炭 charred lotus root node, Nelumbinis Rhizomatis Nodus Carbonisatus)
>
> *bái jí* (白及 bletilla, Bletillae Rhizoma)
>
> *shēng dài zhě shí* (生代赭石 crude hematite, Haematitum Crudum)
>
> *xuán fù huā* (旋覆花 inula flower, Inulae Flos)
>
> *bái máo gēn* (白茅根 imperata, Imperatae Rhizoma)
>
> *xuán shēn* (玄参 scrophularia, Scrophulariae Radix)
>
> *zhī mǔ* (知母 anemarrhena, Anemarrhenae Rhizoma)
>
> *xìng rén* (杏仁 apricot kernel, Armeniacae Semen)

In this case a male patient had bronchiectasis with severe coughing of blood. Every night he had to be taken to the emergency room of a major hospital. When he coughed up blood he had to have an intravenous drip of posterior pituitary hormone in order to stop the bleeding. This continued for several nights in a row. Every night at a certain time, almost as if on cue, he would begin coughing up blood. After taking several packets of the formula described above, varied in accordance with signs, he no longer coughed up blood and could return to a normal work schedule.

3. Damp-Heat Jaundice: For jaundice caused by depressed and steaming damp-heat (yáng jaundice), *zhī zǐ* is combined with medicinals such as *huáng bǎi* (phellodendron), *yīn chén* (virgate wormwood), *shēng dà huáng* (raw rhubarb), and *chē qián zǐ* (plantago seed).

4. Damp-Heat Strangury: When damp-heat pouring downward causes heat strangury with symptoms of frequent urination, burning pain on urination, urine that is yellow or reddish in color, a slimy yellow tongue fur, and a slippery rapid pulse, *zhī zǐ* is combined with medicinals such as:

huáng bǎi (黄柏 phellodendron, Phellodendri Cortex)

mù tōng (木通 trifoliate akebia, Akebiae Trifoliatae Caulis)

huá shí (滑石 talcum, Talcum)

biǎn xù (萹蓄 knotgrass, Polygoni Avicularis Herba)

chē qián zǐ (车前子 plantago seed, Plantaginis Semen)

zé xiè (泽泻 alisma, Alismatis Rhizoma)

zhū líng (猪苓 polyporus, Polyporus)

COMPARISONS

Shēng zhī zǐ (生栀子, raw gardenia) drains fire, whereas *chǎo zhī zǐ* (炒栀子, stir-fried gardenia) and *zhī zǐ tàn* (栀子炭, charred gardenia) stanch bleeding. *Zhī zǐ yī* (栀子衣, gardenia husk) clears heat from the lung and the cutaneous exterior, whereas *zhī zǐ rén* (栀子仁, gardenia seed) clears internal heat and eliminates heart vexation.

Huáng qín (scutellaria)[249] drains fire-heat in the upper and center burners; *huáng lián* (coptis) drains fire-heat in the heart and stomach and it also dries dampness; *huáng bǎi* (phellodendron) drains fire-heat in the lower burner, bladder, and kidney; *zhī zǐ* drains fire-heat in the upper, center, and lower burners.

DOSAGE

The dosage is generally 3–9 g/1–3 qián.

CAUTION

Note that *zhī zǐ* can cause sloppy stool and vacuity diarrhea; thus it should not be used in the absence of a heat pattern.

RESEARCH

Modern research has shown that *zhī zǐ* (gardenia) is cholagogic and promotes the secretion of bile. It has also been shown to have an antibacterial effect on many different kinds of bacteria.

5. 黄柏 **Huáng Bǎi**   Phellodendri Cortex
Phellodendron

Cold in nature and bitter in flavor, *huáng bǎi* (phellodendron) clears heat and dries dampness as well as consolidating the kidney and boosting yīn.

a) *Huáng bǎi* treats damp-heat dysentery in combination with medicinals such as:

> *huáng lián* (黄连 coptis, Coptidis Rhizoma)
> *mù xiāng* (木香 costusroot, Aucklandiae Radix)
> *mǎ chǐ xiàn* (马齿苋 purslane, Portulacae Herba)
> *bái tóu wēng* (白头翁 pulsatilla, Pulsatillae Radix)

b) *Huáng bǎi* treats damp-heat diarrhea when it is combined with medicinals such as:

> *mù xiāng* (木香 costusroot, Aucklandiae Radix)
> *huò xiāng* (藿香 agastache, Agastaches Herba)
> *fú líng* (茯苓 poria, Poria)
> *bái zhú* (白术 white atractylodes, Atractylodis Macrocephalae Rhizoma)

c) *Huáng bǎi* treats damp-heat strangury when it is combined with medicinals such as:

> *mù tōng* (木通 trifoliate akebia, Akebiae Trifoliatae Caulis)
> *shēng dì huáng* (生地黄 dried/fresh rehmannia, Rehmanniae Radix Exsiccata seu Recens)
> *zhú yè* (竹叶 lophatherum, Lophatheri Herba)
> *huá shí* (滑石 talcum, Talcum)
> *biǎn xù* (萹蓄 knotgrass, Polygoni Avicularis Herba)
> *zhū líng* (猪苓 polyporus, Polyporus)

d) Combined with medicinals such as *yīn chén hāo* (virgate wormwood), *zhī zǐ* (gardenia), *chē qián zǐ* (plantago seed), and *shēng dà huáng* (raw rhubarb), it treats jaundice caused by depressed and steaming damp-heat.

e) To treat hemorrhoids with bloody stool, it is combined with medicinals such as:

> *huái jiǎo* (槐角 sophora fruit, Sophorae Fructus)
> *huái huā tàn* (槐花炭 charred sophora flower, Sophorae Flos Carbonisatus)
> *dì yú* (地榆 sanguisorba, Sanguisorbae Radix)
> *fáng fēng* (防风 saposhnikovia, Saposhnikoviae Radix)

f) To treat damp-heat damaging the sinews that manifests as weak-wilting lower limbs and numbness, which in severe cases can produce numbness and tingling or paralysis, it is combined with medicinals such as:

> *cāng zhú* (苍术 atractylodes, Atractylodis Rhizoma)
> *niú xī* (牛膝 achyranthes, Achyranthis Bidentatae Radix)

mù guā (木瓜 chaenomeles, Chaenomelis Fructus)

yǐ mǐ (苡米 coix, Coicis Semen)

Huáng bǎi consolidates the kidney and clears heat as well as boosting yīn; therefore, it is used in conjunction with yīn-enriching medicinals to clear heat and downbear fire in cases of vacuity fire due to yīn vacuity with hyperactivity of yáng. For example, *zhī bǎi dì huáng wán* (Anemarrhena, Phellodendron, and Rehmannia Pill) and *dà bǔ yīn wán* (Major Yīn Supplementation Pill), given below, are both used to treat yīn vacuity effulgent fire resulting in steaming bone consumptive heat, night sweating, dream emission, dry mouth, menstrual block, and flushed cheeks in the afternoon.

Zhī bǎi dì huáng wán 知柏地黄丸   Anemarrhena, Phellodendron, and Rehmannia Pill

---

shú dì huáng (熟地黄 cooked rehmannia, Rehmanniae Radix Praeparata)

shān zhū yú (山茱萸 cornus, Corni Fructus)

shān yào (山药 dioscorea, Dioscoreae Rhizoma)

fú líng (茯苓 poria, Poria)

dān pí (丹皮 moutan, Moutan Cortex)

zé xiè (泽泻 alisma, Alismatis Rhizoma)

zhī mǔ (知母 anemarrhena, Anemarrhenae Rhizoma)

huáng bǎi (黄柏 phellodendron, Phellodendri Cortex)

Dà bǔ yīn wán 大补阴丸   Major Yīn Supplementation Pill

---

dì huáng (地黄 rehmannia, Rehmanniae Radix)

guī bǎn (龟板 tortoise shell, Testudinis Carapax et Plastrum)

zhī mǔ (知母 anemarrhena, Anemarrhenae Rhizoma)

huáng bǎi (黄柏 phellodendron, Phellodendri Cortex)

zhū jǐ suǐ (猪脊髓 pig's spine marrow, Suis Spinae Medulla)

RESEARCH

According to modern research reports, *huáng bǎi* has an antibacterial effect similar to that of *huáng lián* (coptis). It has an inhibitory effect on ameba and *Leishmania*; in addition, it lowers blood pressure and blood sugar levels.

I often find it very effective to use 12–15 g/4–5 qián of *huáng bǎi* or *huáng bǎi tàn* (charred phellodendron) with the following medicinals, varied in accordance with signs, to treat urinary infection or bloody urine:

bái máo gēn (imperata) or *máo gēn tàn* (charred imperata)

dà xiǎo jì (大小蓟 Japanese/field thistle, Cirsii Japonici/Cirsii Herba)

xù duàn tàn (续断炭 charred dipsacus, Dipsaci Radix Carbonisata)

zhū líng (猪苓 polyporus, Polyporus)

fú líng (茯苓 poria, Poria)

mù tōng (木通 trifoliate akebia, Akebiae Trifoliatae Caulis)

shēng dì huáng (生地黄 dried/fresh rehmannia, Rehmanniae Radix Exsiccata seu Recens)

Comparisons

To clear heat and dry dampness, use *shēng huáng bǎi* (raw phellodendron). To consolidate the kidney and clear vacuity heat, use *huáng bǎi* (phellodendron) that has been stir-fried with brine. For bloody urine or bloody stool, use *huáng bǎi tàn* (charred phellodendron).

Dosage

The dosage is generally 3–9 g/1–3 qián; in severe cases, use 12–18 g/4–6 qián.

Caution

In the absence of repletion heat, use with caution.

---

6. 生地黄 Shēng Dì Huáng   Rehmanniae Radix
Dried/Fresh Rehmannia   Exsiccata seu Recens

Also called *shēng dì* 生地. Sweet and slightly bitter in flavor and cold in nature, *shēng dì huáng* (dried/fresh rehmannia) mainly cools the blood and clears heat, and enriches yīn and supplements the kidney.

1. Cooling the Blood and Clearing Heat: *Shēng dì huáng* is sweet, bitter, and cold; it cools the blood and clears heat, as well as cooling the blood and stanching bleeding. It is most commonly used to treat warm heat disease with heat evil invading the construction aspect or the blood aspect. When heat is in the construction aspect, signs will include high fever and, in severe cases, confusion, a tongue body that is red or crimson, dull macules and papules beginning to appear, and a rapid pulse that is slightly thin, but no thirst. If there is heat in the blood aspect, there will be high fever, delirious speech, a purple or crimson tongue with little liquid, outthrust of macules and papules, blood ejection or nosebleed, calmness in the morning with agitation at night, and a fine rapid pulse. For these two conditions, *shēng dì huáng* is used with medicinals such as:

xuán shēn (玄参 scrophularia, Scrophulariae Radix)

lián qiáo (连翘 forsythia, Forsythiae Fructus)

zhī zǐ (栀子 gardenia, Gardeniae Fructus)

yù jīn (郁金 curcuma, Curcumae Radix)

zhú yè xīn (竹叶心 tender lophatherum leaf, Lophatheri Folium Immaturum)[5]

dān pí (丹皮 moutan, Moutan Cortex)

chì sháo (赤芍 red peony, Paeoniae Radix Rubra)

shēng shí gāo (生石膏 crude gypsum, Gypsum Fibrosum Crudum)

xī jiǎo (犀角 rhinoceros horn, Rhinocerotis Cornu)

---

[5] *Zhú yè xīn* (tender lophatherum leaf) is the tender leaf that is, ideally, harvested at dawn. It is primarily used to treat heat in the pericardium that gives rise to delirium. (Ed.)

Combinations of the medicinals listed above include *qīng yíng tāng* (Construction-Clearing Decoction), *huà bān tāng* (Macule-Transforming Decoction), and *xī jiǎo dì huáng tāng* (Rhinoceros Horn and Rehmannia Decoction).

RESEARCH

According to modern research reports, *shēng dì huáng* is a hemostat and coagulant.

2. Enriching Yīn and Supplementing the Kidney: *Shēng dì huáng* enriches yīn and supplements the kidney; it is used for yīn vacuity with heat that gives rise to steaming bone consumptive heat, dry cough, sore and dry throat, phlegm containing blood, heat in the (hearts of the) palms and soles, and night sweats. For this pattern, it is combined with medicinals such as:

dì gǔ pí (地骨皮 lycium root bark, Lycii Cortex)

zhì biē jiǎ (炙鳖甲 mix-fried turtle shell, Trionycis Carapax cum Liquido Frictus Frictus)

dān pí (丹皮 moutan, Moutan Cortex)

qín jiāo (秦艽 large gentian, Gentianae Macrophyllae Radix)

zhī mǔ (知母 anemarrhena, Anemarrhenae Rhizoma)

bái wēi (白薇 black swallowwort, Cynanchi Atrati Radix)

xuán shēn (玄参 scrophularia, Scrophulariae Radix)

tiān dōng (天冬 asparagus, Asparagi Radix)

In addition, in the advanced stage of warm-heat disease, when heat evil has damaged the fluids causing thirst, poor appetite, postmeridian heat vexation, and heat effusion (fever) in the night that abates by the morning, *shēng dì huáng* is used with medicinals such as *mài dōng* (ophiopogon), *yù zhú* (Solomon's seal), *shā shēn* (adenophora/glehnia), *bīng táng* (rock candy), *lí zhī* (pear juice), *xiān ǒu zhī* (lotus root juice), *shēng mài yá* (raw barley sprout), *chǎo gǔ yá* (stir-fried rice sprout), and *xiāng dào yá* (rice sprout) as in *yì wèi tāng* (Stomach-Boosting Decoction), to nourish yīn and engender liquid and to clear heat and boost the stomach.

For vacuous yīn that cannot overcome heat, which results in **dispersion-thirst**[546] (消渴 *xiāo kě*, characterized by thirst with the desire to drink cold fluids but with fluid intake failing to resolve thirst, gradual loss of weight, frequent urination, and a tendency to be hungry), *shēng dì huáng* is often combined with medicinals such as:

shān zhū yú (山茱萸 cornus, Corni Fructus)

shān yào (山药 dioscorea, Dioscoreae Rhizoma)

fú líng (茯苓 poria, Poria)

dān pí (丹皮 moutan, Moutan Cortex)

zé xiè (泽泻 alisma, Alismatis Rhizoma)

wǔ wèi zǐ (五味子 schisandra, Schisandrae Fructus)

tiān huā fěn (天花粉 trichosanthes root, Trichosanthis Radix)

I often achieve good results using large doses of *shēng dì huáng*, *shú dì huáng* (cooked rehmannia), and *shān yào* (dioscorea) combined with medicinals such as *shān zhū yú* (cornus), *fú líng* (poria), *zé xiè* (alisma), *dān pí* (moutan), *wǔ wèi zǐ* (schisandra), and *ròu guì* (cinnamon bark) (do not use too much *ròu guì*; 0.9–2.5 g/ 3–8 fēn is enough), varied in accordance with signs, to treat diabetes mellitus and diabetes insipidus. According to modern research reports, this medicinal has a pronounced hypoglycemic effect.

Comparisons

Shēng dì huáng in Chinese is called "生地 *shēng dì*" for short, and it is used to cool the blood, clear heat, enrich yīn, and engender blood. When char-fried, it is called "*shēng dì tàn* 生地炭," which is used to stanch bleeding in cases of nosebleed, bloody stool, bloody urine, blood ejection, coughing of blood, and flooding and spotting. *Shēng dì huáng* that has been steamed in yellow wine is called *shú dì huáng* (熟地黃, cooked rehmannia); it is used to supplement the kidney and enrich yīn and to nourish blood. *Dì huáng* that is simply dug out of the ground and washed clean is called *xiān shēng dì* (鮮生地, fresh rehmannia); it has "great cold" and is used for warm heat seasonal epidemics in which fire-toxin heat accumulation in the blood causes manic heat (fever), delirious speech, and related symptoms. There is a form called *xì shēng dì* (細生地, thin dried rehmannia) or *xiǎo shēng dì* (小生地, small dried rehmannia), which nourishes yīn and is suitable for advanced-stage heat disease with insufficiency of yīn liquid that causes poor appetite. *Shēng dì huáng* is rich and slimy and has a strong flavor; when taken in large doses or over a long period of time, it can impair the appetite because it is stagnating and slimy. When this happens, it is best to use *xì shēng dì*. Alternatively, one can add *shā rén* (amomum) or stir-fry *shēng dì huáng* with ginger juice.

Combinations

Shēng dì huáng combined with *mài dōng* (ophiopogon) moistens the lung and clears fire; combined with *tiān dōng* (asparagus), it enriches the kidney and down-bears fire; combined with *xuán shēn* (scrophularia), it resolves toxin, clears heat, and cools the blood; combined with *xī jiǎo* (rhinoceros horn), it cools the blood and transforms macules.

Dosage

The dosage is generally 9–15 g/3–5 qián; in severe cases, use 30 g/1 liǎng or even more. When using *xiān shēng dì* the dosage is often 30–60 g/1–2 liǎng.

Caution

Do not use in cases of spleen and stomach vacuity cold or sloppy soft stool. This medicinal is contraindicated for cases of summerheat-damp or oppression in the chest with inability to eat.

7. 犀角 Xī Jiǎo   Rhinocerotis Cornu
Rhinoceros Horn

Xī jiǎo (rhinoceros horn)[6] is cold in nature and bitter and salty in flavor. It primarily clears construction and cools the blood, and also resolves toxin and stabilizes fright.

For warm disease with heat entering the construction aspect, which is characterized by high fever, clouded spirit, delirious speech, and **fright wind**[550] (惊风 *jīng fēng*), one can use *xī jiǎo* combined with medicinals such as:

yù jīn (郁金 curcuma, Curcumae Radix)

tiān zhú huáng (天竹黄 bamboo sugar, Bambusae Concretio Silicea)

xuán shēn (玄参 scrophularia, Scrophulariae Radix)

gōu téng (钩藤 uncaria, Uncariae Ramulus cum Uncis)

líng yáng jiǎo (羚羊角 antelope horn, Saigae Tataricae Cornu)

yuǎn zhì (远志 polygala, Polygalae Radix)

chāng pú (菖蒲 acorus, Acori Tatarinowii Rhizoma)

huáng lián (黄连 coptis, Coptidis Rhizoma)

In cases of warm disease with heat entering the blood aspect, in which heat evil drives the blood causing it to move frenetically and manifesting as blood ejection, nosebleed, coughing of blood, bloody urine, bloody stool, and red macules appearing all over the body, one can use *xī jiǎo* in combination with medicinals such as:

shēng dì huáng (生地黄 dried/fresh rehmannia, Rehmanniae Radix Exsiccata seu Recens)

shēng shí gāo (生石膏 crude gypsum, Gypsum Fibrosum Crudum)

chì sháo (赤芍 red peony, Paeoniae Radix Rubra)

dān pí (丹皮 moutan, Moutan Cortex)

xuán shēn (玄参 scrophularia, Scrophulariae Radix)

bái máo gēn (白茅根 imperata, Imperatae Rhizoma)

xiǎo jì (小蓟 field thistle, Cirsii Herba)

Xī jiǎo is expensive and scarce; it is therefore often used in powder form and taken drenched. In recent years *shuǐ niú jiǎo* (water buffalo horn) and *guǎng xī jiǎo* (African rhinoceros horn) have been substituted. The latter is African rhinoceros horn that has been imported through Guǎngzhōu; in Chinese it is also called *guǎng xī jiǎo* (African rhinoceros horn) and it is relatively inexpensive.[7]

Dosage

The dosage is generally 0.7–1.5 g/2–5 fēn; it is ground into a powder and taken

---

[6]Rhinoceros horn is prohibited from trade since rhinoceros is on the CITES endangered species list. It is typically replaced with *shuǐ niú jiǎo* (水牛角, water buffalo horn) and the dose is increased by tenfold. (Ed.)

[7]Because the rhinoceros is an endangered species, trade in any of its parts is illegal in the United States, and no form of *xī jiǎo* (rhinoceros horn) may be used.

drenched. When using *guǎng xī jiǎo* the dosage is 3–9 g/1–3 qián decocted in water or 1.5–3 g/0.5–1 qián of powder taken drenched. When using *shuǐ niú jiǎo* (water buffalo horn) the dosage is 20–30 g/0.6–1 liǎng; it must be precooked and decocted in water.

---

8. 羚羊角 Líng Yáng Jiǎo
Antelope Horn
Saigae Tataricae Cornu

Líng yáng jiǎo (antelope horn)[8] is salty in flavor and cold in nature. It has three main actions.

1. Clearing Heat and Resolving Toxin: For warm disease, scourge epidemic, or scourge toxin that cause high fever, clouded spirit, delirious speech, and mania, *líng yáng jiǎo* is combined with medicinals such as:

shēng dì huáng (生地黄 dried/fresh rehmannia, Rehmanniae Radix Exsiccata seu Recens)

xuán shēn (玄参 scrophularia, Scrophulariae Radix)

shēng shí gāo (生石膏 crude gypsum, Gypsum Fibrosum Crudum)

hán shuǐ shí (寒水石 glauberite, Gypsum seu Calcitum)

jīn yín huā (金银花 lonicera, Lonicerae Flos)

lián qiáo (连翘 forsythia, Forsythiae Fructus)

huáng lián (黄连 coptis, Coptidis Rhizoma)

dà qīng yè (大青叶 isatis leaf, Isatidis Folium)

yù jīn (郁金 curcuma, Curcumae Radix)

tiān zhú huáng (天竹黄 bamboo sugar, Bambusae Concretio Silicea)

yuǎn zhì (远志 polygala, Polygalae Radix)

chāng pú (菖蒲 acorus, Acori Tatarinowii Rhizoma)

2. Calming the Liver and Extinguishing Wind: For febrile diseases with high fever, convulsions, grinding of the teeth and "hoisted eyes" (吊眼 *dài yǎn*),[552] neck stiffness, forward-staring eyes, hypertonicity of the limbs, child fright wind, and epilepsy of pregnancy (convulsions and grinding of the teeth during pregnancy), *líng yáng jiǎo* is combined with medicinals such as *gōu téng* (uncaria), *quán xiē* (scorpion), *wú gōng* (centipede), *bái sháo* (white peony), *chì sháo* (red peony), *huáng qín* (scutellaria), *bái jí lí* (tribulus), *fáng fēng* (saposhnikovia), *tiān zhú huáng* (bamboo sugar), *dǎn xīng* (bile arisaema), and *shēng dì huáng* (dried/fresh rehmannia). *Gōu téng tāng* (Uncaria Decoction) is a commonly used formula.

Gōu téng tāng 钩藤汤   Uncaria Decoction

líng yáng jiǎo (羚羊角 antelope horn, Saigae Tataricae Cornu)

sāng yè (桑叶 mulberry leaf, Mori Folium)

---

[8]Antelope horn is prohibited from trade since *Saiga tatarica* L. is on the CITES endangered species list. (Ed.)

chuān bèi mǔ (川贝母 Sìchuān fritillaria, Fritillariae Cirrhosae Bulbus)

shēng dì huáng (生地黄 dried/fresh rehmannia, Rehmanniae Radix Exsiccata seu Recens)

gōu téng (钩藤 uncaria, Uncariae Ramulus cum Uncis)

jú huā (菊花 chrysanthemum, Chrysanthemi Flos)

bái sháo (白芍 white peony, Paeoniae Radix Alba)

gān cǎo (甘草 licorice, Glycyrrhizae Radix)

zhú rú (竹茹 bamboo shavings, Bambusae Caulis in Taenia)

fú shén (茯神 root poria, Poria cum Pini Radice)

For excessively exuberant liver fire causing headache and dizziness, *líng yáng jiǎo* is combined with medicinals such as *jú huā* (chrysanthemum), *bái jí lí* (tribulus), *huáng qín* (scutellaria), *màn jīng zǐ* (vitex), *zé xiè* (alisma), *lóng dǎn cǎo* (gentian), *shēng dì huáng* (dried/fresh rehmannia), *shēng dài zhě shí* (crude hematite), and *shēng shí jué míng* (crude abalone shell).

3. Clearing the Liver and Brightening the Eyes: To treat symptoms of liver heat such as clouded vision, sore red swollen eyes, and unclear vision, *líng yáng jiǎo* is combined with medicinals such as:

huáng qín (黄芩 scutellaria, Scutellariae Radix)

huáng lián (黄连 coptis, Coptidis Rhizoma)

zhī zǐ (栀子 gardenia, Gardeniae Fructus)

xuán shēn (玄参 scrophularia, Scrophulariae Radix)

jú huā (菊花 chrysanthemum, Chrysanthemi Flos)

bái jí lí (白蒺藜 tribulus, Tribuli Fructus)

chái hú (柴胡 bupleurum, Bupleuri Radix)

shí hú (石斛 dendrobium, Dendrobii Herba)

dì gǔ pí (地骨皮 lycium root bark, Lycii Cortex)

mù zéi cǎo (木贼草 equisetum, Equiseti Hiemalis Herba)

COMPARISONS

Xī jiǎo (rhinoceros horn)[259] is stronger to cool the blood and resolve toxin than *líng yáng jiǎo*, and it is mainly used for heart heat causing clouded spirit and for blood-heat macules. *Líng yáng jiǎo* cools the liver and extinguishes wind to a greater degree than *xī jiǎo*, and it is mainly used to calm the liver and extinguish wind and to cool the liver and brighten the eyes.

DOSAGE

Líng yáng jiǎo is usually ground into a fine powder and taken drenched in a dosage of 0.7–1.5 g/2–5 fēn each time. If slices of *líng yáng jiǎo* are used, I generally decoct 1.5–3 g/0.5–1 qián separately, then mix with the rest of the decoction.

CAUTION

Do not use *líng yáng jiǎo* in the absence of serious warm heat or scourge toxin, or heat in the liver channel. The major disadvantage of this medicinal is that it is very scarce and expensive.[9]

| **9. 知母 Zhī Mǔ**
Anemarrhena | Anemarrhenae
Rhizoma |

Cold in nature and bitter in flavor,[10] *Zhī mǔ* (anemarrhena) clears heat, enriches yīn, and downbears fire.

Zhī mǔ (anemarrhena) clears heat with cold and bitterness and is effective against effulgent heat evil that causes high fever, sweating, thirst, heart vexation, and a red facial complexion. For this pattern, use it with medicinals such as *shēng shí gāo* (crude gypsum), *shēng gān cǎo* (raw licorice), *tiān huā fěn* (trichosanthes root), *lú gēn* (phragmites), and *huáng qín* (scutellaria). For lung heat with symptoms of cough, yellow sputum, thirst, and constipation, it is combined with medicinals such as:

bèi mǔ (贝母 fritillaria, Fritillariae Bulbus)

guā lóu (瓜蒌 trichosanthes, Trichosanthis Fructus)

huáng qín (黄芩 scutellaria, Scutellariae Radix)

zhī zǐ (栀子 gardenia, Gardeniae Fructus)

shēng shí gāo (生石膏 crude gypsum, Gypsum Fibrosum Crudum)

sāng pí (桑皮 mulberry root bark, Mori Cortex)

xìng rén (杏仁 apricot kernel, Armeniacae Semen)

Most cold and bitter medicinals, including *huáng lián* (coptis), *huáng qín* (scutellaria), *huáng bǎi* (phellodendron), and *zhī zǐ* (gardenia), while they clear heat, also have the disadvantage that they damage yīn and cause transformation to dryness. *Zhī mǔ*, on the other hand, does not have this disadvantage; in fact, it enriches yīn and downbears fire. For symptoms such as yīn vacuity heat, steaming bones and night sweating, seminal emission and yellow urine, vexing heat in the five hearts, pulmonary consumption with cough, and dispersion thirst with intake of fluid, it is often combined with medicinals such as:

dì gǔ pí (地骨皮 lycium root bark, Lycii Cortex)

qín jiāo (秦艽 large gentian, Gentianae Macrophyllac Radix)

shēng dì huáng (生地黄 dried/fresh rehmannia, Rehmanniae Radix Exsiccata seu Recens)

bái sháo (白芍 white peony, Paeoniae Radix Alba)

biē jiǎ (鳖甲 turtle shell, Trionycis Carapax)

---

[9]Certain species of antelope are endangered. This is also an important consideration regarding the use of this medicinal. For further information on the use of products from endangered species in Chinese medicine, contact the World Wildlife Fund (www.worldwildlife.org). (Ed.)

[10]*Běn Cǎo Gāng Mù* (本草纲目 "The Comprehensive Herbal Foundation") cites *zhī mǔ* (anemarrhena) as being acrid and bitter; this draws attention to its capacity to enter the lung channel with acridity. Many modern sources also ascribe sweetness to *zhī mǔ* (anemarrhena), which reflects its supplementing and nourishing nature. (Ed.)

xuán shēn (玄参 scrophularia, Scrophulariae Radix)
huáng bǎi (黄柏 phellodendron, Phellodendri Cortex)
bái wēi (白薇 black swallowwort, Cynanchi Atrati Radix)
mài dōng (麦冬 ophiopogon, Ophiopogonis Radix)

Zhī mǔ is usually stir-fried with brine so that it will move downward into the kidney. If it is stir-fried with yellow wine, it moves upward into the lung.

Comparisons

Huáng bǎi (phellodendron)[254] consolidates the kidney and clears heat; it is used for kidney channel damp-heat, strangury-turbidity, and weakness in the knees. *Zhī mǔ* enriches the kidney and downbears fire; it is used for kidney channel vacuity heat, steaming bones, and dispersion-thirst. *Huáng bǎi* (phellodendron) clears substantial damp-heat in the lower burner, whereas *zhī mǔ* drains rootless fire from the lower burner. Combining the two medicinals increases their ability to enrich the kidney, consolidate the kidney, clear heat, and downbear fire.

Tiān huā fěn (trichosanthes root)[290] and *zhī mǔ* both clear yáng brightness (*yáng míng*) stomach heat. Nevertheless, *tiān huā fěn* boosts the stomach and engenders liquid, while *zhī mǔ* enriches yīn and downbears fire. Some people believe that since *zhī mǔ* is cold, bitter, slippery, and downbearing in nature, frequent use damages the stomach and intestines and causes diarrhea, whereas *tiān huā fěn* is a sweet and cool medicinal that boosts the stomach and engenders liquid, and therefore actually benefits the stomach rather than harming it. Those who hold this view advocate substituting *tiān huā fěn* for *zhī mǔ* in *bái hǔ tāng* (White Tiger Decoction), which is composed of medicinals such as *shēng shí gāo* (crude gypsum), *zhī mǔ* (anemarrhena), *gān cǎo* (licorice), and *gēng mǐ* (non-glutinous rice). I myself, depending on the actual disease pattern, often substitute *tiān huā fěn* in *bái hǔ tāng* (White Tiger Decoction) or use a reduced dose of *zhī mǔ* and add *tiān huā fěn*. I always achieve good results with this method.

Dosage

The dosage is generally 6–9 g/2–3 qián.

Caution

Do not use in cases of kidney yáng vacuity, if both cubit pulses are faint and weak, or if there is sloppy diarrhea.

Research

According to modern research reports, this medicinal has antipyretic properties. It also has a strong antibacterial effect against microorganisms such as *Bacillus typhosus*, *Bacillus dysenteriae*, *Bacillus coli*, *Pseudomonas pyocyanea*, *Staphylococcus*, *Diplococcus pneumoniae*, hemolytic streptococcus, and *Bordatella pertussis*.

10. 大青叶 Dà Qīng Yè   Isatidis Folium
Isatis Leaf

Dà qīng yè (isatis leaf)[11] is bitter in flavor and greatly cold in nature. It mainly clears heat, resolves toxin, and cools the blood.

Dà qīng yè is most commonly used to treat warm disease, scourge epidemic, and scourge toxin that cause high fever, clouded spirit, sore swollen throat, headache and toothache, mouth and tongue sores, maculopapular eruptions, blood ejection or nosebleed, cinnabar toxin [sore], mumps (parotitis), and scarlet fever. For this purpose it is often combined with medicinals such as:

xuán shēn (玄参 scrophularia, Scrophulariae Radix)

shēng dì huáng (生地黄 dried/fresh rehmannia, Rehmanniae Radix Exsiccata seu Recens)

shēng shí gāo (生石膏 crude gypsum, Gypsum Fibrosum Crudum)

zhī mǔ (知母 anemarrhena, Anemarrhenae Rhizoma)

huáng qín (黄芩 scutellaria, Scutellariae Radix)

jīn yín huā (金银花 lonicera, Lonicerae Flos)

lián qiáo (连翘 forsythia, Forsythiae Fructus)

jīng jiè (荆芥 schizonepeta, Schizonepetae Herba)

bò hé (薄荷 mint, Menthae Herba)

dān pí (丹皮 moutan, Moutan Cortex)

guǎng xī jiǎo (广犀角 African rhinoceros horn, Rhinocerotis Cornu Africanum)

For example, in the *zhèng zhì zhǔn shéng* (证治准绳 "The Level-Line of Pattern Identification and Treatment"), *dà qīng tāng* (Isatis Formula) is prescribed for heat toxin macular eruptions.

Dà qīng tāng 大青汤   Isatis Formula

dà qīng yè (大青叶 isatis leaf, Isatidis Folium)

xuán shēn (玄参 scrophularia, Scrophulariae Radix)

shēng shí gāo (生石膏 crude gypsum, Gypsum Fibrosum Crudum)

zhī mǔ (知母 anemarrhena, Anemarrhenae Rhizoma)

mù tōng (木通 trifoliate akebia, Akebiae Trifoliatae Caulis)

gān cǎo (甘草 licorice, Glycyrrhizae Radix)

dì gǔ pí (地骨皮 lycium root bark, Lycii Cortex)

jīng jiè suì (荆芥穗 schizonepeta spike, Schizonepetae Flos)

I find the following formula, varied in accordance with signs, very effectively treats parotitis:

---

[11] Besides *Isatis indigotica* L., *Polygonum tinctorium* AIT. is also an accepted plant for *dà qīng yè* (isatis leaf). The leaf of *Baphicacanthus cusia* (NEES) BREM. (马蓝 *mǎ lán*) is also seen in trade. The latter is considered incorrect. (Ed.)

dà qīng yè (大青叶 isatis leaf, Isatidis Folium) 15 g/5 qián
huáng qín (黄芩 scutellaria, Scutellariae Radix) 6–9 g/2–3 qián
bǎn lán gēn (板蓝根 isatis root, Isatidis Radix) 9 g/3 qián
xuán shēn (玄参 scrophularia, Scrophulariae Radix) 9–12 g/3–4 qián

For warm disease with intense blood-aspect heat toxin causing macular eruptions, nosebleed, and blood ejection, I often get good results using *huà bān tāng* (Macule-Transforming Decoction) with additions.

Huà bān tāng 化斑汤   Macule-Transforming Decoction

---

shēng shí gāo (生石膏 crude gypsum, Gypsum Fibrosum Crudum)
zhī mǔ (知母 anemarrhena, Anemarrhenae Rhizoma)
xuán shēn (玄参 scrophularia, Scrophulariae Radix)
xī jiǎo (犀角 rhinoceros horn, Rhinocerotis Cornu)
gān cǎo (甘草 licorice, Glycyrrhizae Radix)
gēng mǐ (粳米 non-glutinous rice, Oryzae Semen)

Additions:

dà qīng yè (大青叶 isatis leaf, Isatidis Folium)
shēng dì huáng (生地黄 dried/fresh rehmannia, Rehmanniae Radix Exsiccata seu Recens)
dān pí (丹皮 moutan, Moutan Cortex)
chì sháo (赤芍 red peony, Paeoniae Radix Rubra)
chǎo zhī zǐ (炒栀子 stir-fried gardenia, Gardeniae Fructus Frictus)
xiǎo jì (小蓟 field thistle, Cirsii Herba)

According to modern research reports, *dà qīng yè* inhibits or eliminates *Leptospira*. It also has an inhibitory effect on microorganisms such as *Staphylococcus albus*, *Staphylococcus aureus*, alpha streptococcus, *Meningococcus*, and *Diplococcus pneumoniae*. [12]

DOSAGE

The dosage is generally 6–15 g/2–5 qián; for serious conditions, use up to 30 g/ 1 liǎng.

CAUTION

Contraindicated for spleen-stomach vacuity cold.

---

[12]Because of the antimicrobial properties found in this medicinal, modern practitioners often include *dà qīng yè* (isatis leaf) in formulas that treat microbial infections such as pneumonia and hepatitis. (Ed.)

11. 青黛 Qīng Dài   Indigo Naturalis
Indigo

Qīng dài (indigo) is salty in flavor and cold in nature. It is very similiar to *dà qīng yè* (isatis leaf) in its effects, although it has a much stronger blood-cooling effect. Moreover, it disperses phlegm-heat above the diaphram. *Dà qīng yè* (isatis leaf) is processed from the pigment in the dried leaves of *Baphicanthus cusia* (NEES) BREM. (马兰 *mǎ lán*) of the *Acanthacae* family (爵床科 *jué chuáng kē*), *Polygonum tinctorium* AIT. (蓼兰 *liǎo lán*) of the *Polygonaceae* family (蓼科 *liǎo kē*), or *Isatis tinctoria* L. (菘兰 *sōng lán*) of the *Cruciferae* family (十字花科 *shí zì huā kē*).[13] It comes in the form of a fine powder, and is also applied topically.

For frenetic movement of hot blood that causes nosebleed, blood ejection, coughing of blood, as well as warm-heat entering the blood and heat toxin macular eruptions, *qīng dài* (indigo) can be combined with medicinals such as:

shēng dì huáng (生地黄 dried/fresh rehmannia, Rehmanniae Radix Exsiccata seu Recens)

xuán shēn (玄参 scrophularia, Scrophulariae Radix)

dà qīng yè (大青叶 isatis leaf, Isatidis Folium)

bái máo gēn (白茅根 imperata, Imperatae Rhizoma)

shēng shí gāo (生石膏 crude gypsum, Gypsum Fibrosum Crudum)

zhī mǔ (知母 anemarrhena, Anemarrhenae Rhizoma)

dān pí tàn (丹皮炭 charred moutan, Moutan Cortex Carbonisatus)

zhī zǐ tàn (栀子炭 charred gardenia, Gardeniae Fructus Carbonisatus)

ǒu jié tàn (藕节炭 charred lotus root node, Nelumbinis Rhizomatis Nodus Carbonisatus)

To stop nosebleeds, spread a paste of *qīng dài* and *xuè yú tàn* (charred hair) (in a ratio of 2 to 1) on a piece of gauze or absorbent cotton, and stuff up the nose.

For intense liver fire or extreme heat engendering wind causing high fever and convulsions or fright epilepsy with clouded spirit, *qīng dài* is combined with medicinals such as:

dǎn xīng (胆星 bile arisaema, Arisaema cum Bile)

quán xiē (全蝎 scorpion, Scorpio)

tiān zhú huáng (天竹黄 bamboo sugar, Bambusae Concretio Silicea)

yù jīn (郁金 curcuma, Curcumae Radix)

huáng lián (黄连 coptis, Coptidis Rhizoma)

yuǎn zhì (远志 polygala, Polygalae Radix)

chāng pú (菖蒲 acorus, Acori Tatarinowii Rhizoma)

gōu téng (钩藤 uncaria, Uncariae Ramulus cum Uncis)

---

[13] *Qīng dài* (indigo) is principally made from the leaves of *Polygonum tinctorium* AIT. Typically the leaves are soaked and mixed in a solution with limestone. The dregs are dried and ground to a fine powder. (Ed.)

For lung heat cough with phlegm that is sticky, formed into lumps, and not easily expectorated, use *qīng dài* to disperse heat phlegm above the diaphram. For this purpose it is often combined with *gé fěn* (mactra clamshell powder), a combination known as *dài gé sǎn* (Indigo and Clamshell Powder). The dosage is 0.9–1.5 g/3–5 fēn, which is taken drenched with a decoction each time.

Qīng dài is also used as a **laryngeal insufflation**[556] (吹喉 *chuī hòu*) to treat sores in the throat or a red, swollen, painful, and putrefied throat. For example:

Qīng dài sǎn[14] 青黛散   Indigo Powder

---

yá xiāo (牙硝 horse-tooth niter, Nitrum Equidens) 1.8 g/6 fēn

qīng dài (青黛 indigo, Indigo Naturalis) 1.8 g/6 fēn

zhū shā (朱砂 cinnabar, Cinnabaris) 1.8 g/6 fēn

huáng lián (黄连 coptis, Coptidis Rhizoma) 9 g/3 qián

huáng bǎi (黄柏 phellodendron, Phellodendri Cortex) 9 g/3 qián

xióng huáng (雄黄 realgar, Realgar) 0.9 g/3 fēn

niú huáng (牛黄 bovine bezoar, Bovis Calculus) 0.9 g/3 fēn

péng shā (硼砂 borax, Borax) 0.9 g/3 fēn

bīng piàn (冰片 borneol, Borneolum) 0.3 g/1 fēn

Grind this formula into a fine powder and insufflate into the throat. For the pain and swelling of parotitis, use *qīng dài* mixed in cool drinking water to disperse swelling and relieve pain.

COMPARISONS

Dà qīng yè (isatis leaf)[266] clears heat toxins from the heart and stomach; it is used mainly for scourge epidemic heat mania. *Qīng dài* drains depressed fire in the liver channel; it is used for fright epilepsy and heat macules.

DOSAGE

The dosage is generally 0.9–4.5 g/3 fēn–1.5 qián. Decoct wrapped in gauze. If taken drenched with decoction medicine, the dosage is 0.3–0.6 g/1–2 fēn or 1.0 g/3 fēn.

CAUTION

Contraindicated for center burner vacuity cold and yīn vacuity tidal fever.

---

[14]There are many versions of *qīng dài sǎn* (Indigo Powder). Omitting the *zhū shā* (cinnabar) and *xióng huáng* (realgar) also yields an effective formula. For internal applications, natural *bīng piàn* (borneol) must be used. For mumps, mix with water and apply to the swollen glands; when the paste dries, brush off the powder and re-apply the paste. This procedure can be repeated several times a day. Some practitioners prefer to use vinegar to make the paste. (Ed.)

12. 板蓝根 Bǎn Lán Gēn   Isatidis Radix
Isatis Root

Bǎn lán gēn (isatis root)[15] is cold in nature and bitter in flavor. Its main actions are to clear heat and cool the blood, and to resolve toxin and disinhibit the throat.

1. Massive Head Scourge[557] (大头温 *dà tóu wēn*)[16]: When wind-heat scourge toxin invades the blood aspect, causing redness and swelling on the head, heat [effusion] (fever), sore swollen throat, or, in severe cases, clouded spirit and delirious speech, one can use this medicinal to downbear heart fire, clear stomach heat, cool the blood, and resolve scourge toxin. For this purpose it is often combined with medicinals such as:

huáng lián (黄连 coptis, Coptidis Rhizoma)

niú bàng zǐ (牛蒡子 arctium, Arctii Fructus)

xuán shēn (玄参 scrophularia, Scrophulariae Radix)

lián qiáo (连翘 forsythia, Forsythiae Fructus)

huáng qín (黄芩 scutellaria, Scutellariae Radix)

chái hú (柴胡 bupleurum, Bupleuri Radix)

mǎ bó (马勃 puffball, Lasiosphaera seu Calvatia)

2. Seasonal Epidemic Maculopapular Eruptions: *Bǎn lán gēn* is used for seasonal epidemic (contagious, infectious, or seasonal heat diseases) contagions with warm toxin entering the blood and intense heat in construction-blood, presenting as generalized heat [effusion] (fever), vexation and agitation, thirst, headache, sore pharynx, nosebleeds, macular or papular eruptions, and a crimson and dark-purple tongue. For such conditions, use *bǎn lán gēn* combined with medicinals such as:

jīn yín huā (金银花 lonicera, Lonicerae Flos)

lián qiáo (连翘 forsythia, Forsythiae Fructus)

bò hé (薄荷 mint, Menthae Herba)

niú bàng zǐ (牛蒡子 arctium, Arctii Fructus)

xuán shēn (玄参 scrophularia, Scrophulariae Radix)

shēng dì huáng (生地黄 dried/fresh rehmannia, Rehmanniae Radix Exsiccata seu Recens)

dān pí (丹皮 moutan, Moutan Cortex)

shēng shí gāo (生石膏 crude gypsum, Gypsum Fibrosum Crudum)

guǎng xī jiǎo (广犀角 African rhinoceros horn, Rhinocerotis Cornu Africanum)

3. Sore Swollen Throat: For wind-heat toxin fire invading the throat, causing headache, heat [effusion] (fever), thirst, constipation, a red swollen throat that is

---

[15] *Bǎn lán gēn* (isatis root) should come from *Isatis indigotica* FORT. *Baphicacanthus cusia* (NEES) BREM. is commonly seen in southern China and foreign markets. (Ed.)

[16] Massive head scourge is a type of warm toxin also known as "massive head wind" (大头风 *dà tóu fēng*) or "massive head cold damage" (大头伤寒 *dà tóu shāng hán*). It is attributable to contraction of wind-warmth seasonal toxin invading the lung and stomach and is characterized by red and swollen face and head and by a sore swollen throat. (Au.)

hot and sore, or single and double baby moths[542] (hemilateral or bilateral swollen tonsils), one can use this medicinal to clear heat, cool the blood, and resolve toxin. For this purpose it is often combined with medicinals such as:

huáng qín (黄芩 scutellaria, Scutellariae Radix)

zhī zǐ (栀子 gardenia, Gardeniae Fructus)

shēng dì huáng (生地黄 dried/fresh rehmannia, Rehmanniae Radix Exsiccata seu Recens)

xuán shēn (玄参 scrophularia, Scrophulariae Radix)

bò hé (薄荷 mint, Menthae Herba)

niú bàng zǐ (牛蒡子 arctium, Arctii Fructus)

shè gān (射干 belamcanda, Belamcandae Rhizoma)

jǐn dēng lóng (锦灯笼 lantern plant calyx, Physalis Calyx seu Fructus)[271]

lián qiáo (连翘 forsythia, Forsythiae Fructus)

jīn yín huā (金银花 lonicera, Lonicerae Flos)

shēng dà huáng (生大黄 raw rhubarb, Rhei Radix et Rhizoma Crudi)

Comparisons

Dà qīng yè (isatis leaf)[264] and *bǎn lán gēn* both clear heat, cool the blood, and resolve toxin; however, *dà qīng yè* has much more pronounced blood-cooling, macular-transforming, and toxin-resolving effects. *Bǎn lán gēn* disinhibits the throat and treats massive head scourge (大头瘟 *dà tóu wēn*) much more effectively than *dà qīng yè*.

Dosage

The dosage is generally 4.5–9 g/1.5 qián–3 qián or 12 g/4 qián.

Caution

This medicinal is inappropriate in cases of spleen-stomach vacuity cold.

Research

According to experimental research and clinical reports, *bǎn lán gēn* has an inhibitory effect on *Bacillus typhosus, hemolytic streptococcus, Bacillus coli, Bacillus paratyphosus, Bacillus dysenteriae,* and *Staphylococcus.* This medicinal is also very effective for treating infectious parotitis. For this, take 8–10 g/2.5–3 qián as a raw powder or in pressed tablet form, swallowed with warm water, every four hours. Continue for three or four days. For epidemic encephalitis B (Japanese encephalitis), 6–9 g/2–3 qián of *bǎn lán gēn*, administered every two hours, is very effective. This medicinal is also effective against both influenza and measles. *Bǎn lán gēn* injection fluid is effective in treating both icteric hepatitis and chronic hepatitis.

13. 山豆根 Shān Dòu Gēn

Bushy Sophora

Sophorae
Tonkinensis Radix

Shān dòu gēn (bushy sophora) is bitter in flavor and cold in nature. Its main actions are to drain fire, resolve toxin, and disinhibit the throat. It is often used to treat sore red swollen throat.

For fire-heat flaming upward and heat toxin rising and invading the throat, causing a red swollen throat with pain and difficulty swallowing, use this medicinal to drain fire and clear heat, resolve toxin and disperse swelling. For this purpose it is often combined with medicinals such as *xuán shēn* (scrophularia), *mài dōng* (ophiopogon), *jīn yín huā* (lonicera), *jié gěng* (platycodon), *gān cǎo* (licorice), *bò hé* (mint), and *jǐn dēng lóng* (lantern plant calyx). For acute throat wind (which includes severe acute tonsillitis), clenched jaw, and inability to swallow food or drink, use 15 g/5 qián of *shān dòu gēn* in combination with 12 g/4 qián of *jié gěng* (platycodon) and 12 g/4 qián of *bái yào zǐ* (cepharantha). In these cases, quickly administering this decoction is effective.

For lung heat cough, *shān dòu gēn* is combined with medicinals such as *huáng qín* (scutellaria), *guā lóu* (trichosanthes), *bèi mǔ* (fritillaria), *zhī mǔ* (anemarrhena), *jié gěng* (platycodon), and *xuán shēn* (scrophularia).

a) Combined with *shè gān* (belamcanda),[272] *shān dòu gēn* treats binding stagnation of phlegm-heat in the throat that causes swelling and pain in the throat.

b) Combined with *bǎn lán gēn* (isatis root),[268] it treats intense toxic heat that causes putrefying sore throat.

c) Combined with *huái jiǎo* (sophora fruit) and *huái huā* (sophora flower), it treats painful bleeding hemorrhoids.

Comparisons

Bǎn lán gēn (isatis root)[268] mainly treats warmth toxin swelling under the chin, and red, putrifying throat, whereas *shān dòu gēn* treats fire toxin flaming upward and causing a red swollen throat.

Mǎ bó (puffball)[293] treats sore throat and tends to lightly diffuse lung heat to vent heat evil outwards; *shān dòu gēn* treats sore throat, but tends to drain heat and resolve toxin, as well as downbear fire and disperse swelling; *shè gān* (belamcanda) treats sore throat and is most effective at clearing heat, dispersing phlegm, and dissipating binds. It mainly treats phlegm-heat binding stagnation and red and swollen tonsils.

Research

According to modern research reports, *shān dòu gēn* is effective in treating cancerous tumors. Some people have also reported that *shān dòu gēn* is effective against naso-pharyngeal cancer.

DOSAGE

The dosage is generally 3–9 g/1–3 qián. In cases of spleen-stomach vacuity cold or diarrhea, this medicinal is inappropriate.

---

14. 锦灯笼 Jǐn Dēng Lóng
Lantern Plant Calyx

Physalis Calyx seu Fructus

Also called *jīn dēng* 金灯.[17] Cold in nature and bitter in flavor, *jǐn dēng lóng* (lantern plant calyx) clears heat and resolves toxin, and dissipates fire and disperses swelling. It is used primarily to clear lung heat.

For lung heat cough with signs such as copious thick yellow phlegm and a sore swollen throat, *jǐn dēng lóng* is used to clear and dissipate lung heat in combination with medicinals such as:

guā lóu (瓜蒌 trichosanthes, Trichosanthis Fructus)

huáng qín (黄芩 scutellaria, Scutellariae Radix)

zhī mǔ (知母 anemarrhena, Anemarrhenae Rhizoma)

xuán shēn (玄参 scrophularia, Scrophulariae Radix)

jié gěng (桔梗 platycodon, Platycodonis Radix)

shān dòu gēn (山豆根 bushy sophora, Sophorae Tonkinensis Radix)

I often use it in combination with the following medicinals to treat acute tonsillitis:

shēng dì huáng (生地黄 dried/fresh rehmannia, Rehmanniae Radix Exsiccata seu Recens)

xuán shēn (玄参 scrophularia, Scrophulariae Radix)

jīng jiè (荆芥 schizonepeta, Schizonepetae Herba)

bò hé (薄荷 mint, Menthae Herba)

jīn yín huā (金银花 lonicera, Lonicerae Flos)

lián qiáo (连翘 forsythia, Forsythiae Fructus)

jié gěng (桔梗 platycodon, Platycodonis Radix)

huáng qín (黄芩 scutellaria, Scutellariae Radix)

shān dòu gēn (山豆根 bushy sophora, Sophorae Tonkinensis Radix)

shè gān (射干 belamcanda, Belamcandae Rhizoma)

My experience in treating tonsillitis is as follows:

a) If the tonsils are red, swollen, and enlarged, use *shè gān* (belamcanda).

b) If the throat is red and sore, but the tonsils are not particularly swollen, use *shān dòu gēn* (bushy sophora).

---

[17] *Jǐn dēng lóng* (lantern plant calyx) is also known as *guà jīn dēng* 挂金灯 and *suān jiāng shí* 酸浆实. In *Shén Nóng Běn Cǎo* (神农本草 "The Divine Husbandman's Herbal Foundation") it is recommended for treatment of difficult delivery. In modern use it primarily addresses lung-heat sore throat and heat-strangury disorders. (Ed.)

c) If the voice is also hoarse, use *niú bàng zǐ* (arctium) and *chán tuì* (cicada molting).

d) If the neck [the area of the lymph glands] is also red and swollen, use *mǎ bó* (puffball), and *bǎn lán gēn* (isatis root).

e) If the tonsils suppurate and there is evidence of putrefaction, use *qīng dài* (indigo), and *bǎn lán gēn* (isatis root), or *qīng dài sǎn* (Indigo Powder) as a laryngeal insufflation (the complete formula is on page 267, under *qīng dài* (indigo)).

f) For enlarged tonsils that do not easily shrink (are resistant to treatment), use *bái jiāng cán* (silkworm) in addition to *shè gān* (belamcanda).

Jǐn dēng lóng is added to each of the formulas described above; it is very effective for sore, swollen throats. It is important to pay attention to the condition of the whole body and vary the formula in accordance with signs.

DOSAGE

The dosage is generally 3–6 g/1–2 qián; in severe cases, one may use up to 9 g/ 3 qián. In the absence of fire-heat sore throat (either generalized heat signs or local redness and swelling), do not use this medicinal.

---

15. 射干 Shè Gān
Belamcanda
Belamcandae Rhizoma

Shè gān (belamcanda) is cold in nature and bitter in flavor. Its main actions are to clear heat and resolve toxin, and to disperse phlegm and dissipate binds.

1. **Sore Swollen Throat:** For phlegm and heat binding together and blocking the throat, causing a sore, swollen throat, phlegm that is not easily expectorated, phlegm that sounds like the rasping of a saw, and difficulty breathing, use this medicinal to clear lung-stomach phlegm-heat, to disperse swelling and dissipate binds, and to disinhibit the throat. For this purpose it is often combined with medicinals such as *shān dòu gēn* (bushy sophora), *jié gěng* (platycodon), *gān cǎo* (licorice), *xuán shēn* (scrophularia), *lián qiáo* (forsythia), *huáng qín* (scutellaria), and *jǐn dēng lóng* (lantern plant calyx). *Shè gān* (belamcanda) is a primary medicinal for treating throat impediment and sore throat.

2. **Lung Heat Panting and Cough and Phlegm Rale in the Throat:** When lung heat phlegm bind manifests as panting and cough and a frog rale in the throat, use this medicinal to clear the lung and disperse phlegm. For this purpose it is often combined with medicinals such as:

má huáng (麻黄 ephedra, Ephedrae Herba)

bàn xià (半夏 pinellia, Pinelliae Rhizoma)

huáng qín (黄芩 scutellaria, Scutellariae Radix)

xì xīn (细辛 asarum, Asari Herba)

kuǎn dōng huā (款冬花 coltsfoot, Farfarae Flos)

zĭ wăn (紫菀 aster, Asteris Radix)

xìng rén (杏仁 apricot kernel, Armeniacae Semen)

guā lóu (瓜蔞 trichosanthes, Trichosanthis Fructus)

bái guŏ (白果 ginkgo, Ginkgo Semen)

3. Concretions, Conglomerations, Strings, and Aggregations in the Abdomen (癥瘕痃癖 *zhēng jiă xián pì:* For accumulated phlegm and static blood in the abdomen that binds and forms strings and aggregations (including hepatosplenomegaly), use this medicinal to dissipate blood and disperse phlegm, and to open binds and disperse accumulations. For this purpose it is often made into pills in combination with medicinals such as:

biē jiă (鳖甲 turtle shell, Trionycis Carapax)

shén qū (神曲 medicated leaven, Massa Medicata Fermentata)

é zhú (莪术 curcuma rhizome, Curcumae Rhizoma)

shān zhā hé (山楂核 crataegus pit, Crataegi Endocarpium et Semen)

zhì shān jiă (炙山甲 mix-fried pangolin scales, Manis Squama cum Liquido Fricta)

shēng mŭ lì (生牡蛎 crude oyster shell, Ostreae Concha Cruda)

shēng dà huáng (生大黄 raw rhubarb, Rhei Radix et Rhizoma Crudi)

zhĭ shí (枳实 unripe bitter orange, Aurantii Fructus Immaturus)

hóng huā (红花 carthamus, Carthami Flos)

táo rén (桃仁 peach kernel, Persicae Semen)

dāng guī (当归 Chinese angelica, Angelicae Sinensis Radix)

chì sháo (赤芍 red peony, Paeoniae Radix Rubra)

huáng lián (黄连 coptis, Coptidis Rhizoma)

bái zhú (白术 white atractylodes, Atractylodis Macrocephalae Rhizoma)

bīng láng (槟榔 areca, Arecae Semen)

Comparisons

Shān dòu gēn (bushy sophora)[270] drains fire and clears heat to a greater extent than *shè gān*, but *shè gān* disperses phlegm and dissipates binds to a greater extent than *shān dòu gēn*. *Mă bó* (puffball) clears and dissipates lung heat and thereby disinhibits the throat; it is used for nondiffusion of lung qì that results in cough, sore throat, and loss of voice. *Shè gān* drains repletion heat in the chest, and disperses phlegm and dissipates binds to disinhibit the throat; it is used for exuberant heat and phlegm bind causing cough, swollen throat, and **frog rale in the throat**[551] (喉中有水鸡声 *hóu zhōng yŏu shuĭ jī shēng*).

Research

According to modern research reports, *shè gān* eliminates the exudate associated with upper respiratory tract infections. It also relieves pain and acts as an antipyretic.

Dosage

The dosage is generally 2.5–4.5 g/8 fēn–1.5 qián; in severe cases, one can use 6–9 g/2–3 qián. The dosage should not be too large.

CAUTION

This medicinal is contraindicated for spleen-stomach vacuity cold and pregnant women.

---

16. 金银花 Jīn Yín Huā   Lonicerae Flos
Lonicera

Also called *yín huā* 银花 and *rěn dōng huā* 忍冬花. Sweet in flavor and cold in nature, *jīn yín huā* (lonicera) is a frequently used heat-clearing toxin-resolving medicinal.

1. **Resolving the Exterior and Clearing Heat:** For initial-stage warm disease with evil in the defense aspect and heat in the upper burner that presents as generalized heat [effusion], headache, thirst, cough, dry throat, and a rapid floating pulse, use this medicinal to clear and dissipate upper burner wind-heat, and to resolve the exterior and clear heat. For this purpose it is often combined with medicinals such as:

> *lián qiáo* (连翘 forsythia, Forsythiae Fructus)
>
> *niú bàng zǐ* (牛蒡子 arctium, Arctii Fructus)
>
> *jīng jiè* (荆芥 schizonepeta, Schizonepetae Herba)
>
> *bò hé* (薄荷 mint, Menthae Herba)
>
> *dòu chǐ* (豆豉 fermented soybean, Sojae Semen Praeparatum)

2. **Clearing Heat and Resolving Toxin:** For congestion of toxic heat in the blood aspect causing welling-abscesses, swellings and sores; redness, swelling, heat, and pain; and in severe cases, ulcerations, use this medicinal to clear blood heat and resolve sore toxin. For this purpose it is often combined with medicinals such as *lián qiáo* (forsythia), *chì sháo* (red peony), *dāng guī wěi* (Chinese angelica tail), *jú huā* (chrysanthemum), *mò yào* (myrrh), *rǔ xiāng* (frankincense), *tiān huā fěn* (trichosanthes root), and *gān cǎo* (licorice). *Jīn yín huā* (lonicera), in combination with other medicinals varied in accordance with signs, is used to treat all welling-abscesses (痈 *yōng*), sores (疮 *chuāng*), scab (疥 *jiè*), and lichen (癣 *xiǎn*), as well as syphillitic sores.

3. **Clearing Heat and Checking Dysentery:** For heat toxin collecting and stagnating in the center burner causing heat [effusion] and abdominal pain, stool containing pus and blood, and tenesmus, this medicinal is used to clear heat and resolve toxin. For this purpose it is often combined with medicinals such as:

> *dāng guī* (当归 Chinese angelica, Angelicae Sinensis Radix)
>
> *bái sháo* (白芍 white peony, Paeoniae Radix Alba)
>
> *gé gēn* (葛根 pueraria, Puerariae Radix)
>
> *huáng lián* (黄连 coptis, Coptidis Rhizoma)
>
> *mù xiāng* (木香 costusroot, Aucklandiae Radix)
>
> *bái tóu wēng* (白头翁 pulsatilla, Pulsatillae Radix)
>
> *chì sháo* (赤芍 red peony, Paeoniae Radix Rubra)
>
> *gān cǎo* (甘草 licorice, Glycyrrhizae Radix)

According to modern research, this medicinal has an antibacterial effect on the following types of bacteria: *Bacillus dysenteriae*, *Bacillus typhosus*, *Bacillus coli*, *Bordatella pertussis*, *Staphylococcus*, and *Diplococcus pneumoniae*. Therefore, it is used for acute bacterial dysentery that presents as a heat pattern. For this purpose it is often combined with medicinals such as:

huáng lián (黄连 coptis, Coptidis Rhizoma)

huáng qín (黄芩 scutellaria, Scutellariae Radix)

bái sháo (白芍 white peony, Paeoniae Radix Alba)

gé gēn (葛根 pueraria, Puerariae Radix)

mù xiāng (木香 costusroot, Aucklandiae Radix)

mǎ chǐ xiàn (马齿苋 purslane, Portulacae Herba)

To treat the onset of lobar pneumonia, use this medicinal in combination with medicinals such as *xìng rén* (apricot kernel), *lián qiáo* (forsythia), *niú bàng zǐ* (arctium), *jié gěng* (platycodon), and *bò hé* (mint) (See point 2. Clearing Heat and Resolving Toxin, above). For a disease condition that has converted into lung-heat cough and panting, it is combined with medicinals such as:

má huáng (麻黄 ephedra, Ephedrae Herba)

shēng shí gāo (生石膏 crude gypsum, Gypsum Fibrosum Crudum)

xìng rén (杏仁 apricot kernel, Armeniacae Semen)

shēng gān cǎo (生甘草 raw licorice, Glycyrrhizae Radix Cruda)

lián qiáo (连翘 forsythia, Forsythiae Fructus)

huáng qín (黄芩 scutellaria, Scutellariae Radix)

zhī mǔ (知母 anemarrhena, Anemarrhenae Rhizoma)

bò hé (薄荷 mint, Menthae Herba)

Dosage

The dosage is generally 6–12 g/2–4 qián; in special cases, use up to 30–60 g/ 1–2 liǎng.

Caution

This medicinal is inappropriate for vacuity cold diarrhea and sores exuding clear pus without heat toxin.

Addendum

Jīn yín téng (lonicera stem and leaf) and *jīn yín huā* (lonicera) are similar in their natures and flavors. Therefore, if *jīn yín huā* (lonicera) is unavailable one can substitute *jīn yín téng* (lonicera stem and leaf). Nevertheless, the effects of the stem are slightly less than the effects of the flower; therefore, the dosage should accordingly be increased to 15–30 g/5 qián–1 liǎng. *Jīn yín téng* (lonicera stem and leaf) also frees the channels and quickens the network vessels, and disperses wind-heat from the channels and network vessels. I often use it to treat acute arthritis that manifests as hot, swollen, and painful joints. For this purpose I often combine it with medicinals such as:

wēi líng xiān (威灵仙 clematis, Clematidis Radix)

qín jiāo (秦艽 large gentian, Gentianae Macrophyllae Radix)

qiāng huó (羌活 notopterygium, Notopterygii Rhizoma et Radix)

dú huó (独活 pubescent angelica, Angelicae Pubescentis Radix)

huáng bǎi (黄柏 phellodendron, Phellodendri Cortex)

chì sháo (赤芍 red peony, Paeoniae Radix Rubra)

cāng zhú (苍术 atractylodes, Atractylodis Rhizoma)

fáng jǐ (防己 fangji, Stephaniae Tetrandrae Radix)

mù guā (木瓜 chaenomeles, Chaenomelis Fructus)

tòu gǔ cǎo (透骨草 speranskia/balsam, Speranskiae seu Impatientis Herba)

hóng huā (红花 carthamus, Carthami Flos)

---

17. 连翘 Lián Qiáo   Forsythiae Fructus
Forsythia

Cold in nature and bitter and acrid in flavor, *lián qiáo* (forsythia) is a frequently used heat-clearing toxin-resolving medicinal.

1. Clearing Heart Fire: *Lián qiáo* is used for various conditions in which fire affects the heart:

a) Warm-heat disease heat evil entering the heart: The signs of this pattern include high fever, clouded spirit, delirious speech, and vexation and agitation. Combine *lián qiáo* with medicinals such as:

xuán shēn (玄参 scrophularia, Scrophulariae Radix)

mài dōng (麦冬 ophiopogon, Ophiopogonis Radix)

zhú yè juǎn xīn (竹叶卷心 tender lophatherum leaf, Lophatheri Folium Immaturum)

lián zǐ xīn (莲子心 lotus plumule, Nelumbinis Plumula)

tiān zhú huáng (天竹黄 bamboo sugar, Bambusae Concretio Silicea)

yù jīn (郁金 curcuma, Curcumae Radix)

huáng lián (黄连 coptis, Coptidis Rhizoma)

guǎng xī jiǎo (广犀角 African rhinoceros horn, Rhinocerotis Cornu Africanum)

b) Fire in the heart channel spreading heat to the small intestine: This pattern manifests as painful voidings of hot urine, strangury-turbidity, frequent urination, and painful urination. Combine *lián qiáo* with medicinals such as:

shēng dì huáng (生地黄 dried/fresh rehmannia, Rehmanniae Radix Exsiccata seu Recens)

mù tōng (木通 trifoliate akebia, Akebiae Trifoliatae Caulis)

zhū líng (猪苓 polyporus, Polyporus)

zé xiè (泽泻 alisma, Alismatis Rhizoma)

biǎn xù (萹蓄 knotgrass, Polygoni Avicularis Herba)

fú líng (茯苓 poria, Poria)

huá shí (滑石 talcum, Talcum)

c) Heart fire flaming upward: The signs of this pattern include sore red swollen eyes, sore swollen throat, and mouth and tongue sores. Combine *lián qiáo* with medicinals such as:

jīn yín huā (金银花 lonicera, Lonicerae Flos)

chì sháo (赤芍 red peony, Paeoniae Radix Rubra)

huáng qín (黄芩 scutellaria, Scutellariae Radix)

shēng shí gāo (生石膏 crude gypsum, Gypsum Fibrosum Crudum)

shēng dì huáng (生地黄 dried/fresh rehmannia, Rehmanniae Radix Exsiccata seu Recens)

xuán shēn (玄参 scrophularia, Scrophulariae Radix)

2. Resolving Sore-Toxin: *Lián qiáo* clears heat and dissipates binds, and resolves toxin and expels pus. For toxic heat gathering and binding causing various forms of sore-toxin and swollen welling-abscesses, it is combined with medicinals such as:

jīn yín huā (金银花 lonicera, Lonicerae Flos)

jú huā (菊花 chrysanthemum, Chrysanthemi Flos)

chì sháo (赤芍 red peony, Paeoniae Radix Rubra)

hóng huā (红花 carthamus, Carthami Flos)

dì dīng (地丁 violet, Violae Herba)

pú gōng yīng (蒲公英 dandelion, Taraxaci Herba)

Because *lián qiáo* is often used to treat various forms of sore-toxin, welling-abscesses, and boils, physicians of the past had the experience-based understanding that it was the "essential medicine for sore-sufferers."

3. Dissipating Warm Evil: For initial-stage warm-heat disease with warm-heat toxic evil in the defense aspect and heat in the upper burner causing generalized heat [effusion], headache, thirst, slight aversion to cold or absence of aversion to cold, slight cough, a sore throat, and a rapid floating pulse, this medicinal is used to clear and dissipate upper burner heart and lung heat evil. For example, the formula below is used for this condition.

Yín qiáo sǎn 银翘散	Lonicera and Forsythia Powder

lián qiáo (连翘 forsythia, Forsythiae Fructus)

jīn yín huā (金银花 lonicera, Lonicerae Flos)

jié gěng (桔梗 platycodon, Platycodonis Radix)

bò hé (薄荷 mint, Menthae Herba)

zhú yè (竹叶 lophatherum, Lophatheri Herba),

jīng jiè suì (荆芥穗 schizonepeta spike, Schizonepetae Flos)

dàn dòu chǐ (淡豆豉 fermented soybean (unsalted), Sojae Semen Praeparatum)

niú bàng zǐ (牛蒡子 arctium, Arctii Fructus)

lú gēn (芦根 phragmites, Phragmitis Rhizoma)

gān cǎo (甘草 licorice, Glycyrrhizae Radix)

If there is pronounced cough, *lián qiáo* may be used in a combination such as *sāng jú yǐn* (Mulberry Leaf and Chrysanthemum Beverage).

Sāng jú yǐn 桑菊饮	Mulberry Leaf and Chrysanthemum Beverage

lián qiáo (连翘 forsythia, Forsythiae Fructus)
sāng yè (桑叶 mulberry leaf, Mori Folium)
jú huā (菊花 chrysanthemum, Chrysanthemi Flos)
xìng rén (杏仁 apricot kernel, Armeniacae Semen)
bò hé (薄荷 mint, Menthae Herba)
jié gěng (桔梗 platycodon, Platycodonis Radix)
gān cǎo (甘草 licorice, Glycyrrhizae Radix)
lú gēn (芦根 phragmites, Phragmitis Rhizoma)

COMPARISONS

Jīn yín huā (lonicera)[274] also dissipates wind-heat; therefore its ability to up-bear, dissipate, and outthrust is more pronounced than that of *lián qiáo*. *Lián qiáo* also dissipates depressed and bound fire in the blood; therefore it has a more pronounced ability to disperse swelling and dissipate binds than *jīn yín huā*.

Pú gōng yīng (dandelion)[279] has a greater effect on clove-sore toxin than *lián qiáo*, but *lián qiáo* has a more pronounced ability to clear upper burner heart-lung fire and heat than *pú gōng yīng*.

On the basis of their experience, physicians of the past believed that *lián qiáo* that includes the "heart" (i.e., the seed) tends to enter the heart channel; therefore, when treating heat entering the pericardium in warm disease, *lián qiáo* is usually used with the seed. *Lián qiáo xīn* (forsythia seed) is cold in nature and bitter in flavor. It primarily enters the heart channel. In prescriptions to clear heart fire, it is used to guide medicinals to the heart channel to attack the evil.

COMBINATIONS

a) *Lián qiáo* and *lián zǐ xīn* (lotus plumule)[177] are used together to enter the heart channel.

b) When combined with *jīn yín huā* (lonicera),[274] *lián qiáo* clears heat and resolves toxin and also dissipates wind-heat.

c) When combined with *chì xiǎo dòu* (rice bean), it clears heat and disinhibits dampness.

d) When combined with *jīng jiè* (schizonepeta)[15] and *bò hé* (mint),[30] it resolves the exterior with coolness and acridity.

DOSAGE

The dosage is generally 6–9 g/2–3 qián; in special cases one can use up to 15–30 g/5 qián–1 liǎng.

CAUTION

This medicinal is inappropriate if there is cold in the large intestine and sloppy diarrhea, or for **yīn flat-abscesses**[569] (阴疽 *yīn jū*) that are neither hot nor painful.

Research

According to modern research reports, this medicinal has an antibacterial effect on the following: *Staphylococcus aureus*, *Bacillus dysenteriae*, *Bacillus typhosus*, *Bacillus coli*, *Pseudomonas pyocyanea*, and *Diplococcus pneumoniae*. It has also been shown to have an antimycotic effect.

---

18. 蒲公英 Pú Gōng Yīng   Taraxaci Herba
Dandelion

Also called *gōng yīng* 公英. Cold in nature and bitter in flavor, *pú gōng yīng* (dandelion) clears heat and resolves toxin, disperses welling-abscesses, and dissipates binds.

In external medicine, it is often used to treat **mammary welling-abscesses**[557] (乳痈 *rǔ yōng*), **intestinal welling-abscesses**[554] (肠痈 *cháng yōng*), clove sores, swollen boils, and swollen welling-abscesses.[18] In internal medicine, it is often used to treat heat dysentery, warmth toxin, parotitis, and tonsillitis. For this purpose it is often combined with medicinals such as:

jīn yín huā (金银花 lonicera, Lonicerae Flos)

lián qiáo (连翘 forsythia, Forsythiae Fructus)

huáng qín (黄芩 scutellaria, Scutellariae Radix)

huáng lián (黄连 coptis, Coptidis Rhizoma)

dà qīng yè (大青叶 isatis leaf, Isatidis Folium)

chì sháo (赤芍 red peony, Paeoniae Radix Rubra)

xuán shēn (玄参 scrophularia, Scrophulariae Radix)

shān dòu gēn (山豆根 bushy sophora, Sophorae Tonkinensis Radix)

I often use 15–30 g/5 qián–1 liǎng of *pú gōng yīng* in combination with the following to treat acute mastitis:

guā lóu (瓜蒌 trichosanthes, Trichosanthis Fructus) 30 g/1 liǎng

bái zhǐ (白芷 Dahurian angelica, Angelicae Dahuricae Radix) 6–9 g/2–3 qián

lián qiáo (连翘 forsythia, Forsythiae Fructus) 9 g/3 qián

zhì shān jiǎ (炙山甲 mix-fried pangolin scales, Manis Squama cum Liquido Fricta) 6 g/2 qián

chì sháo (赤芍 red peony, Paeoniae Radix Rubra) 12 g/4 qián

hóng huā (红花 carthamus, Carthami Flos) 9 g/3 qián

zào jiǎo cì (皂角刺 gleditsia thorn, Gleditsiae Spina) 4.5 g/1.5 qián

xià kū cǎo (夏枯草 prunella, Prunellae Spica) 9 g/3 qián

If the welling-abscess has already broken and ulcerated, leave out the *shān jiǎ* (pangolin scales), *zào jiǎo cì* (gleditsia thorn), *tiān huā fěn* (trichosanthes root), and

---

[18]When using *pú gōng yīng* (dandelion) as a poultice, the freshly picked medicinal is pounded into a pulp. For mammary welling-abscesses, the addition of *máng xiāo* (mirabilite) is also effective. (Ed.)

dāng guī (Chinese angelica). I get good results with this formula and recommend it to readers.

COMPARISONS

Dì dīng (violet)[280] has more pronounced effects for cooling the blood and resolving toxin than *pú gōng yīng*, but *pú gōng yīng* dissipates binds and disperses swelling more effectively than *dì dīng*. These two medicinals are often used together.

Bái jiàng cǎo (patrinia)[22] clears heat and expels pus, and tends to be used to treat intestinal welling-abscesses, including appendicitis. *Pú gōng yīng* clears heat and resolves toxin, and tends to be used to treat mammary welling-abscesses (mastitis).

Yú xīng cǎo (houttuynia) clears heat and resolves toxin; its acridity enters the lung. It diffuses and disperses binds and tends to be used to treat pulmonary welling-abscesses as well as lung infections. *Pú gōng yīng* enters the liver and stomach channels; it disperses swelling and dissipates binds, and tends to be used to treat mammary welling-abscesses and breast lumps. For treating breast lumps, the formula given above for mammary welling-abscesses may be supplemented with *shēng mǔ lì* (crude oyster shell) 30 g/1 liǎng, *xuán shēn* (scrophularia) 15–24 g/ 5–8 qián, and *dà bèi mǔ* (Zhejiang fritillaria) 9 g/3 qián.

DOSAGE

The dosage is generally 9–25 g/3–8 qián; use 30–60 g/1–2 liǎng in severe cases. *Pú gōng yīng* is pounded into a pulp and applied topically to treat mammary welling-abscesses, clove sores, and swollen welling-abscesses.

CAUTION

This medicinal is contraindicated for yīn flat-abscesses or enduring festering sores.

RESEARCH

According to modern research, this medicinal has an inhibitory effect on *Staphylococcus aureus*, *Bacillus coli*, and *Bacillus dysenteria*.

---

19. 地丁 Dì Dīng   Violae Herba
Violet

Also called *zǐ huā dì dīng* 紫花地丁.[19] Cold in nature and bitter and acrid in flavor, *dì dīng* (violet) clears heat and resolves toxin, and cools the blood and disperses swelling. In external medicine, it is often used for treating clove-sore toxin, swollen welling-abscesses, **innominate toxin swellings**[553] (无名肿毒 *wú míng zhǒng dú*), and malign sores. It is often used with medicinals such as:

pú gōng yīng (蒲公英 dandelion, Taraxaci Herba)

---

[19] *Viola yedoensis* MAK. is the correct species for this medicinal. *Viola patrinii* DC. (白花地丁 *bái huā dì dīng*) and *Viola japonica* LANGS. (犁头草 *lí tóu cǎo*) are frequently sold as *dì dīng* (violet). (Ed.)

jīn yín huā (金银花 lonicera, Lonicerae Flos)

lián qiáo (连翘 forsythia, Forsythiae Fructus)

jú huā (菊花 chrysanthemum, Chrysanthemi Flos)

chì sháo (赤芍 red peony, Paeoniae Radix Rubra)

dāng guī wěi (当归尾 Chinese angelica tail, Angelicae Sinensis Radicis Extremitas)

In internal medicine, *dì dīng* is often combined with medicinals such as *jīn yín huā* (lonicera), *lián qiáo* (forsythia), *dà qīng yè* (isatis leaf), *xuán shēn* (scrophularia), *shēng dì huáng* (dried/fresh rehmannia), *dān pí* (moutan), *chì sháo* (red peony), *huáng qín* (scutellaria), and *huáng lián* (coptis) to treat conditions due to toxic-heat in the blood and construction, which include warmth toxin, epidemic toxin, macular eruptions, and manic agitation. This medicinal is also used for bacterial infections that cause high fever, vexation, and agitation.

Dì dīng (violet) is combined with *jīn yín huā* (lonicera), *tiān kuí* (semiaquilegia), *pú gōng yīng* (dandelion), and *yě jú huā* (wild chrysanthemum flower) to make *wǔ wèi xiāo dú yǐn* (Five-Ingredient Toxin-Dispersing Beverage), a commonly used formula for all toxic-sores and swollen welling-abscesses that is used especially for clove-sore toxin. This may be used as a base formula and modified in accordance with signs.

Comparisons

Pú gōng yīng (dandelion)[280] dissipates binds and disperses swelling; it is effective in treating mammary welling-abscesses. *Dì dīng* cools the blood and resolves toxin; it is effective in treating clove-sore toxin.

Research

According to modern research reports, this medicinal has a broad antibacterial effect.

Dosage

The dosage is generally 9–15 g/3–5 qián; use 30–60 g/1–2 liǎng in severe cases.

Caution

This medicinal is inappropriate for yīn flat-abscesses with no heat signs.

---

20. 龙胆草 Lóng Dǎn Cǎo   Gentianae Radix
Gentian

Cold in nature and bitter in flavor, *lóng dǎn cǎo* (gentian) clears and drains liver and gallbladder heat and fire, and it eliminates lower burner damp-heat.

1. Clearing and Draining Liver and Gallbladder Heat and Fire: This medicinal is used to treat repletion heat fire evil in both the liver and gallbladder channels that causes dizziness, distention and pain in the head, rib-side pain, bitter taste in the mouth, deafness, swelling of the ear, thirst, yellow urine, scant urine, and jaundice. For such cases, use *lóng dǎn xiè gān tāng* (Gentian Liver-Draining Decoction).

Lóng dǎn xiè gān tāng 龙胆泻肝汤   Gentian Liver-Draining Decoction

---

> *lóng dǎn cǎo* (龙胆草 gentian, Gentianae Radix)
>
> *huáng qín* (黄芩 scutellaria, Scutellariae Radix)
>
> *zhī zǐ* (栀子 gardenia, Gardeniae Fructus)
>
> *zé xiè* (泽泻 alisma, Alismatis Rhizoma)
>
> *mù tōng* (木通 trifoliate akebia, Akebiae Trifoliatae Caulis)
>
> *chē qián zǐ* (车前子 plantago seed, Plantaginis Semen)
>
> *dāng guī* (当归 Chinese angelica, Angelicae Sinensis Radix)
>
> *chái hú* (柴胡 bupleurum, Bupleuri Radix)
>
> *shēng dì huáng* (生地黄 dried/fresh rehmannia, Rehmanniae Radix Exsiccata
> seu Recens)
>
> *gān cǎo* (甘草 licorice, Glycyrrhizae Radix)

This prescription is commonly used in the clinic and is very effective for clearing and draining liver and gallbladder damp-heat. For treating infectious hepatitis that presents as liver and gallbladder damp-heat, adding *lóng dǎn cǎo* to a prescription based on pattern identification is sometimes helpful in reducing transaminase levels.

2. Clearing and Eliminating Lower Burner Damp-Heat: *Lóng dǎn cǎo* enters the liver channel, and since the liver controls the lower burner, it treats damp-heat in the liver channel that causes symptoms such as damp itching and burning pain in the genitals, eczema of the external genitals, and urethral pain; frequent, burning urination; scant urine, and bloody urine. For this purpose it is combined with medicinals such as:

> *huáng bǎi* (黄柏 phellodendron, Phellodendri Cortex)
>
> *zé xiè* (泽泻 alisma, Alismatis Rhizoma)
>
> *shí wéi* (石韦 pyrrosia, Pyrrosiae Folium)
>
> *biǎn xù* (萹蓄 knotgrass, Polygoni Avicularis Herba)
>
> *mù tōng* (木通 trifoliate akebia, Akebiae Trifoliatae Caulis)
>
> *kǔ shēn* (苦参 flavescent sophora, Sophorae Flavescentis Radix)
>
> *zhú yè* (竹叶 lophatherum, Lophatheri Herba),
>
> *fú líng* (茯苓 poria, Poria)

For damp-heat pouring downward causing red, swollen feet and knees, and leg qi[556] (脚气 *jiǎo qì*) swelling with exudate, it is combined with medicinals such as *niú xī* (achyranthes), *mù guā* (chaenomeles), *huáng bǎi* (phellodendron), *cāng zhú* (atractylodes), *bīng láng* (areca), *fáng jǐ* (fangji), *rěn dōng téng* (lonicera stem and leaf), and *chì sháo* (red peony).

3. Increasing the Appetite: If used in small amounts, such as 0.6–1.0 g/ 2–3 fēn, *lóng dǎn cǎo* stimulates stomach secretions, increases the appetite, and aids digestion. However, if larger doses are used, its cold and bitterness harms the stomach and can cause nausea and vomiting, or dizziness with no desire for food and drink.

4. Clearing the Liver and Brightening the Eyes: For fire-heat in the liver and gallbladder that invades upwards to the eyes, causing redness, swelling and pain in the eyes, proud flesh due to blood stasis, aversion to light, and excess eye secretions, *lóng dǎn cǎo* is used in combination with medicinals such as:

mù zéi cǎo (木贼草 equisetum, Equiseti Hiemalis Herba)

jú huā (菊花 chrysanthemum, Chrysanthemi Flos)

cǎo jué míng (草决明 fetid cassia, Cassiae Semen)

jīng jiè (荆芥 schizonepeta, Schizonepetae Herba)

màn jīng zǐ (蔓荆子 vitex, Viticis Fructus)

huáng qín (黄芩 scutellaria, Scutellariae Radix)

DOSAGE

The dosage is generally 0.6–6.0 g/2 fēn–2 qián.

CAUTION

This medicinal is contraindicated for spleen-stomach vacuity and diarrhea.[20]

---

21. 苦参 Kǔ Shēn
Flavescent Sophora
Sophorae Flavescentis Radix

Kǔ shēn (flavescent sophora) is cold in nature and bitter in flavor. It clears heat, dries dampness, and kills worms. It is often used for depressed or hidden damp-heat and for skin diseases.

For depressed and stagnant damp-heat causing dysentery, jaundice, yellow or white vaginal discharge, *kǔ shēn* is used with medicinals such as:

huáng bǎi (黄柏 phellodendron, Phellodendri Cortex)

mù xiāng (木香 costusroot, Aucklandiae Radix)

fú líng (茯苓 poria, Poria)

chē qián zǐ (车前子 plantago seed, Plantaginis Semen) (wrapped in cloth)

bái sháo (白芍 white peony, Paeoniae Radix Alba)

yīn chén (茵陈 virgate wormwood, Artemisiae Scopariae Herba)

yǐ mǐ (苡米 coix, Coicis Semen)

lóng dǎn cǎo (龙胆草 gentian, Gentianae Radix)

For damp-heat brewing and binding causing eczema, urticaria (hives), and damp sores[545] (湿疮 *shī chuāng*) of the skin, *kǔ shēn* is used in combination with medicinals such as:

lián qiáo (连翘 forsythia, Forsythiae Fructus)

chì sháo (赤芍 red peony, Paeoniae Radix Rubra)

fáng fēng (防风 saposhnikovia, Saposhnikoviae Radix)

bái xiǎn pí (白藓皮 dictamnus, Dictamni Cortex)

---

[20]Chinese studies suggest that large doses or prolonged use of *lóng dǎn cǎo* (gentian) can damage the stomach and cause diarrhea and discomfort. (Ed.)

hóng huā (红花 carthamus, Carthami Flos)

huáng bǎi (黄柏 phellodendron, Phellodendri Cortex)

chán tuì (蝉蜕 cicada molting, Cicadae Periostracum)

I often get very good results using *kǔ shēn* in the following combination to treat the more stubborn cases of urticaria.

kǔ shēn (苦参 flavescent sophora, Sophorae Flavescentis Radix)

bái xiǎn pí (白藓皮 dictamnus, Dictamni Cortex)

chì sháo (赤芍 red peony, Paeoniae Radix Rubra)

hóng huā (红花 carthamus, Carthami Flos)

sāng zhī (桑枝 mulberry twig, Mori Ramulus)

fáng fēng (防风 saposhnikovia, Saposhnikoviae Radix)

lián qiáo (连翘 forsythia, Forsythiae Fructus)

zào jiǎo cì (皂角刺 gleditsia thorn, Gleditsiae Spina)

zhì shān jiǎ (炙山甲 mix-fried pangolin scales, Manis Squama cum Liquido Fricta)

chán tuì (蝉蜕 cicada molting, Cicadae Periostracum)

shé tuì (蛇蜕 snake slough, Serpentis Periostracum) 0.3–0.6 g/1–2 fēn[21]

Combinations

Kǔ shēn in combination with *jú huā* (chrysanthemum) brightens the eyes and stops tearing. Combined with *mài dōng* (ophiopogon), it allays thirst and engenders liquid. Combined with *yīn chén* (virgate wormwood) and *chē qián zǐ* (plantago seed), it treats damp-heat jaundice. Combined with *huái huā* (sophora flower), it treats descent of blood with the stool and heat dysentery. With a small amount of *má huáng* (ephedra) as an "assistant," it treats generalized itchy papules.

Decocted and used as a wash in combination with medicinals such as *pí xiāo* (impure mirabilite), *kǔ liàn pí* (chinaberry bark), and *huái huā* (sophora flower), *kǔ shēn* treats painful hemorrhoids, anal sores, and genital sores.[22]

Comparisons

Xuán shēn (scrophularia)[129] cools the blood and enrichs yīn, and clears heat and downbears fire; it tends to be used for pain and swelling of the throat. *Kǔ shēn* (flavescent sophora) cools the blood and drains fire, and clears heat and dries dampness; it tends to be used to treat eczema and urticaria.

Dosage

The dosage is generally 6–9 g/2–3 qián; for skin diseases, one can sometimes use 15–30 g/5 qián–1 liǎng.

Caution

Kǔ shēn is contraindicated for liver-kidney vacuity cold. There is a saying that taken over extended periods or in numerous large doses, *kǔ shēn* may damage the

---

[21]While this medicinal should be used within this dosage range, the others are more variable. (Ed.)

[22]*Kǔ shēn* (flavescent sophora) has many uses in external medicine. Besides those mentioned here, it is included in washes for eczema and in douches that address vaginal itching. (Ed.)

kidney and cause pain or heaviness in the lumbar area. I mention this for your reference.

RESEARCH

According to modern research reports, *kǔ shēn* has pronounced diuretic properties and is effective in eliminating *trichomonas vaginalis*. It also has an inhibitory effect on various kinds of skin fungi.

---

22. 胡黄连 Hú Huáng Lián   Picrorhizae Rhizoma
Picrorhiza

Hú huáng lián (picrorhiza) is cold in nature and bitter in flavor. It mainly disperses gān accumulation and abates **taxation heat**[565] (劳热 *láo rè*).

For children who, owing to inattention to proper diet or to the presence of parasitic disease, have damage to the spleen and stomach that affects digestion and gradually leads to gān accumulation (enlarged abdominal veins, poor appetite, emaciated limbs, low-grade fever, dry knotting hair, and enlarged spleen), *hú huáng lián* is used with medicinals such as:

  jiāo sān xiān (焦三仙 scorch-fried three immortals, Tres Immortales Usti)
  bīng láng (槟榔 areca, Arecae Semen)
  chǎo jī nèi jīn (炒鸡内金 stir-fried gizzard lining, Galli Gigeriae Endothelium Corneum Frictum)
  mù xiāng (木香 costusroot, Aucklandiae Radix)
  chǎo lái fú zǐ (炒莱菔子 stir-fried radish seed, Raphani Semen Frictum)
  zhǐ shí (枳实 unripe bitter orange, Aurantii Fructus Immaturus)
  bái zhú (白术 white atractylodes, Atractylodis Macrocephalae Rhizoma)
  dì gǔ pí (地骨皮 lycium root bark, Lycii Cortex)
  shǐ jūn zǐ (使君子 quisqualis, Quisqualis Fructus)

It is also used for damp-heat dysentery for which it is often combined with medicinals such as:

  mù xiāng (木香 costusroot, Aucklandiae Radix)
  bīng láng (槟榔 areca, Arecae Semen)
  bái sháo (白芍 white peony, Paeoniae Radix Alba)
  dāng guī (当归 Chinese angelica, Angelicae Sinensis Radix)
  bái tóu wēng (白头翁 pulsatilla, Pulsatillae Radix)

For yīn vacuity taxation heat with symptoms of heat [effusion] (fever), heat in the (hearts of the) palms and soles, emaciation, and reddening of both cheeks, *hú huáng lián* is used with medicinals such as:

  dì gǔ pí (地骨皮 lycium root bark, Lycii Cortex)
  bái wēi (白薇 black swallowwort, Cynanchi Atrati Radix)
  bǎi bù (百部 stemona, Stemonae Radix)
  shā shēn (沙参 adenophora/glehnia, Adenophorae seu Glehniae Radix)

qīng hāo (青蒿 sweet wormwood, Artemisiae Annuae Herba)

zhì biē jiǎ (炙鳖甲 mix-fried turtle shell, Trionycis Carapax cum Liquido Frictus)

qín jiāo (秦艽 large gentian, Gentianae Macrophyllae Radix)

shēng dì huáng (生地黄 dried/fresh rehmannia, Rehmanniae Radix Exsiccata seu Recens)

xuán shēn (玄参 scrophularia, Scrophulariae Radix)

If this combination of medicinals is modified on the basis of pattern identification, it will achieve good results in the treatment of tubercular low-grade fever.

This medicinal is most often used in pediatrics, where it is commonly prescribed for generalized heat [effusion] (fever), **fright wind**[550] (惊风 *jīng fēng*), and **gān accumulation**[551] (疳积 *gān jī*).

Hú huáng lián is very effective for treating clouded vision and red eyes caused by liver channel wind-heat. For this it is ground into a fine powder, mixed with breast milk, and applied topically to the eyes.[23]

I have achieved good results in treating infectious hepatitis and chronic liver dysfunction in children of eight or nine years by using *hú huáng lián* combined with medicinals such as:

jī nèi jīn (鸡内金 gizzard lining, Galli Gigeriae Endothelium Corneum)

chái hú (柴胡 bupleurum, Bupleuri Radix)

huáng qín (黄芩 scutellaria, Scutellariae Radix)

hóng huā (红花 carthamus, Carthami Flos)

jiāo sān xiān (焦三仙 scorch-fried three immortals, Tres Immortales Usti)

bīng láng (槟榔 areca, Arecae Semen)

chǎo lái fú zǐ (炒莱菔子 stir-fried radish seed, Raphani Semen Frictum)

chén pí (陈皮 tangerine peel, Citri Reticulatae Pericarpium)

bàn xià (半夏 pinellia, Pinelliae Rhizoma)

lú huì (芦荟 aloe, Aloe) 0.15 g/0.5 fēn

COMPARISONS

Chuān huáng lián (Sìchuān coptis)[246] clears heat and drains fire; it tends to be used for exuberant damp-heat toxin, dysentery, sore-toxin, and other repletion heat patterns. *Hú huáng lián* is mainly used for yīn-vacuity heat [effusion] (fever), child gān accumulation, and fright wind.

DOSAGE

The dosage is generally 3–9 g/1–3 qián.

CAUTION

This medicinal is contraindicated for externally contracted heat [effusion] (fever) and for spleen-stomach vacuity cold.

---

[23]This application may not be appropriate in Western practices. (Ed.)

23. 芦根 Lú Gēn   Phragmitis Rhizoma
Phragmites

Sweet in flavor and cold in nature, *lú gēn* (phragmites) clears heat and engenders liquid.

1. **Clearing Heat and Resolving Thirst:** Because *lú gēn* is sweet in flavor, it engender fluids. Because it is cold in nature, it clears heat and downbears fire. In the upper burner, it clears lung heat; in the center burner, it clears stomach fire; in the lower burner, it disinhibits urine and conducts heat out through the urine. Therefore, for initial-stage warm heat disease with symptoms such as heat [effusion] (fever), thirst, slight cough, and headache, *lú gēn* is combined with medicinals such as *sāng yè* (mulberry leaf), *jú huā* (chrysanthemum), *lián qiáo* (forsythia), and *bò hé* (mint), as in the formula *sāng jú yǐn* (Mulberry Leaf and Chrysanthemum Beverage) from *wēn bìng tiáo biàn* (温病条辨 "Systematized Identification of Warm Diseases").

Sāng jú yǐn 桑菊饮   Mulberry Leaf and Chrysanthemum Beverage

>   *sāng yè* (桑叶 mulberry leaf, Mori Folium)
>   *jú huā* (菊花 chrysanthemum, Chrysanthemi Flos)
>   *xìng rén* (杏仁 apricot kernel, Armeniacae Semen)
>   *lián qiáo* (连翘 forsythia, Forsythiae Fructus)
>   *bò hé* (薄荷 mint, Menthae Herba)
>   *jié gěng* (桔梗 platycodon, Platycodonis Radix)
>   *gān cǎo* (甘草 licorice, Glycyrrhizae Radix)
>   *lú gēn* (芦根 phragmites, Phragmitis Rhizoma)

In warm disease, when heat enters the qì aspect and damages liquid, causing symptoms such as high fever, sweating, thirst with intake of fluids, short voidings of reddish urine, and vexation and agitation, it is combined with medicinals such as:

>   *shēng shí gāo* (生石膏 crude gypsum, Gypsum Fibrosum Crudum)
>   *zhī mǔ* (知母 anemarrhena, Anemarrhenae Rhizoma)
>   *gān cǎo* (甘草 licorice, Glycyrrhizae Radix)
>   *gēng mǐ* (粳米 non-glutinous rice, Oryzae Semen)
>   *tiān huā fěn* (天花粉 trichosanthes root, Trichosanthis Radix)

2. **Clearing Lung Heat:** For wind-heat invading the lung that causes lung heat cough, yellow phlegm, thirst, itchy throat, and oppression in the chest (in severe cases, possibly phlegm containing blood), *lú gēn* is combined with medicinals such as:

>   *xìng rén* (杏仁 apricot kernel, Armeniacae Semen)
>   *jié gěng* (桔梗 platycodon, Platycodonis Radix)
>   *jīn yín huā* (金银花 lonicera, Lonicerae Flos)
>   *shēng shí gāo* (生石膏 crude gypsum, Gypsum Fibrosum Crudum)

zhī mǔ (知母 anemarrhena, Anemarrhenae Rhizoma)

guā lóu (瓜蒌 trichosanthes, Trichosanthis Fructus)

niú bàng zǐ (牛蒡子 arctium, Arctii Fructus)

dà qīng yè (大青叶 isatis leaf, Isatidis Folium)

huáng qín (黄芩 scutellaria, Scutellariae Radix)

chǎo zhī zǐ (炒栀子 stir-fried gardenia, Gardeniae Fructus Frictus)

For lobar pneumonia, the combination above can be modified to treat specific signs.

a) If there is also aversion to cold, chest pain and fullness, and absence of sweating, add *jīng jiè* (schizonepeta), *bò hé* (mint), and *sū yè* (perilla leaf) or *má huáng* (ephedra).

b) If there is also alternating heat and cold, and chest and rib-side pain, fullness, and distention, add *chái hú* (bupleurum) and *qīng hāo* (sweet wormwood).

c) If there is also red face, vigorous heat [effusion] (fever), thirst, and sweating, double the *shí gāo* (gypsum) and *lú gēn* (phragmites) and add *lián qiáo* (forsythia).

d) If there is phlegm containing relatively large amounts of blood, add *shēng ǒu jié* (raw lotus root node), *bái máo gēn* (imperata), and *bái jí* (bletilla).

When a person who usually has internal amassment of toxic heat in the lung contracts an external evil that fetters and blocks the skin and [body] hair, it causes nondiffusion of the lung qì so that toxic heat does not dissipate. As a result, depression and congestion [of the heat] transforms [fluids] into pus and forms a lung welling-abscess (pulmonary abscess). This disease is characterized by symptoms such as fullness in the chest, chest pain, cough, heat [effusion] (fever), phlegm containing blood, and rotten, fishy-smelling phlegm. In such cases, *lú gēn* is used with medicinals such as *shēng yǐ mǐ* (raw coix), *táo rén* (peach kernel), and *dōng guā zǐ* (wax gourd seed). Generally, in the early stage, add *jīng jiè* (schizonepeta), *jīn yín huā* (lonicera), *lián qiáo* (forsythia), and *huáng qín* (scutellaria); in the middle stage, when there is purulent and copious phlegm, add *jié gěng* (platycodon), *bái jí* (bletilla), and *tián tíng lì* (descurainia); and in the advanced stage, when the phlegm has already been expelled, add *shā shēn* (adenophora/glehnia), *tiān huā fěn* (trichosanthes root), and *shēng huáng qí* (raw astragalus).

3. Clearing the Lung and Outthrusting Papules: For initial-stage measles in children, use 30–60 g/1–2 liǎng of *lú gēn* decocted in water until about a teacup remains. Divide and administer several times throughout the day. One may also add an equal amount of *xī hé liǔ* (tamarisk) and decoct both medicinals together in water. This decoction has the functions of clearing and draining lung heat and allowing the measles to come out more easily.

COMPARISONS

Lú gēn (phragmites) is divided into two types: *gān lú gēn* (dried phragmites) and *xiān lú gēn* (fresh phragmites). Generally speaking, *xiān lú gēn* has a more pronounced effect of clearing heat, engendering liquid, clearing the lung, and outthrusting papules, but if it is unavailable *gān lú gēn* may be used instead.[24]

---

[24]The exported item is dried *lú gēn* (phragmites). (Ed.)

Tiān huā fěn (trichosanthes root)[290] tends to enter the stomach channel, clear stomach heat, engender liquid, and allay thirst. It also resolves toxin, disperses swelling, expels pus, and engenders flesh. *Lú gēn* tends to enter the lung channel, clear and diffuse lung heat, treat **pulmonary welling-abscess**[560] (肺痈 *fèi yōng*), and outthrust measles.

Dosage

The dosage is generally 9–30 g/3 qián–1 liǎng. If the fresh medicinal is used, the dosage is 15–60 g/5 qián–2 liǎng.

---

24. 竹叶 Zhú Yè   Lophatheri Herba
Lophatherum

Also called *dàn zhú yè* 淡竹叶.[25] Sweet and bland in flavor and cold in nature, *zhú yè* (lophatherum) clears heat and eliminates vexation, and disinhibits urine and percolates dampness.

For heart channel fire or upper burner repletion heat causing symptoms such as vexation and insomnia, *zhú yè* is combined with medicinals such as *dòu chǐ* (fermented soybean) and *zhī zǐ rén* (gardenia seed).

In warm-heat disease, when heat evil enters the heart and causes clouded spirit and delirious speech, *zhú yè* is combined with medicinals such as *lián zǐ xīn* (lotus plumule), *lián qiào* (forsythia), *yù jīn* (curcuma), *tiān zhú huáng* (bamboo sugar), *chāng pú* (acorus), and *yuǎn zhì* (polygala). Modern animal experiments have demonstrated that *dàn zhú yè* has an antipyretic effect.

When damp-heat in the small intestine and heart manifests with symptoms such as a red-tipped tongue, yellow or reddish urine, and roughness and pain in the urethra, *zhú yè* is combined with medicinals such as:

mù tōng (木通 trifoliate akebia, Akebiae Trifoliatae Caulis)

shēng dì huáng (生地黄 dried/fresh rehmannia, Rehmanniae Radix Exsiccata seu Recens)

zhū líng (猪苓 polyporus, Polyporus)

zé xiè (泽泻 alisma, Alismatis Rhizoma)

dēng xīn (灯心 juncus, Junci Medulla)

huáng bǎi (黄柏 phellodendron, Phellodendri Cortex)

---

[25]This medicinal, which is the leaf of *Lophatherum gracile* Brongn., should properly be known as *dàn zhú yè* (lophatherum). It is often called *zhú yè* 竹叶, but this is also the name of *zhú yè* (black bamboo leaf), which is the leaf of *Phyllostachys nigra* (Lodd.) Munro. While *Phyllostachys nigra* is a bamboo, *Lophatherum gracile* is not. The two medicinals are confused both in China and abroad. The strength of *zhú yè* (black bamboo leaf) is in clearing heart heat and engendering liquid, especially for contraction of heat patterns. *Dàn zhú yè* (lophatherum) is most often used to clear heat and disinhibit urine in the treatment of strangury or mouth sores; it conducts heart heat out through the urine. (Ed.)

Comparisons

Dēng xīn (juncus) and *zhú yè* both clear the heart and disinhibit water. However, *dēng xīn* tends to treat the five stranguries, roughness and pain in the urethra, and inhibited urination, while *zhú yè* tends to treat vexation heat in the heart that is accompanied by a red tongue, reddish urine, and inhibited urination. Whereas *dēng xīn* also enters the lung, *zhú yè* mainly enters the heart.

Dàn zhú yè belongs to the Gramineae; it is not (as the name suggests) the leaf of a true bamboo. This point should not be confused.

Dosage

The dosage is generally 1.5–4.5 g/5 fēn–1.5 qián; in special cases, use up to 9 g/ 3 qián.

---

25. 天花粉 Tiān Huā Fěn   Trichosanthis Radix
Trichosanthes Root

Also called *huā fěn* 花粉 and *guā lóu gēn* 瓜蔞根. Sweet in flavor and cold in nature, *tiān huā fěn* (trichosanthes root) clears heat, engenders liquid, resolves toxin, and expels pus. It is commonly used in both internal and external medicine.

1. **Heat Disease Damaging Liquid:** For warm heat disease with intense heat evil that damages the fluids, causing symptoms such as dry lips, thirst, red tongue with scant liquid, and vexation, *tiān huā fěn* is combined with medicinals such as *mài dōng* (ophiopogon), *shí hú* (dendrobium), *yù zhú* (Solomon's seal), *shēng dì huáng* (dried/fresh rehmannia), and *xuán shēn* (scrophularia).

2. **Dispersion-Thirst:** Dispersion-thirst is characterized by symptoms such as thirst with intake of fluids, intake of fluid failing to resolve thirst, drinking several times the amount of water that a normal person drinks, drinking large amounts of water, copious urine, rapid hungering and increased appetite, and gradual emaciation. *Tiān huā fěn* is sweet and sour; it engenders liquid and also allays thirst and eliminates vexation. When treating dispersion-thirst, it is often combined with medicinals such as:

shēng dì huáng (生地黃 dried/fresh rehmannia, Rehmanniae Radix Exsiccata seu Recens)

shān zhū yú (山茱萸 cornus, Corni Fructus)

shān yào (山藥 dioscorea, Dioscoreae Rhizoma)

mài dōng (麥冬 ophiopogon, Ophiopogonis Radix)

wǔ wèi zǐ (五味子 schisandra, Schisandrae Fructus)

dān pí (丹皮 moutan, Moutan Cortex)

zhī mǔ (知母 anemarrhena, Anemarrhenae Rhizoma)

shēng shí gāo (生石膏 crude gypsum, Gypsum Fibrosum Crudum)

On the basis of tradition, I often use a similar combination to treat diabetes mellitus, diabetes insipidus, hyperthyroidism, and other diseases that have thirst as the primary presenting symptom. One should determine and modify the formula in accordance with pattern identification.

3. Swelling of Welling-Abscesses and Sore Toxin: *Tiān huā fěn* clears heat and resolves toxin, expels pus and disperses swelling, and is often used for mammary welling-abscesses[557] (乳痈 *rǔ yōng*). For this purpose it is often combined with medicinals such as:

guā lóu (瓜蒌 trichosanthes, Trichosanthis Fructus)

bái zhǐ (白芷 Dahurian angelica, Angelicae Dahuricae Radix)

bèi mǔ (贝母 fritillaria, Fritillariae Bulbus)

lòu lú (漏芦 rhaponticum, Rhapontici Radix)

pú gōng yīng (蒲公英 dandelion, Taraxaci Herba)

For swollen welling-abscesses[567] (痈 *yōng*), it is combined with medicinals such as *lián qiáo* (forsythia), *jīn yín huā* (lonicera), *chì sháo* (red peony), *dāng guī wěi* (Chinese angelica tail), *zhì shān jiǎ* (mix-fried pangolin scales), and *zào jiǎo cì* (gleditsia thorn). For treating boils[543] (疖 *jié*) and sores, it is combined with medicinals such as:

lián qiáo (连翘 forsythia, Forsythiae Fructus)

rěn dōng téng (忍冬藤 lonicera stem and leaf, Lonicerae Caulis)

gān cǎo jié (甘草节 resinous licorice root, Glycyrrhizae Radix Resinosa)

dì dīng (地丁 violet, Violae Herba)

chì sháo (赤芍 red peony, Paeoniae Radix Rubra)

Comparisons

Shí hú (dendrobium)[134] and *tiān huā fěn* both engender liquid and allay thirst, but *shí hú* has a more pronounced ability to enrich kidney yīn and brighten the eyes, whereas *tiān huā fěn* has a greater ability to clear fire and nourish stomach yīn.

Tiān dōng (asparagus)[133] and *mài dōng* (ophiopogon)[131] also nourish yīn, engender liquid, and allay thirst, but they are sticky in nature and easily clog the stomach (influencing appetite and digestion). In contrast, *tiān huā fěn* engenders liquid and allays thirst, as well as boosting the stomach.

Dosage

The dosage is generally 9–15 g/3–5 qián. When treating dispersion-thirst, one can sometimes use up to 30 g/1 liǎng.

Caution

Do not use this medicinal with *wū tóu* (wild aconite) or *fù zǐ* (aconite). This medicinal is contraindicated for patients with spleen-stomach vacuity cold.

26. 败酱草 Bài Jiàng Cǎo   Patriniae Herba
Patrinia

Acrid and bitter in flavor and slightly cold in nature, *bài jiàng cǎo* (patrinia)[26] quickens stasis, disperses swelling, and expels pus. In the treatment of intestinal welling-abscesses[554] (肠痈 *cháng yōng*, appendicitis), it is often combined with medicinals such as *lián qiáo* (forsythia), *shēng dà huáng* (raw rhubarb), *mǔ dān pí* (moutan), *dōng guā zǐ* (wax gourd seed), *chì sháo* (red peony), and *yuán míng fěn* (refined mirabilite).

For blood stasis causing abdominal pain, abdominal distention, or lumps in the abdomen, *bài jiàng cǎo* is combined with medicinals such as:

dāng guī (当归 Chinese angelica, Angelicae Sinensis Radix)
chì sháo (赤芍 red peony, Paeoniae Radix Rubra)
hóng huā (红花 carthamus, Carthami Flos)
yán hú suǒ (延胡索 corydalis, Corydalis Rhizoma)
mù xiāng (木香 costusroot, Aucklandiae Radix)
wǔ líng zhī (五灵脂 squirrel's droppings, Trogopteri Faeces)
táo rén (桃仁 peach kernel, Persicae Semen)
sān léng (三棱 sparganium, Sparganii Rhizoma)

I have used this medicinal in the following combination to treat a patient with an appendix that had burst and formed an abscess that had persisted for a relatively long time:

shēng yǐ mǐ (生苡米 raw coix, Coicis Semen Crudum)
jīn yín huā (金银花 lonicera, Lonicerae Flos)
lián qiáo (连翘 forsythia, Forsythiae Fructus)
zhì fù piàn (制附片 sliced processed aconite, Aconiti Radix Lateralis
    Praeparata Secta)
wū yào (乌药 lindera, Linderae Radix)
bái sháo (白芍 white peony, Paeoniae Radix Alba)
dāng guī (当归 Chinese angelica, Angelicae Sinensis Radix)
wǔ líng zhī (五灵脂 squirrel's droppings, Trogopteri Faeces)
táo rén (桃仁 peach kernel, Persicae Semen)

COMPARISONS

Pú gōng yīng (dandelion)[279] is most effective in treating mammary welling-abscesses, while *bài jiàng cǎo* is most effective in treating intestinal welling-abscesses.

DOSAGE

The dosage is generally 9–15 g/3–5 qián; in severe cases, one may use up to 30 g/ 1 liǎng.

---

[26]Most of what is used for *bài jiàng cǎo* (patrinia) in the West is *Thlaspi arvense* L., but *Patrinia scabiosaefolia* FISCH. (黄花败酱草 *huáng huā bài jiàng cǎo*) and *Patrinia villosa* JUSS. (白花败酱草 *bái huā bài jiàng cǎo*) are preferred. (Ed.)

CAUTION

Ths medicinal is contraindicated for cold-pattern abdominal pain.

| 27. 马勃 Mǎ Bó | Lasiosphaera seu |
| Puffball | Calvatia |

Mǎ bó (puffball) is acrid in flavor and neutral in nature. It mainly clears lung heat and treats sore throat.

For heat in the lung channel causing a sore, swollen throat or a dry nose and throat, *mǎ bó* is combined with medicinals such as *lián qiáo* (forsythia), *jīng jiè* (schizonepeta), *shān dòu gēn* (bushy sophora), *shè gān* (belamcanda), *huáng qín* (scutellaria), *bò hé* (mint), and *xuán shēn* (scrophularia). For scourge toxin that causes soreness and swelling in the larynx, neck, and cheeks, *mǎ bó* is used with medicinals such as:

bǎn lán gēn (板蓝根 isatis root, Isatidis Radix)

lián qiáo (连翘 forsythia, Forsythiae Fructus)

niú bàng zǐ (牛蒡子 arctium, Arctii Fructus)

bò hé (薄荷 mint, Menthae Herba)

jīng jiè (荆芥 schizonepeta, Schizonepetae Herba)

xuán shēn (玄参 scrophularia, Scrophulariae Radix)

bái jiāng cán (白僵蚕 silkworm, Bombyx Batryticatus)

jié gěng (桔梗 platycodon, Platycodonis Radix)

I usually find this formula effective for infectious parotitis, modifying it according to the pattern identified.

Mǎ bó is also used for lung heat causing coughing of blood, nosebleed, and related symptoms. For this purpose it is often combined with *huáng qín tàn* (charred scutellaria), *bái máo gēn* (imperata), *shēng ǒu jié* (raw lotus root node), and *shēng cè bǎi* (raw biota leaf). Ground into a powder and applied topically, *mǎ bó* stanches bleeding due to external injury.[27]

For wind-heat invading the lung causing cough, loss of voice, and related symptoms, *mǎ bó* is combined with medicinals such as *jīng jiè* (schizonepeta), *bò hé* (mint), *xìng rén* (apricot kernel), *niú bàng zǐ* (arctium), *chán tuì* (cicada molting), *qián hú* (peucedanum), and *jǐn dēng lóng* (lantern plant calyx).

Mǎ bó treats massive head scourge. It is used in *pǔ jì xiāo dú yǐn* (Universal Salvation Toxin-Dispersing Beverage):

---

[27]As an example, sterilized *mǎ bó* (puffball) powder is used to stanch post-surgical bleeding in China. (Ed.)

Pǔ jì xiāo dú yǐn 普济消毒饮	Universal Salvation Toxin-Dispersing Beverage

mǎ bó (马勃 puffball, Lasiosphaera seu Calvatia)

lián qiáo (连翘 forsythia, Forsythiae Fructus)

bò hé (薄荷 mint, Menthae Herba)

niú bàng zǐ (牛蒡子 arctium, Arctii Fructus)

jīng jiè suì (荆芥穗 schizonepeta spike, Schizonepetae Flos)

bái jiāng cán (白僵蚕 silkworm, Bombyx Batryticatus)

huáng lián (黄连 coptis, Coptidis Rhizoma)

huáng qín (黄芩 scutellaria, Scutellariae Radix)

xuán shēn (玄参 scrophularia, Scrophulariae Radix)

bǎn lán gēn (板蓝根 isatis root, Isatidis Radix)

jié gěng (桔梗 platycodon, Platycodonis Radix)

gān cǎo (甘草 licorice, Glycyrrhizae Radix)

shēng má (升麻 cimicifuga, Cimicifugae Rhizoma)

chái hú (柴胡 bupleurum, Bupleuri Radix)

It should be noted that some practitioners leave out *shēng má* (cimicifuga) and *chái hú* (bupleurum).

DOSAGE

The dosage is generally 1.5–6 g/5 fēn–2 qián. For scourge toxin, massive head scourge, or other severe conditions, use up to 15 g/5 qián or even more.[28]

---

28. 蚤休 Zǎo Xiū   Paridis Rhizoma
Paris

Also called *cǎo hé chē* 草河车, *jīn xiàn chóng lóu* 金线重楼, and *qī yè yī zhī huā* 七叶一枝花. Bitter in flavor, slightly cold in nature, and possessing minor toxicity, *zǎo xiū* (paris) is commonly used to clear heat and resolve toxin.

1. **Sore Swollen Throat:** For toxic heat in the stomach and lung causing sore swollen throat, single [baby] moth red swollen tonsils (tonsils swollen on one side), and double [baby] moth red swollen tonsils (both sides), *zǎo xiū* is combined with medicinals such as:

lián qiáo (连翘 forsythia, Forsythiae Fructus)

huáng qín (黄芩 scutellaria, Scutellariae Radix)

shēng dì huáng (生地黄 dried/fresh rehmannia, Rehmanniae Radix Exsiccata seu Recens)

xuán shēn (玄参 scrophularia, Scrophulariae Radix)

chì sháo (赤芍 red peony, Paeoniae Radix Rubra)

---

[28] Generally, *mǎ bó* (puffball) is wrapped before it is placed in a pot for decoction; this prevents the powder from making the decoction unpalatable. (Ed.)

shè gān (射干 belamcanda, Belamcandae Rhizoma)

shān dòu gēn (山豆根 bushy sophora, Sophorae Tonkinensis Radix)

bò hé (薄荷 mint, Menthae Herba)

jǐn dēng lóng (锦灯笼 lantern plant calyx, Physalis Calyx seu Fructus)

2. Clove-Sore Toxin: For toxic heat in the blood causing various forms of toxin sores, swollen welling-abscesses, clove-sore toxin, and malign sores, *zǎo xiū* is often combined with medicinals such as *jīn yín huā* (lonicera), *lián qiáo* (forsythia), *chì sháo* (red peony), *dāng guī wěi* (Chinese angelica tail), *hóng huā* (carthamus), *tiān huā fěn* (trichosanthes root), *zhì shān jiǎ* (mix-fried pangolin scales), *dì dīng* (violet), *pú gōng yīng* (dandelion), and *yě jú huā* (wild chrysanthemum flower). *Běn Cǎo Gāng Mù* (本草纲目 "The Comprehensive Herbal Foundation") records the following folk saying: "[I am] *qī yè yī zhī huā* 七叶一枝花. The deep mountains are my home. If one encounters welling-abscesses and flat-abscesses, reach out and pick me." This saying makes it clear that this medicinal is very effective for welling-abscesses and sore toxin.[29] When combined with *xià kū cǎo* (prunella) it is used to treat tuberculosis of the lymph nodes.

RESEARCH

According to modern research, *zǎo xiū* has an antibacterial effect. It has also been used experimentally in treating malginant tumors.[30]

COMPARISONS

Zǎo xiū resolves and dispels toxins to a greater degree than *pú gōng yīng* (dandelion),[279] *dì dīng* (violet),[280] *jīn yín huā* (lonicera),[274] and other similar medicinals; therefore, for diseases in which a great deal of toxin is involved, this medicinal is commonly used to resolve toxin and protect the heart. The intention is to prevent toxic qì from invading the heart.

DOSAGE

The dosage is generally 6–9 g/2–3 qián. Larger doses can produce side-effects such as nausea and vomiting, although this reaction is generally not dangerous. According to tradition, it is believed that if toxin is present in the body, nausea and vomiting easily occur. After vomiting, however, the toxin can internally disperse. One must analyze the specific condition of the patient and act accordingly.

---

[29]For the treatment of welling- and flat-abscesses, many classical texts recommend an external application of *zǎo xiū* (paris) powder mixed with vinegar. (Ed.)

[30]*Zǎo xiū* (paris) is most commonly used in formulas that treat cancers of the throat, prostate, and breast. (Ed.)

29. 鸦胆子 Yā Dǎn Zǐ   Bruceae Fructus
Brucea

Yā dǎn zǐ (brucea)[31] is cold in nature and bitter in flavor. It is mainly used for intermittent dysentery, heat accumulation dysentery, and tertian malaria.[32]

Intermittent dysentery[553] (休息痢 *xiū xī lì*) refers to dysentery that is symptomatic for a time and then is in remission for a time; it is active for a time and then rests, in repeating cycles. This is very difficult to cure and may go on for up to a year or two. Amebic dysentery is included within this category of dysentery. When the dysentery is active, use the following method. Remove the shell from ten to twenty pieces of *yā dǎn zǐ* and place the seeds within *lóng yǎn ròu* (longan flesh). Squeeze them into several small pills and take with warm water on an empty stomach. If it is not cured after one administration, wait two or three days and take it again. Try this two or three times in a row. When the dysentery is "resting" (in remission), administer medicinals that regulate the spleen and stomach to support right qì and strengthen the patient's resistance.

For heat evil accumulation and stagnation causing dysentery with stool that looks like crataegus (hawthorn) paste (i.e., red), *yā dǎn zǐ* is combined with medicinals such as *huáng lián* (coptis), *mù xiāng* (costusroot), *zhǐ shí* (unripe bitter orange), *bái sháo* (white peony), and *bīng láng* (areca). When administering this decoction, also give five to ten pieces of *yā dǎn zǐ* (i.e., five fruits).

For tertian malaria remove the shell from five to ten pieces of *yā dǎn zǐ*, grind the seeds, and place into capsules. Take the capsules three times per day for three to five days in a row.

RESEARCH

According to modern research reports, this medicinal eliminates ameba, plasmodium, intestinal parasites, and trichomonas vaginalis.

Yā dǎn zǐ rén (brucea seed) may be pounded to a pulp and applied topically to erode warts and corns; applied in this fashion, it causes them to fall off.[33]

DOSAGE

The dosage is generally five to ten pieces, taken three times per day. Alternatively, ten to twenty pieces may be taken each time at intervals of two to three days. According to traditional experience, physicians believed that the dosage of *yā dǎn zǐ* for young people could be based on their age: one piece for each year. Nevertheless, it should be wrapped in *lóng yǎn ròu* (longan flesh) before swallowing. If a

---

[31] *Yā dǎn zǐ* (brucea) is also called *kǔ shēn zǐ* 苦参子, although it has no botanical relation to the medicinal *kǔ shēn* (苦参, flavescent sophora). (Ed.)

[32] Tertian malaria, 间日疟 *jiān rì nuè*: See footnote on page 508. (Ed.)

[33] When using the pounded seeds to treat warts or corns, carefully protect the surrounding skin with tape before applying the paste. (Ed.)

large amount is administered in modern capsules, it will cause abdominal pain and diarrhea.[34]

CAUTION

Contraindicated for vacuity cold dysentery.

---

30. 漏芦 Lòu Lú   Rhapontici Radix
Rhaponticum

Cold in nature and bitter and salty in flavor, *lòu lú* (rhaponticum) clears heat and resolves toxin, and also **frees milk**[550] (通乳 *tōng rǔ*, i.e., induce or enhance the flow of milk).

Lòu lú (rhaponticum) is most commonly used to treat mammary welling-abscesses. When treating mammary welling-abscesses that have not yet ruptured, it is often combined with medicinals such as *guā lóu* (trichosanthes), *bái zhǐ* (Dahurian angelica), *pú gōng yīng* (dandelion), *lián qiáo* (forsythia), and *zào jiǎo cì* (gleditsia thorn). For treating **mammary welling-abscesses**[557] (乳痈 *rǔ yōng*) that have already ruptured, omit *zào jiǎo cì* (gleditsia thorn) and add *tiān huā fěn* (trichosanthes root) and *dāng guī* (Chinese angelica).

For postpartum women with lactation problems such as **scant breast milk**[561] (乳汁少 *rǔ zhī shǎo*) or **breast milk stoppage**[543] (乳汁不下 *rǔ zhī bù xià*), *lòu lú* is combined with medicinals such as:

lù lù tōng (路路通 liquidambar fruit, Liquidambaris Fructus)

wáng bù liú xíng (王不留行 vaccaria, Vaccariae Semen)

zhì shān jiǎ (炙山甲 mix-fried pangolin scales, Manis Squama cum Liquido Fricta)

tiān huā fěn (天花粉 trichosanthes root, Trichosanthis Radix)

tōng cǎo (通草 rice-paper plant pith, Tetrapanacis Medulla)

COMPARISONS

Guā lóu (trichosanthes)[320] treats mammary welling-abscesses because it is effective in loosening the chest and dissipating binds, clearing heat, and transforming phlegm; *pú gōng yīng* (dandelion)[279] treats mammary welling-abscesses because it is effective in clearing heat and resolving toxin, as well as dispersing welling-abscesses and dissipating binds; *lòu lú* treats mammary welling-abscesses because it is effective in draining heat and resolving toxin, freeing milk, and disinhibiting the channels.

DOSAGE

The dosage is generally 6–9 g/2–3 qián.

---

[34] *Yā dǎn zǐ* (brucea) is caustic and extremely irritating to the mucous membranes and thus should be wrapped in *lóng yǎn ròu* (longan flesh) before ingestion. This medicinal is sometimes decocted to use as an enema or douche. Its caustic properties are not present in decocted form. (Ed.)

31. 夏枯草 Xià Kū Cǎo   Prunellae Spica
Prunella

Bitter in flavor and cold in nature, *xià kū cǎo* (prunella) calms liver yáng and dissipates binding depression.

1. Liver Yáng Headache: For ascendant hyperactivity of liver yáng causing distention and pain in the head, dizziness, and flowery vision, use this medicinal to clear liver fire and calm liver yáng. For this purpose it is often combined with medicinals such as:

jú huā (菊花 chrysanthemum, Chrysanthemi Flos)

bái jí lí (白蒺藜 tribulus, Tribuli Fructus)

shēng dài zhě shí (生代赭石 crude hematite, Haematitum Crudum)

huáng qín (黄芩 scutellaria, Scutellariae Radix)

shēng mǔ lì (生牡蛎 crude oyster shell, Ostreae Concha Cruda)

bái sháo (白芍 white peony, Paeoniae Radix Alba)

shēng dì huáng (生地黄 dried/fresh rehmannia, Rehmanniae Radix Exsiccata seu Recens)

zé xiè (泽泻 alisma, Alismatis Rhizoma)

dì gǔ pí (地骨皮 lycium root bark, Lycii Cortex)

For hypertension patients who present with ascendant hyperactivity of liver yáng, one can also use this formula varied in accordance with signs. According to modern research reports, *xià kū cǎo* lowers blood pressure and acts as a diuretic.

2. Scrofula and Phlegm Nodes: For scrofula[562] (瘰疬 *luǒ lì*) and phlegm nodes[559] (痰核 *tán hé*) on both sides of the neck (including tuberculosis of the lymph nodes) that are caused by binding depression of liver qì with phlegm and qì congealing and gathering, *xià kū cǎo* is used to soothe liver depression, moderate liver fire, dissipate binds, and disperse phlegm. For this purpose it is often combined with medicinals such as:

shēng mǔ lì (生牡蛎 crude oyster shell, Ostreae Concha Cruda)

xuán shēn (玄参 scrophularia, Scrophulariae Radix)

huáng qín (黄芩 scutellaria, Scutellariae Radix)

hǎi zǎo (海藻 sargassum, Sargassum)

bèi mǔ (贝母 fritillaria, Fritillariae Bulbus)

bǎi bù (百部 stemona, Stemonae Radix)

chái hú (柴胡 bupleurum, Bupleuri Radix)

chì sháo (赤芍 red peony, Paeoniae Radix Rubra)

For breast lumps,[35] it is combined with medicinals such as:

guā lóu (瓜蒌 trichosanthes, Trichosanthis Fructus)

bái zhǐ (白芷 Dahurian angelica, Angelicae Dahuricae Radix)

pú gōng yīng (蒲公英 dandelion, Taraxaci Herba)

---

[35] *Xià kū cǎo* (prunella) is also frequently found in formulas for treating breast cancer. (Ed.)

lòu lú (漏芦 rhaponticum, Rhapontici Radix)

For parotitis (mumps), it is combined with medicinals such as *bǎn lán gēn* (isatis root), *mǎ bó* (puffball), *niú bàng zǐ* (arctium), and *dà qīng yè* (isatis leaf). *Xià kū cǎo gāo* (夏枯草膏 Prunella Paste) is also available from pharmacies.

According to modern research, this medicinal has an inhibitory effect on *Bacillus dysenteriae* and *Mycobacterium tuberculosis*.

3. Eyeball Pain at Night: The liver governs the eyes; thus liver and kidney yīn vacuity or exuberance of liver yáng can cause eye pain. The defining characteristic of this condition is that although the eyeball appears normal (it is neither red nor swollen), the patient feels distending pain or spastic pain in the afternoon or evening. *Xià kū cǎo* is specifically effective for relieving "eyeball pain at night." I often use this medicinal to treat [simple] eyeball pain or [eyeball pain] from glaucoma or hypertension manifesting as "eyeball pain at night" in combination with medicinals such as:

cǎo jué míng (草决明 fetid cassia, Cassiae Semen)
shēng shí jué míng (生石决明 crude abalone shell, Haliotidis Concha Cruda)
bái jí lí (白蒺藜 tribulus, Tribuli Fructus)
shí hú (石斛 dendrobium, Dendrobii Herba)
dì gǔ pí (地骨皮 lycium root bark, Lycii Cortex)
huáng qín (黄芩 scutellaria, Scutellariae Radix)
shēng dì huáng (生地黄 dried/fresh rehmannia, Rehmanniae Radix Exsiccata seu Recens)
xuán shēn (玄参 scrophularia, Scrophulariae Radix)

I find that this combination is always effective. For chronic pain with blood vacuity, one may add *dāng guī* (Chinese angelica) and *bái sháo* (white peony).

Comparisons

Xuán shēn (scrophularia)[129] treats scrofula; it tends to enrich yīn and downbear fire and to resolve toxin and dissipate binds. *Xià kū cǎo* also treats scrofula; it tends to calm the liver and resolve depression, clear heat and dissipate binds.

Jú huā (chrysanthemum) and *xià kū cǎo* both treat headache, but *jú huā* tends to dissipate wind-heat, whereas *xià kū cǎo* tends to calm the liver and clear heat.

Dosage

The dosage is generally 9 g/3 qián; in certain severe cases one may use up to 15 g/5 qián.

32. 草决明 Cǎo Jué Míng   Cassiae Semen
Fetid Cassia

Salty in flavor and slightly cold in nature,[36] *cǎo jué míng* (fetid cassia)[37] is a commonly used medicinal for clearing heat and brightening the eyes.[38]

Cǎo jué míng clears liver-gallbladder depressed heat. When depressed liver-gallbladder heat causes sore, red swollen eyes, headache, dizziness, and aversion to light and tearing, *cǎo jué míng* is combined with medicinals such as:

jú huā (菊花 chrysanthemum, Chrysanthemi Flos)

màn jīng zǐ (蔓荆子 vitex, Viticis Fructus)

huáng qín (黄芩 scutellaria, Scutellariae Radix)

bái jí lí (白蒺藜 tribulus, Tribuli Fructus)

qīng xiāng zǐ (青葙子 celosia, Celosiae Semen)

mù zéi cǎo (木贼草 equisetum, Equiseti Hiemalis Herba)

Taken over a long period of time, *cǎo jué míng* brightens the eyes. I often use it to treat liver and kidney insufficiency that causes clouded vision, decreased visual acuity, dry eyes, and twitching of the eyes (including retinitis and degeneration of the optical nerve) in combination with medicinals such as the following:

shēng dì huáng (生地黄 dried/fresh rehmannia, Rehmanniae Radix Exsiccata seu Recens)

shí hú (石斛 dendrobium, Dendrobii Herba)

dāng guī (当归 Chinese angelica, Angelicae Sinensis Radix)

bái sháo (白芍 white peony, Paeoniae Radix Alba)

huáng qín (黄芩 scutellaria, Scutellariae Radix)

tóng jí lí (潼蒺藜 complanate astragalus seed, Astragali Complanati Semen)

bái jí lí (白蒺藜 tribulus, Tribuli Fructus)

dì gǔ pí (地骨皮 lycium root bark, Lycii Cortex)

jú huā (菊花 chrysanthemum, Chrysanthemi Flos)

gǒu qǐ zǐ (枸杞子 lycium, Lycii Fructus)

shēng shí jué míng (生石决明 crude abalone shell, Haliotidis Concha Cruda)

yè míng shā (夜明砂 bat's droppings, Verspertilionis Faeces)

According to modern research, this medicinal contains substances similar to vitamin A.

---

[36]Many sources additionally describe the flavor of *cǎo jué míng* (fetid cassia) as bitter and sweet. (Ed.)

[37]The name *cǎo jué míng* 草决明 literally means "herb decisive clarity." "Decisive clarity" appears to be a reference to the eye-brightening action of this medicinal. The word "herb" distinguishes it from *shí jué míng* (石决明, abalone shell),[335] another eye-brightening medicinal, whose Chinese name literally means "stone decisive clarity." (Ed.)

[38]*Cǎo jué míng* (fetid cassia) is also said to moisten the intestine and free the stool. Thus, it is used to treat dry-stool constipation, especially in the aged. (Ed.)

Cǎo jué míng is helpful for patients with hypertension and accompanying symptoms, such as clouded vision, red eyes, and dry stool. For this purpose, crush approximately 6 g/2 qián, decoct or infuse in water, and use as a tea, once per day. It is also combined with *jú huā* (chrysanthemum) and *xià kū cǎo* (prunella) for this purpose. According to modern research reports, *cǎo jué míng* lowers blood pressure.

Comparisons

Màn jīng zǐ[34] treats bilateral headaches and is most effective for pain in the temporal and zygomatic region; it tends to dissipate wind and brighten the eyes. *Cǎo jué míng* (fetid cassia) also treats bilateral headache, but it is most effective for treating pain around the Greater Yáng (*tài yáng*) point; it tends to clear the liver and brighten the eyes.

Mù zéi cǎo (equisetum) abates eye screens (目翳 *mù yì*) and brightens the eyes, whereas *cǎo jué míng* clears liver heat and brightens the eyes.

Dosage

The dosage is generally 3–9 g/1–3 qián; it should be crushed and decocted.[39]

---

33. 青葙子 Qīng Xiāng Zǐ
Celosia

Celosiae
Semen

Bitter in flavor and slightly cold in nature, *qīng xiāng zǐ* (celosia) is commonly used in ophthalmology. It treats liver channel toxic heat surging upwards causing red sore swollen eyes, eye screens (目翳 *mù yì*), aversion to light, and tearing. For this purpose it is commonly combined with medicinals such as:

jú huā (菊花 chrysanthemum, Chrysanthemi Flos)

xià kū cǎo (夏枯草 prunella, Prunellae Spica)

huáng qín (黄芩 scutellaria, Scutellariae Radix)

mù zéi cǎo (木贼草 equisetum, Equiseti Hiemalis Herba)

sāng yè (桑叶 mulberry leaf, Mori Folium)

màn jīng zǐ (蔓荆子 vitex, Viticis Fructus)

lóng dǎn cǎo (龙胆草 gentian, Gentianae Radix)

huáng lián (黄连 coptis, Coptidis Rhizoma)

Qīng xiāng zǐ dissipates wind and clears heat and also dissipates wind and relieves itching; thus for liver channel wind-heat causing headache, dizziness, red eyes, eye distention, clouded vision, and hypertension, it is often combined with medicinals such as:

lóng dǎn cǎo (龙胆草 gentian, Gentianae Radix)

huáng qín (黄芩 scutellaria, Scutellariae Radix)

shēng dài zhě shí (生代赭石 crude hematite, Haematitum Crudum)

---

[39] This medicinal is very difficult to crush unless it is first dry-fried. A grinder is necessary to grind it when unprocessed. (Ed.)

    shēng shí jué míng (生石决明 crude abalone shell, Haliotidis Concha Cruda)

    cǎo jué míng (草决明 fetid cassia, Cassiae Semen)

    shēng dì huáng (生地黄 dried/fresh rehmannia, Rehmanniae Radix Exsiccata seu Recens)

    chì sháo (赤芍 red peony, Paeoniae Radix Rubra)

    jú huā (菊花 chrysanthemum, Chrysanthemi Flos)

    gōu téng (钩藤 uncaria, Uncariae Ramulus cum Uncis)

For itchy skin due to wind-heat, *qīng xiāng zǐ* is combined with medicinals such as *bái xiǎn pí* (dictamnus), *chán tuì* (cicada molting), *fáng fēng* (saposhnikovia), *bò hé* (mint), *zhī zǐ yī* (gardenia husk), and *kǔ shēn* (flavescent sophora).

DOSAGE

The dosage is generally 3–9 g/1–3 qián.

CAUTION

This medicinal has the effect of enlarging the pupils and should not be used if the patient has an eye disease that causes dilated pupils.

---

34. 密蒙花 Mì Méng Huā   Buddleja Flos
Buddleia

Sweet in flavor and slightly cold in nature, *mì méng huā* (buddleia)[40] is a commonly used medicinal in ophthalmology that abates screens and brightens the eyes.

Mì méng huā clears liver channel vacuity heat and brightens the eyes. It is often used for **clear-eye blindness**[544] (青盲 *qīng máng*), clouded vision, excessive tearing, excessive eye secretions, and gān qì attacking the eyes in children. For these conditions, it is combined with medicinals such as:

    bái jí lí (白蒺藜 tribulus, Tribuli Fructus)

    jú huā (菊花 chrysanthemum, Chrysanthemi Flos)

    cǎo jué míng (草决明 fetid cassia, Cassiae Semen)

    shí jué míng (石决明 abalone shell, Haliotidis Concha)

    qiāng huó (羌活 notopterygium, Notopterygii Rhizoma et Radix)

    gǔ jīng cǎo (谷精草 eriocaulon, Eriocauli Flos)

Mì méng huā disperses red vessels in the eyes and eliminates eye screens; for this purpose it is combined with medicinals such as:

    mù zéi cǎo (木贼草 equisetum, Equiseti Hiemalis Herba)

    sāng yè (桑叶 mulberry leaf, Mori Folium)

    xià kū cǎo (夏枯草 prunella, Prunellae Spica)

---

[40] *Edgeworthia chrysantha* LINDL., a visually more pleasing medicinal, is frequently substituted for *Buddleja officinalis* MAXIM. *Buddleja* is dull brown in color with multiple small clusters of flower buds on a single stem, while *Edgeworthia* is characterized by a single bright-yellow (and sometimes yellow-green) bud cluster on a stem. (Ed.)

jú huā (菊花 chrysanthemum, Chrysanthemi Flos)

yè míng shā (夜明砂 bat's droppings, Verspertilionis Faeces)

chán tuì (蝉蜕 cicada molting, Cicadae Periostracum)

It also expels wind in the eye to treat itching of the eyeball, for which I often achieve good results by combining it with medicinals such as:

màn jīng zǐ (蔓荆子 vitex, Viticis Fructus)

fáng fēng (防风 saposhnikovia, Saposhnikoviae Radix)

chì sháo (赤芍 red peony, Paeoniae Radix Rubra)

jú huā (菊花 chrysanthemum, Chrysanthemi Flos)

jīng jiè (荆芥 schizonepeta, Schizonepetae Herba)

bò hé (薄荷 mint, Menthae Herba)(a small amount)

DOSAGE

The dosage is generally 3–9 g/1–3 qián.

---

35. 夜明砂 Yè Míng Shā
Bat's Droppings
Vespertilionis
Faeces

Cold in nature and acrid in flavor, *yè míng shā* (bat's droppings) is commonly used to brighten the eyes and to disperse screens and obstructions. It clears heat in the blood aspect of the liver channel and dissipates static blood.

For liver heat causing clouded vision, night blindness, and glaucoma, *yè míng shā* is combined with medicinals such as:

cǎo jué míng (草决明 fetid cassia, Cassiae Semen)

shēng dì huáng (生地黄 dried/fresh rehmannia, Rehmanniae Radix Exsiccata seu Recens)

gǒu qǐ zǐ (枸杞子 lycium, Lycii Fructus)

jú huā (菊花 chrysanthemum, Chrysanthemi Flos)

gǔ jīng cǎo (谷精草 eriocaulon, Eriocauli Flos)

mì méng huā (密蒙花 buddleia, Buddleja Flos)

shēng shí jué míng (生石决明 crude abalone shell, Haliotidis Concha Cruda)

bái jí lí (白蒺藜 tribulus, Tribuli Fructus)

huáng qín (黄芩 scutellaria, Scutellariae Radix)

Yè míng shā dissipates static blood and disperses gān accumulation. For internal obstructions (内障 *nèi zhàng*) within the eye or **external screens**[549] (外翳 *wài yì*) that cause blindness, chronic aversion to light, and eye gān in children, it is combined with medicinals such as:

mì méng huā (密蒙花 buddleia, Buddleja Flos)

cǎo jué míng (草决明 fetid cassia, Cassiae Semen)

wàng yuè shā (望月砂 hare's droppings, Lepi Faeces)[41]

mù zéi cǎo (木贼草 equisetum, Equiseti Hiemalis Herba)

ruí rén (蕤仁 prinsepia, Prinsepiae Nux)[42]

yáng gān (羊肝 goat's or sheep's liver, Caprae seu Ovis Iecur)

jī gān (鸡肝 chicken's liver, Galli Iecur)

DOSAGE

The dosage is generally 2.5–9 g/8 fēn–3 qián.

---

36. 丹皮 **Dān Pí**   Moutan Cortex
Moutan

Originally called *mǔ dān pí* 牡丹皮 in Chinese. *Dān pí* (moutan) is acrid and bitter in flavor and cold in nature. It cools the blood and quickens the blood.

1. Cooling the Blood: The blood-cooling effect of *dān pí* is further subdivided into two functions: cooling the blood and stanching bleeding, and cooling the blood and eliminating steaming bone.

a) Cooling the blood and stanching bleeding: *Dān pí* is used for heat in the blood aspect causing blood ejection, nosebleed, coughing of blood, bloody urine, profuse menstruation, and maculopapular eruptions. For these conditions, it is combined with medicinals such as:

shēng dì huáng (生地黄 dried/fresh rehmannia, Rehmanniae Radix Exsiccata seu Recens)

xuán shēn (玄参 scrophularia, Scrophulariae Radix)

guǎng xī jiǎo (广犀角 African rhinoceros horn, Rhinocerotis Cornu Africanum)

chì sháo (赤芍 red peony, Paeoniae Radix Rubra)

zhī mǔ (知母 anemarrhena, Anemarrhenae Rhizoma)

shēng shí gāo (生石膏 crude gypsum, Gypsum Fibrosum Crudum)

dà qīng yè (大青叶 isatis leaf, Isatidis Folium)

máo gēn (茅根 imperata, Imperatae Rhizoma)

xiān hè cǎo (仙鹤草 agrimony, Agrimoniae Herba)

dì yú tàn (地榆炭 charred sanguisorba, Sanguisorbae Radix Carbonisata)

zōng tàn (棕炭 charred trachycarpus, Trachycarpi Petiolus Carbonisatus)

b) Cooling the blood and eliminating steaming bone: For yīn vacuity blood heat causing steaming bone consumptive heat [effusion] (fever), absence of sweating, thirst, and menstrual block, *dān pí* can be used to clear latent blood heat

---

[41] *Wàng yuè shā* (hare's droppings) is the stool of the hare *Lepus tolai* PALLAS. The medicinal is acrid and cold, and it brightens the eyes and kills worms. It is primarily used in the treatment of eye screens, gān diseases, and hemorrhoids. The dosage is 3–9 g/1–3 qián in decoction. (Ed.)

[42] *Ruí rén* (prinsepia) is the inner kernel of the fruit of *Prinsepia uniflora* BATAL. It is primarily used to treat eye disorders. Sweet and cold, it dispels wind, disperses heat, nourishes the liver, and brightens the eyes. The dosage is 4.5–9 g/1.5–3 qián in decoctions. (Ed.)

and thereby cool the blood and eliminate steaming bone. For this purpose it is often combined with medicinals such as *qīng hāo* (sweet wormwood), *biē jiǎ* (turtle shell), *dì gǔ pí* (lycium root bark), *sāng bái pí* (mulberry root bark), *xuán shēn* (scrophularia), and *qín jiāo* (large gentian).[43]

2. Quickening the Blood: The blood-quickening effect is also subdivided into two different uses: quickening the blood and transforming stasis, and quickening the blood and dispelling welling-abscesses.

a) Quickening the blood and transforming stasis: For collected blood stasis causing menstrual block and concretion lumps in the abdomen, use *dān pí* to dissipate static blood and transform concretion lumps. For this purpose it is often combined with the following medicinals, as in *mǔ dān pí sǎn* (Moutan Powder), recorded in *Fù Rén Liáng Fāng* (妇人良方 "Good Remedies for Women"):

Mǔ dān pí sǎn 牡丹皮散   Moutan Powder

---

dān pí (丹皮 moutan, Moutan Cortex)
dāng guī wěi (当归尾 Chinese angelica tail, Angelicae Sinensis Radicis Extremitas)
chì sháo (赤芍 red peony, Paeoniae Radix Rubra)
yán hú suǒ (延胡索 corydalis, Corydalis Rhizoma)
niú xī (牛膝 achyranthes, Achyranthis Bidentatae Radix)
sān léng (三棱 sparganium, Sparganii Rhizoma)
é zhú (莪术 curcuma rhizome, Curcumae Rhizoma)
guì xīn (桂心 shaved cinnamon bark, Cinnamomi Cortex Rasus)
hóng huā (红花 carthamus, Carthami Flos)

b) Quickening the blood and dispersing welling-abscesses: In treating an initial-stage **intestinal welling-abscess**[554] (肠痈 *cháng yōng*, acute appendicitis), when it has not yet suppurated and the patient has symptoms of heat [effusion] (fever), vomiting, and lower right abdomen pain, use *dān pí* to dissipate static blood and disperse the swollen welling-abscess. For this purpose, it is often combined with the following medicinals, as in *dà huáng mǔ dān pí tāng* (Rhubarb and Moutan Decoction), which is recorded in *Jīn Guì Yào Lüè* (金匮要略 "Essential Prescriptions of the Golden Coffer").

Dà huáng mǔ dān pí tāng 大黄牡丹皮汤   Rhubarb and Moutan Decoction

---

mǔ dān pí (牡丹皮 moutan, Moutan Cortex)
dà huáng (大黄 rhubarb, Rhei Radix et Rhizoma)
máng xiāo (芒硝 mirabilite, Natrii Sulfas)
táo rén (桃仁 peach kernel, Persicae Semen)

---

[43]Since acrid medicinals promote perspiration, *dān pí* (moutan) is used for steaming-bone conditions in which sweating is absent. *Dì gǔ pí* (lycium root bark) is sweet and cold and thus can be used to treat these conditions when they present with sweating. Note that despite an ancient prohibition, *dān pí* (moutan) is nowadays sometimes used even when sweating is present. (Ed.)

dōng guā zǐ (冬瓜子 wax gourd seed, Benincasae Semen)

chì sháo (赤芍 red peony, Paeoniae Radix Rubra)

COMPARISONS

Dì gǔ pí (lycium root bark)[306] tends to treat steaming bone consumptive heat [effusion] (fever) with sweating; *mǔ dān pí* tends to treat steaming bone consumptive heat [effusion] (fever) with an absence of sweating. *Dì gǔ pí* also drains latent heat in the lung, whereas *mǔ dān pí* mainly drains latent heat in the blood.

Huáng bǎi (phellodendron)[254] and *dān pí* both expel heat from the kidney. *Huáng bǎi* is bitter; it consolidates the kidney and downbears evil fire in the kidney. *Dān pí* is acrid, cool, and moistening; it clears dryness and fire in the kidney.

PROCESSING

To cool the blood and stanch bleeding, *dān pí* should be char-fried. To cool the blood and clear heat, or to quicken the blood and transform stasis, the raw form should be used.

DOSAGE

The dosage is generally 4.5–9 g/1.5–3 qián.

CAUTION

This medicinal is contraindicated for spleen-stomach vacuity cold diarrhea.

RESEARCH

According to modern research reports, *dān pí* inhibits bacterial growth and is both antipyretic and hypotensive. It also causes the endometrium of the uterus to be suffused with blood and promotes menstruation.

---

37. 地骨皮 Dì Gǔ Pí   Lycii Cortex
Lycium Root Bark

Dì gǔ pí (lycium root bark) is sweet and slightly bitter in flavor and cold in nature. It mainly drains lung fire and clears vacuity heat.

1. **Lung Heat Cough:** For heat in the lung channel that is depressed and transforms into fire, causing cough, rapid breathing, yellow phlegm, thirst, and in severe cases cough with blood-flecked phlegm, generalized heat [effusion] (fever), nosebleeds (especially in children), a red tongue, and a rapid pulse, use *dì gǔ pí* to clear and drain lung channel fire-heat. For this purpose it is often combined with medicinals such as:

sāng bái pí (桑白皮 mulberry root bark, Mori Cortex)

shēng gān cǎo (生甘草 raw licorice, Glycyrrhizae Radix Cruda)

huáng qín (黄芩 scutellaria, Scutellariae Radix)

shēng shí gāo (生石膏 crude gypsum, Gypsum Fibrosum Crudum)

bèi mǔ (贝母 fritillaria, Fritillariae Bulbus)

zhī mǔ (知母 anemarrhena, Anemarrhenae Rhizoma)

If there is also constipation and dry stool, add *shēng dà huáng* (raw rhubarb), *guā lóu* (trichosanthes), and *xìng rén ní* (crushed apricot kernel). *Qián yǐ xiè bái sǎn* (Qián-Yǐ White-Draining Powder) is a very effective formula for lung heat cough in children.

Qián yǐ xiè bái sǎn 钱乙泻白散   Qián-Yǐ White-Draining Powder

---

dì gǔ pí (地骨皮 lycium root bark, Lycii Cortex)

sāng bái pí (桑白皮 mulberry root bark, Mori Cortex)

shēng gān cǎo (生甘草 raw licorice, Glycyrrhizae Radix Cruda)

gēng mǐ (粳米 non-glutinous rice, Oryzae Semen)

2. Steaming Bone Consumptive Heat [Effusion] (Fever): Use *dì gǔ pí* to cool the blood and abate vacuity heat when effulgent yīn vacuity fire and blood vacuity internal heat give rise to **postmeridian tidal heat [effusion]**[559] (下午潮热 *xià wǔ cháo rè*), reddening of both cheeks, night sweating, thirst, heat in the (hearts of the) palms and soles, vexation and agitation, dry cough (with blood-flecked phlegm, in severe cases), a thin red tongue, and a fine rapid pulse. It is very effective in treating steaming bone with sweating, for which it is often combined with medicinals such as:

shēng dì huáng (生地黄 dried/fresh rehmannia, Rehmanniae Radix Exsiccata seu Recens)

biē jiǎ (鳖甲 turtle shell, Trionycis Carapax)

tiān dōng (天冬 asparagus, Asparagi Radix)

mài dōng (麦冬 ophiopogon, Ophiopogonis Radix)

ē jiāo (阿胶 ass hide glue, Asini Corii Colla)

yín chái hú (银柴胡 stellaria, Stellariae Radix)

shā shēn (沙参 adenophora/glehnia, Adenophorae seu Glehniae Radix)

xuán shēn (玄参 scrophularia, Scrophulariae Radix)

zhī mǔ (知母 anemarrhena, Anemarrhenae Rhizoma)

3. Dispersion-Thirst with Vexation and Heat: Because *dì gǔ pí* cools the blood and clears heat, it is used for internal heat dispersion-thirst, great thirst with fluid intake, intake of fluid failing to resolve thirst, and heat vexation in the heart. It is combined with medicinals such as:

shēng dì huáng (生地黄 dried/fresh rehmannia, Rehmanniae Radix Exsiccata seu Recens)

tiān huā fěn (天花粉 trichosanthes root, Trichosanthis Radix)

zhī mǔ (知母 anemarrhena, Anemarrhenae Rhizoma)

shēng shí gāo (生石膏 crude gypsum, Gypsum Fibrosum Crudum)

shēng shān yào (生山药 raw dioscorea, Dioscoreae Rhizoma Crudum)

wǔ wèi zǐ (五味子 schisandra, Schisandrae Fructus)

gǒu qǐ zǐ (枸杞子 lycium, Lycii Fructus)

zé xiè (泽泻 alisma, Alismatis Rhizoma)

mài dōng (麦冬 ophiopogon, Ophiopogonis Radix)

yù zhú (玉竹 Solomon's seal, Polygonati Odorati Rhizoma)

shēng huáng qí (生黄芪 raw astragalus, Astragali Radix Cruda)

Building on the experience described above, I often add *dì gǔ pí* to an appropriate formula, when it is appropriate in accordance with the patttern identified, to treat diabetes mellitus manifesting as dispersion-thirst. I also often use this medicinal combined with *zé xiè* (alisma) to treat hypertension (primarily diastolic hypertension) that presents with blood heat and liver effulgence and invariably find it to be effective.

RESEARCH

According to modern research reports, *dì gǔ pí* has a modest ability to lower blood sugar; it also acts as an antipyretic and hypotensive.

4. Blood Heat Bleeding: Use this medicinal to treat heat in the blood aspect causing coughing of blood, nosebleed, bloody urine, and related symptoms. If the fresh medicinal is available, crush it to extract the juice and drink one-half teacup to one teacup of the juice. If the fresh medicinal is not available, one may use a water decoction. For coughing of blood and nosebleed, the juice (or decoction) should be taken after meals; for bloody urine and blood ejection, it should be taken before meals. For this purpose, *dì gǔ pí* is also combined with medicinals such as:

shēng dì huáng (生地黄 dried/fresh rehmannia, Rehmanniae Radix Exsiccata seu Recens)

máo gēn (茅根 imperata, Imperatae Rhizoma)

ǒu jié (藕节 lotus root node, Nelumbinis Rhizomatis Nodus)

cè bǎi yè (侧柏叶 arborvitae leaf, Platycladi Cacumen)

dà jì (大蓟 Japanese thistle, Cirsii Japonici Herba seu Radix)

xiǎo jì (小蓟 field thistle, Cirsii Herba)

huáng qín tàn (黄芩炭 charred scutellaria, Scutellariae Radix Carbonisata)

dān pí tàn (丹皮炭 charred moutan, Moutan Cortex Carbonisatus)

COMPARISONS

Sāng bái pí (mulberry root bark)[445] clears lung heat and drains lung fire; it primarily enters the qì aspect. *Dì gǔ pí* drains lung fire and clears blood heat; it primarily enters the blood aspect. These two medicinals are often used together to clear both the qì and the blood.

DOSAGE

The dosage is generally 3–9 g/1–3 qián.

CAUTION

This medicinal is not appropriate in the absence of blood-aspect heat if there is center burner vacuity cold. It is also inappropriate if there is blood-aspect heat with simultaneous external contraction.

38. 紫草　Zǐ Cǎo
Arnebia/Lithospermum

Arnebiae/Lithospermi Radix

Sweet and slightly bitter in flavor and cold in nature, *zǐ cǎo* (arnebia/lithospermum)[44] cools and quickens the blood, outthrusts papules and macules, clears heat and resolves toxin, and frees the stool.

1. Clearing and Quickening the Blood; Outthrusting Papules and Macules: *Zǐ cǎo* cools the blood, quickens the blood, resolves toxin, and outthrusts papules in cases of measles or maculopapular eruptions due to effulgent heat toxin in the blood that presents as generalized heat [effusion] (fever), thirst, dry stool, and macules or papules that fail to erupt or that erupt but incompletely. For this purpose it is often combined with medicinals such as *bò hé* (mint), *niú bàng zǐ* (arctium), *chán tuì* (cicada molting), *jié gěng* (platycodon), and *lián qiáo* (forsythia). If there are macules and papules that erupt but that are dark or purple, as well as constipation and bound stool, use *zǐ cǎo* to cool the blood, quicken the blood, and free the stool, in combination with medicinals such as:

chì sháo (赤芍 red peony, Paeoniae Radix Rubra)

dān pí (丹皮 moutan, Moutan Cortex)

dà qīng yè (大青叶 isatis leaf, Isatidis Folium)

chán tuì (蝉蜕 cicada molting, Cicadae Periostracum)

lián qiáo (连翘 forsythia, Forsythiae Fructus)

The combination of 3–6 g/1–2 qián of *zǐ cǎo* and 1.5–3 g/5 fēn–1 qián of *gān cǎo* (licorice) prevents measles. Decoct with water, and take once per day for three to seven days in a row. According to some reports, when people who had been exposed to measles patients were given this decoction within five days of exposure, it was more than 90% effective at preventing the disease. Nevertheless, some people still believe that its effectiveness in preventing measles is still not confirmed, and we must await further observations. I hope that practitioners everywhere will research this question.

2. Dispersing Swelling and Resolving Toxin, and Freeing the Stool: Most swollen welling-abscesses and sores are due to depressed blood-aspect heat toxin and present with symptoms such as tidal reddening, swelling, distention, scorching hot pain, and bound stool. In such cases, use *zǐ cǎo* to cool the blood and resolve toxin, and to quicken the blood and disperse swelling; for this purpose it is often combined with medicinals such as *jīn yín huā* (lonicera), *lián qiáo* (forsythia), *dāng guī wěi* (Chinese angelica tail), *chì sháo* (red peony), *hóng huā* (carthamus), and *zào jiǎo cì* (gleditsia thorn). (If the abscess has already ruptured, do not use *zào jiǎo cì*.) Another very effective treatment is to use the following formula, mixed with white vinegar and sesame oil. Boil the formula into a paste and apply topically.

---

[44] *Zǐ cǎo* (紫草, arnebia/lithospermum) is often referred to as *zǐ cǎo gēn* 紫草根 and *zǐ shēn* 紫参. Two types are available: *yìng zǐ cǎo* (硬紫草, lithospermum) and *ruǎn zǐ cǎo* (软紫草, arnebia). (Ed.)

Yù hóng gāo 玉红膏	Jade and Red Paste

> *zǐ cǎo* (紫草 arnebia/lithospermum, Arnebiae/Lithospermi Radix)
> *bái là* (白腊 white wax, Cera Alba)
> *má yóu* (麻油 sesame oil, Sesami Oleum)
> *dāng guī* (当归 Chinese angelica, Angelicae Sinensis Radix)
> *xuè jié* (血竭 dragon's blood, Daemonoropis Resina)
> *qīng fěn* (轻粉 calomel, Calomelas)
> *bái zhǐ* (白芷 Dahurian angelica, Angelicae Dahuricae Radix)
> *gān cǎo* (甘草 licorice, Glycyrrhizae Radix)

Commercially available products include *zǐ cǎo yóu* (Arnebia/Lithospermum Oil) (*zǐ cǎo* and *zhí wù yóu* (vegetable oil) in a 1:2 ratio that has been soaked for 7–10 days), and *zǐ cǎo gāo* (Arnebia/Lithospermum Paste), which is a 10% paste that uses 15% lanolin and 85% petroleum jelly as a base. These are both commonly used to treat dermatitis, scalds and burns, eczema, otitis media, vaginitis, and cervicitis.

Because *zǐ cǎo* cools the blood and frees the stool, it is added to the appropriate base formula for cases of bound stool and constipation due to toxic heat in the blood aspect.

RESEARCH

According to modern research reports, this medicinal excites the heart and has a moderate antipyretic effect.

DOSAGE

The dosage is generally 3–9 g/1–3 qián.

CAUTION

Regardless of presence of maculopapular eruptions or sore-toxin, if the stool is thin and watery, this medicinal should not be used. It is also inappropriate in cases of stomach and intestinal vacuity cold with sloppy diarrhea.

39. 银柴胡 Yín Chái Hú   Stellariae Radix
Stellaria

Yín chái hú (stellaria) is sweet and slightly bitter in flavor and slightly cold in nature. Its main effects are cooling the blood and clearing vacuity heat.

1. **Steaming Bone Taxation Heat:** For effulgent yīn vacuity fire and steaming bone taxation heat, causing tidal heat [effusion] (fever), steaming bones and night sweating, heat in the (hearts of the) palms and soles, vexation thirst, a yellow-white face with red cheeks, and a fine rapid pulse, use *yín chái hú* in combination with medicinals such as *hú huáng lián* (picrorhiza), *qín jiāo* (large gentian), *shēng dì huáng* (dried/fresh rehmannia), *biē jiǎ* (turtle shell), *dì gǔ pí* (lycium root bark),

xuán shēn (scrophularia), *qīng hāo* (sweet wormwood), and *zhī mǔ* (anemarrhena). A commonly used formula for this purpose is the following:

Qīng gǔ sǎn 清骨散	Bone-Clearing Powder

yín chái hú (银柴胡 stellaria, Stellariae Radix)

hú huáng lián (胡黄连 picrorhiza, Picrorhizae Rhizoma)

qín jiāo (秦艽 large gentian, Gentianae Macrophyllae Radix)

biē jiǎ (鳖甲 turtle shell, Trionycis Carapax)

dì gǔ pí (地骨皮 lycium root bark, Lycii Cortex)

qīng hāo (青蒿 sweet wormwood, Artemisiae Annuae Herba)

zhī mǔ (知母 anemarrhena, Anemarrhenae Rhizoma)

gān cǎo (甘草 licorice, Glycyrrhizae Radix)

2. Gān Accumulation with Heat [Effusion] (Fever): This medicinal may be used for children with poor digestion or worm accumulation that causes a distended and enlarged abdomen, yellow face and emaciated flesh, withered head hair and body hair, and low-grade fever or heat [effusion] (fever) in the afternoon or evening with fever being most pronounced in the rib-side and abdomen. This condition is gān accumulation with heat [effusion] (fever), and it is treated by combining *yín chái hú* with medicinals such as:

dì gǔ pí (地骨皮 lycium root bark, Lycii Cortex)

hú huáng lián (胡黄连 picrorhiza, Picrorhizae Rhizoma)

shān zhā (山楂 crataegus, Crataegi Fructus)

shén qū (神曲 medicated leaven, Massa Medicata Fermentata)

mài yá (麦芽 barley sprout, Hordei Fructus Germinatus)

shǐ jūn zǐ (使君子 quisqualis, Quisqualis Fructus)

bīng láng (槟榔 areca, Arecae Semen)

jī nèi jīn (鸡内金 gizzard lining, Galli Gigeriae Endothelium Corneum)

COMPARISONS

Běi chái hú (northern bupleurum), which is usually known simply as *chái hú* (bupleurum),[37] abates heat and is mainly used to resolve lesser yáng channel repletion heat. *Yín chái hú* also abates heat, but is primarily used to abate vacuity heat in the yīn aspect.

Qīng hāo (sweet wormwood) enters the liver and gallbladder and clears liver-gallbladder vacuity heat. It is also effective for lingering warm-heat that resembles both exterior and interior patterns and that is similar to both vacuity and repletion patterns (i.e., cannot be clearly classified as either one). *Yín chái hú* enters the liver and stomach. It clears liver and stomach vacuity heat and abates gān disease heat [effusion].

DOSAGE

The dosage is generally 2.5–9 g/8 fēn–3 qián.

40. 白薇 Bái Wēi
Black Swallowwort

Cynanchi Atrati
Radix

Bái wēi (black swallowwort)[45] is slightly bitter in flavor and cold in nature. It mainly clears heat, cools the blood, and boosts yīn. It is often used to treat low-grade fever due to vacuity heat.

1. Low-Grade Fever Due to Damage to Yīn in Febrile Disease: In the recovery stage of warm-heat disease, when high fever abates after causing damage to yīn-liquid that prevents right qì from recovering immediately, there is often residual heat that manifests in low-grade fever, thirst, heat effusion (fever) at night that abates at dawn, postmeridian low-grade fever, and poor appetite. In such cases, *bái wēi* is combined with medicinals such as:

dì gŭ pí (地骨皮 lycium root bark, Lycii Cortex)

zhī mŭ (知母 anemarrhena, Anemarrhenae Rhizoma)

qīng hāo (青蒿 sweet wormwood, Artemisiae Annuae Herba)

dān pí (丹皮 moutan, Moutan Cortex)

shā shēn (沙参 adenophora/glehnia, Adenophorae seu Glehniae Radix)

tiān huā fĕn (天花粉 trichosanthes root, Trichosanthis Radix)

What is described above is the most commonly used clinical application. In addition, *bái wēi* is also used for heat entering the construction aspect in warm-heat disease patterns and for high fever in blood-aspect patterns. *Bái wēi* is an excellent medicinal for treating warm-heat diseases because it enters the yáng brightness (*yáng míng*) channel (as well as the controlling and thoroughfare vessels), cools the blood, clears heat, boosts the stomach, and engenders liquid. It is combined with medicinals such as:

shēng dì huáng (生地黄 dried/fresh rehmannia, Rehmanniae Radix Exsiccata seu Recens)

xuán shēn (玄参 scrophularia, Scrophulariae Radix)

shēng shí gāo (生石膏 crude gypsum, Gypsum Fibrosum Crudum)

chì sháo (赤芍 red peony, Paeoniae Radix Rubra)

zhī mŭ (知母 anemarrhena, Anemarrhenae Rhizoma)

dān pí (丹皮 moutan, Moutan Cortex)

dà qīng yè (大青叶 isatis leaf, Isatidis Folium)

lián qiáo (连翘 forsythia, Forsythiae Fructus)

guăng xī jiăo (广犀角 African rhinoceros horn, Rhinocerotis Cornu Africanum)

Even for the onset of warm disease, when signs include a red tongue, dry mouth, and aversion to wind, and possibly headache, one may add this medicinal to acrid, cool formulas that resolve the surface. For example, it is combined with medicinals

---

[45] *Bái wēi* (black swallowwort), which should be the root of *Cynanchum atratum* BGE., is frequently substituted by the whole plant of *Gerbera piloselloides* CASS. What is sold as *bái qián* (白前, willowleaf swallowwort)[435] is often the root of *Cynanchum atratum*. (Ed.)

such as *jīn yín huā* (lonicera), *niú bàng zǐ* (arctium), *bò hé* (mint), and *jú huā* (chrysanthemum).

2. Antepartum and Postpartum Heat Vexation: For pregnant women with heat vexation, enuresis, and painful voidings of hot urine, *bái wēi* is combined with *bái sháo* (white peony), *huáng qín* (scutellaria), and *huáng bǎi* (phellodendron) because it enters the controlling and thoroughfare vessels and clears heat from the blood aspect. For postpartum women who, due to excessive blood loss, have blood vacuity heat [effusion] (fever), vexation and derangement, and nausea and vomiting, *bái wēi* is combined with medicinals such as *zhú rú* (bamboo shavings), *huò xiāng* (agastache), *qīng hāo* (sweet wormwood), and *chén pí* (tangerine peel).

Because this medicinal enters the controlling vessel, I often add it to prescriptions, formulated for the identified pattern, to treat red urine, strangury pain, cystitis, and prostatitis due to blood heat; this invariably achieves good results.

COMPARISONS

Qīng hāo (sweet wormwood)[313] clears liver-gallbladder vacuity heat, abates bone steaming with an absence of sweating, treats heat in the bone, and conducts heat evil from the yīn aspect up to the qì aspect so that it can leave the body. *Bái wēi* clears gastrointestinal vacuity heat and treats low-grade fever of unclear etiology. It also clears blood heat in the thoroughfare and controlling vessels.

Bái liǎn (ampelopsis) eliminates blood heat. It tends to be used to resolve toxin and treat sores and to close open sores. *Bái wēi* eliminates blood heat and tends to be used to abate vacuity heat.

DOSAGE

The dosage is generally 4.5–12 g/1.5–5 qián. In severe cases, use up to 15 g/ 5 qián.

CAUTION

Do not use this medicinal in the absence of blood-aspect heat, or in the presence of gastrointestinal vacuity cold or diarrhea.

---

41. 青蒿 Qīng Hāo
Sweet Wormwood

Artemisiae Annuae Herba

Qīng hāo (sweet wormwood)[46] is cold in nature and bitter in flavor, and possesses a cool and aromatic smell. Its main use is as a heat-clearing medicinal and it clears, cools, and resolves summerheat.

1. Clearing Vacuity Heat: *Qīng hāo* clears and eliminates latent heat in the yīn aspect. It is used in the recovery stage of warm-heat disease, when evil heat has damaged yīn and there is residual heat failing to clear from the yīn-aspect, which is marked by heat [effusion] (fever) in the night that abates by the morning

---

[46]*Artemisia annua* L. is the most commonly used type of *qīng hāo* (sweet wormwood); it is specifically referred to as *huáng qīng hāo* 黄青蒿. (Ed.)

and dry mouth with a red tongue.[47] For this purpose it is often combined with *zhī mǔ* (anemarrhena), *biē jiǎ* (turtle shell), *dān pí* (moutan), and *shēng dì huáng* (dried/fresh rehmannia), as in *qīng hǎo biē jiǎ tāng* (Sweet Wormwood and Turtle Shell Decoction), which is recorded in Wú Jú-Tōng's *Wēn Bìng Tiáo Biàn* (温病条辨 "Systematized Identification of Warm Diseases").

2. Steaming Bone Taxation Heat [Effusion] (Fever): For effulgent yīn vacuity fire causing steaming bone taxation heat, night sweating, cough, phlegm containing blood, reddening of the cheeks, heart vexation, and heat [effusion] on the palms and soles, use *qīng hǎo* to clear latent fire in the blood, eliminate yīn-aspect latent heat, and abate steaming bone taxation heat [effusion] (fever). For this purpose it is often combined with medicinals such as:

biē jiǎ (鳖甲 turtle shell, Trionycis Carapax)

qín jiāo (秦艽 large gentian, Gentianae Macrophyllae Radix)

zhī mǔ (知母 anemarrhena, Anemarrhenae Rhizoma)

dì gǔ pí (地骨皮 lycium root bark, Lycii Cortex)

hú huáng lián (胡黄连 picrorhiza, Picrorhizae Rhizoma)

shēng dì huáng (生地黄 dried/fresh rehmannia, Rehmanniae Radix Exsiccata seu Recens)

dān pí (丹皮 moutan, Moutan Cortex)

bái wēi (白薇 black swallowwort, Cynanchi Atrati Radix)

dāng guī (当归 Chinese angelica, Angelicae Sinensis Radix)

3. Malaria with Cold and Heat: For warm-heat disease with a disease evil latent in the lesser yáng (*shào yáng*) channel that causes alternating cold and heat, or malaria with [aversion to] cold and heat [effusion] occuring at set periods, *qīng hǎo* can be used to enter the liver and gallbladder channels and to clear and outthrust evil heat. For this purpose it is often combined with medicinals such as:

huáng qín (黄芩 scutellaria, Scutellariae Radix)

yù jīn (郁金 curcuma, Curcumae Radix)

chāng pú (菖蒲 acorus, Acori Tatarinowii Rhizoma)

jīn yín huā (金银花 lonicera, Lonicerae Flos)

zhú rú (竹茹 bamboo shavings, Bambusae Caulis in Taenia)

zhǐ qiào (枳壳 bitter orange, Aurantii Fructus)

bàn xià (半夏 pinellia, Pinelliae Rhizoma)

To treat malaria with cold and heat occurring at set periods, this medicinal is combined with the formula below, with the addition of *bīng láng* (areca) and *cǎo guǒ* (tsaoko).

---

[47]This pattern of post-illness nighttime heat effusion (fever) and early morning cool results from the continued presence of deep-lying heat in the inner body. At night, the body's yáng qì naturally sinks inward, combines with the deep-lying heat, and gives rise to inner-body heat. In the early morning, when the yáng qì of the body returns to the outer body, the heat naturally recedes without the occurrence of a sweat. This pattern is typically treated with *qīng hǎo biē jiǎ tāng* (Sweet Wormwood and Turtle Shell Decoction). (Ed.)

Xiǎo chái hú tāng 小柴胡汤	Minor Bupleurum Decoction

chái hú (柴胡 bupleurum, Bupleuri Radix)

huáng qín (黄芩 scutellaria, Scutellariae Radix)

bàn xià (半夏 pinellia, Pinelliae Rhizoma)

dǎng shēn (党参 codonopsis, Codonopsis Radix)

gān cǎo (甘草 licorice, Glycyrrhizae Radix)

shēng jiāng (生姜 fresh ginger, Zingiberis Rhizoma Recens)

dà zǎo (大枣 jujube, Jujubae Fructus)

In recent years, there have been some reports that untreated *qīng hāo* ground into a dry powder and made into tablets is effective in treating malaria. One should take 3.75 g/1.25 qián three to four hours before an episode and continue for five or six days in a row. This is effective against most types of malaria, with an effectiveness rate of up to 81.8%. Nevertheless, it is somewhat less effective against pernicious malaria.[48]

4. **Resolving Summerheat-Heat:** *Qīng hāo* transforms turbidity with aroma and clears summerheat and repels foulness. For summer-season summerheat, generalized heat [effusion] (fever) without sweating, cumbersome and fatigued limbs, and oppression in the chest, it is often combined with medicinals such as:

huò xiāng (藿香 agastache, Agastaches Herba)

pèi lán (佩兰 eupatorium, Eupatorii Herba)

dà dòu juǎn (大豆卷 dried soybean sprout, Sojae Semen Germinatum)

huá shí (滑石 talcum, Talcum)

tōng cǎo (通草 rice-paper plant pith, Tetrapanacis Medulla)

In addition, *qīng hāo* clears heat from the liver and gallbladder, brightens the eyes, and abates jaundice. It is used to treat liver fire flaming upwards that causes clouded vision, red eyes, and aversion to light, for which it is combined with medicinals such as:

jú huā (菊花 chrysanthemum, Chrysanthemi Flos)

shí jué míng (石决明 abalone shell, Haliotidis Concha)

cǎo jué míng (草决明 fetid cassia, Cassiae Semen)

huáng qín (黄芩 scutellaria, Scutellariae Radix)

zhī zǐ (栀子 gardenia, Gardeniae Fructus)

For depressed and steaming damp-heat in the gallbladder channel causing jaundice, heat [effusion] (fever), reddish urine, or scant urine, it is combined with medicinals such as *yīn chén* (virgate wormwood), *chē qián zǐ* (plantago seed), *huáng bǎi* (phellodendron), and *zhī zǐ* (gardenia).

COMPARISONS

Dì gǔ pí (lycium root bark)[306] drains liver-kidney vacuity heat, abates steaming

---

[48]Pernicious malaria, 恶性疟 *è xìng nüè*: See footnote on page 508. (Ed.)

bone with sweating, and clears latent heat in the lung. *Qīng hāo* clears liver-gallbladder vacuity heat, abates steaming bone with absence of sweating, and eliminates persistent warm-heat.

Chái hú (bupleurum)[37] harmonizes the exterior and interior; it mainly treats evil in the lesser yáng (*shào yáng*) with alternating cold and heat. *Qīng hāo* clears liver-gallbladder vacuity heat and treats lingering warm-heat with signs such as alternating cold and heat, signs that resemble exterior and interior patterns, and signs that belong to both vacuity and repletion patterns. It also treats fever in the night that abates by the morning and persists over a long period of time.

Dosage

The dosage is generally 3–9 g/1–3 qián; in especially severe cases, use 12–25 g/4–8 qián.

Caution

This medicinal is contraindicated for internal vacuity cold, sloppy diarrhea, or postpartum qì vacuity.

---

42. 白头翁 Bái Tóu Wēng   Pulsatillae Radix
Pulsatilla

Bitter in flavor and cold in nature, *bái tóu wēng* (pulsatilla)[49] drains stomach and large intestinal evil heat and is often used to treat dysentery. It also resolves toxin.

For gastrointestinal heat toxin accumulation and stagnation that gives rise to stool containing pus and blood (copious blood and scant pus), tenesmus, abdominal pain, and frequent defecation, *bái tóu wēng* can be used to clear large intestinal evil heat and to free large intestinal accumulation and stagnation. For this purpose it is often combined with medicinals such as:

huáng lián (黃连 coptis, Coptidis Rhizoma)
huáng bǎi (黃柏 phellodendron, Phellodendri Cortex)
qín pí (秦皮 ash, Fraxini Cortex)
mù xiāng (木香 costusroot, Aucklandiae Radix)
bīng láng (槟榔 areca, Arecae Semen)
bái sháo (白芍 white peony, Paeoniae Radix Alba)

In combination with medicinals such as *dì yú* (sanguisorba), *huái huā tàn* (charred sophora flower), *huáng qín tàn* (charred scutellaria), and *chǎo huái jiǎo* (stir-fried sophora fruit), *bái tóu wēng* treats heat in the large intestine causing descent of blood with the stool and hemorrhoids with descent of blood.

---

[49] *Bái tóu wēng* (pulsatilla), which should be the root of *Pulsatilla chinensis* (Bge.) Reg., is often represented in southern China by the above-ground portion of *Polycarpaea corymbosa* (L.) Lam. Unfortunately, it is this latter medicinal that is often exported to Táiwān, Hongkong, and the West. (Ed.)

COMPARISONS

Huáng lián (coptis)[246] and *bái tóu wēng* both treat dysentery, but *huáng lián* clears heat, also dries dampness, and is most effective for damp-heat dysentery; *bái tóu wēng* primarily clears large intestinal blood heat and is most effective for heat dysentery with descent of blood. *Huáng lián* is best for bacterial dysentery; *bái tóu wēng* is best for amebic dysentery.

DOSAGE

The dosage is generally 3–9 g/1–3 qián.

CAUTION

This medicinal is contraindicated for enduring dysentery due to vacuity cold.

---

43. 秦皮 Qín Pí   Fraxini Cortex
Ash

Qín pí (ash) is bitter and slightly astringent in flavor and cold in nature.

1. **Clearing Heat and Treating Dysentery:** *Qín pí* is used to treat damp-heat dysentery with symptoms such as stool containing pus and blood, tenesmus, slimy yellow tongue fur, dry mouth with no desire to drink large quantities, and slippery pulse. This pattern occurs most often during the transition between summer and autumn. For this pattern, *qín pí* is used in combination with medicinals such as:

huáng lián (黄连 coptis, Coptidis Rhizoma)
huáng bǎi (黄柏 phellodendron, Phellodendri Cortex)
bái tóu wēng (白头翁 pulsatilla, Pulsatillae Radix)
mù xiāng (木香 costusroot, Aucklandiae Radix)
bīng láng (槟榔 areca, Arecae Semen)
bái sháo (白芍 white peony, Paeoniae Radix Alba)
dāng guī (当归 Chinese angelica, Angelicae Sinensis Radix)
hòu pò (厚朴 officinal magnolia bark, Magnoliae Officinalis Cortex)
zhǐ shí (枳实 unripe bitter orange, Aurantii Fructus Immaturus)
fú líng (茯苓 poria, Poria)

2. **Clearing the Liver and Brightening the Eyes:** For fire in the liver channel that attacks upwards into the eyes, causing red, swollen, and painful eyes, sensation of heat in the eyes, aversion to light and the sun, visual obstructions, and tearing on exposure to wind, use *qín pí sǎn* (Ash Powder), which is recorded in *Zhèng Zhì Zhǔn Zhéng* (证治准绳 "The Level-Line of Pattern Identification and Treatment"):

Qín pí sǎn 秦皮散   Ash Powder

---

qín pí (秦皮 ash, Fraxini Cortex)

huá shí (滑石 talcum, Talcum)

huáng lián (黄连 coptis, Coptidis Rhizoma)

Use all the medicinals in equal proportions, grind into a fine powder, and decoct 5 fēn each time in water, boiling it several times. Throw out the dregs and use the clear liquid as a wash when it cools to room temperature.[50]

Combine *qín pí* with medicinals such as *jú huā* (chrysanthemum), *bò hé* (mint), *sāng yè* (mulberry leaf), *huáng qín* (scutellaria), *mù zéi cǎo* (equisetum), and *cǎo jué míng* (fetid cassia) to make an internal formula for simultaneous use.

RESEARCH

According to modern research reports, *qín pí* is effective against diseases such as rheumatoid arthritis and rheumatic myositis. It has been shown to markedly increase uric acid in the urine of patients with rheumatoid conditions.

COMPARISONS

Bái tóu wēng (pulsatilla)[316] treats dysentery and tends to clear heat and cool the blood, whereas *qín pí* treats dysentery and tends to clear heat and astringe the intestines.

DOSAGE

The dosage is generally 3–9 g/1–3 qián.

---

44. 白藓皮 Bái Xiǎn Pí   Dictamni Cortex
Dictamnus

Bái xiǎn pí (dictamnus) is bitter in flavor and cold in nature. It mainly dispels dampness and disinhibits the joints.

This medicinal is most commonly used to treat depressed and stagnant damp-heat presenting with symptoms such as itching skin sores, eczema, scrotal eczema, scab and lichen, and wind sores. For these conditions, it is combined with medicinals such as:

jīn yín huā (金银花 lonicera, Lonicerae Flos)

lián qiáo (连翘 forsythia, Forsythiae Fructus)

jīng jiè (荆芥 schizonepeta, Schizonepetae Herba)

huáng bǎi (黄柏 phellodendron, Phellodendri Cortex)

cāng zhú (苍术 atractylodes, Atractylodis Rhizoma)

kǔ shēn (苦参 flavescent sophora, Sophorae Flavescentis Radix)

hóng huā (红花 carthamus, Carthami Flos)

chì sháo (赤芍 red peony, Paeoniae Radix Rubra)

zhì shān jiǎ (炙山甲 mix-fried pangolin scales, Manis Squama cum Liquido Fricta)

---

[50] All eye washes must be strained carefully through filter paper before they are used to prevent particles from entering the eye. (Ed.)

fú líng (茯苓 poria, Poria)

I myself often use the following formula, varied in accordance with signs and the concrete situation, to treat stubborn cases of urticaria, and I find it very effective.

bái xiǎn pí (白藓皮 dictamnus, Dictamni Cortex) 30 g/1 liǎng

kǔ shēn (苦参 flavescent sophora, Sophorae Flavescentis Radix) 15–30 g/5 qián–1 liǎng

jīng jiè (荆芥 schizonepeta, Schizonepetae Herba) 9 g/3 qián

fáng fēng (防风 saposhnikovia, Saposhnikoviae Radix) 9 g/3 qián

lián qiáo (连翘 forsythia, Forsythiae Fructus) 12 g/4 qián

chì sháo (赤芍 red peony, Paeoniae Radix Rubra) 15 g/5 qián

hóng huā (红花 carthamus, Carthami Flos) 9 g/3 qián

chán tuì (蝉蜕 cicada molting, Cicadae Periostracum) 6 g/2 qián

fú líng (茯苓 poria, Poria) 9 g/3 qián

shé tuì (蛇蜕 snake slough, Serpentis Periostracum) 0.3 g/1 fēn

zhì shān jiǎ (炙山甲 mix-fried pangolin scales, Manis Squama cum Liquido Fricta) 6 g/2 qián

Bái xiǎn pí is also used for swollen, painful joints due to damp-heat, for which it is often combined with medicinals such as *wēi líng xiān* (clematis), *huáng bǎi* (phellodendron), *mù guā* (chaenomeles), *cāng zhú* (atractylodes), *fáng jǐ* (fangji), *yǐ mǐ* (coix), and *sōng jié* (knotty pine wood).

For women with damp-heat pouring downward that causes pudendal damp itch or red and white vaginal discharge, use *bái xiǎn pí* in combination with medicinals such as:

fú líng (茯苓 poria, Poria)

zé xiè (泽泻 alisma, Alismatis Rhizoma)

cāng zhú (苍术 atractylodes, Atractylodis Rhizoma)

huáng bǎi (黄柏 phellodendron, Phellodendri Cortex)

kǔ shēn (苦参 flavescent sophora, Sophorae Flavescentis Radix)

niú xī (牛膝 achyranthes, Achyranthis Bidentatae Radix)

Based on the experience of past physicians that this medicinal treats wind jaundice (yellowing) and acute jaundice (yellowing), I have used *bái xiǎn pí* with medicinals such as those listed below, varied in accordance with signs, to treat acute infectious icteric hepatitis that has not responded to large doses of *yīn chén* (virgate wormwood):

chái hú (柴胡 bupleurum, Bupleuri Radix)

huáng qín (黄芩 scutellaria, Scutellariae Radix)

zé xiè (泽泻 alisma, Alismatis Rhizoma)

chē qián zǐ (车前子 plantago seed, Plantaginis Semen)

huáng bǎi (黄柏 phellodendron, Phellodendri Cortex)

qín jiāo (秦艽 large gentian, Gentianae Macrophyllae Radix)

jiāo sān xiān (焦三仙 scorch-fried three immortals, Tres Immortales Usti)

This combination is very effective against hepatitis when it manifests as depressed and steaming damp-heat that causes severe jaundice.

RESEARCH

According to modern research reports, *bái xiǎn pí* has varying inhibitory effects on many kinds of cutaneous fungus. The liquid extracted from soaking this medicinal resolves heat.

DOSAGE

The dosage is generally 3–9 g/1–3 qián; in severe cases, use up to 15–24 g/ 5–8 qián, or even 30 g/1 liǎng.

CAUTION

This medicinal is contraindicated for vacuity cold in the lower part of the body.

---

45. 瓜蒌 Guā Lóu   Trichosanthis Fructus
Trichosanthes

Also called *guā lóu* 栝楼, *quán guā lóu* 全瓜蒌, *guā lóu shí* 瓜蒌实, and *guā lóu bǐng* 瓜蒌饼 in Chinese, *guā lóu* (trichosanthes) is sweet and slightly bitter in flavor and cold in nature. It flushes depressed heat from the chest, disperses bound phlegm from the lung channel, and clears fire from the upper burner. Its main actions are to clear heat and transform phlegm, loosen the chest and downbear qì, moisten the intestines and free the stool, and treat mammary welling-abscesses (including acute mastitis).

1. Clearing Heat and Transforming Phlegm: For lung heat with copious phlegm, which is marked by symptoms such as cough, copious yellow phlegm that is sticky and difficult to expectorate, oppression in the chest, hasty breathing, thirst, and a slimy yellow tongue fur, use *guā lóu* with medicinals such as:

zhī mǔ (知母 anemarrhena, Anemarrhenae Rhizoma)

bèi mǔ (贝母 fritillaria, Fritillariae Bulbus)

huáng qín (黄芩 scutellaria, Scutellariae Radix)

jié gěng (桔梗 platycodon, Platycodonis Radix)

sāng pí (桑皮 mulberry root bark, Mori Cortex)

dì gǔ pí (地骨皮 lycium root bark, Lycii Cortex)

pí pá yè (枇杷叶 loquat leaf, Eriobotryae Folium)

For dry cough with scant phlegm, thirst, dry lips, dry throat, dry stool, and a dry yellow tongue fur due to lung heat damaging the fluids or dryness-heat in the lung, use *guā lóu* to clear heat and moisten dryness. For this purpose it is often combined with medicinals such as *mài dōng* (ophiopogon), *shā shēn* (adenophora/glehnia), *zhī mǔ* (anemarrhena), *lí pí* (pear peel), *pí pá yè* (loquat leaf), *xuán shēn* (scrophularia), and *shēng dì huáng* (dried/fresh rehmannia).

2. Loosening the Chest and Downbearing Qì: For phlegm-turbidity stagnating and binding in the chest and causing signs such as stifling oppression and pain, heart pain stretching through to the back, and back pain stretching through to the heart, combine *guā lóu* with medicinals such as:

xiè bái (薤白 Chinese chive, Allii Macrostemonis Bulbus)

zhǐ shí (枳实 unripe bitter orange, Aurantii Fructus Immaturus)

bīng láng (槟榔 areca, Arecae Semen)

hóng huā (红花 carthamus, Carthami Flos)

tán xiāng (檀香 sandalwood, Santali Albi Lignum)

wǔ líng zhī (五灵脂 squirrel's droppings, Trogopteri Faeces)

jiāo shān zhā (焦山楂 scorch-fried crataegus, Crataegi Fructus Ustus)

dān shēn (丹参 salvia, Salviae Miltiorrhizae Radix)

For external contraction that has been inappropriately treated with precipitation causing stomach duct pain with hardness and glomus, aversion to pressure, and stifling sensation and pain in the chest, use *xiǎo xiàn xiōng tāng* (Minor Chest Bind Decoction):

Xiǎo xiàn xiōng tāng 小陷胸汤   Minor Chest Bind Decoction

---

guā lóu (瓜蒌 trichosanthes, Trichosanthis Fructus)

huáng lián (黄连 coptis, Coptidis Rhizoma)

bàn xià (半夏 pinellia, Pinelliae Rhizoma)

3. Moistening the Intestines and Freeing the Stool: In addition to moistening the lung and transforming phlegm, *guā lóu* also moistens the large intestine and frees the stool. Use *guā lóu rén* (trichosanthes seed) or *quán guā lóu* (trichosanthes) to moisten the intestines and free the stool when treating dry and bound stool due to heat in the large intestine and lung, damage to fluids, enduring illness, or insufficient fluids in the elderly. I often add the following medicinals to formulas for constipation due to the patterns described above:

guā lóu (瓜蒌 trichosanthes, Trichosanthis Fructus) 30 g/1 liǎng

táo rén ní (桃仁泥 crushed peach kernel, Persicae Semen Tusum) 9 g/3 qián

xìng rén ní (杏仁泥 crushed apricot kernel, Armeniacae Semen Tusum)
    9 g/3 qián

bīng láng (槟榔 areca, Arecae Semen) 9 g/3 qián

For elderly or weak patients suffering from dry, bound stool with no bowel movements for several days and for whom offensive precipitation with *dà huáng* (rhubarb) would be inappropriate, use 30 g/1 liǎng of *guā lóu* and 1.5–4.5 g/0.5–1.5 qián of *yuán míng fěn* (refined mirabilite). Pound the two medicinals together until the *guā lóu rén* have been broken open, decoct, and drink or add to the decoction prescribed for the presenting pattern. This combination is both safe and reliable for freeing the stool. When necessary for the pathocondition, it may be used with *dà huáng* (rhubarb).

4. Dispersing Mammary Welling-Abscesses: For inhibited postpartum flow of milk, milk accumulation transforming into heat, or toxic heat brewing and forming a welling-abscess, causing symptoms such as redness, swelling, and pain in the breasts, aversion to cold, and heat [effusion] (fever), use 30 g/1 liǎng of *guā lóu* combined with medicinals such as:

bái zhǐ (白芷 Dahurian angelica, Angelicae Dahuricae Radix)

dāng guī (当归 Chinese angelica, Angelicae Sinensis Radix)

rǔ xiāng (乳香 frankincense, Olibanum)

mò yào (没药 myrrh, Myrrha)

lòu lú (漏芦 rhaponticum, Rhapontici Radix)

jīn yín huā (金银花 lonicera, Lonicerae Flos)

pú gōng yīng (蒲公英 dandelion, Taraxaci Herba)

zhì shān jiǎ (炙山甲 mix-fried pangolin scales, Manis Squama cum Liquido Fricta)

Guā lóu pí (trichosanthes rind) tends to loosen the chest and downbear qì; *guā lóu rén* (trichosanthes seed) tends to downbear phlegm and treat intestinal welling-abscesses. An example of the latter use is *qiān jīn mǔ dān pí sǎn* (Thousand Gold Pieces Moutan Powder).

Qiān jīn mǔ dān pí sǎn 千金牡丹皮散   Thousand Gold Pieces Moutan Powder

guā lóu rén (瓜蒌仁 trichosanthes seed, Trichosanthis Semen)

mǔ dān pí (牡丹皮 moutan, Moutan Cortex)

shēng yǐ mǐ (生苡米 raw coix seed, Coicis Semen Crudum)

táo rén (桃仁 peach kernel, Persicae Semen)

This formula is used for acute intestinal welling-abscesses (including appendicitis). *Quán guā lóu* (trichosanthes) tends to loosen the chest and downbear qì, moisten the intestines and free the stool, and to treat mammary welling-abscesses.

I once treated a 70-year-old woman suffering from lung cancer with the following formula:

guā lóu (瓜蒌 trichosanthes, Trichosanthis Fructus) 30 g/1 liǎng

chuān jiāo mù (川椒目 zanthoxylum seed, Zanthoxyli Semen) 5 g/2 qián

sāng pí (桑皮 mulberry root bark, Mori Cortex) 9 g/3 qián

sū zǐ (苏子 perilla fruit, Perillae Fructus) 10 g/3 qián

tíng lì zǐ (葶苈子 lepidium/descurainia, Lepidii/Descurainiae Semen) 9 g/3 qián

chǎo lái fú zǐ (炒莱菔子 stir-fried radish seed, Raphani Semen Frictum) 9 g/3 qián

bàn xià (半夏 pinellia, Pinelliae Rhizoma) 9 g/3 qián

huà jú hóng (化橘红 red Huàzhōu pomelo peel, Citri Grandis Exocarpium Rubrum) 10 g/3 qián

fú líng (茯苓 poria, Poria) 15 g/5 qián

zhū líng (猪苓 polyporus, Polyporus) 12 g/4 qián

chē qián zǐ (车前子 plantago seed, Plantaginis Semen) (wrapped) 12 g/4 qián

bái jí lí (白蒺藜 tribulus, Tribuli Fructus) 10 g/3 qián

guì zhī (桂枝 cinnamon twig, Cinnamomi Ramulus) 5 g/2 qián

There was fluid accumulation in her left pleural cavity. The first affiliated hospital of a certain medical college had run tests and determined that she had hydrothorax and numerous cancer cells. Her family thought she was already in the final stage and was preparing for her death. It was completely unexpected when, after taking 15 packets of the above formula, the patient showed marked improvement. (Sometimes the formula was modified slightly to adjust the treatment to the presenting symptoms.) She was no longer coughing or wheezing and she could comfortably lie in a supine posture or on either side. For about one month prior to this, she had been unable to lie down comfortably and needed to sit up and lie on one side, or prop herself up with pillows and blankets. Her appetite also increased after this first round of medicinals. After 30–50 more packets, she felt that her symptoms had disappeared, and she was able to walk by herself, stroll, sun herself in the hospital garden, and take care of her daily needs. Half a year later, I went to visit her and found that she was still doing well; she was as healthy as she had been before her illness. According to modern research, *guā lóu* and *zhū líng* (polyporus) both have anti-cancer effects and perhaps this was a factor in her recovery. Unfortunately, for reasons related to my work, I was unable to follow up on this case later.

DOSAGE

The dosages are generally as follows: *guā lóu pí* (trichosanthes rind) 6–12 g/ 2–4 qián; *guā lóu rén* (trichosanthes seed) 6–15 g/2–5 qián; *quán guā lóu* (trichosanthes) 9–30 g/3 qián–1 liǎng.

CAUTION

This medicinal is inappropriate for vacuity cold diarrhea. It should also not be used with *fù zǐ* (aconite) or *wū tóu* (wild aconite).

---

46. 葶苈子 Tíng Lì Zǐ
Lepidium/Descurainia
Lepidii/Descurainiae Semen

Acrid and bitter in flavor and cold in nature, *tíng lì zǐ* (lepidium/descurainia)[51] drains the lung, downbears qì, expels phlegm-rheum, and disperses water swelling.

1. **Draining the Lung and Downbearing Qì:** For congested lung qì that fails to perform its function of depurative downbearing, resulting in qì counterflow with panting, or cough with copious phlegm, use *tíng lì zǐ* with medicinals such as *sū zǐ* (perilla fruit), *bàn xià* (pinellia), *pí pá yè* (loquat leaf), *xìng rén* (apricot kernel), and *bái qián* (willowleaf swallowwort). For depressed heat forming welling-abscesses in the lung, use it in combination with medicinals such as:

---

[51] *Tíng lì zǐ* (葶苈子, lepidium/descurainia) is *Descurainia sophia* (L.) SCHUR; *kǔ tíng lì zǐ* (苦葶苈子, lepidium) is *Lepidium apetalum* WILLD. The former is also called *nán* 南 (southern) *tíng lì zǐ* 葶苈子 and the latter, *běi* 北 (northern) *tíng lì zǐ* 葶苈子. The two are very similar in appearance with the exception that the northern kind is larger. Whereas the northern variety is 0.1–0.15 cm long and 0.05–0.1 cm wide, the southern variety is only 0.08–0.12 cm long and about 0.05 cm wide. (Ed.)

jīn yín huā (金银花 lonicera, Lonicerae Flos)

lián qiáo (连翘 forsythia, Forsythiae Fructus)

xiān lú gēn (鲜芦根 fresh phragmites, Phragmitis Rhizoma Recens)

shēng yǐ mǐ (生苡米 raw coix, Coicis Semen Crudum)

dōng guā zǐ (冬瓜子 wax gourd seed, Benincasae Semen)

táo rén (桃仁 peach kernel, Persicae Semen)

2. Expelling Phlegm-Rheum and Dispersing Water Swelling: *Tíng lì zǐ* enters the lung channel to downbear and drain lung qì. It also enters the bladder channel to disinhibit water. It is therefore used to treat congested and stagnant lung qì, poor qì transformation, and inhibited water qì that cause phlegm turbidity and water-rheum, which in turn impair the lung qì's function of depurative downbearing, producing signs such as cough and panting, copious phlegm, phlegm rale in the throat, chest and rib-side distention and oppression, panting with inability to lie down, and generalized water swelling or water swelling of the face and around the eyes. For this pattern, it is combined with medicinals such as:

dà zǎo (大枣 jujube, Jujubae Fructus)

fáng jǐ (防己 fangji, Stephaniae Tetrandrae Radix)

jiāo mù (椒目 zanthoxylum seed, Zanthoxyli Semen)

dà huáng (大黄 rhubarb, Rhei Radix et Rhizoma)

xìng rén (杏仁 apricot kernel, Armeniacae Semen)

fú líng (茯苓 poria, Poria)

bèi mǔ (贝母 fritillaria, Fritillariae Bulbus)

mù tōng (木通 trifoliate akebia, Akebiae Trifoliatae Caulis)

Tíng lì zǐ (lepidium/descurainia) is also called *kǔ tíng lì* (lepidium). It is very potent and takes effect very quickly; in draining the lung it also easily damages the stomach. For this reason, it is often combined with *dà zǎo* (jujube) in order to protect the center qì. There is also a medicinal called *tián tíng lì* (descurainia), which has effects similar to *kǔ tíng lì* (lepidium); however, its medicinal strength is much more moderate and it drains the lung without damaging the stomach. It is suitable for treating elderly people or vacuity patients.

COMPARISONS

Dà huáng (rhubarb)[45] drains blood block and also flushes and drains bound heat in the intestines. *Tíng lì zǐ* drains qì block and also disperses and expels water accumulation in the bladder.

According to modern research reports, *tíng lì zǐ* strengthens the heart and acts as a diuretic. Some researchers have also reported that taking 1–2 g of it three times per day after meals treats chronic, primary pulmonary heart disease, and stimulates the heart after cardiac failure.

DOSAGE

The dosage is generally 2.5–6 g/1–2 qián; for severe cases, use up to 10 g/3 qián.

Caution

Contraindicated for lung vacuity and during pregnancy.

---

47. 天竹黄 Tiān Zhú Huáng Bamboo Sugar		Bambusae Concretio Silicea

Sweet in flavor and cold in nature, *tiān zhú huáng* (bamboo sugar) has a special ability to clear heat and phlegm from the heart channel, open the orifices and arouse the spirit, and sweep phlegm and stabilize fright.

For febrile disease characterized by clouded spirit due to high fever (heat evil entering the heart), copious phlegm, and delirious speech, combine *tiān zhú huáng* with medicinals such as *lián qiáo* (forsythia), *shēng shí gāo* (crude gypsum), *zhī mǔ* (anemarrhena), *xuán shēn* (scrophularia), *yuǎn zhì* (polygala), *chāng pú* (acorus), *chén dǎn xīng* (old bile arisaema), *zhú yè juǎn xīn* (tender lophatherum leaf), and *huáng lián* (coptis). If the patient also presents with convulsions of the limbs and bruxism (grinding of the teeth) due to phlegm and heat engendering wind, add medicinals such as:

gōu téng (钩藤 uncaria, Uncariae Ramulus cum Uncis)

quán xiē (全蝎 scorpion, Scorpio)

wú gōng (蜈蚣 centipede, Scolopendra)

yù jīn (郁金 curcuma, Curcumae Radix)

xī jiǎo (犀角 rhinoceros horn, Rhinocerotis Cornu)

líng yáng jiǎo fěn (羚羊角粉 antelope horn powder, Saigae Tataricae Cornu Pulveratum) (take drenched)

To treat children with lung heat causing cough and panting, as well as copious phlegm, use *tiān zhú huáng* with medicinals such as *guā lóu* (trichosanthes), *zhī mǔ* (anemarrhena), *huáng qín* (scutellaria), *bèi mǔ* (fritillaria), and *pí pá yè* (loquat leaf). For childhood phlegm-heat fright wind marked by copious phlegm in the throat, **hoisted eyes**[552] (吊眼 *diào yǎn*), forward-staring eyes, clenched jaw, and convulsions of the limbs, use it in combination with medicinals such as *dǎn xīng* (bile arisaema), *xióng huáng* (realgar), *niú huáng* (bovine bezoar), *zhū shā* (cinnabar), *shè xiāng* (musk), *yù jīn* (curcuma), *bái jiāng cán* (silkworm), *fú líng* (poria), *chán tuì* (cicada molting), and *quán xiē* (scorpion). *Niú huáng zhèn jīng wán* (Bovine Bezoar Fright-Settling Pill) and *bào lóng wán* (Dragon-Embracing Pill) are examples of this use that are available in prepared form.

For **wind strike**[568] (中风 *zhòng fēng*) with loss of speech, phlegm-drool congestion, deviated eyes and mouth, and hemiplegia, use *tiān zhú huáng* in combination with medicinals such as:

bái jiāng cán (白僵蚕 silkworm, Bombyx Batryticatus)

tiān má (天麻 gastrodia, Gastrodiae Rhizoma)

dǎn xīng (胆星 bile arisaema, Arisaema cum Bile)

shí jué míng (石决明 abalone shell, Haliotidis Concha)

quán xiē (全蝎 scorpion, Scorpio)

guā lóu (瓜蒌 trichosanthes, Trichosanthis Fructus)

sāng zhī (桑枝 mulberry twig, Mori Ramulus)

hóng huā (红花 carthamus, Carthami Flos)

gōu téng (钩藤 uncaria, Uncariae Ramulus cum Uncis)

COMPARISONS

Dǎn xīng (bile arisaema)[361] tends to flush and disperse heat-phlegm from the lung, spleen, and liver channels, whereas *tiān zhú huáng* tends to clear and sweep heat-phlegm from the heart channel.

Chuān bèi mǔ (Sìchuān fritillaria)[436] moistens dryness and transforms phlegm in the lung channel, whereas *tiān zhú huáng* stabilizes fright and eliminates phlegm from the heart channel.

DOSAGE

The dosage is generally 2.5–9 g/1–3 qián.

---

48. 竹茹 Zhú Rú
Bamboo Shavings

Bambusae
Caulis in Taenia

Sweet in flavor and slightly cold in nature, *zhú rú* (bamboo shavings) clears heat and eliminates vexation, transforms phlegm, and checks retching.

For heat in the stomach causing retching counterflow and heart vexation, immediate vomiting of ingested food, a yellow tongue fur, thirst, and a rapid pulse, combine *zhú rú* with medicinals such as *huáng lián* (coptis), *jú pí* (tangerine peel), *bàn xià* (pinellia), and *fú líng* (poria). For center burner phlegm-heat ascending counterflow and causing nausea and vomiting, rib-side distention, fright palpitations and sleeplessness, center burner vexation and derangement, hiccups, bitter taste in the mouth, vomitus in the form of turbid phlegm-like sticky fluid or that is foul-smelling, use *wēn dǎn tāng* (Gallbladder-Warming Decoction) with the addition of *huáng qín* (scutellaria) and *pí pá yè* (loquat leaf).

Wēn dǎn tāng 温胆汤   Gallbladder-Warming Decoction

---

zhú rú (竹茹 bamboo shavings, Bambusae Caulis in Taenia)

zhǐ shí (枳实 unripe bitter orange, Aurantii Fructus Immaturus)

bàn xià (半夏 pinellia, Pinelliae Rhizoma)

jú pí (橘皮 tangerine peel, Citri Reticulatae Pericarpium)

fú líng (茯苓 poria, Poria)

gān cǎo (甘草 licorice, Glycyrrhizae Radix)

For stomach vacuity with heat causing retching counterflow and vexation, *zhú rú* is the most suitable medicinal. Its sweet flavor harmonizes the stomach; its cold nature clears heat. For this condition, use *jú pí zhú rú tāng* (Tangerine Peel and Bamboo Shavings Decoction) from *Jīn Guì Yào Lüè* (金匮要略 "Essential Prescriptions of the Golden Coffer").

Jú pí zhú rú tāng 橘皮竹茹汤   Tangerine Peel and Bamboo Shavings Decoction

---

zhú rú (竹茹 bamboo shavings, Bambusae Caulis in Taenia)

jú pí (橘皮 tangerine peel, Citri Reticulatae Pericarpium)

dǎng shēn (党参 codonopsis, Codonopsis Radix)

gān cǎo (廿草 licorice, Glycyrrhizae Radix)

dà zǎo (大枣 jujube, Jujubae Fructus)

To treat **malign obstruction**[557] (遏阻 *è zǔ*, i.e., morning sickness) in pregnancy causing vomiting and vexation, *zhú rú* is often combined with medicinals such as:

huáng qín (黄芩 scutellaria, Scutellariae Radix)

jú pí (橘皮 tangerine peel, Citri Reticulatae Pericarpium)

fú líng (茯苓 poria, Poria)

sū gěng (苏梗 perilla stem, Perillae Caulis)

zhú yè (竹叶 lophatherum, Lophatheri Herba)

COMPARISONS

Zhú yè (lophatherum)[289] clears upper burner heat and vexation, cools the heart, and disinhibits water. *Zhú rú* clears center burner heat and vexation, harmonizes the stomach, and checks vomiting.

Bàn xià (pinellia)[359] is warm and drying; it checks retching by transforming dampness and phlegm. *Zhú rú* is sweet and cold; it checks retching by dispersing heat and phlegm.

Pí pá yè (loquat leaf)[446] clears heat from the lung and stomach; it tends to be used for wind-heat repletion fire causing cough and vomiting. *Zhú rú* clears heat from the lung and stomach; it tends to be used for vacuity heat phlegm turbidity causing vexation and retching counterflow.

The dosage is generally 4.5–9 g/1.5 qián–3 qián.

---

49. 竹沥 Zhú Lì   Bambusae Succus
Bamboo Sap

Sweet, slightly bitter, and acrid in flavor and cold in nature, *zhú lì* (bamboo sap)[52] is a very important medicinal for dispelling phlegm. It has a unique ability to dispel phlegm and turbidity from the channels and network vessels, the limbs, and **outside the membrane within the skin**[559] (皮里膜外 *pí lǐ mó wài*).

---

[52] *Zhú lì* (bamboo sap) is not readily available in the West. It is usually replaced in formulas by *tiān zhú huáng* (bamboo sugar). Note that *zhú lì* is a liquid and, when available, is usually packaged in glass vials. (Ed.)

1. Wind Strike with Loss of Speech and Hemiplegia: For liver wind stirring internally and wind-phlegm harassing the upper body causing wind strike, which manifests in collapse, loss of consciousness, clenched jaw, phlegm accompanied by a gurgling sound, hemiplegia, and difficult speech, use 9–30 g/3 qián–1 liǎng of *zhú lì* (mixed with 2–3 drops of *shēng jiāng zhī* (ginger juice)); take it drenched with a decoction prescribed for the individual pattern. If the patient is unable to swallow, this combination is administered through a nasal feeding tube. If the spirit-mind has already become clear again (i.e., the patient has regained consciousness), but there is still hemiplegia or lack of control over the limbs due to phlegm turbidity obstructing the channels and network vessels and disrupting the flow of qì and blood, use this medicinal to dispel phlegm turbidity from the channels and network vessels of the limbs and from outside the membrane within the skin. For this purpose it should be taken drenched with an appropriate decoction medicine. It is most effective when taken with several drops of *shēng jiāng zhī*. I often achieve good results in treating hemiplegia caused by cerebral thrombosis by using 15–60 g/ 5 qián–2 liǎng of *zhú lì* (mixed with several drops of *shēng jiāng zhī*) in combination with medicinals such as:

> *sāng zhī* (桑枝 mulberry twig, Mori Ramulus)
>
> *hóng huā* (红花 carthamus, Carthami Flos)
>
> *chì sháo* (赤芍 red peony, Paeoniae Radix Rubra)
>
> *chuān xiōng* (川芎 chuanxiong, Chuanxiong Rhizoma)
>
> *dāng guī wěi* (当归尾 Chinese angelica tail, Angelicae Sinensis Radicis Extremitas)
>
> *táo rén* (桃仁 peach kernel, Persicae Semen)
>
> *zhì shān jiǎ* (炙山甲 mix-fried pangolin scales, Manis Squama cum Liquido Fricta)
>
> *dì lóng* (地龙 earthworm, Pheretima)
>
> *dǎn xīng* (胆星 bile arisaema, Arisaema cum Bile)
>
> *gōu téng* (钩藤 uncaria, Uncariae Ramulus cum Uncis)
>
> *guā lóu* (瓜蒌 trichosanthes, Trichosanthis Fructus)
>
> *bàn xià* (半夏 pinellia, Pinelliae Rhizoma)

2. Fright-Wind in Children or Mania and Withdrawal Pattern in Adults: For children with congested phlegm-heat harassing upwards to the clear orifices and phlegm-heat producing wind, which results in symptoms such as fright wind convulsions, grinding of the teeth and **hoisted eyes**[552] (吊眼 *diào yǎn*), and ejection of phlegm-drool with bubbles, use *zhú lì* to clear phlegm-heat from the heart and stomach, thus extinguishing wind by transforming phlegm. For this purpose, 3–6 g/1–2 qián of this medicinal is poured into the mouth or taken drenched with a decoction.

In adults, when liver qì depression transforms into heat and phlegm-heat clouds the orifices of the heart, which causes changes in consciousness that possibly include cursing and hitting others, climbing on roofs and walls, laughing and crying alone, and talking to oneself, use *zhú lì* to clear heat and transform phlegm, lubricate the intestines and free the stool, and clear phlegm-heat from the heart and stomach. For this purpose it is often combined with medicinals such as:

yù jīn (郁金 curcuma, Curcumae Radix)

tiān zhú huáng (天竹黄 bamboo sugar, Bambusae Concretio Silicea)

chāng pú (菖蒲 acorus, Acori Tatarinowii Rhizoma)

yuǎn zhì (远志 polygala, Polygalae Radix)

xiāng fù (香附 cyperus, Cyperi Rhizoma)

shēng dài zhě shí (生代赭石 crude hematite, Haematitum Crudum)

qīng méng shí (青礞石 chlorite, Chloriti Lapis)

dǎn xīng (胆星 bile arisaema, Arisaema cum Bile)

shēng tiě luò (生铁落 iron flakes, Ferri Frusta)

huáng lián (黄连 coptis, Coptidis Rhizoma)

huáng qín (黄芩 scutellaria, Scutellariae Radix)

dà huáng (大黄 rhubarb, Rhei Radix et Rhizoma)

3. Heat Entering the Pericardium: For patients with febrile diseases who suddenly present with coma during the high-fever stage of the disease and who have phlegm with gurgling sounds, delirious speech, and vexation and agitation, use *zhú lì* to clear and transform phlegm and heat in the chest and heart channel. For this purpose it is often combined with medicinals such as:

niú huáng (牛黄 bovine bezoar, Bovis Calculus)

guǎng xī jiǎo (广犀角 African rhinoceros horn, Rhinocerotis Cornu Africanum)

shēng dì huáng (生地黄 dried/fresh rehmannia, Rehmanniae Radix Exsiccata seu Recens)

xuán shēn (玄参 scrophularia, Scrophulariae Radix)

yù jīn (郁金 curcuma, Curcumae Radix)

huáng lián (黄连 coptis, Coptidis Rhizoma)

lián qiáo xīn (连翘心 forsythia seed, Forsythiae Semen)

yuǎn zhì (远志 polygala, Polygalae Radix)

chāng pú (菖蒲 acorus, Acori Tatarinowii Rhizoma)

In recent years, *zhú lì* has been used to treat infectious encephalitis B and epidemic cerebrospinal meningitis that present with the symptoms described above. In such cases, 0.6–1.2 g/2–4 fēn of *zhú lì* (bamboo sap) is given with *ān gōng niú huáng wán* (Peaceful Palace Bovine Bezoar Pill) through a feeding tube in the nose. This combination has proven useful for dispelling phlegm, clearing heat, and arousing the spirit.

COMPARISONS

Bái jiè zǐ (white mustard)[364] expels phlegm from outside the membrane within the skin, but it is warm in nature, whereas *zhú lì* is cold in nature and is particularly able to expel phlegm from the channels and network vessels.

Tiān zhú huáng (bamboo sugar) and *zhú lì* both clear heat and phlegm from the heart. But the former tends to be drying, whereas the latter has a lubricating, disinhibiting nature.

Zhú lì is cold and lubricating, and so it is best to add several drops of *shēng jiāng zhī* (ginger juice)[28] to each liáng. This addition increases its ability to move through the channels and network vessels, move through the limbs, and to expel phlegm from outside the membrane within the skin. It also prevents the stomach from being damaged by too much cold.

The dosage is generally 9–30 g/3 qián–1 liǎng; in severe cases, use up to 60 g/2 liǎng.[53]

CAUTION

This medicinal is contraindicated for cold phlegm, cold cough, a weak stomach with poor digestion, and sloppy diarrhea.

---

50. 昆布　Kūn Bù Kelp	Laminariae/Eckloniae Thallus

Salty in flavor and cold in nature, *kūn bù* (kelp) softens hardness and dissipates binds, and transforms phlegm and disperses accumulations.

Kūn bù (kelp) is used for phlegm and qì binding and gathering that causes scrofula, goiter, and tumors of the neck (including tubercular lymphadenitis of the neck and thyroid gland tumors). For these conditions it is combined with medicinals such as:

xuán shēn (玄参 scrophularia, Scrophulariae Radix)

shēng mǔ lì (生牡蛎 crude oyster shell, Ostreae Concha Cruda)

xià kū cǎo (夏枯草 prunella, Prunellae Spica)

bèi mǔ (贝母 fritillaria, Fritillariae Bulbus)

huáng qín (黄芩 scutellaria, Scutellariae Radix)

chì sháo (赤芍 red peony, Paeoniae Radix Rubra)

hóng huā (红花 carthamus, Carthami Flos)

bǎi bù (百部 stemona, Stemonae Radix)

hǎi zǎo (海藻 sargassum, Sargassum)

To treat glomus[551] (痞 *pǐ*), aggregations[542] (癖 *pǐ*), and concretions and conglomerations[544] (癥瘕 *zhēng jiǎ*) in the abdomen (including hepatosplenomegaly, pelvic cysts, and tumors) caused by phlegm and food stagnation or long-term blood stasis, combine *kūn bù* with medicinals such as the following to disperse and dissipate accumulations and lumps:

zhì biē jiǎ (炙鳖甲 mix-fried turtle shell, Trionycis Carapax cum Liquido Frictus)

shēng mǔ lì (生牡蛎 crude oyster shell, Ostreae Concha Cruda)

xiāng fù (香附 cyperus, Cyperi Rhizoma)

cǎo hóng huā (草红花 carthamus, Carthami Flos)

---

[53]This medicinal is usually mixed into a decoction just before it is imbibed.　(Ed.)

zhì shān jiǎ (炙山甲 mix-fried pangolin scales, Manis Squama cum Liquido Fricta)

jiāo shén qū (焦神曲 scorch-fried medicated leaven, Massa Medicata Fermentata Usta)

shān zhā hé (山楂核 crataegus pit, Crataegi Endocarpium et Semen)

dāng guī (当归 Chinese angelica, Angelicae Sinensis Radix)

táo rén (桃仁 peach kernel, Persicae Semen)

sān léng (三棱 sparganium, Sparganii Rhizoma)

é zhú (莪术 curcuma rhizome, Curcumae Rhizoma)

Research

According to modern research reports, this medicinal is used for hyperthyroid and goiter due to iodine deficiency.

Comparisons

Hǎi zǎo (sargassum)[331] and *kūn bù* have very similar effects, the main difference being that the former has a relatively moderate medicinal strength, whereas the latter is much more fierce and is also lubricating and disinhibiting. There is a saying that taking large amounts of medicinals like these would cause one to become thin. I myself have advised obese patients with arteriosclerosis and high cholesterol to eat a lot of *hǎi dài* (eelgrass) and have found that it definitely assists the treatment.

Dosage

The dosage is generally 6–9 g/2–3 qián.

Caution

This medicinal is inappropriate for patients with spleen-stomach vacuity cold or gathering and accumulations due to cold phlegm.

---

51. 海藻 Hǎi Zǎo
Sargassum

Sargassum

Bitter and salty in flavor and cold in nature, *hǎi zǎo* (sargassum) is the same in action as *kūn bù* (kelp), except that it has a moderate medicinal strength and the additional action of disinhibiting water. It is mainly used to dissipate scrofula, for which it is combined with medicinals such as *lián qiáo* (forsythia), *chén pí* (tangerine peel), *qīng pí* (unripe tangerine peel), *bàn xià* (pinellia), *xià kū cǎo* (prunella), *tiān nán xīng* (arisaema), *huáng qín* (scutellaria), *xuán shēn* (scrophularia), *shēng mǔ lì* (crude oyster shell), and *niú bàng zǐ* (arctium). It is also used to treat goiter and tumors of the neck, for which it is combined with medicinals such as:

kūn bù (昆布 kelp, Laminariae/Eckloniae Thallus)

chuān xiōng (川芎 chuanxiong, Chuanxiong Rhizoma)

xià kū cǎo (夏枯草 prunella, Prunellae Spica)

dāng guī (当归 Chinese angelica, Angelicae Sinensis Radix)

bái zhǐ (白芷 Dahurian angelica, Angelicae Dahuricae Radix)

xì xīn (细辛 asarum, Asari Herba)

guān guì (官桂 quilled cinnamon, Cinnamomi Cortex Tubiformis)

shēng mǔ lì (生牡蛎 crude oyster shell, Ostreae Concha Cruda)

xiāng fù (香附 cyperus, Cyperi Rhizoma)

dǎn xīng (胆星 bile arisaema, Arisaema cum Bile)

Comparisons

Hǎi dài (eelgrass) also softens hardness and dissipates scrofula, but its medicinal strength is much less than that of *hǎi zǎo* or *kūn bù* (kelp).

Dosage

The dosage is generally 6–12 g/2–4 qián.

Caution

This medicinal is inappropriate in cases of spleen-stomach vacuity cold. It should not be combined with *gān cǎo* (licorice).[54]

---

52. 代赭石 Dài Zhě Shí   Haematitum
Hematite

Bitter and sweet in flavor and cold in nature, *dài zhě shí* (hematite) stabilizes counterflow, downbears fire, calms the liver, and nourishes the blood.

1. Stabilizing Counterflow: For stomach qì ascending counterflow that causes vomiting, eructation (a symptom that is less severe than hiccup, but more severe than belching), stomach fullness that causes qì counterflow, glomus and oppression in the stomach duct that will not go down, or, in severe cases, **stomach reflux**[564] (反胃 *fǎn wèi*) and **dysphagia-occlusion**[548] (噎膈 *yē gé*), use *dài zhě shí* in combination with medicinals such as:

xuán fù huā (旋覆花 inula flower, Inulae Flos)

bàn xià (半夏 pinellia, Pinelliae Rhizoma)

shēng jiāng (生姜 fresh ginger, Zingiberis Rhizoma Recens)

dà zǎo (大枣 jujube, Jujubae Fructus)

bīng láng (槟榔 areca, Arecae Semen)

gōng dīng xiāng (公丁香 clove, Caryophylli Flos)

sū gěng (苏梗 perilla stem, Perillae Caulis)

For patients who are elderly, or who have enduring illness or weak stomach qì, remove *bīng láng* (areca) from the above formula and add *dǎng shēn* (codonopsis). For cases of dysphagia-occlusion, add *shā shēn* (adenophora/glehnia), *bèi mǔ* (fritillaria), *shān cí gū* (cremastra/pleione), and *chǔ tóu kāng* (rice husk). For stomach reflux, add *fù zǐ* (aconite), *ròu guì* (cinnamon bark), and *dāo dòu zǐ* (sword bean).

---

[54]This prohibition dates back to ancient times. It is one of the **eighteen clashes**[548] (十八反 *shí bā fǎn*). (Ed.)

2. Downbearing Fire: *Dài zhĕ shí* downbears fire, cools the blood, and stanches bleeding. For fire-heat causing **frenetic movement of the blood**[550] (血热妄行 *xuè rè wàng xíng*) that results in nosebleeds, blood ejection, coughing of blood, bloody stool, and uterine bleeding, it is combined with medicinals such as:

> *shēng dì huáng* (生地黄 dried/fresh rehmannia, Rehmanniae Radix Exsiccata seu Recens)
>
> *dān pí* (丹皮 moutan, Moutan Cortex)
>
> *zhī zĭ* (栀子 gardenia, Gardeniae Fructus)
>
> *xuán shēn* (玄参 scrophularia, Scrophulariae Radix)
>
> *ē jiāo* (阿胶 ass hide glue, Asini Corii Colla)
>
> *bái máo gēn* (白茅根 imperata, Imperatae Rhizoma)
>
> *dà jì* (大蓟 Japanese thistle, Cirsii Japonici Herba seu Radix)
>
> *xiăo jì* (小蓟 field thistle, Cirsii Herba)

For bloody stool, add *huái huā tàn* (charred sophora flower) and *dì yú tàn* (charred sanguisorba). For uterine bleeding, add *zōng tàn* (charred trachycarpus), *ài yè tàn* (charred mugwort), and *xù tàn* (charred dipsacus).

3. Calming the Liver: When ascendant hyperactivity of liver yáng causes headache or dizziness, use *dài zhĕ shí* in combination with medicinals such as *jú huā* (chrysanthemum), *bái jí lí* (tribulus), *gōu téng* (uncaria), *huáng qín* (scutellaria), and *tiān má* (gastrodia). For liver fire surging upward or liver qì depression with enduring depression transforming into heat and resulting in rashness, impatience, irascibility, distention in the head, oppression in the chest, insomnia, and in severe cases yelling, cursing, or fighting, use large doses of *dài zhĕ shí* to tranquilize the patient, and to calm the liver and clear heat. For this purpose it is often combined with medicinals such as:

> *huáng qín* (黄芩 scutellaria, Scutellariae Radix)
>
> *huáng lián* (黄连 coptis, Coptidis Rhizoma)
>
> *tiān zhú huáng* (天竹黄 bamboo sugar, Bambusae Concretio Silicea)
>
> *dăn xīng* (胆星 bile arisaema, Arisaema cum Bile)
>
> *xiāng fù* (香附 cyperus, Cyperi Rhizoma)
>
> *shēng mŭ lì* (生牡蛎 crude oyster shell, Ostreae Concha Cruda)
>
> *shēng tiĕ luò* (生铁落 iron flakes, Ferri Frusta)

For fright, epilepsy, convulsions, and related patterns, one may add this medicinal to decoctions formulated for the pattern in order to calm the liver and to settle and stabilize. According to modern research reports, this medicinal has a tranquilizing effect on the central nervous system.

4. Nourishing the Blood: *Dài zhĕ shí* enters the blood aspect of the liver channel (the liver stores blood) and of the pericardium channel (the heart governs the blood). It has a sweet and bitter flavor and is cold in nature. It clears heat as well as nourishing the blood; therefore, it is used for blood heat that causes blood ejection, nosebleed, and coughing of blood that lead to blood vacuity flusteredness and yellow face. For these conditions, use *dài zhĕ shí* in combination with medicinals such as:

bái sháo (白芍 white peony, Paeoniae Radix Alba)

dāng guī (当归 Chinese angelica, Angelicae Sinensis Radix)

shēng dì huáng (生地黄 dried/fresh rehmannia, Rehmanniae Radix Exsiccata seu Recens)

shú dì huáng (熟地黄 cooked rehmannia, Rehmanniae Radix Praeparata)

shā shēn (沙参 adenophora/glehnia, Adenophorae seu Glehniae Radix)

yù zhú (玉竹 Solomon's seal, Polygonati Odorati Rhizoma)

lóng yǎn ròu (龙眼肉 longan flesh, Longan Arillus)

chén pí (陈皮 tangerine peel, Citri Reticulatae Pericarpium)

Although this medicinal nourishes the blood and engenders blood, the dosage should not be too high. According to modern research reports, this medicinal contains iron and when taken internally has an astringent effect on the intestinal wall and a protective effect on the intestinal mucosa. Once it enters the blood stream, it promotes the production of red blood cells and hemochrome.

COMPARISONS

Xuán fù huā (inula flower)[211] enters the qì aspect, downbears lung and stomach qì, expels phlegm turbidity, and checks counterflow retching. *Dài zhě shí* enters the blood aspect, suppresses and downbears liver and stomach qì counterflow, clears heat and nourishes the blood, and checks vomiting and spontaneous bleeding.

Chì shí zhī (halloysite) is warm and astringent, and therefore checks enduring dysentery, bloody stool, and flooding and spotting. It tends to be used for bleeding in the lower body. *Dài zhě shí* is a heavy-settling, bitter, cold medicinal; it checks vomiting and stops flooding and spotting. It is used to treat bleeding in both the upper and lower body.

Cí shí (loadstone) pulls down lesser yīn (*shào yīn*) kidney fire that is flaming upward and conducts lung qì into the kidney. It therefore is used to supplement the kidney to promote qì absorption. *Dài zhě shí* settles reverting yīn (*jué yīn*) liver channel counterflow and expels heat from the blood vessels. It is therefore used to nourish the blood and settle the liver.

Dài zhě shí, when used raw, downbears fire, calms the liver, settles counterflow, cools the blood, and clears heat. When it is used calcined, it has the additional quality of being astringent; thus it is used to stanch bleeding and check diarrhea. Currently, *shēng dài zhě shí* (crude hematite) is the most commonly used form in clinical practice. Occasionally, one encounters patients who need to take *dài zhě shí* but cannot take it because they have sloppy stool. In such cases, use *duàn zhě shí* (calcined hematite) instead. The dosage of *shēng dài zhě shí* (crude hematite) is somewhat larger, whereas the dosage of *duàn zhě shí* (calcined hematite) should be somewhat smaller.

The dosage is generally 9–30 g/3 qián–1 liǎng; in severe cases, use up to 60–90 g/ 2–3 liǎng. The dosage for *duàn zhě shí* (calcined hematite) is generally 6–15 g/ 2–5 qián.[55]

CAUTION

This medicinal is contraindicated for gastrointestinal vacuity cold and pregnant women.

---

53. 石决明 Shí Jué Míng   Haliotidis Concha
Abalone Shell

Salty in flavor and cool in nature, *shí jué míng* (abalone shell) calms the liver and subdues yáng, boosts yīn and brightens the eyes. It is the most commonly used medicinal for treating insufficiency of liver yīn and ascendant hyperactivity of liver yáng.

1. **Headache and Dizziness:** For liver-kidney yīn vacuity causing ascendant hyperactivity of liver yáng that presents with symptoms such as headache, hemilateral headache, dizzy head, dizzy vision, insomnia, rashness, irascibility, and booming heat [effusion] (轰热 *hōng rè*, recurrent episodes of a sudden feeling of heat that quickly dissipates), which includes hypertensive patients with these symptoms, *shí jué míng* is used to nourish liver yīn and subdue liver yáng. It is often combined with medicinals such as:

shēng dài zhě shí (生代赭石 crude hematite, Haematitum Crudum)

shēng dì huáng (生地黄 dried/fresh rehmannia, Rehmanniae Radix Exsiccata seu Recens)

shēng bái sháo (生白芍 raw white peony, Paeoniae Radix Alba Cruda)

huáng qín (黄芩 scutellaria, Scutellariae Radix)

xiāng fù (香附 cyperus, Cyperi Rhizoma)

xià kū cǎo (夏枯草 prunella, Prunellae Spica)

jú huā (菊花 chrysanthemum, Chrysanthemi Flos)

tiān má (天麻 gastrodia, Gastrodiae Rhizoma)

gōu téng (钩藤 uncaria, Uncariae Ramulus cum Uncis)

sāng jì shēng (桑寄生 mistletoe, Taxilli Herba)

niú xī (牛膝 achyranthes, Achyranthis Bidentatae Radix)

zé xiè (泽泻 alisma, Alismatis Rhizoma)

bái jí lí (白蒺藜 tribulus, Tribuli Fructus)

For patients with neurasthenia who also present with the symptoms described above, I often prescribe the following formula, which I have tentatively named *yì shén tāng* (Spirit-Compensating Decoction).

---

[55] It is best to purchase *dài zhě shí* (hematite) as a powder or use the calcined medicinal because it is almost impossible to crush it to size in a standard crushing mortar. *Dài zhě shí* should be predecocted. (Ed.)

Yì shén tāng 挹神汤   Spirit-Compensating Decoction

shēng shí jué míng (生石决明 crude abalone shell, Haliotidis Concha Cruda)
    15–45 g/5 qián–1.5 liǎng (predecoct)

shēng dài zhě shí (生代赭石 crude hematite, Haematitum Crudum)
    25–45 g/8 qián–1.5 liǎng (predecoct)

shēng dì huáng (生地黄 dried/fresh rehmannia, Rehmanniae Radix Exsiccata
    seu Recens) 12 g/4 qián

shēng bái sháo (生白芍 raw white peony, Paeoniae Radix Alba Cruda)
    12 g/4 qián

xiāng fù (香附 cyperus, Cyperi Rhizoma) 9 g/3 qián

huáng qín (黄芩 scutellaria, Scutellariae Radix) 9 g/3 qián

bái jí lí (白蒺藜 tribulus, Tribuli Fructus) 12 g/4 qián

jú huā (菊花 chrysanthemum, Chrysanthemi Flos) 9 g/3 qián

yuǎn zhì (远志 polygala, Polygalae Radix) 9 g/3 qián

yè jiāo téng (夜交藤 flowery knotweed stem, Polygoni Multiflori Caulis)
    15–30 g/5 qián–1 liǎng

I have observed 55 cases that were treated with this as the base formula, with modifications made in accordance with signs. Of these 55 cases, 8 completely recovered, 8 were basically cured, 17 showed marked improvement, 19 showed improvement, and only 3 showed no improvement in symptoms. This formula is certainly effective and is also used for menopausal symptoms.

2. Visual Obstructions: For fire in the liver channel that gives rise to sore red swollen eyes, aversion to light, or eye screens and obstructions, use *shí jué míng* to clear liver heat and brighten the eyes. For this purpose it is often combined with medicinals such as:

sāng yè (桑叶 mulberry leaf, Mori Folium)

jú huā (菊花 chrysanthemum, Chrysanthemi Flos)

màn jīng zǐ (蔓荆子 vitex, Viticis Fructus)

huáng qín (黄芩 scutellaria, Scutellariae Radix)

shēng dì huáng (生地黄 dried/fresh rehmannia, Rehmanniae Radix Exsiccata
    seu Recens)

mù zéi cǎo (木贼草 equisetum, Equiseti Hiemalis Herba)

cǎo jué míng (草决明 fetid cassia, Cassiae Semen)

For liver-kidney yīn vacuity and ascendant hyperactivity of liver yáng causing distention in the head, eye pain, loss of visual acuity, internal obstruction (内障 *nèi zhàng*), or glaucoma, it is used to nourish liver yīn, clear liver heat, and brighten the eyes. For this purpose it is often combined with medicinals such as:

shēng dì huáng (生地黄 dried/fresh rehmannia, Rehmanniae Radix Exsiccata
    seu Recens)

shú dì huáng (熟地黄 cooked rehmannia, Rehmanniae Radix Praeparata)

dì gǔ pí (地骨皮 lycium root bark, Lycii Cortex)

shí hú (石斛 dendrobium, Dendrobii Herba)

tù sī zǐ (菟丝子 cuscuta, Cuscutae Semen)

shān zhū yú (山茱萸 cornus, Corni Fructus)

wǔ wèi zǐ (五味子 schisandra, Schisandrae Fructus)

gǒu qǐ zǐ (枸杞子 lycium, Lycii Fructus)

jú huā (菊花 chrysanthemum, Chrysanthemi Flos)

yè míng shā (夜明砂 bat's droppings, Verspertilionis Faeces)

zhī mǔ (知母 anemarrhena, Anemarrhenae Rhizoma)

For blindness or unclear vision at night, it is combined with medicinals such as *zhū gān* (pig's liver), *yáng gān* (goat's or sheep's liver), *cāng zhú* (atractylodes), and *cǎo jué míng* (fetid cassia).

Used raw, *shí jué míng* has a much greater ability to nourish liver yīn, clear liver heat, and subdue and downbear liver yáng. After it is calcined, its ability to subdue and downbear and to clear heat is diminished; thus, *shēng shí jué míng* (crude abalone shell) is used more frequently in the clinic.

COMPARISONS

Mǔ lì (oyster shell)[171] subdues yáng and also enters the kidney channel; it mainly treats floating yáng straying to the exterior. *Shí jué míng* subdues yáng and enters the liver channel; it subdues and downbears liver yáng harassing upwards. *Mǔ lì* is astringent; *shí jué míng* is downbearing.

Zhēn zhū mǔ (mother-of-pearl)[163] subdues yáng and tends to nourish the heart and quiet the spirit. *Shí jué míng* subdues yáng, and tends to nourish the liver, subdue, and downbear. Its ability to subdue and downbear is much more pronounced than that of *zhēn zhū mǔ*.

DOSAGE

The dosage is generally 9–45 g/3 qián–1.5 liǎng. When using the calcined form, the dosage is usually 9–20 g/3–7 qián.

Lecture Seven
Warm & Hot Medicinals
温热药 *Wēn Rè Yào*

This lecture deals with medicinals that are warm or hot in nature and that dispel cold evil. An old axiom of therapy is "treat cold by warming" (寒者温之 *hán zhě wēn zhī*), which means use warm and hot medicinals to treat cold patterns. When cold evil is in the exterior, it must be treated with warm acrid exterior-resolving medicinals, which have been discussed in Lecture Two, Effusing and Dissipating Medicinals. When cold evil is in the interior, it is treated with warm and hot medicinals. Because medicinals that dispel cold evil can also assist the yáng qì of the human body, we can see that, from the point of view of supporting right (扶正 *fú zhèng*), warm and hot medicinals are also supplementing (i.e., yáng-supplementing) medicinals. They are also frequently used in combination with supplementing medicinals. Thus these two groups of medicinals should be viewed in relation to each other.

1. 附子 Fù Zǐ	Aconiti Radix
Aconite	Lateralis Praeparata

Also called *chuān fù zǐ* 川附子, literally "Sìchuān aconite," because the best is produced in the Province of Sìchuān. *Fù zǐ* is acrid and sweet in flavor, hot in nature, and toxic. It returns yáng and stems counterflow, expels cold and dries dampness, and warms and assists kidney yáng. Mobile rather than static in nature, it reaches into the interior and out to the exterior; it upbears and downbears. For any congealed and **intractable cold**[554] (痼冷 *gù lěng*) and for impediment binding in the bowels and viscera, sinews and bones, channels and network vessels, and blood vessels, *fù zǐ* has an opening, freeing, warming, and dissipating action. Whenever yáng qì is on the verge of desertion, marked by icy-cold limbs due to reverse-flow, cold dripping sweat, or **oily expiration sweating**[549] (绝汗 *jué hàn*), *fù zǐ* returns yáng and stems counterflow and immediately rescues the patient from danger.

1. **Returning Yáng and Stemming Counterflow:** When heart-kidney yáng is vacuous and on the verge of expiration or when great vomiting, great precipitation, or great sweating gives rise to yáng vacuity verging on desertion, critical signs

of vacuity cold that appear include faint pulse verging on expiration, reverse-flow of the limbs, and icy-cold extremities. Such conditions are treated by quickly giving 9–15 g/3–5 qián of *fù zǐ* to return yáng and expel cold, stimulate the yáng qì of the body, and strengthen the life force. For this *fù zǐ* is often combined with 9 g/ 3 qián of *gān jiāng* (dried ginger) and 6 g/2 qián of *zhì gān cǎo* (mix-fried licorice) to make *sì nì tāng* (Counterflow Cold Decoction); alternatively, *fù zǐ* is combined with 9–15 g/3–5 qián or even up to 30 g/1 liǎng of *rén shēn* (ginseng) to make *shēn fù tāng* (Ginseng and Aconite Decoction). Both these formulas return yáng and stem counterflow. Generally, *sì nì tāng* (Counterflow Cold Decoction) is used for patterns arising from internal cold, while *shēn fù tāng* (Ginseng and Aconite Decoction) is used for conditions arising from dual vacuity of qì and blood. If there is also great dripping sweat, one can add 9 g/3 qián each of *mài dōng* (ophiopogon) and *wǔ wèi zǐ* (schisandra). I frequently use *fù zǐ* in emergency treatment of various forms of shock and usually find it works best combined with *rén shēn* (ginseng), *mài dōng* (ophiopogon), *wǔ wèi zǐ* (schisandra), etc. If the patient cannot take the medicine orally, it can be administered by nasal feed. See also *rén shēn* (ginseng) on page 89 and *gān jiāng* (dried ginger) on page 348. When these medicinals are used in the treatment of shock, it is important to pay attention to pattern identification.

2. Expelling Cold and Drying Dampness: When wind, cold, and dampness invade the body, they cause stagnant qì and congealing blood. The signs of this are joint pain, muscular pain, numbness or heaviness of sinews and bones, and inhibited bending and stretching of the knee and elbow. The pain is exacerbated by damp, rainy, yīn-type weather. To treat such conditions, *fù zǐ* is used for its cold-expelling and dampness-drying qualities and is often combined with medicinals such as:

qiāng huó (羌活 notopterygium, Notopterygii Rhizoma et Radix)

dú huó (独活 pubescent angelica, Angelicae Pubescentis Radix)

wēi líng xiān (威灵仙 clematis, Clematidis Radix)

sāng jì shēng (桑寄生 mistletoe, Taxilli Herba)

qín jiāo (秦艽 large gentian, Gentianae Macrophyllae Radix)

chì sháo (赤芍 red peony, Paeoniae Radix Rubra)

zhì shān jiǎ (炙山甲 mix-fried pangolin scales, Manis Squama cum Liquido Fricta)

sōng jié (松节 knotty pine wood, Pini Nodi Lignum)

cāng zhú (苍术 atractylodes, Atractylodis Rhizoma)

dāng guī (当归 Chinese angelica, Angelicae Sinensis Radix)

When the spleen is invaded by cold, manifesting in signs such as abdominal pain, diarrhea, clear thin stool, cold extremities, and lack of warmth in the abdomen, use *fù zǐ* for the same action of expelling cold and drying dampness. For such cases, it is often combined with medicinals such as *gān jiāng* (dried ginger), *bái zhú* (white atractylodes), *dǎng shēn* (codonopsis), *fú líng* (poria), and *zhì gān cǎo* (mix-fried licorice).

3. Warming and Assisting Kidney Yáng: Debilitation of kidney yáng can take the form of a decrease in sexual function, which manifests as impotence in men and uterine cold infertility in women. *Fù zǐ* supplements the kidney and assists yáng, thereby strengthening sexual function. It is often combined with medicinals such as:

> lù jiǎo jiāo (鹿角胶 deerhorn glue, Cervi Cornus Gelatinum)
>
> shú dì huáng (熟地黄 cooked rehmannia, Rehmanniae Radix Praeparata)
>
> ròu guì (肉桂 cinnamon bark, Cinnamomi Cortex)
>
> tù sī zǐ (菟丝子 cuscuta, Cuscutae Semen)
>
> gǒu qǐ zǐ (枸杞子 lycium, Lycii Fructus)
>
> dāng guī (当归 Chinese angelica, Angelicae Sinensis Radix)
>
> bā jǐ tiān (巴戟天 morinda, Morindae Officinalis Radix)
>
> shēng ài yè (生艾叶 raw mugwort, Artemisiae Argyi Folium Crudum)
>
> yáng qǐ shí (阳起石 actinolite, Actinolitum)
>
> fú líng (茯苓 poria, Poria)

In Chinese medicine, it is believed that kidney yáng is the original yáng of the human body, the primal motor force of all life activity. Thus to warm and assist kidney yáng is also to boost original yáng. *Fù zǐ* is used to treat debilitation of kidney yáng that causes cold pain in the lumbus and knees, impotence, seminal cold, pain in the umbilical region, profuse urination at night, cold feet and limp knees, little thought of food and drink, fifth-watch diarrhea, fatigued spirit and fear of cold, and weak right cubit pulse. When supplementing kidney yīn, it is often used in combination with medicinals such as *shú dì huáng* (cooked rehmannia), *shān zhū yú* (cornus), *shān yào* (dioscorea), and *ròu guì* (cinnamon bark), as the following two examples show:

Bā wèi dì huáng wán 八味地黄丸   Eight-Ingredient Rehmannia Pill

> shú dì huáng (熟地黄 cooked rehmannia, Rehmanniae Radix Praeparata)
>
> shān zhū yú (山茱萸 cornus, Corni Fructus)
>
> shān yào (山药 dioscorea, Dioscoreae Rhizoma)
>
> dān pí (丹皮 moutan, Moutan Cortex)
>
> fú líng (茯苓 poria, Poria)
>
> zé xiè (泽泻 alisma, Alismatis Rhizoma)
>
> fù zǐ (附子 aconite, Aconiti Radix Lateralis Praeparata)
>
> ròu guì (肉桂 cinnamon bark, Cinnamomi Cortex)

Yòu guī yǐn 右归饮   Right-Restoring [Life Gate] Beverage

> shú dì huáng (熟地黄 cooked rehmannia, Rehmanniae Radix Praeparata)
>
> shān zhū yú (山茱萸 cornus, Corni Fructus)
>
> shān yào (山药 dioscorea, Dioscoreae Rhizoma)
>
> gǒu qǐ zǐ (枸杞子 lycium, Lycii Fructus)
>
> dù zhòng (杜仲 eucommia, Eucommiae Cortex)
>
> fù zǐ (附子 aconite, Aconiti Radix Lateralis Praeparata)
>
> ròu guì (肉桂 cinnamon bark, Cinnamomi Cortex)

gān cǎo (甘草 licorice, Glycyrrhizae Radix)

RESEARCH

According to modern research reports, *fù zǐ* (aconite) has a cardiotonic effect.

COMPARISONS

Ròu guì (cinnamon bark)[339] assists kidney yáng, warms the lower burner, and conducts upward floating fire down to the kidney (i.e., conducts fire to the origin). *Fù zǐ* returns yáng qì, frees the twelve channels, and restores dissipated original yáng (kidney yáng) on the verge of expiration.

Bái fù zǐ (typhonium)[368] is the tuber of a different plant. It is like *fù zǐ* (aconite) in shape (though smaller), and in Chinese is therefore called 白附子 *bái fù zǐ*, "white aconite." Tending to ascend, it dispels wind and dries phlegm, and is used to treat wind-phlegm diseases of the head and face, such as "hoisted line wind" (吊线风 *diào xiàn fēng*, neuroparalysis of the face with deviated eyes and mouth). *Chuān fù zǐ* returns yáng and expels cold, and assists kidney yáng. *Bái fù zǐ* (typhonium) has no power to assist kidney yáng.

Different processed forms of *fù zǐ* are known by a variety of names: *pào fù zǐ* (blast-fried aconite), *dàn fù piàn* (desalted sliced aconite), *hēi fù piàn* (black sliced aconite), and *bái fù piàn* (white sliced aconite). There are two slight distinctions in therapeutic effect. The most commonly used form, *pào fù zǐ* (blast-fried aconite), also called *hēi fù piàn* (black sliced aconite), has ample medicinal strength and is quick acting. *Dàn fù piàn* (desalted sliced aconite), also called *bái fù piàn* (white sliced aconite), has milder medicinal strength.[1]

In addition, there is *chuān wū* (aconite root), which comes from the same plant as *fù zǐ* (aconite) and is similar in nature, flavor, and action; indeed some pharmacies today do not distinguish between the two. Traditionally, however, physicians used *fù zǐ* to warm the kidney and assist yáng and used *chuān wū* to free impediment and dispel wind. See *wū tóu* (wild aconite), page 371.

COMBINATIONS

Fù zǐ combined with *rén shēn* (ginseng) and *shān zhū yú* (cornus) treats sweating desertion with collapse of yáng. Combined with *shú dì huáng* (cooked rehmannia) and *dāng guī* (Chinese angelica), its blood-engendering power is increased. Combined with *ròu guì* (cinnamon bark), it can supplement and assist kidney yáng.

---

[1]Soaking *fù zǐ* (aconite) with different substances and for different lengths of time produces *hēi fù piàn* (黑附片, black sliced aconite), *yán fù piàn* (盐附片, salted aconite), *bái fù piàn* (白附片, white sliced aconite), and *dàn fù piàn* (淡附片, desalted sliced aconite). *Hēi fù piàn* (黑附片, black sliced aconite) is dark brown (described as the color of strong tea) with a dark outer bark. *Yán fù piàn* (盐附片, salted aconite) is characterized by its salty taste and salt crystals on its surface. *Bái fù piàn* (白附片, white sliced aconite) is light yellow with no present outer bark, and, by the way, it is this *bái fù piàn* that is often sold as *bái fù zǐ* (白附子, typhonium). *Dàn fù piàn* (淡附片, desalted sliced aconite) is bland in taste; the books do not describe its appearance (and I have never seen it). *Pào fù zǐ* (炮附子, blast-fried aconite) is not *hēi fù piàn* (黑附片, black sliced aconite), but is cleaned *fù zǐ* (aconite) that is blast-fried in sand until it puffs and becomes black. *Dàn fù piàn* (淡附片, desalted sliced aconite) is not *bái fù zǐ* (白附子, typhonium), but is *yán fù piàn* (盐附片, salted sliced aconite) that is soaked to remove the salt and then soaked again with licorice and black beans. (Ed.)

Combined with *guì zhī* (cinnamon twig), *bái sháo* (white peony), and *huáng qí* (astragalus), it treats yáng vacuity spontaneous sweating.

DOSAGE

The dosage is generally 1.5–9 g/5 fēn–3 qián.

CAUTION

This medicinal is contraindicated for patterns other than vacuity-cold and cold-damp. Patients with **heat reversal**[552] (热厥 *rè jué*) can die instantly after taking it. It is contraindicated for pregnancy. Generally, it is not combined with the following[2]:

bàn xià (半夏 pinellia, Pinelliae Rhizoma)

guā lóu (瓜蒌 trichosanthes, Trichosanthis Fructus)

bèi mǔ (贝母 fritillaria, Fritillariae Bulbus)

bái jí (白及 bletilla, Bletillae Rhizoma)

bái liǎn (白蔹 ampelopsis, Ampelopsis Radix)

---

2. 肉桂 Ròu Guì   Cinnamomi Cortex
Cinnamon Bark

Acrid and sweet in flavor and hot in nature, *ròu guì* (cinnamon bark) warms and supplements kidney yáng, warms the center and expels cold, and diffuses the blood vessels. It is turbid, thick, congealing, and downbearing in nature; it is static rather than mobile. It tends to warm the lower burner and helps the yáng qì of the kidney, traditionally called the "life gate fire" (命门之火 *mìng mén zhī huǒ*). It also promotes qì absorption in the kidney and conducts fire to the origin.

1. **Warming and Supplementing Kidney Yáng:** Insufficiency of kidney yáng can cause impotence and **seminal cold**[562] (精冷 *jīng lěng*) in men and persistent infertility in women. *Ròu guì* (cinnamon bark) is combined with different medicinals for these two applications:

Men

lù róng (鹿茸 velvet deerhorn, Cervi Cornu Pantotrichum)

shú dì huáng (熟地黄 cooked rehmannia, Rehmanniae Radix Praeparata)

tù sī zǐ (菟丝子 cuscuta, Cuscutae Semen)

gǒu qǐ zǐ (枸杞子 lycium, Lycii Fructus)

tóng jí lí (潼蒺藜 complanate astragalus seed, Astragali Complanati Semen)

shān zhū yú (山茱萸 cornus, Corni Fructus)

fù zǐ (附子 aconite, Aconiti Radix Lateralis Praeparata)

ròu cōng róng (肉苁蓉 cistanche, Cistanches Herba)

bā jǐ tiān (巴戟天 morinda, Morindae Officinalis Radix)

shān yào (山药 dioscorea, Dioscoreae Rhizoma)

---

[2]These prohibitions are from the **eighteen clashes**[548] (十八反 *shí bā fǎn*). (Ed.)

fú líng (茯苓 poria, Poria)

zé xiè (泽泻 alisma, Alismatis Rhizoma)

Women

dāng guī (当归 Chinese angelica, Angelicae Sinensis Radix)

shú dì huáng (熟地黄 cooked rehmannia, Rehmanniae Radix Praeparata)

bái sháo (白芍 white peony, Paeoniae Radix Alba)

chuān xiōng (川芎 chuanxiong, Chuanxiong Rhizoma)

xiāng fù (香附 cyperus, Cyperi Rhizoma)

shēng ài yè (生艾叶 raw mugwort, Artemisiae Argyi Folium Crudum)

fù zǐ (附子 aconite, Aconiti Radix Lateralis Praeparata)

zǐ shí yīng (紫石英 fluorite, Fluoritum)

wú yú (吴萸 evodia, Evodiae Fructus)

wū yào (乌药 lindera, Linderae Radix)

Kidney yáng vacuity also causes **inhibited urination**[553] (小便不利 *xiǎo biàn bù lì*) and in severe cases even water swelling. In the treatment of such conditions, *ròu guì* is combined with medicinals such as *shú dì huáng* (cooked rehmannia), *shān yào* (dioscorea), *niú xī* (achyranthes), *shān zhū yú* (cornus), *fú líng* (poria), *dān pí* (moutan), *zé xiè* (alisma), *fù zǐ* (aconite), and *chē qián zǐ* (plantago seed) to form *jì shēng shèn qì wán* (Life Saver Kidney Qì Pill). See also "2. Warming and Assisting Kidney Yáng" in the section describing *fù zǐ* (aconite), page 339.

2. Warming the Center and Expelling Cold: For pain in the heart [region] and abdomen, abdominal distention, cold pain in the smaller abdomen, cold mounting (寒疝 *shàn*), or menstrual pain due to contraction of cold qì, *ròu guì* can be used in combination with medicinals such as *gāo liáng jiāng* (lesser galangal), *xiāng fù* (cyperus), *wú yú* (evodia), *xiǎo huí xiāng* (fennel), *wū yào* (lindera), *dīng xiāng* (clove), and *chén xiāng* (aquilaria). Spleen-kidney yáng vacuity affects movement and transformation in the center burner, and causes vacuity cold diarrhea with clear thin stool, in severe cases containing **untransformed food**[566] (完谷不化 *wán gǔ bù huà*). In this case, *ròu guì* may be combined with medicinals such as:

dǎng shēn (党参 codonopsis, Codonopsis Radix)

bái zhú (白术 white atractylodes, Atractylodis Macrocephalae Rhizoma)

fú líng (茯苓 poria, Poria)

zhì gān cǎo (炙甘草 mix-fried licorice, Glycyrrhizae Radix cum Liquido Fricta)

gān jiāng (干姜 dried ginger, Zingiberis Rhizoma)

fù zǐ (附子 aconite, Aconiti Radix Lateralis Praeparata)

bǔ gǔ zhī (补骨脂 psoralea, Psoraleae Fructus)

ròu dòu kòu (肉豆蔻 nutmeg, Myristicae Semen)

hē zǐ (诃子 chebule, Chebulae Fructus)

wǔ wèi zǐ (五味子 schisandra, Schisandrae Fructus)

I often combine *ròu guì* with medicinals such as:

fù zǐ (附子 aconite, Aconiti Radix Lateralis Praeparata)

dǎng shēn (党参 codonopsis, Codonopsis Radix)

bái zhú (白术 white atractylodes, Atractylodis Macrocephalae Rhizoma)

fú líng (茯苓 poria, Poria)

mù xiāng (木香 costusroot, Aucklandiae Radix)

bǔ gǔ zhī (补骨脂 psoralea, Psoraleae Fructus)

wú zhū yú (吴茱萸 evodia, Evodiae Fructus)

ròu dòu kòu (肉豆蔻 nutmeg, Myristicae Semen)

wǔ wèi zǐ (五味子 schisandra, Schisandrae Fructus)

hē zǐ (诃子 chebule, Chebulae Fructus)

chǎo shān yào (炒山药 stir-fried dioscorea, Dioscoreae Rhizoma Frictum)

zào xīn tǔ (灶心土 oven earth, Terra Flava Usta) (This ingredient is decocted in water and then the resulting decoction is used to cook the rest of the ingredients.)

This combination, varied in accordance with signs, is effective in treating diseases such as chronic dysentery and chronic enteritis that manifest in vacuity-cold diarrhea.

According to modern research, the volatile oils contained in *ròu guì* are a moderate stimulant and strengthen digestive function, expel accumulated gas in the digestive tract, and relieve cramping pain in the stomach and intestines.

3. Freeing the Blood Vessels: Blood flows in the vessels; cold causes congelation and impairs flow, whereas warmth promotes free flow. Qì and blood vacuity, cold evil stagnation, and poor flow of blood and qì can cause yīn flat-abscesses or cold and pain in the fingers or toes, or blackening and putrefaction of the finger and toe joints that in severe cases gives rise to sloughing. In Chinese medicine, this is traditionally called "sloughing flat-abscess"[563] (脱骨疽 *tuō gǔ jū*); and in modern medicine, it is called obliterating phlebitis. For this purpose use *ròu guì* to warm and free the blood vessels, usually combining it with medicinals such as *shú dì huáng* (cooked rehmannia) and *má huáng* (ephedra) (crushed together), *bái jiè zǐ* (white mustard), *lù jiǎo jiāo* (deerhorn glue), *fù piàn* (sliced aconite), *hóng huā* (carthamus), *gān jiāng* (dried ginger), *xì xīn* (asarum), and *guì zhī* (cinnamon twig) When owing to qì and blood vacuity, the welling- or flat-abscess fails to close after rupturing, use *shí quán dà bǔ tāng* (Perfect Major Supplementation Decoction):

Shí quán dà bǔ tāng 十全大补汤   Perfect Major Supplementation Decoction

---

ròu guì (肉桂 cinnamon bark, Cinnamomi Cortex)

dǎng shēn (党参 codonopsis, Codonopsis Radix)

huáng qí (黄芪 astragalus, Astragali Radix)

bái zhú (白术 white atractylodes, Atractylodis Macrocephalae Rhizoma)

fú líng (茯苓 poria, Poria)

dāng guī (当归 Chinese angelica, Angelicae Sinensis Radix)

bái sháo (白芍 white peony, Paeoniae Radix Alba)

chuān xiōng (川芎 chuanxiong, Chuanxiong Rhizoma)

shú dì huáng (熟地黄 cooked rehmannia, Rehmanniae Radix Praeparata)

zhì gān cǎo (炙廿草 mix-fried licorice, Glycyrrhizae Radix cum Liquido Fricta)

According to modern research, this medicinal causes vasodilation, both centrally and peripherally, and enhances blood circulation.

4. Conducting Fire to the Origin: When in debilitation of kidney yáng, traditionally called "insufficiency of the true fire of the life gate" (命门真火不足 *mìng mén zhēn huǒ bù zú*), vacuous yáng strays upward and manifests in a red face, vacuity panting, putting forth of oily sweat,[3] cold feet and knees, and a vacuous pulse without root,[4] as well as a slightly weak cubit pulse, this is upcast yáng in which there is true cold and false heat. This pattern requires swift treatment with *ròu guì* (cinnamon bark) to conduct fire to the origin and to promote qì absorption in the kidney. For this purpose, *ròu guì* is often combined with medicinals such as *shú dì huáng* (cooked rehmannia), *shān zhū yú* (cornus), *wǔ wèi zǐ* (schisandra), *rén shēn* (ginseng), *fù zǐ* (aconite), *duàn lóng gǔ* (calcined dragon bone), and *duàn mǔ lì* (calcined oyster shell). For kidney fire floating upward that manifests in upper body heat signs, such as dry mouth, sore throat, and toothache (marked by no redness or swelling of the gums, and by pain that grows worse at night and stretches into the cheeks), together with lower body cold, such as lumbar pain, cold legs and feet, sloppy stool, and weak cubit pulse, use *ròu guì* in order to conduct fire to the origin; it is usually combined with medicinals such as *xuán shēn* (scrophularia), *xù duàn* (dipsacus), *niú xī* (achyranthes), *shú dì huáng* (cooked rehmannia), *zhī mǔ* (anemarrhena), *xì xīn* (asarum), and *sāng jì shēng* (mistletoe). For this purpose, 0.9–2.5 g/3–8 fēn of *ròu guì* is sufficient.

COMPARISONS

Fù zǐ (aconite)[339] acts rapidly to treat yīn cold patterns in which yáng qì is about to dissipate (i.e., it returns yáng and stems counterflow, 回阳救逆 *huí yáng jiù nì*). For this reason, it is traditionally said to "rescue the yáng in yīn" (救阴中之 阳 *jiù yīn zhōng zhī yáng*). *Ròu guì* (cinnamon bark), being harmonious, moderate, turbid, and thick, supplements insufficiency of true fire in the lower burner and kidney (i.e., it warms and supplements kidney yáng). It also conducts fire to the origin in order to extinguish rootless fire. For this reason it is also traditionally said to "rescue the yáng in yáng" (救阳中之阳 *jiù yáng zhōng zhī yáng*). Emergency medicines usually include *fù zǐ* (aconite), while supplementing medicines usually contain *ròu guì* (cinnamon bark).

Gān jiāng (dried ginger)[348] warms the center and expels cold. It tends to enter the qì aspect of the spleen channel and also return yáng and free the vessels, as well as freeing heart yáng. *Ròu guì* (cinnamon bark) also warms the center and expels cold, but it tends to enter the blood aspect of the kidney channel, repress the liver and support the spleen, as well as promote the interaction of the heart and kidney.

---

[3]Putting forth of oily sweat, 汗出如油 *hàn chū rú yóu*: Sweating with sticky oily sweat that does not run easily; observed in yáng collapse vacuity desertion patterns.

[4]Vacuous pulse without root, 脉虚无根 *mài xū wú gēn*: A vacuous pulse is large and forceless; a pulse without root is forceless particularly at the deep level.

QUALITY

Good quality *ròu guì* with full medicinal strength is called *zǐ yóu guì* (purple oil cinnamon). When its rough outer bark is scraped off, the thin layer of inner bark that remains is called *guì xīn* (shaved cinnamon bark). It is not too drying and is suitable for assisting heart yáng and promoting the interaction of the heart and kidney. Young bark is called *guān guì* (quilled cinnamon). Weak in strength and dry in nature, it is suitable for warming the center and drying dampness. Generally, these forms are referred to as *ròu guì*.

I often enhance *liù wèi dì huáng tāng* (Six-Ingredient Rehmannia Decoction) (see below) with the addition of 0.9–2 g/3–7 fēn of *ròu guì* (best to use *zǐ yóu guì*). This combination is brewed in 1–2 thermos flasks of water and left to cool. This, taken as a tea, treats diabetes mellitus with thirst and drinking of fluids. If patients drink this decoction whenever they experience thirst, it will gradually alleviate the signs and reduce fluid intake. As this happens, the amount of water used to make the decoction is reduced. When fluid intake is reduced to virtually normal, the same formula is taken as a decoction, one packet a day. This method is often very effective, and I recommend it to readers. Note that I sometimes add 6–9 g/ 2–3 qián of *wǔ wèi zǐ* (schisandra) to the formula.

Liù wèi dì huáng tāng 六味地黄汤	Six-Ingredient Rehmannia Decoction

shú dì huáng (熟地黄 cooked rehmannia, Rehmanniae Radix Praeparata) 60 g/2 liǎng (or use 30 g/1 liǎng each of *shú dì huáng* (cooked rehmannia) and *shēng dì huáng* (dried/fresh rehmannia))

shān yào (山药 dioscorea, Dioscoreae Rhizoma) 60 g/2 liǎng

shān zhū yú (山茱萸 cornus, Corni Fructus) 9 g/3 qián

fú líng (茯苓 poria, Poria) 9 g/3 qián

dān pí (丹皮 moutan, Moutan Cortex) 9 g/3 qián

zé xiè (泽泻 alisma, Alismatis Rhizoma) 6 g/2 qián

DOSAGE

The dosage of *ròu guì* is generally 0.6–4.5 g/2 fēn–1.5 qián. In especially severe cases, use 9–15 g/3–5 qián.[5]

CAUTION

This medicinal is contraindicated for effulgent yīn vacuity fire and damage to liquid in heat (febrile) diseases. It is also contraindicated for pregnancy. It should not be used with *chì shí zhī* (halloysite).

---

[5]The dosage when taken as a powder and mixed into a cooked decoction is 0.5–1.5 g/2–5 fēn per dose. (Ed.)

3. 干姜 Gān Jiāng   Zingiberis Rhizoma
Dried Ginger

Gān jiāng (dried ginger) is acrid in flavor and hot in nature. Its main actions are to warm the center and dissipate cold and to return yáng and free the vessels. It conducts blood-aspect medicinals into the qì aspect of the blood and engenders blood. It conducts *fù zǐ* (aconite) into the kidney to dispel cold and return yáng. It also warms and assists the yáng qì of the heart and lung.

1. **Abdominal Pain and Diarrhea:** When spleen-stomach vacuity cold or cold evil affects movement and transformation of the spleen and stomach and causes cold pain in the stomach duct and abdomen with a liking for heat and pressure, or vomiting or diarrhea with clear thin vomitus/stool, *gān jiāng* can be used to warm the center and dissipate cold. For this purpose it is often combined with medicinals such as *dǎng shēn* (codonopsis), *bái zhú* (white atractylodes), *zhì gān cǎo* (mix-fried licorice), *huò xiāng* (agastache), *wú yú* (evodia), *fú líng* (poria), and *chén pí* (tangerine peel). For cold pain in the chest and abdomen, great cold, retching, vomiting, and inability to eat, cold qì surging upward in the abdomen, and pain in the upper and lower body, *gān jiāng* is combined with *chuān jiāo* (zanthoxylum), *rén shēn* (ginseng) (or *dǎng shēn*), and *yí táng* (malt sugar); these ingredients form *dà jiàn zhōng tāng* (Major Center-Fortifying Decoction) from *Jīn Guì Yào Lüè* (金匮要略 "Essential Prescriptions of the Golden Coffer").

2. **Yáng-Collapse Vacuity Desertion:** People with weak health and yáng vacuity have low resistance. If they contract an exuberant cold evil that invades the bowels and viscera and causes a faint pulse verging on expiration, counterflow cold of the limbs, cold sweat that soaks the clothing, and clear thin stool containing **untransformed food**[566] (完谷不化 *wán gǔ bù huà*), or if excessive use of effusing and dissipating medicinals gives rise to great dripping sweat, counterflow cold of the limbs, and a low body temperature, then these are patterns of yáng qì on the verge of desertion due either to cold evil damaging yáng, or to yáng collapse due to great sweating. Treat with swift administration of *gān jiāng*, usually in combination with *fù zǐ* (aconite) and *gān cǎo* (licorice), to return yáng and free the vessels. This formula is *sì nì tāng* (Counterflow Cold Decoction) from *Shāng Hán Lùn* (伤寒论 "On Cold Damage"). For vacuous or elderly patients, add *dǎng shēn* (codonopsis) (or *rén shēn*). For incessant cold sweating, add *mài dōng* (ophiopogon), *wǔ wèi zǐ* (schisandra), *shān zhū yú* (cornus), etc.

3. **Cold Phlegm Cough and Panting:** When owing to yáng qì vacuity, water-damp fails to transform and gathers to form rheum, then water-rheum and cold phlegm invade the lung and manifest in signs such as cough, ejection of thin bubbly phlegm, panting, fear of cold, dizzy head, no desire to drink water, and other signs that easily occur during winter time. For this pattern *gān jiāng* is combined with *xì xīn* (asarum) and *wǔ wèi zǐ* (schisandra) to form what is known as the "ginger, asarum, and schisandra method," which has the effects of warming the lung, opening the lung, and closing the lung. These three medicinals are often

added to appropriate decoction medicines. An example of this method is the formula *xiǎo qīng lóng tāng* (Minor Green-Blue Dragon Decoction).

Xiǎo qīng lóng tāng 小青龙汤   Minor Green-Blue Dragon Decoction

> *má huáng* (麻黄 ephedra, Ephedrae Herba)
>
> *guì zhī* (桂枝 cinnamon twig, Cinnamomi Ramulus)
>
> *bái sháo* (白芍 white peony, Paeoniae Radix Alba)
>
> *gān cǎo* (甘草 licorice, Glycyrrhizae Radix)
>
> *bàn xià* (半夏 pinellia, Pinelliae Rhizoma)
>
> *gān jiāng* (干姜 dried ginger, Zingiberis Rhizoma)
>
> *xì xīn* (细辛 asarum, Asari Herba)
>
> *wǔ wèi zǐ* (五味子 schisandra, Schisandrae Fructus)

COMPARISON

Xiè bái (Chinese chive)[214] is acrid and bitter, warm and lubricating; it enters the heart channel, frees qì stagnation, and assists chest yáng in the treatment of chest impediment (pain in the heart and chest that reaches into the back). *Gān jiāng*, by contrast, is warm and acrid; it enters the spleen channel, but also enters the heart and lung, and assists yáng and supplements heart qì.

Pào jiāng tàn (blast-fried ginger) is used to warm the channels and stanch bleeding. It tends to be used to treat cold in the smaller abdomen and spleen-kidney cold. *Gān jiāng* tends to be used to treat cold in the stomach duct, the umbilical region, and the heart and lung.

DOSAGE

The dosage is generally 0.9–6 g/3 fēn–2 qián. *Pào jiāng tàn* (blast-fried ginger) is used in quantities of 0.6–3 g/2 fēn–1 qián.

CAUTION

Inappropriate for insufficiency of essence blood and heat evil in the interior.

---

4. 吴茱萸 **Wú Zhū Yú**   Evodiae Fructus
Evodia

Wú zhū yú (evodia) is acrid and bitter in flavor and hot in nature. It warms the stomach and dissipates cold, courses the liver and dries the spleen, and warms the kidney and treats mounting.

1. Stomach Pain and Acid Vomiting: For stomach cold pain, acid swallowing[541] (吞酸 *tūn suān*), vomiting, and fullness in the chest, use *wú zhū yú* to warm the stomach and dissipate cold and to downbear counterflow and check vomiting. For this purpose it is combined with medicinals such as *shēng jiāng* (fresh ginger), *bàn xià* (pinellia), *gāo liáng jiāng* (lesser galangal), *huò xiāng* (agastache), and *shā rén* (amomum). For acid vomiting[541] (吐酸 *tu suān*) and stomach pain due to liver qì depression transforming into heat with liver heat invading the stomach, *wú zhū* *yú* has the effect of coursing the liver. It is combined with *huáng lián* (coptis) (using five times the weight of *huáng lián* to *wú zhū yú*) to form *zuǒ jīn wán* (Left-Running Metal Pill).

2. Spleen-Kidney Vacuity Diarrhea: *Wú zhū yú* is used for spleen-kidney vacuity cold causing diarrhea with signs such as rumbling and pain in the abdomen at daybreak heralding sudden diarrhea, as well as aching lumbus and cold legs, and a liking for warmth in the abdomen. Warm and acrid, *wú zhū yú* enters the kidney and dissipates cold qì in the lower abdomen. For this pattern it is often combined with *bǔ gǔ zhī* (psoralea), *wǔ wèi zǐ* (schisandra), and *ròu dòu kòu* (nutmeg) to form *sì shén wán* (Four Spirits Pill). These four medicinals provide a basic formula that is very effective when combined with other medicinals and varied according to signs. For chronic enteritis and other disorders of intestinal function, I often use *sì shén wán* (Four Spirits Pill) with the addition of medicinals such as *chǎo bái zhú* (stir-fried white atractylodes), *fú líng* (poria), *dǎng shēn* (codonopsis), *mù xiāng* (costusroot), *tǔ chǎo bái sháo* (earth-fried white peony), *bīng láng* (areca), *chǎo huáng bǎi* (stir-fried phellodendron), and *zào xīn tǔ* (oven earth) (decocted first and used to cook the other ingredients). By varying the ingredients in accordance with signs, I usually gain satisfactory results.

3. Mounting Pain: For mounting pain (疝痛 *shàn tòng*) with painful sagging of the testicles due to liver-kidney cold qì, *wú zhū yú* is combined with medicinals such as:

wū yào (乌药 lindera, Linderae Radix)

qīng pí (青皮 unripe tangerine peel, Citri Reticulatae Pericarpium Viride)

chuān liàn zǐ (川楝子 toosendan, Toosendan Fructus)

jú hé (橘核 tangerine pip, Citri Reticulatae Semen)·

xiǎo huí xiāng (小茴香 fennel, Foeniculi Fructus)

ròu guì (肉桂 cinnamon bark, Cinnamomi Cortex)

lì zhī hé (荔枝核 litchee pit, Litchi Semen)

4. Menstrual Pain: For delayed menstruation, scant black menstrual flow, and menstrual abdominal pain due to uterine cold, combine *wú zhū yú* with medicinals such as:

chuān xiōng (川芎 chuanxiong, Chuanxiong Rhizoma)

dāng guī (当归 Chinese angelica, Angelicae Sinensis Radix)

hóng huā (红花 carthamus, Carthami Flos)

táo rén (桃仁 peach kernel, Persicae Semen)

xiāng fù (香附 cyperus, Cyperi Rhizoma)

xiǎo huí xiāng (小茴香 fennel, Foeniculi Fructus)

niú xī (牛膝 achyranthes, Achyranthis Bidentatae Radix)

shú dì huáng (熟地黄 cooked rehmannia, Rehmanniae Radix Praeparata)

ròu guì (肉桂 cinnamon bark, Cinnamomi Cortex)

According to modern research, *wú zhū yú* has the effect of promoting uterine contractions.

COMPARISONS

Bàn xià (pinellia)[359] checks vomiting due to disharmony of stomach qì and dampness in the center burner. *Wú zhū yú*, by contrast, checks vomiting due to spleen-stomach vacuity cold and counterflow qì ascent.

Chuān jiāo (zanthoxylum)[351] tends to treat debilitation of the kidney fire and counterflow ascent of kidney channel cold qì. *Wú zhū yú*, on the other hand, treats turbid yīn failing to bear downward and liver channel counterflow qì ascent. It also conducts heat downward (it is used to treat mouth and tongue sores due to upflaming vacuity fire).

Shān zhū yú (cornus)[124] enriches the yīn humor of the reverting yīn (*jué yīn*) (liver) channel. It warms the liver and supplements the kidney; it checks vacuity sweating and seminal emission. By contrast, *wú zhū yú* opens reverting yīn (*jué yīn*) qì depression,[6] warms the kidney and spleen, precipitates counterflow qì, and checks cold retching.

DOSAGE

The dosage is generally 0.9–6 g /3 fēn–2 qián; in especially severe cases, use 9 g/ 3 qián.

CAUTION

Contraindicated for any dryness-heat pattern.

---

5. 川椒 Chuān Jiāo
Zanthoxylum

Zanthoxyli
Pericarpium

Including

▷ *Chuān jiāo mù* (川椒目 zanthoxylum seed, Zanthoxyli Semen)

Acrid in flavor and hot in nature, *chuān jiāo* (zanthoxylum)[7] warms the center and dispels cold, precipitates qì, and kills worms.

1. Stomach Pain and Abdominal Pain: In patterns of stomach pain and abdominal pain due to cold, with cold qì in the stomach causing distention, *chuān jiāo* is combined with *gān jiāng* (dried ginger), *dǎng shēn* (codonopsis) (or *rén shēn* (ginseng)), *yí táng* (malt sugar),[8] *gāo liáng jiāng* (lesser galangal), and *xiāng fù*

---

[6] "Opens reverting yīn qì depression" is a reference to the use of this medicinal in the treatment of cold stasis in the liver channel. (Ed.)

[7] This medicinal is the husk of the ripe fruit of *Zanthoxylum bungeanum* MAXIM. or *Zanthoxylum schinifolium* SIEB. ET ZUCC. (*Z. avicennai* LAM. DC. and *Z. simulans* HANCE are also used). It is acrid and hot and some sources say it bears a slight toxicity. It is also called *huā jiāo* 花椒. The seed of the fruit is called *chuān jiāo mù* 川椒目, and modern books list it as bitter, cold, and toxic. This latter medicinal is mostly used to treat fluid accumulation in the lungs that gives rise to asthmatic breathing or water accumulation in the abdomen that presents as drum distention. (Ed.)

[8] These four medicinals—*chuān jiāo* (zanthoxylum), *gān jiāng* (dried ginger), *rén shēn* (ginseng), and *yí táng* (malt sugar)—form *dà jiàn zhōng tāng* (Major Center-Fortifying Decoction). (Au.)

(cyperus). According to the findings of animal experiments, *chuān jiāo* contains volatile oils that in small quantities produce a lasting increase in intestinal tissue peristalsis and in larger quantities inhibit it.

2. Roundworm: For roundworm that causes vomiting and pain in the stomach duct and abdomen, *chuān jiāo* is combined with medicinals such as *wū méi* (mume), *huáng lián* (coptis), *huáng bǎi* (phellodendron), *xì xīn* (asarum), *guì zhī* (cinnamon twig), *fù zǐ* (aconite), *gān jiāng* (dried ginger), and *dāng guī* (Chinese angelica) to form *wū méi wán* (Mume Pill) from *Shāng Hán Lùn* (伤寒论 "On Cold Damage").

3. External Wash for Eczema: *Chuān jiāo* is decocted to make an external wash for the treatment of eczema and wind-damp pain in the limbs.[9]

Jiāo mù (zanthoxylum seed) is acrid and bitter in flavor and cold in nature. It enters the kidney and moves water, disinhibits urine, disperses water swelling, and eliminates water-rheum. It is often combined with medicinals such as:

fú líng pí (茯苓皮 poria skin, Poriae Cutis)

dà fù pí (大腹皮 areca husk, Arecae Pericarpium)

bīng láng (槟榔 areca, Arecae Semen)

chì xiǎo dòu (赤小豆 rice bean, Phaseoli Semen)

zé xiè (泽泻 alisma, Alismatis Rhizoma)

mù tōng (木通 trifoliate akebia, Akebiae Trifoliatae Caulis)

In the past, I have used *jiāo mù guā lóu tāng* (Zanthoxylum Seed and Trichosanthes Decoction) from *Yī Chún Shèng Yì* (医醇賸义 "Enriching the Meaning of the Wine of Medicine") to treat cases of exudative pleurisy with fluid collecting in the chest. It is very effective. I often use variations of the following prescription:

chuān jiāo mù (川椒目 zanthoxylum seed, Zanthoxyli Semen) 9 g/3 qián

quán guā lóu (全瓜蒌 trichosanthes, Trichosanthis Fructus) 30 g/1 liǎng

sāng bái pí (桑白皮 mulberry root bark, Mori Cortex) 12 g/4 qián

tíng lì zǐ (葶苈子 lepidium/descurainia, Lepidii/Descurainiae Semen) 9 g/3 qián

zé xiè (泽泻 alisma, Alismatis Rhizoma) 12 g/4 qián

zhū líng (猪苓 polyporus, Polyporus) 15 g/5 qián

fú líng (茯苓 poria, Poria) 15 g/5 qián

chē qián zǐ (车前子 plantago seed, Plantaginis Semen) 12 g/4 qián (cloth-wrapped)

xìng rén (杏仁 apricot kernel, Armeniacae Semen) 9 g/3 qián

bái jí lí (白蒺藜 tribulus, Tribuli Fructus) 9 g/3 qián

zhǐ qiào (枳壳 bitter orange, Aurantii Fructus) 9 g/3 qián

dōng guā pí (冬瓜皮 wax gourd rind, Benincasae Exocarpium) 30 g/1 liǎng

guì zhī (桂枝 cinnamon twig, Cinnamomi Ramulus) 4.5 g/1.5 qián

---

[9]One such formula is *kǔ shēn* (flavescent sophora) 30 g, *dì fū zǐ* (kochia) 16 g, *shé chuáng zǐ* (cnidium seed) 12 g, and *huā jiāo* (zanthoxylum) 10 g. This combination comes from the *Shí Yòng Zhōng Cǎo Yào Wài Zhì Fǎ Dà Quán* (实用中草药外治法大全 "Complete Compendium of External Treatment Methods Using Chinese Medicinals and Herbal Medicines"). (Ed.)

Dosage

The dosage is generally 1.5–4.5 g/5 fēn–1.5 qián. The dosage of *chuān jiāo mù* (zanthoxylum seed) is slightly larger.

Caution

Contraindicated for effulgent yīn vacuity fire.

---

6. 小茴香 **Xiǎo Huí Xiāng**   Foeniculi Fructus
Fennel

Acrid in flavor and warm in nature, *xiǎo huí xiāng* (fennel) warms the kidney and dispels cold, as well as moving qì and opening the stomach. It is a major medicine for mounting qì pain (疝气痛 *shàn qì tòng*).

When cold in the lower burner causes liver and kidney counterflow qì that manifests in small intestinal mounting qì, lesser-abdominal pain, sagging distention in the smaller abdomen, pain, swelling, and distention of the testicles, or unilateral sagging of the testicles with pulling pain, this can be treated by combining *xiǎo huí xiāng* with medicinals such as *wū yào* (lindera), *jú hé* (tangerine pip), *wú yú* (evodia), *qīng pí* (unripe tangerine peel), *chǎo chuān liàn zǐ* (stir-fried toosendan), *lì zhī hé* (litchee pit), *mù xiāng* (costusroot), and *hú lú bā* (fenugreek). In the past, I have varied this formula in accordance with signs to treat tuberculosis of the testis and chronic orchitis, with good results. According to modern research, *xiǎo huí xiāng* contains anysaldehide, which has been shown to increase dihydrostreptomycin in experimental tuberculosis in guinea pigs.

Xiǎo huí xiāng enters the lower burner, warming the channels and dissipating cold, so it also treats delayed menstruation, abdominal pain during menstruation, liking for warmth in the abdomen, and black menstrual flow with clots. For this purpose it is often combined with medicinals such as:

dāng guī (当归 Chinese angelica, Angelicae Sinensis Radix)

shú dì huáng (熟地黄 cooked rehmannia, Rehmanniae Radix Praeparata)

chuān xiōng (川芎 chuanxiong, Chuanxiong Rhizoma)

bái sháo (白芍 white peony, Paeoniae Radix Alba)

chǎo chuān liàn zǐ (炒川楝子 stir-fried toosendan, Toosendan Fructus Frictus)

yán hú suǒ (延胡索 corydalis, Corydalis Rhizoma)

wǔ líng zhī (五灵脂 squirrel's droppings, Trogopteri Faeces)

nán hóng huā (南红花 carthamus, Carthami Flos)

Xiǎo huí xiāng also moves qì and opens the stomach. For signs such as pain due to cold qì in the stomach and qì counterflow with retching and vomiting, it is combined with medicinals such as *bàn xià* (pinellia), *shēng jiāng* (fresh ginger), *wú yú* (evodia), *fú líng* (poria), and *mù xiāng* (costusroot). For indigestion, poor appetite, and persistent bloating and distention after eating due to stomach cold, it is combined with medicinals such as:

mài yá (麦芽 barley sprout, Hordei Fructus Germinatus)

chén pí (陈皮 tangerine peel, Citri Reticulatae Pericarpium)

xiāng dào yá (香稻芽 rice sprout, Oryzae Fructus Germinatus)

chǎo shén qū (炒神曲 stir-fried medicated leaven, Massa Medicata Fermentata Fricta)

shā rén (砂仁 amomum, Amomi Fructus)

mù xiāng (木香 costusroot, Aucklandiae Radix)

COMPARISONS

Both *hú lú bā* (fenugreek)[358] and *xiǎo huí xiāng* warm the kidney, dissipate cold, and treat mounting, but *hú lú bā* tends to be used for enduring intractable cold, while *xiǎo huí xiāng* tends to be used for simple cold of recent onset.

Both *wú zhū yú*[349] and *xiǎo huí xiāng* (fennel) treat cold mounting, but while *wú zhū yú* tends to warm the liver, *xiǎo huí xiāng* tends to warm the kidney.

PROCESSING

Xiǎo huí xiāng used raw tends to rectify qì; stir-fried with brine, it tends to warm the kidney.[10]

DOSAGE

The dosage is generally 0.25–9 g/0.8 fēn–3 qián.

CAUTION

Contraindicated for yīn vacuity with heat.

---

7. 丁香 Dīng Xiāng   Caryophylli Flos
Clove

Including

  ▷ *Mǔ dīng xiāng* (母丁香 clove fruit, Caryophylli Fructus)

Dīng xiāng (clove) is acrid in flavor and warm in nature. It has a strong aroma.

1. **Warming the Stomach:** For cold-pattern stomach duct pain and cold-type abdominal pain, abdominal distention, and acid swallowing on exposure to cold, use *dīng xiāng* to warm the spleen and stomach and to rectify qì and downbear counterflow. It is often combined with medicinals such as *mù xiāng* (costusroot), *shā rén* (amomum), *chén pí* (tangerine peel), *huò xiāng* (agastache), *gāo liáng jiāng* (lesser galangal), and *bīng láng* (areca).

2. **Downbearing Counterflow:** *Dīng xiāng* warms the stomach and downbears counterflow qì to treat hiccup or vomiting due to cold evil invading the stomach and preventing the normal downbearing of stomach qì. It is a major medicine for treating cold-pattern hiccup or vomiting. It is often combined with medicinals

---

[10]Salt, being cold in nature, clears heat and cools the blood; being salty in flavor, it enters the kidney and softens hardness. It also improves flavors and acts as a preservative. Stir-frying with brine is a common method of processing medicinals that supplement the kidney, secure essence, treat mounting qì, and drain kidney fire, such as *bǔ gǔ zhī* (psoralea), *xiǎo huí xiāng* (fennel), *zhī mǔ* (anemarrhena), *huáng bǎi* (phellodendron), and *zé xiè* (alisma). (Ed.)

such as *shì dì* (persimmon calyx), *xuán fù huā* (inula flower), *wú yú* (evodia), and *huò xiāng gěng* (agastache stem). For cold strike hiccup in the elderly or in enduring illness, add *rén shēn* (ginseng) (or *dǎng shēn*), *chén pí* (tangerine peel), *zhú rú* (bamboo shavings), and *shēng jiāng* (fresh ginger). For cold-pattern vomiting, *dīng xiāng* can be combined with medicinals such as:

wú yú (吴萸 evodia, Evodiae Fructus)

bàn xià (半夏 pinellia, Pinelliae Rhizoma)

shēng jiāng (生姜 fresh ginger, Zingiberis Rhizoma Recens)

gāo liáng jiāng (高良姜 lesser galangal, Alpiniae Officinarum Rhizoma)

chén pí (陈皮 tangerine peel, Citri Reticulatae Pericarpium)

3. Warming the Kidney: For insufficiency of kidney yáng that causes genital cold or impotence, *dīng xiāng* is used to warm the kidney and assist yáng. For this it is combined with medicinals such as:

shú dì huáng (熟地黄 cooked rehmannia, Rehmanniae Radix Praeparata)

shān zhū yú (山茱萸 cornus, Corni Fructus)

ròu guì (肉桂 cinnamon bark, Cinnamomi Cortex)

fù zǐ (附子 aconite, Aconiti Radix Lateralis Praeparata)

shān yào (山药 dioscorea, Dioscoreae Rhizoma)

bā jǐ tiān (巴戟天 morinda, Morindae Officinalis Radix)

fú líng (茯苓 poria, Poria)

yín yáng huò (淫羊藿 epimedium, Epimedii Herba)

COMPARISONS

A distinction is made between *gōng dīng xiāng* (公丁香, clove) and *mǔ dīng xiāng* (母丁香, clove fruit). They are similar in nature and flavor, although the former tends to be quicker acting, and the latter tends to maintain its strength longer. The two are often used together.

Shì dì (persimmon calyx)[210] shares with *dīng xiāng* the ability to treat hiccup, but is bitter and warm, and downbears qì, while *dīng xiāng* warms the stomach with acridity and aroma and downbears counterflow.

Dīng xiāng shù pí (clove bark), sometimes called 丁皮 *dīng pí* in Chinese, treats cold pain in the region of the heart and abdomen. For this purpose it is used as a substitute for *dīng xiāng*.

DOSAGE

The dosage is generally 0.9–3 g/3 fēn–1 qián. In especially severe cases, somewhat larger doses may be used.

CAUTION

Inappropriate for insufficiency of stomach liquid and center burner dryness-heat.

---

8. 高良姜 Gāo Liáng Jiāng   Alpiniae Officinarum

Lesser Galangal   Rhizoma

Including

> *Hóng dòu kòu* (红豆蔻 galangal fruit, Galangae Fructus)

Acrid in flavor and hot in nature, *gāo liáng jiāng* (lesser galangal) warms the stomach and dissipates cold, and disperses food.

Gāo liáng jiāng treats cold pain in the stomach duct, stomach cold vomiting, center burner cold-type abdominal pain or spleen-stomach vacuity cold that causes diarrhea, and stomach cold food stagnation. For cold-type stomach pain, it is often combined with medicinals such as *xiāng fù* (cyperus), *wú yú* (evodia), *shā rén* (amomum), *huò xiāng* (agastache), and *shén qū* (medicated leaven). For cold-type vomiting, it is often combined with medicinals such as *bàn xià* (pinellia), *shēng jiāng* (fresh ginger), *dīng xiāng* (clove), *fú líng* (poria), and *sū zǐ* (perilla fruit). For cold-type abdominal pain, it is combined with medicinals such as *dāng guī* (Chinese angelica), *chǎo bái sháo* (stir-fried white peony), *guì zhī* (cinnamon twig), and *pào jiāng* (blast-fried ginger). For cold-type diarrhea, it is combined with medicinals such as *mù xiāng* (costusroot), *fú líng* (poria), *zé xiè* (alisma), *ròu guì* (cinnamon bark), *chǎo shān yào* (stir-fried dioscorea), and *qiàn shí* (euryale). For stomach cold food stagnation, it is combined with medicinals such as:

shā rén (砂仁 amomum, Amomi Fructus)

jiāo sān xiān (焦三仙 scorch-fried three immortals, Tres Immortales Usti)

chǎo bīng láng (炒槟榔 stir-fried areca, Arecae Semen Frictum)

cǎo dòu kòu (草豆蔻 Katsumada's galangal seed, Alpiniae Katsumadai Semen)

chǎo jī nèi jīn (炒鸡内金 stir-fried gizzard lining, Galli Gigeriae Endothelium
     Corneum Frictum)

Gāo liáng jiāng figures in two old empirical formulas. One is *liáng fù wán* (Lesser Galangal and Cyperus Pill), a combination of *gāo liáng jiāng* and *xiāng fù* (cyperus) that is used for stomach pain. The other is *gāo liáng jiāng tāng* (Lesser Galangal Decoction), which contains *gāo liáng jiāng*, *hòu pò* (officinal magnolia bark), *dāng guī* (Chinese angelica), *guì xīn* (shaved cinnamon bark), and *shēng jiāng* (fresh ginger) and is used for gastrointestinal colic (gripping pain in the stomach or intestines). Both formulas are effective and are commonly used in clinical practice.

COMPARISONS

Gān jiāng (dried ginger)[348] has a center-warming action that focuses on the spleen and is used to warm spleen cold in the treatment of cold pain in the umbilical region. *Gāo liáng jiāng* has a center-warming action that focuses on the stomach and is used to dissipate stomach cold in the treatment of cold pain in the stomach duct and abdomen.

Shēng jiāng (fresh ginger)[28] is more acrid than it is warm. It is effective in reaching the outer body and the exterior. It dispels external cold and also checks vomiting and retching. *Gāo liáng jiāng* is more warm than it is acrid. Its strength lies in warming the center and penetrating the interior; it dissipates internal cold and relieves pain.

Hóng dòu kòu (galangal fruit), the fruit of a related plant,[11] warms the lung and dissipates cold, arouses the spleen and dries dampness, and disperses food and resolves liquor. To treat pneumosilicosis that manifests in lung-stomach cold, cough with ejection of white phlegm, and stomach duct pain, I find it clinically effective to combine *hóng dòu kòu* with the following:

gān jiāng (干姜 dried ginger, Zingiberis Rhizoma)
gān cǎo (甘草 licorice, Glycyrrhizae Radix)
kuǎn dōng huā (款冬花 coltsfoot, Farfarae Flos)
zǐ wǎn (紫菀 aster, Asteris Radix)
sū zǐ (苏子 perilla fruit, Perillae Fructus)
wú yú (吴萸 evodia, Evodiae Fructus)
xìng rén (杏仁 apricot kernel, Armeniacae Semen)
fú líng (茯苓 poria, Poria)
xiāng fù (香附 cyperus, Cyperi Rhizoma)
bàn xià (半夏 pinellia, Pinelliae Rhizoma)

Dosage

The dosage is generally 2.5–9 g/8 fēn–3 qián.

Caution

Contraindicated for vomiting and diarrhea, or stomach pain due to heat.

---

9. 艾叶 Aì Yè   Artemisiae Argyi
Mugwort   Folium

Aì yè (mugwort) is bitter and acrid in flavor and warm in nature. There are different clinical uses for *shēng aì yè* (raw mugwort) and *aì yè tàn* (charred mugwort).

1. **Warming the Center and Dispelling Cold:** *Aì yè* warms the center and dispels cold; it warms the uterus, regulates menstruation, and quiets the fetus. For cold pain in the abdomen, smaller-abdominal cold pain, uterine cold, persistent failure to conceive, and vacuity-cold–type menstrual pain, it is combined with medicinals such as:

dāng guī (当归 Chinese angelica, Angelicae Sinensis Radix)
gān jiāng (干姜 dried ginger, Zingiberis Rhizoma)
chǎo bái sháo (炒白芍 stir-fried white peony, Paeoniae Radix Alba Fricta)
ròu guì (肉桂 cinnamon bark, Cinnamomi Cortex)
xiǎo huí xiāng (小茴香 fennel, Foeniculi Fructus)

---

[11]*Hóng dòu kòu* 红豆蔻 is the fruit of *Alpinia galanga* Willd. It is acrid and warm and is attributed with the actions of warming the center, dispersing cold, moving qì, and relieving pain. It treats cold pain in the abdomen, vomiting, lack of appetite, and diarrhea when these symptoms are from cold-damp. (Ed.)

wú yú (吴萸 evodia, Evodiae Fructus)

xiāng fù (香附 cyperus, Cyperi Rhizoma)

2. Stanching Bleeding: When char-fried, *ài yè* is called *ài yè tàn* (charred mugwort), or simply *ài tàn* 艾炭 in Chinese, and it is used to stanch bleeding. This form is effective for lower origin vacuity cold that causes profuse menstruation, flooding and spotting (uterine bleeding), and, in pregnancy, contraction of cold that causes pain in the abdomen and stirring fetus. *Ài yè tàn* is combined with medicinals such as:

dāng guī (当归 Chinese angelica, Angelicae Sinensis Radix)

bái sháo (白芍 white peony, Paeoniae Radix Alba)

shú dì huáng (熟地黄 cooked rehmannia, Rehmanniae Radix Praeparata)

ē jiāo (阿胶 ass hide glue, Asini Corii Colla)

zōng tàn (棕炭 charred trachycarpus, Trachycarpi Petiolus Carbonisatus)

yì mǔ cǎo (益母草 leonurus, Leonuri Herba)

sāng jì shēng (桑寄生 mistletoe, Taxilli Herba)

xù duàn tàn (续断炭 charred dipsacus, Dipsaci Radix Carbonisata)

Ài yè that is pounded to a fluffy consistency is called "moxa floss." Although this has the same action as *ài yè*, it is superior. Moxa floss is also made into the moxa rolls and moxa cones used in acumoxatherapy.

Dosage

The dosage for *ài yè* is generally 2.5–6 g/8 fēn–2 qián. When used to stanch bleeding, the dosage of *ài yè tàn* (charred mugwort) is 15–30 g/5 qián–1 liǎng.

Caution

Ài yè is inappropriate for yīn vacuity with blood heat.

---

10. 胡芦巴 Hú Lú Bā   Trigonellae Semen
Fenugreek

Bitter in flavor and greatly warm in nature, *hú lú bā* (fenugreek) warms and supplements kidney yáng, and dissipates cold and eliminates dampness. It is most commonly used to treat mounting qì (疝气 *shàn qì*) cold pain.

When liver-kidney vacuity cold causes mounting qì pain, painful sagging of the testicles, smaller-abdominal mounting-conglomeration (小腹疝瘕 *shào fù shàn jiǎ*), and pain, swelling, and cold of the testicles, use *hú lú bā* combined with medicinals such as the following:

xiǎo huí xiāng (小茴香 fennel, Foeniculi Fructus)

wú zhū yú (吴茱萸 evodia, Evodiae Fructus)

chǎo jú hé (炒橘核 stir-fried tangerine pip, Citri Reticulatae Semen Frictum)

wū yào (乌药 lindera, Linderae Radix)

chuān liàn zǐ (川楝子 toosendan, Toosendan Fructus)

ròu guì (肉桂 cinnamon bark, Cinnamomi Cortex)

qīng pí (青皮 unripe tangerine peel, Citri Reticulatae Pericarpium Viride)

In the past I have used the above formula, varied in accordance with signs, in the treatment of tuberculosis of the testis, chronic orchitis, or epididymitis with painful sagging but no redness and heat. It is very effective as long as there is no redness, swelling, or heat.

For cramping gastrointestinal pain due to contraction of cold or coolness, use this medicinal combined with:

gāo liáng jiāng (高良姜 lesser galangal, Alpiniae Officinarum Rhizoma)

xiāng fù (香附 cyperus, Cyperi Rhizoma)

mù xiāng (木香 costusroot, Aucklandiae Radix)

gān jiāng (干姜 dried ginger, Zingiberis Rhizoma)

wú yú (吴萸 evodia, Evodiae Fructus)

COMPARISON

Xiǎo huí xiāng (fennel) and *hú lú bā* both treat mounting; however, the former tends to move qì and dissipate cold, while the latter tends to warm the kidney and dissipate cold.

DOSAGE

The dosage is generally 3–9 g/1–3 qián.

CAUTION

Contraindicated for hyperactivity of yáng due to yīn vacuity.

---

11. 半夏 Bàn Xià   Pinelliae Rhizoma
Pinellia

Acrid in flavor and warm in nature,[12] *bàn xià* (pinellia)[13] dries dampness and transforms phlegm, fortifies the spleen and stomach, harmonizes the center and downbears qì, and checks vomiting and retching.

1. **Drying Dampness and Transforming Phlegm:** The spleen governs movement and transformation of water-damp. When dampness is not moved and transformed, phlegm may be engendered. Thus, it is said that "the spleen is the source of phlegm formation." a) When exuberant dampness and copious phlegm impair depurative downbearing of the lung, which manifests in cough, oppression in the chest, coughing up of copious thin white phlegm that is easily expectorated, a thick slimy white tongue fur, and a slippery pulse, use *bàn xià* combined with medicinals such as *jú hóng* (red tangerine peel), *fú líng* (poria), *sū zǐ* (perilla fruit), *tiān nán xīng* (arisaema), *chǎo lái fú zǐ* (stir-fried radish seed), and *xìng*

---

[12]Most sources also state that the prepared rhizome of *Pinellia ternata* is slightly toxic. (Ed.)

[13]The rhizome of *Pinellia ternata* (THUNB.) Breit. is the correct medicinal, however a frequently used substitute for it is the rhizome of *Typhonium flagelliforme*, which is called *shuǐ bàn xià* 水半夏. (Ed.)

rén (apricot kernel). b) For center burner vacuity cold in which water-rheum fails to transform and invades the lung, producing signs such as cough, coughing and spitting of thin, clear, possibly foamy phlegm, and fear of cold in the chest and back, use *bàn xià* combined with medicinals such as *sū zǐ* (perilla fruit), *jú hóng* (red tangerine peel), *guì zhī* (cinnamon twig), *zhū líng* (polyporus), *fú líng* (poria), *bái zhú* (white atractylodes), *gān jiāng* (dried ginger), *xì xīn* (asarum), and *wǔ wèi zǐ* (schisandra). The spleen is averse to dampness, and *bàn xià* dries dampness and transforms phlegm, so it also fortifies the spleen and stomach.

2. Harmonizing the Center and Downbearing Qì: For excessively exuberant center burner damp turbidity that gives rise to fullness and oppression in the stomach duct, and qì counterflow with retching and vomiting, use *bàn xià* combined with medicinals such as *jiāng zhú rú* (ginger-processed bamboo shavings), *dīng xiāng* (clove), *wú zhū yú* (evodia), *huò xiāng* (agastache), *shēng jiāng* (fresh ginger), *chén pí* (tangerine peel), and *fú líng* (poria). In the past, I have had good results combining *bàn xià* with *shēng dài zhě shí* (crude hematite), *xuán fù huā* (inula flower), *shēng dà huáng* (raw rhubarb), *shēng gān cǎo* (raw licorice), *guā lóu* (trichosanthes), *bīng láng* (areca), and *táo rén ní* (crushed peach kernel), varying the ingredients in accordance with signs, to treat stubborn neurogenic vomiting.

Combinations

1) Combined with medicinals such as *shēng jiāng* (fresh ginger), *gān jiāng* (dried ginger), *fù zǐ* (aconite), *cāng zhú* (atractylodes), and *jú hóng* (red tangerine peel), *bàn xià* treats cold phlegm. 2) Combined with *zào jiǎo* (gleditsia), *tiān má* (gastrodia), and *tiān nán xīng* (arisaema), it treats wind-phlegm. 3) Combined with *zhú lì* (bamboo sap) and *bái jiè zǐ* (white mustard), it treats phlegm in the channels and network vessels, in the limbs, and between the skin and its inner membrane, i.e., it is used for wind strike (stroke) and hemiplegia.

Processing

Bàn xià processed with ginger is called *jiāng bàn xià* (姜半夏, ginger-processed pinellia), which tends to be used to treat vomiting. *Qīng bàn xià* (清半夏, purified pinellia), which is processed with *bái fán* (alum), and *fǎ bàn xià* (法半夏, pro formula pinellia), which is processed with *gān cǎo* (licorice), tend to be used to transform phlegm and to dry dampness and fortify the spleen and stomach. *Bàn xià qū* (半夏曲, pinellia leaven) transforms phlegm and also aids digestion.[14]

---

[14]There are many processing methods for *bàn xià* (pinellia). *Jiāng bàn xià* (ginger-processed pinellia) is prepared by soaking unprocessed *bàn xià* in water and then cooking it in a decoction of ginger, usually with the addition of *bái fán* (alum). *Qīng bàn xià* (purified pinellia) is made by soaking *bàn xià* in a solution of *bái fán*, then slicing and drying it. There are many ways to produce *fǎ bàn xià* (pro formula pinellia); most involve soaking unprocessed *bàn xià* in water and then draining it and cooking it at least once in a decoction of *gān cǎo* (licorice). A solution of *shí huī* (limestone) is added and the medicinal is soaked for several days and then dried and sliced. *Bái fán* is often added in such methods. (Ed.)

RESEARCH

According to modern research reports, *bàn xià* acts on the central nervous system to inhibit vomiting and also has an antitussive effect.[15]

DOSAGE

The dosage is generally 3–9 g/1–3 qián.

CAUTION

Contraindicated for all forms of yīn vacuity, shortage of blood, and insufficiency of the fluids, as well as in the presence of a red tongue without fur, and in the final stages of pregnancy. It should not be combined with *wū tóu* (wild aconite).

---

12. 天南星 **Tiān Nán Xīng**   Arisaematis Rhizoma
Arisaema

Bitter and acrid in flavor and warm in nature, *tiān nán xīng* (arisaema) dispels wind-phlegm. There are two different processed forms that have different clinical applications.

1. *Zhì nán xīng* (制南星, processed arisaema) is arisaema processed with *shēng jiāng* (fresh ginger). It is mainly used for wind-phlegm harassing the upper body that causes dizziness; for wind strike with collapse, deviated eyes and mouth, stiff tongue and inability to speak, and the gurgling sound of phlegm; and for **fright wind**[550] (惊风 *jīng fēng*), epilepsy, and lockjaw. *Zhì nán xīng* dries phlegm and dispels wind-phlegm from the channels and network vessels. It is combined with different medicinals for different purposes:

For dizziness

tiān má (天麻 gastrodia, Gastrodiae Rhizoma)

bái zhú (白术 white atractylodes, Atractylodis Macrocephalae Rhizoma)

bàn xià (半夏 pinellia, Pinelliae Rhizoma)

fú líng (茯苓 poria, Poria)

jú huā (菊花 chrysanthemum, Chrysanthemi Flos)

bái jí lí (白蒺藜 tribulus, Tribuli Fructus)

For wind strike

sāng zhī (桑枝 mulberry twig, Mori Ramulus)

hóng huā (红花 carthamus, Carthami Flos)

táo rén (桃仁 peach kernel, Persicae Semen)

chì sháo (赤芍 red peony, Paeoniae Radix Rubra)

zhì shān jiǎ (炙山甲 mix-fried pangolin scales, Manis Squama cum Liquido Fricta)

---

[15] *Bàn xià* (pinellia) is commonly used nowadays in small doses in the first trimester of pregnancy to treat nausea and vomiting associated with morning sickness. A typical formula is *bàn xià xiè xīn tāng* (Pinellia Heart-Draining Decoction). Given the downbearing nature of this medicinal, however, it must be used with great care. (Ed.)

dì lóng (地龙 earthworm, Pheretima)

guā lóu (瓜蒌 trichosanthes, Trichosanthis Fructus)

gōu téng (钩藤 uncaria, Uncariae Ramulus cum Uncis)

chén pí (陈皮 tangerine peel, Citri Reticulatae Pericarpium)

For fright wind or epilepsy

yù jīn (郁金 curcuma, Curcumae Radix)

quán xiē (全蝎 scorpion, Scorpio)

tiān zhú huáng (天竹黄 bamboo sugar, Bambusae Concretio Silicea)

yuǎn zhì (远志 polygala, Polygalae Radix)

chāng pú (菖蒲 acorus, Acori Tatarinowii Rhizoma)

zhū shā (朱砂 cinnabar, Cinnabaris)

bái jiāng cán (白僵蚕 silkworm, Bombyx Batryticatus)

For lockjaw

bái fù zǐ (白附子 typhonium, Typhonii Rhizoma)

qiāng huó (羌活 notopterygium, Notopterygii Rhizoma et Radix)

fáng fēng (防风 saposhnikovia, Saposhnikoviae Radix)

wú gōng (蜈蚣 centipede, Scolopendra)

2. *Dǎn xīng* (胆星, bile arisaema) (or *dǎn nán xīng* 胆南星) is arisaema prepared with ox bile.[16] The ox bile makes it cold in nature so that it sweeps phlegm as well as clearing heat. *Dǎn xīng* is used for phlegm-heat giving rise to epilepsy, child fright wind, and wind strike, with signs such as generalized heat [effusion] (fever), yellow tongue fur, constipation, thick yellow phlegm, and a slippery rapid pulse. For this purpose it is often combined with medicinals such as:

guā lóu (瓜蒌 trichosanthes, Trichosanthis Fructus)

tiān zhú huáng (天竹黄 bamboo sugar, Bambusae Concretio Silicea)

yù jīn (郁金 curcuma, Curcumae Radix)

chāng pú (菖蒲 acorus, Acori Tatarinowii Rhizoma)

yuǎn zhì (远志 polygala, Polygalae Radix)

huáng lián (黄连 coptis, Coptidis Rhizoma)

niú huáng (牛黄 bovine bezoar, Bovis Calculus)

xióng huáng (雄黄 realgar, Realgar)

zhū shā (朱砂 cinnabar, Cinnabaris)

shēng dà huáng (生大黄 raw rhubarb, Rhei Radix et Rhizoma Crudi)

zhú lì (竹沥 bamboo sap, Bambusae Succus)

COMPARISONS

Bàn xià (pinellia)[359] transforms phlegm; it is acrid but static. While it is mainly used to dry damp phlegm and to fortify the spleen and stomach, it also checks retching. By contrast, *zhì nán xīng* (processed arisaema) transforms phlegm; it is acrid but not static. It is mainly used to transform channel and network vessel wind-phlegm in the treatment of wind strike and lockjaw.

---

[16] *Dǎn nán xīng* (bile arisaema) is sometimes treated with bile from the gallbladder of pigs (and, more rarely, goats or sheep) instead of bovine bile. (Ed.)

SPECIAL USES

To treat cerebral thrombosis and cerebral embolism manifesting as exuberant phlegm, I often use *zhì nán xīng* (processed arisaema) variously combined according to the signs with the following:

bàn xià (半夏 pinellia, Pinelliae Rhizoma)

fú líng (茯苓 poria, Poria)

guā lóu (瓜蒌 trichosanthes, Trichosanthis Fructus)

tiān zhú huáng (天竹黄 bamboo sugar, Bambusae Concretio Silicea)

zhú lì (竹沥 bamboo sap, Bambusae Succus)

sāng zhī (桑枝 mulberry twig, Mori Ramulus)

yuǎn zhì (远志 polygala, Polygalae Radix)

táo rén (桃仁 peach kernel, Persicae Semen)

hóng huā (红花 carthamus, Carthami Flos)

gōu téng (钩藤 uncaria, Uncariae Ramulus cum Uncis)

jú huā (菊花 chrysanthemum, Chrysanthemi Flos)

chì sháo (赤芍 red peony, Paeoniae Radix Rubra)

dì lóng (地龙 earthworm, Pheretima)

zhì shān jiǎ (炙山甲 mix-fried pangolin scales, Manis Squama cum Liquido Fricta)

For epilepsy and child fright wind, I usually get good results using *dǎn xīng* (bile arisaema) variously combined according to signs with the following:

yù jīn (郁金 curcuma, Curcumae Radix)

bái zhú (白术 white atractylodes, Atractylodis Macrocephalae Rhizoma)

bàn xià (半夏 pinellia, Pinelliae Rhizoma)

huáng lián (黄连 coptis, Coptidis Rhizoma)

quán xiē (全蝎 scorpion, Scorpio)

tiān zhú huáng (天竹黄 bamboo sugar, Bambusae Concretio Silicea)

chāng pú (菖蒲 acorus, Acori Tatarinowii Rhizoma)

yuǎn zhì (远志 polygala, Polygalae Radix)

huà jú hóng (化橘红 red Huàzhōu pomelo peel, Citri Grandis Exocarpium Rubrum)

fú líng (茯苓 poria, Poria)

wú gōng (蜈蚣 centipede, Scolopendra)

bái jiāng cán (白僵蚕 silkworm, Bombyx Batryticatus)

xiāng fù (香附 cyperus, Cyperi Rhizoma)

DOSAGE

The dosage for *zhì nán xīng* (processed arisaema) is generally 3–6 g/1–2 qián. In severe cases, use up to 9 g/3 qián. *Dǎn xīng* (bile arisaema) is usually used in slightly smaller doses, but it is used in similar doses to those above.

CAUTION

Contraindicated for yīn vacuity with dry phlegm and in pregnancy.

Research

According to modern research reports, animal studies show that *tiān nán xīng* has marked expectorant, analgesic, antispasmodic, and sedative properties.

13. 白芥子 Bái Jiè Zǐ   Sinapis Albae Semen
White Mustard

Acrid in flavor and warm in nature, *bái jiè zǐ* (white mustard)[17] disinhibits qì and sweeps phlegm, and disperses swelling and dissipates binds.

Bái jiè zǐ disinhibits lung qì and transforms cold phlegm and water-rheum. It treats cold phlegm and water-rheum that gathers and binds in the chest and rib-side, impairing the diffusion and depuration of the lung and causing qì counterflow, which manifests in panting, cough, oppression in the chest, and rib-side pain. For this purpose it is combined with *chǎo lái fú zǐ* (stir-fried radish seed), *chǎo sū zǐ* (stir-fried perilla fruit), *tíng lì zǐ* (lepidium/descurainia), *bàn xià* (pinellia), *chén pí* (tangerine peel), and *fú líng* (poria). Another formula is *kòng xián dān* (Drool-Controlling Elixir) from *Sān Yīn Fāng* (三因方 "Three Causes Formulary"), which contains 3 g/1 qián of *gān suì* (kansui), 3 g/1 qián of *dà jǐ* (euphorbia/knoxia), and 6 g/2 qián of *bái jiè zǐ* (white mustard). The ingredients are ground together to a fine powder, mixed with water, and formed into pills each the size of a *wú tóng zǐ* (firmiana seed). Take ten pills at a time (or take more or less depending on the condition). This pill treats panting and pain in both rib-sides.

Bái jiè zǐ dispels cold phlegm gathering and binding between the skin and its inner membrane and in the rib-sides. When cold phlegm stagnates and binds, it can cause swellings known as **yīn flat-abscesses**[569] (阴疽 *yīn jū*), which are characterized by the absence of any change in skin color, absence of heat, absence of pain, and that do not move easily. For these swellings, use *yáng hé tāng* (Harmonious Yáng Decoction):

Yáng hé tāng 阳和汤	Harmonious Yáng Decoction

bái jiè zǐ (白芥子 white mustard, Sinapis Albae Semen) 6 g/2 qián

ròu guì (肉桂 cinnamon bark, Cinnamomi Cortex) 3 g/1 qián

shú dì huáng (熟地黄 cooked rehmannia, Rehmanniae Radix Praeparata) 30 g/1 liǎng

má huáng (麻黄 ephedra, Ephedrae Herba) 1.5 g/5 fēn (crushed along with the *shú dì huáng*)

pào jiāng (炮姜 blast-fried ginger, Zingiberis Rhizoma Praeparatum) 1.5 g/5 fēn

---

[17] *Bái jiè zǐ* (white mustard), as the name implies, should be white. Most of what is used in trade is actually *huáng jiè zǐ* (mustard seed) (*Brassica Juncea* (L.) Czern. et Coss). It is very similar in appearance to *bái jiè zǐ* (white mustard), but is yellow in color with some seeds bearing a brown hue. (Ed.)

lù jiǎo jiāo (鹿角胶 deerhorn glue, Cervi Cornus Gelatinum) 9 g/3 qián

shēng gān cǎo (生甘草 raw licorice, Glycyrrhizae Radix Cruda) 3 g/1 qián

These ingredients are brewed with water to produce a decoction to which a little *bái jiǔ* (white liquor) is added before taking. I have had good results using variations of this formula to treat obliterating phlebitis of the lower extremities. For phlegm turbidity or water-rheum collecting in the rib-side that produces cough with rib-side pain and shortness of breath, which in severe cases prevents the patient from lying flat, use *bái jiè zǐ* combined with medicinals such as:

guā lóu (瓜蒌 trichosanthes, Trichosanthis Fructus)

chuān jiāo mù (川椒目 zanthoxylum seed, Zanthoxyli Semen)

bàn xià (半夏 pinellia, Pinelliae Rhizoma)

chén pí (陈皮 tangerine peel, Citri Reticulatae Pericarpium)

sāng bái pí (桑白皮 mulberry root bark, Mori Cortex)

zhū líng (猪苓 polyporus, Polyporus)

fú líng (茯苓 poria, Poria)

xìng rén (杏仁 apricot kernel, Armeniacae Semen)

sū zǐ (苏子 perilla fruit, Perillae Fructus)

bái jí lí (白蒺藜 tribulus, Tribuli Fructus)

tíng lì zǐ (葶苈子 lepidium/descurainia, Lepidii/Descurainiae Semen)

guì zhī (桂枝 cinnamon twig, Cinnamomi Ramulus)

Comparisons

Sū zǐ (perilla fruit)[364] downbears qì and transforms phlegm. *Lái fú zǐ* (radish seed)[212] moves qì and disperses phlegm. *Bái jiè zǐ* warms the lung and sweeps phlegm.

Tíng lì zǐ (lepidium/descurainia)[323] is bitter and cold; it drains the lung and moves water, and tends to treat phlegm or water in the chest and diaphragm. *Bái jiè zǐ* is warm and acrid; it disinhibits qì and sweeps phlegm, and tends to eliminate phlegm between the skin and its inner membrane and in the rib-sides.

Special Uses

Bái jiè zǐ is also ground to a powder and applied topically.[18] In the past I have used it to treat peripheral neuroparalysis of the face by mixing it with enough strong tea to make a paste and smearing it on a piece of cloth cut to the required size and applied to the affected area for 4–8 hours. At the same time, the patient should take a decoction medicine appropriate for the pattern (see *bái fù zǐ* (typhonium), page 368). One packet of the decoction medicine is taken each day, and the topical application of *bái jiè zǐ* is performed once every two or three days. The effect is enhanced by pricking the mucous membrane of the buccal surface of the mouth at eight or nine spots on the affected side to allow slight bleeding.

Dosage

The dosage is generally 3–9 g/1–3 qián.

---

[18]When applied externally, *bái jiè zǐ* (white mustard) can irritate the skin and cause blistering. The blistering can leave small scars or a discolored area. (Ed.)

CAUTION

Contraindicated for cough due to lung vacuity with heat and in any form of yīn vacuity internal heat.

RESEARCH

According to modern research, *bái jiè zǐ* used externally dilates the capillary blood vessels, so it is a stimulant to the skin and mucous membrane. Consumed in large quantities, it decreases cardiac volume and rate.

---

14. 皂角 Zào Jiǎo   Gleditsiae Fructus
Gleditsia

Including

> ▷ *Zào jiǎo cì* (皂角刺 gleditsia thorn, Gleditsiae Spina)

Also called *zào jiá* 皂荚. Acrid and salty in flavor and warm in nature,[19] *zào jiǎo* (gleditsia) is a powerful phlegm-dispelling medicine. It also has the effect of opening the orifices and tracking down wind.

For wind strike with failure to recognize people and clenched jaw, use *zào jiǎo*—optionally adding an equal measure of *xì xīn* (asarum)—ground to a powder and blown into the nose to make the patient sneeze. After sneezing, the orifices of the lung will be free, qì and blood will flow smoothly, and treatment with acupuncture or medicinals will be more effective. If the patient does not sneeze, this is a sign that qì and blood are blocked and that the condition is hard to treat. For patients with strong constitutions, phlegm-drool congestion, and gurgling sound of phlegm in the throat, one can also use 30 g/1 liǎng of *zào jiǎo mò* (gleditsia powder) mixed with 15 g/5 qián of *bái fán mò* (alum powder). This is taken in doses of 3 g/ 1 qián, mixed with water and poured into the patient's mouth. This has the effect of thinning the drool and downbearing the phlegm, or in some cases, it will cause the patient to discharge a little thin drool. After this initial treatment, a decoction medicine tailored to the patient's pattern is given.

Zào jiǎo taken internally disperses phlegm accumulations, breaks concretions and binds, and precipitates wind constipation (bound stool in wind strike patients). For copious phlegm blocking the airways, cough with copious phlegm, or sticky white phlegm that is difficult to expectorate, grind *zào jiǎo* (made crisp through processing) to a powder, mix with honey, and form into pills the size of *wú tóng zǐ* (firmiana seed). This is taken in doses of three pills at a time, three or four times a day, and is known as *zào jiá wán* (Gleditsia Fruit Pill) from *Jīn Guì Yào Lüè* (金匮 要略 "Essential Prescriptions of the Golden Coffer"). For the same condition, one can also combine *zào jiǎo* with *sū zǐ* (perilla fruit), *bàn xià* (pinellia), *jú hóng* (red tangerine peel), *fú líng* (poria), *lái fú zǐ* (radish seed), and *xìng rén* (apricot kernel). For phlegm accumulation binding in a lump in the abdomen causing concretions

---

[19] *Zào jiǎo* (gleditsia) is considered to be slightly toxic. It is primarily used in pills and powders and generally is not decocted. (Ed.)

or aggregations, combine it with medicinals such as *zhǐ shí* (unripe bitter orange), *bái zhú* (white atractylodes), *shēng mǔ lì* (crude oyster shell), *zhì biē jiǎ* (mix-fried turtle shell), *táo rén* (peach kernel), *hóng huā* (carthamus), *sān léng* (sparganium), *é zhú* (curcuma rhizome), *shān zhā hé* (crataegus pit), and *zhì shān jiǎ* (mix-fried pangolin scales). For wind strike with exuberant phlegm and bound stool with absence of defecation for several days, make a decoction from *zào jiǎo* combined with medicinals such as *guā lóu* (trichosanthes) and *táo rén ní* (crushed peach kernel).

COMPARISONS

Zào jiǎo cì (gleditsia thorn) has actions broadly similar to those of *zào jiǎo* (gleditsia), but it quickens blood and dissipate binds and it is often used to treat welling- and flat-abscesses (痈疽 *yōng jū*) that have not ruptured, for which it is combined with medicinals such as *dāng guī wěi* (Chinese angelica tail), *chì sháo* (red peony), *hóng huā* (carthamus), *tiān huā fěn* (trichosanthes root), *jīn yín huā* (lonicera), *lián qiáo* (forsythia), *chén pí* (tangerine peel), and *zhì shān jiǎ* (mix-fried pangolin scales). I often use *zào jiǎo cì* combined with *bái jí lí* (tribulus), because *zào jiǎo cì* quickens the blood, transforms phlegm, and dissipates binds, while *bái jí lí* enters the liver channel, moves liver qì, and conducts *zào jiǎo cì* into the liver channel. I further combine these two medicinals to treat rib-side pain, hepatomegaly, and abdominal distention from infectious hepatitis. For this, I combine them with medicinals that regulate the liver and rectify qì, harmonize the stomach and aid digestion, and quicken stasis, such as:

chái hú (柴胡 bupleurum, Bupleuri Radix)

huáng qín (黄芩 scutellaria, Scutellariae Radix)

bàn xià (半夏 pinellia, Pinelliae Rhizoma)

chuān liàn zǐ (川楝子 toosendan, Toosendan Fructus)

wǔ líng zhī (五灵脂 squirrel's droppings, Trogopteri Faeces)

hóng huā (红花 carthamus, Carthami Flos)

jiāo sān xiān (焦三仙 scorch-fried three immortals, Tres Immortales Usti)

liú jì nú (刘寄奴 anomalous artemisia, Artemisiae Anomalae Herba)

jiāo bīng láng (焦槟榔 scorch-fried areca, Arecae Semen Ustum)

This formula, varied according to the signs, produces good results after 20–50 packets of the formula are taken.

Bái jiè zǐ (white mustard),[364] being acrid and penetrating, enters the area **outside the membrane within the skin**[559] (皮里膜外 *pí lǐ mó wài*) as well as the chest and rib-side where it warms and transforms phlegm binds. *Zào jiǎo*, being acrid and salty, disperses phlegm binds and is used for exuberant phlegm with cough, wind strike with exuberant phlegm, and phlegm-accumulation lumps in the abdomen.

DOSAGE

The dosage is generally 0.9–3 g/3 fēn–1 qián. *Zào jiǎo cì* (gleditsia thorn) is used in doses of 3–9 g/1–3 qián.

CAUTION

Contraindicated for vacuity patterns with phlegm, welling-abscesses and sores that have already ruptured, and pregnant women.

---

15. 白附子 Bái Fù Zǐ   Typhonii Rhizoma
Typhonium

Acrid in flavor and warm in nature, *bái fù zǐ* (typhonium)[20] dispels wind, transforms phlegm, and expels cold-damp. It is often used to treat wind-phlegm.

1. Wind Strike with Deviated Eyes and Mouth: When the head and face are assailed by wind-cold, which causes channel vessel hypertonicity, and wind-phlegm obstructs the channels and network vessels, causing deviation of the mouth and eyes, this can be treated by using *bái fù zǐ* combined with *bái jiāng cán* (silkworm) and *quán xiē* (scorpion) to form *qiān zhèng sǎn* (Pull Aright Powder). I frequently treat facial paralysis (Bell's palsy) using *qiān zhèng sǎn* (Pull Aright Powder) with additions such as the following:

bái zhǐ (白芷 Dahurian angelica, Angelicae Dahuricae Radix)

jīng jiè (荆芥 schizonepeta, Schizonepetae Herba)

fáng fēng (防风 saposhnikovia, Saposhnikoviae Radix)

hóng huā (红花 carthamus, Carthami Flos)

tiān nán xīng (天南星 arisaema, Arisaematis Rhizoma)

bái jiè zǐ (白芥子 white mustard, Sinapis Albae Semen)

zào jiǎo cì (皂角刺 gleditsia thorn, Gleditsiae Spina)

táo rén (桃仁 peach kernel, Persicae Semen)

sū mù (苏木 sappan, Sappan Lignum)

A tip worth remembering is that the effect of the decoction medicine is invariably enhanced if a hot pack made by placing the dregs of the decoction inside a bag is applied to the affected side of the face.

2. Lockjaw with Stiff Neck, Rigidity of the Limbs, Convulsions, Arched-Back Rigidity, and Clenched Jaw: For such conditions, *bái fù zǐ* is combined with medicinals such as:

bái zhǐ (白芷 Dahurian angelica, Angelicae Dahuricae Radix)

tiān nán xīng (天南星 arisaema, Arisaematis Rhizoma)

tiān má (天麻 gastrodia, Gastrodiae Rhizoma)

qiāng huó (羌活 notopterygium, Notopterygii Rhizoma et Radix)

fáng fēng (防风 saposhnikovia, Saposhnikoviae Radix)

chán tuì (蝉蜕 cicada molting, Cicadae Periostracum)

quán xiē (全蝎 scorpion, Scorpio)

---

[20] *Bái fù zǐ* (Typhonium) should be prepared from the tuber of *Typhonium giganteum* ENGL. In and outside of China, *bái fù piàn* 白附片 (*Aconitum coreanum* (LÉVL.) RAIPAICS) is commonly used as a substitute. (Ed.)

wú gōng (蜈蚣 centipede, Scolopendra)

gōu téng (钩藤 uncaria, Uncariae Ramulus cum Uncis)

3. Headache and Hemilateral Headache: When cold-damp or wind-phlegm produces headache or hemilateral headache, *bái fù zǐ* upbears and dissipates with warmth and acridity. Its nature is to move upward, and it enters the yáng brightness (*yáng míng*) channel and penetrates the head and face to expel cold-damp and to dispel wind-phlegm. *Bái fù zǐ* is frequently combined with medicinals such as *bái zhǐ* (Dahurian angelica), *chuān xiōng* (chuanxiong), *bàn xià* (pinellia), *tiān má* (gastrodia), *màn jīng zǐ* (vitex), and *fáng fēng* (saposhnikovia) for headaches.

COMPARISONS

Chuān fù zǐ (aconite) expels wind-cold-damp and tends to enter the kidney channel; it warms and assists kidney yáng. *Bái fù zǐ* dispels wind-phlegm cold-damp and tends to enter the stomach channel; it treats wandering wind of the face.

Bái jiāng cán (silkworm) tends to be used to treat wind-heat phlegm bind and throat impediment[566] (喉痹 *hóu bì*) with swollen throat. *Bái fù zǐ* tends to be used to treat wind-phlegm cold-damp and all diseases of the upper body and of the head and face.

DOSAGE

The dosage is generally 2.5–6 g/8 fēn–2 qián, but in severe conditions one may use up to 9 g/3 qián.

CAUTION

Contraindicated for repletion heat wind strike or fire-heat invading the upper body.

---

16. 硫黄 Liú Huáng   Sulphur
Sulfur

Sour in flavor, hot in nature, and toxic, *liú huáng* (sulfur) strongly supplements kidney yáng. It also courses and disinhibits the large intestine, and, being hot in nature, though not drying, it is used to treat vacuity constipation in the elderly (yáng vacuity with bound stool).

Liú huáng is taken internally for debilitation of kidney yáng that leads to cold extremities with a lack of strength, impotence, and genital cold (which in extreme cases can become fulminant expiration of yáng qì, where life is about to expire); it is combined with medicinals such as:

shú dì huáng (熟地黄 cooked rehmannia, Rehmanniae Radix Praeparata)

shān zhū yú (山茱萸 cornus, Corni Fructus)

bā jǐ tiān (巴戟天 morinda, Morindae Officinalis Radix)

yín yáng huò (淫羊藿 epimedium, Epimedii Herba)

ròu cōng róng (肉苁蓉 cistanche, Cistanches Herba)

bǔ gǔ zhī (补骨脂 psoralea, Psoraleae Fructus)

ròu guì (肉桂 cinnamon bark, Cinnamomi Cortex)

fù zǐ (附子 aconite, Aconiti Radix Lateralis Praeparata)

rén shēn (人参 ginseng, Ginseng Radix)

For elderly patients or those with chronic vacuity in whom there is lower burner yáng vacuity, blockage of stool and urine, a lack of force in the large intestine, and bound stool that fails to descend, use *liú huáng* combined with *bàn xià* (pinellia), *ròu cōng róng* (cistanche), *dāng guī* (Chinese angelica), and *shú dì huáng* (cooked rehmannia) to assist yáng and free the stool. Physicians of former times used *bàn liú wán* (Pinellia and Sulfur Pill), which contains *bàn xià* and *liú huáng*, to treat vacuity constipation in the elderly. In the past I have used 0.9–1.5 g/3–5 fēn of *liú huáng*, taken with decoction medicine, twice a day, to specifically treat an inability to pass stool in paraplegics with chronic myelitis affecting the lower extremities and have achieved satisfactory effects. One should consider using the prescription below.

shú dì huáng (熟地黄 cooked rehmannia, Rehmanniae Radix Praeparata)
    30–45 g/1–1.5 liǎng

shān zhū yú (山茱萸 cornus, Corni Fructus) 9 g/3 qián

dāng guī (当归 Chinese angelica, Angelicae Sinensis Radix) 12 g/4 qián

ròu cōng róng (肉苁蓉 cistanche, Cistanches Herba) 15–25 g/5–8 qián

táo rén ní (桃仁泥 crushed peach kernel, Persicae Semen Tusum) 12 g/4 qián

bā jǐ tiān (巴戟天 morinda, Morindae Officinalis Radix) 12 g/4 qián

yín yáng huò (淫羊藿 epimedium, Epimedii Herba) 12 g/4 qián

ròu guì (肉桂 cinnamon bark, Cinnamomi Cortex) 6–9 g/2–3 qián

bàn xià (半夏 pinellia, Pinelliae Rhizoma) 9 g/3 qián

shēng dà huáng (生大黄 raw rhubarb, Rhei Radix et Rhizoma Crudi)
    9 g/3 qián (this is used when *dà huáng* (rhubarb) has already been used
    and the stool has not been passed)

bīng láng (槟榔 areca, Arecae Semen) 9 g/3 qián

Decoct with water; divide 1.8–3 g/6 fēn–1 qián of *liú huáng* into two parts and take drenched with the decoction. This formula is varied in accordance with signs.

Liú huáng applied topically can treat skin diseases such as scab (*jiè*), lichen (*xuǎn*), and **damp sores**[545] (湿疮 *shī chuāng*). It is frequently used as an oil paste, a wash, or a skin rub.[21]

DOSAGE

The dosage is generally 0.6–2.5 g/2 fēn–8 fēn. It is often taken in pill form or ground to a powder that is then taken drenched with the decoction medicine.

---

[21]*liú huáng gāo* (Sulfur Paste) is one example. This paste, used to treat damp eczema and scabies, is made by combining 10% (by weight) *liú huáng* (sulfur) with 90% petroleum jelly (a non-petroleum substitute can be used). (Ed.)

CAUTION

This medicinal is toxic, so it should not be taken in excessively large doses or over extended periods of time. One must be careful to avoid poisonings.

17. 乌头 **Wū Tóu**
Wild Aconite
Aconiti Kusnezoffii Radix

Distinction is made between two kinds of *wū tóu* (wild aconite). The kind grown in Sìchuān is called *chuān wū tóu* (川乌头, aconite root) or *chuān wū* (for the other type see "*Fù zǐ* (附子, aconite)," page 339). Wild varieties and those grown anywhere else in China are referred to as *cǎo wū tóu* 草乌头 or *cǎo wū* 草乌. *Chuān wū tóu* (aconite root) is acrid, very hot, and highly toxic. Its actions and contraindications are similar to those of *fù zǐ* (aconite); therefore, please see that section as they will not be repeated here.

Cǎo wū tóu (wild aconite) is also acrid, very hot, and highly toxic. Its primary actions are to track (down) wind and overcome dampness, eliminate cold and free impediment, and break accumulations and dissipate binds. It also frees stubborn phlegm in order to treat stubborn sores, and has anesthetic and analgesic actions. Its power to attack toxin with toxin (以毒攻毒 *yǐ dú gōng dú*)[22] is greater than that of *chuān wū* (aconite root) and *fù zǐ* (aconite).

Cǎo wū tóu is combined with medicinals such as *sāng jì shēng* (mistletoe), *dú huó* (pubescent angelica), *xù duàn* (dipsacus), *niú xī* (achyranthes), *wēi líng xiān* (clematis), *shēn jīn cǎo* (ground pine), *qiān nián jiàn* (homalomena), *fù piàn* (sliced aconite), and *gǔ suì bǔ* (drynaria) to treat patterns of wind-cold that cause low back, leg, joint, or flesh pain, that make it difficult to walk, and that are intractable and do not respond to treatment. Combined with *chuān wū* (aconite root), *rǔ xiāng* (frankincense), *mò yào* (myrrh), *sāng zhī* (mulberry twig), *guì zhī* (cinnamon twig), *fáng fēng* (saposhnikovia), *chuān xiōng* (chuanxiong), *hóng huā* (carthamus), *dì lóng* (earthworm), *zhì shān jiǎ* (mix-fried pangolin scales), and *dà hēi dòu* (black soybean), it is used for paralysis from stroke, shaking hands and feet, and inhibited speech.

Cǎo wū tóu is frequently used to make medicinal wine. For example, place 6 g/ 2 qián each of *cǎo wū tóu* (wild aconite), *chuān wū* (aconite root), *wū méi* (mume), *jīn yín huā* (lonicera), *gān cǎo* (licorice), and *hóng huā* (carthamus) in 1 jīn of *bái jiǔ* (white liquor) and steep for 20 days; one can also add 50 g/1.7 liǎng each of *hóng táng* (brown sugar) and *bái táng* (white sugar). Take 5 ml three times a day. This medicinal wine treats wind-cold-damp that gives rise to joint pain, lumbar and leg pain, rheumatic arthritis, rheumatoid arthritis, and similar diseases, as long as there are no heat signs.

---

[22]Attack toxin with toxin, 以毒攻毒 *yǐ dú gōng dú*: Poisonous things can overcome other poisonous things, a notion commonly applied in Chinese medicine. (Ed.)

For intractable cases of head wind, headache, or wind-phlegm headache, combine *căo wū tóu* with equal doses of *chuān wū* (aconite root), *chì xiăo dòu* (rice bean), *cāng zhú* (atractylodes), *chuān xiōng* (chuanxiong), *shēng jiāng* (fresh ginger), *huò xiāng* (agastache), *rŭ xiāng* (frankincense), *shè xiāng* (musk) (a small amount), and *pèi lán* (eupatorium). Grind to a fine powder. Use water in which scallions were boiled to make the powder into pills each the size of a *lǜ dòu* (mung bean). Take the pills twice a day, after meals, with a decoction made from 1.5 g/ 0.5 qián of *bò hé* (mint). Take 1.5–3 g/5 fēn–1 qián of the pills at a time. At the same time, one can take several of the pills, dissolve them in warm water, and apply the liquid to the Greater Yáng point and the forehead. (Note: avoid getting the medicinal solution in the eyes.) This method is invariably effective.

RESEARCH

According to modern research, *chuān wū tóu* (aconite root) and *căo wū tóu* (wild aconite) both contain aconitine, which has definite anti-cancer effects. As a result, these medicinals have been used as anti-cancer medicinals.

When I use this medicinal to treat cancer, it is generally part of the classical prescription *xiăo jīn dān* (Minor Golden Elixir), which is traditionally a ready-prepared medicine. This goes with a decoction medicine that is chosen on the basis of pattern identification and treatment differentiation. The prescription and processing method for *xiăo jīn dān* (Minor Golden Elixir) are given below:

>*căo wū tóu* (草乌头 wild aconite, Aconiti Kusnezoffii Radix) 46 g/1.5 liăng (mix-fried in water with *gān căo* and *jīn yín huā*)
>
>*bái jiāo xiāng* (白胶香 liquidambar, Liquidambaris Resina) 46 g/ 1.5 liăng[23]
>
>*wŭ líng zhī* (五灵脂 squirrel's droppings, Trogopteri Faeces) (mix-fried with vinegar) 46 g/1.5 liăng
>
>*dì lóng ròu* (地龙肉 earthworm, Pheretima) 46 g/1.5 liăng
>
>*mù biē zĭ* (木鳖子 momordica, Momordicae Semen) (remove peel) 46 g/1.5 liăng
>
>*rŭ xiāng* (乳香 frankincense, Olibanum) (mix-fried with vinegar) 23 g/8 qián
>
>*mò yào* (没药 myrrh, Myrrha) (mix-fried with vinegar) 23 g/8 qián
>
>*dāng guī* (当归 Chinese angelica, Angelicae Sinensis Radix) 23 g/8 qián
>
>*xiāng mò* (香墨 ink, Atramentum) 3.7 g/1 qián

Grind all the ingredients to a fine powder. Grind into this 9.4 g/3 qián of *shè xiāng* (musk), mixing thoroughly until evenly distributed. Then mix 94 g/3 liăng of white wheat flour into a paste and let it cool. Thoroughly mix the medicinal powder into the paste so it is distributed evenly. Form this mixture into pills and dry in the shade. Each dry pill should weigh approximately 0.63 g. Take two pills, twice a day, with warm water or warm *huáng jiŭ* (yellow wine). This pill is used for scrofular tuberculosis, mammary sores, mammary welling-abscesses, hard, painful swellings, and early-stage yīn abscesses.

---

[23]*Bái jiāo xiāng* (白胶香, liquidambar) is also called 枫脂香 *fēng zhī xiāng*.

I have given patients *xiǎo jīn dān* (Minor Golden Elixir) (2–3 pills, or 1 pill if the pills are 1.5 g/5 fēn) twice a day with a decoction medicine, chosen in accordance with the principle of pattern identification as the basis for determining treatment, to treat cervical lymph granuloma, breast cancer (early stage), and stomach cancer. (The pills may be swallowed with the decoction or taken separately.) This method achieves a definite effect, not only relieving the subjective symptoms, but also causing any hard binds to soften or reduce in size. In some cases, these binds may dissipate completely. Unfortunately, patients were too few and the duration of treatment was not long enough to permit a systematic study offering useful conclusions. I merely offer my experience.

DOSAGE

The dosage is generally 0.6–3 g/2 fēn–1 qián. Slightly more is used in severe cases.

CAUTION

Contraindications and points for attention are the same as for *fù zǐ* (aconite), as explained on page 339.[24]

---

[24]Like *fù zǐ* (aconite), this medicinal should be pre-decocted. (Ed.)

Lecture Eight
Blood-Quickening Stasis-Transforming Medicinals
活血化瘀药 *Huó Xuè Huà Yū Yào*

Generally speaking, medicinals that quicken the blood and transform stasis can treat any disease or symptom caused by static blood or loss of smooth blood circulation. Nevertheless, when using medicinals that quicken the blood and transform stasis, one must consider the etiology of the static blood as well as all the other relevant factors. Therefore, one must flexibly combine the principles of identifying patterns as the basis for determining treatment with a holistic consideration [of the problem], comprehensive analysis, the requirements of the particular condition, and the selection of medicinals appropriate to the pattern.

In addition, more than a few of the medicinals that quicken the blood and transform stasis also stanch bleeding; therefore it is important to pay attention to the processing and combining of these medicinals. Moreover, readers may wish to refer to Lecture Nine, where blood-stanching medicinals are discussed, since some of those medicinals also have blood-moving effects.

Medicinals that quicken the blood and transform stasis are sometimes also used to treat diseases without static blood, in which case they increase the movement of qì and blood in order to achieve the goal of curing illness. The following sayings are examples from the precious experience of past physicians: "To treat wind, first treat the blood; when blood moves, the wind naturally disappears" (治风先治血, 血行风自灭 *zhì fēng xiān zhì xuè, xuè xíng fēng zì miè*); "quicken the blood to outthrust papules" (活血透疹 *huó xuè tòu zhěn*); and "quicken the blood to resolve toxin" (活血解毒 *huó xuè jiě dú*). From this we can see that our understanding of medicinals that quicken the blood and transform stasis should not be too narrow or static.

1. 川芎 **Chuān Xiōng**   Chuanxiong Rhizoma
Chuanxiong

Chuān xiōng (chuanxiong) was originally known as *xiōng qióng* 芎藭, but because Sìchuān Province produces the greatest quantities and the highest quality of this medicinal, it is commonly known as *chuān xiōng* (chuanxiong). *Chuān xiōng*, which is acrid in flavor and warm in nature, moves the qì and quickens the blood, tracks down wind, and opens depression. It is a medicinal for the qì within the blood. It ascends to the head and descends to the sea of blood. It is acrid, warming, mobile, and pentrating; it presses forward and is penetrating without containing.

1. **Moving Qì and Quickening the Blood:** Qì stagnation in the blood that inhibits movement of blood can cause menstrual irregularities, **menstrual block**[557] (经 闭 *jīng bì*), abdominal pain during menstruation, difficult delivery, or retention of the placenta. This medicinal enters the blood to move qì, and when the qì moves, the blood is quickened. For this purpose it is often combined with medicinals such as *dāng guī* (Chinese angelica), *sháo yào* (peony), *hóng huā* (carthamus), *yì mǔ cǎo* (leonurus), *shú dì huáng* (cooked rehmannia), *xiāng fù* (cyperus), and *ài yè* (mugwort). This medicinal may be used in pregnancy, before labor, or after delivery; it is commonly used in gynecology. I often use it for postpartum blood stasis and qì stagnation that causes pain in the smaller abdomen or for pain in the lesser or smaller abdomen that has persisted for many days after birth, or for irregular menstrual cycles. For this one should use the following formula.

Shēng huà tāng 生化汤   Engendering Transformation Decoction

---

chuān xiōng (川芎 chuanxiong, Chuanxiong Rhizoma) 6–9 g/2–3 qián

dāng guī (当归 Chinese angelica, Angelicae Sinensis Radix) 9 g/3 qián

hóng huā (红花 carthamus, Carthami Flos) 3 g/1 qián

táo rén (桃仁 peach kernel, Persicae Semen) 3 g/1 qián

pào jiāng (炮姜 blast-fried ginger, Zingiberis Rhizoma Praeparatum) 1.5–2.5 g/5–8 fēn

With the addition of:

yì mǔ cǎo (益母草 leonurus, Leonuri Herba) 9–15 g/3–5 qián

wǔ líng zhī (五灵脂 squirrel's droppings, Trogopteri Faeces) 9 g/3 qián

yán hú suǒ (延胡索 corydalis, Corydalis Rhizoma) 6 g/2 qián

If this formula is varied in accordance with signs, it will certainly achieve good results.

In internal medicine, for blood stasis and qì stagnation that causes various forms of pain with fixed location, *chuān xiōng* is often combined with medicinals such as:

hóng huā (红花 carthamus, Carthami Flos)

táo rén (桃仁 peach kernel, Persicae Semen)

wǔ líng zhī (五灵脂 squirrel's droppings, Trogopteri Faeces)

rǔ xiāng (乳香 frankincense, Olibanum)

mò yào (没药 myrrh, Myrrha)

2. Drying Dampness and Tracking Down Wind: For joint and limb pain, numbness, or hypertonicity of the arms and legs that arises when wind-cold-damp coagulates in the blood, and the blood stagnates and fails to move as normal, one can use *chuān xiōng* to enter the blood and move the qì. When the qì moves, the blood is quickened; when the blood moves, wind-cold is dispersed. This medicinal also dries damp evil in the blood and therefore can be used for any impediment pattern due to wind-cold-damp. An example of this is the formula below:

Sān bì tāng 三痹汤   Three Impediment Decoction

dǎng shēn (党参 codonopsis, Codonopsis Radix)

huáng qí (黄芪 astragalus, Astragali Radix)

chuān xiōng (川芎 chuanxiong, Chuanxiong Rhizoma)

dāng guī (当归 Chinese angelica, Angelicae Sinensis Radix)

bái sháo (白芍 white peony, Paeoniae Radix Alba)

shēng dì huáng (生地黄 dried/fresh rehmannia, Rehmanniae Radix Exsiccata seu Recens)

dù zhòng (杜仲 eucommia, Eucommiae Cortex)

niú xī (牛膝 achyranthes, Achyranthis Bidentatae Radix)

guì xīn (桂心 shaved cinnamon bark, Cinnamomi Cortex Rasus)

xì xīn (细辛 asarum, Asari Herba)

qín jiāo (秦艽 large gentian, Gentianae Macrophyllae Radix)

dú huó (独活 pubescent angelica, Angelicae Pubescentis Radix)

fáng fēng (防风 saposhnikovia, Saposhnikoviae Radix)

In the Qīng Dynasty, Zhāng Shí-Wǎn (张石顽) recorded a similar formula by the same name, *sān bì tāng* (Three Impediment Decoction). In his version, *shēng dì huáng* (dried/fresh rehmannia), *dù zhòng* (eucommia), *niú xī* (achyranthes), *qín jiāo* (large gentian), and *dú huó* (pubescent angelica) were subtracted, while *fáng jǐ* (fangji), *bái zhú* (white atractylodes), and *wū tóu* (wild aconite) were added. One should choose the formula most suited to the identified pattern. When wind-cold invades the head and causes qì and blood stagnation and blockage, resulting in headache or hemilateral headache, use this medicinal to ascend to the head and eyes, dissipate wind, and course the exterior. For this purpose it is often combined with medicinals such as *bái zhǐ* (Dahurian angelica), *qiāng huó* (notopterygium), *fáng fēng* (saposhnikovia), *xì xīn* (asarum), and *bò hé* (mint), as in *chuān xiōng chá tiáo sǎn* (Tea-Blended Chuanxiong Powder). If there is concurrent wind-heat, add medicinals such as *jú huā* (chrysanthemum), *màn jīng zǐ* (vitex), *jīng jiè* (schizonepeta), *bò hé* (mint), *huáng qín* (scutellaria), and *jīn yín huā* (lonicera). This medicinal enters the liver and gallbladder channels and is therefore used as a channel conductor when treating hemilateral headache.

3. Opening Depression and Regulating the Liver: The liver controls storage of the blood and employs the qì. Both qì and blood depression affect the smooth flow of qì and blood in the liver channel, which can cause symptoms such as oppression in the chest, rib-side pain, hemilateral distention and pain in the head, and menstrual irregularities. In such cases, *chuān xiōng* can be used to resolve depression with acridity and dispersion (the liver functions best under conditions of acridity and dispersion). For this purpose it is often combined with medicinals such as:

xiāng fù (香附 cyperus, Cyperi Rhizoma)

chái hú (柴胡 bupleurum, Bupleuri Radix)

bái sháo (白芍 white peony, Paeoniae Radix Alba)

chuān liàn zǐ (川楝子 toosendan, Toosendan Fructus)

dāng guī (当归 Chinese angelica, Angelicae Sinensis Radix)

sū gěng (苏梗 perilla stem, Perillae Caulis)

zhǐ qiào (枳壳 bitter orange, Aurantii Fructus)

When *chuān xiōng* is added to blood-supplementing formulas, it moves blood stagnation and moves damp qì in the blood. An example of this use is *sì wù tāng* (Four Agents Decoction), which contains *shú dì huáng* (cooked rehmannia), *bái sháo* (white peony), *dāng guī* (Chinese angelica), and *chuān xiōng*. In this formula, *chuān xiōng* moves the blood and disperses damp qì to mitigate the sticky, slimy, and clogging effects of *shú dì huáng* (cooked rehmannia) and *bái sháo* (white peony). It also assists blood-supplementing medicinals in fully expressing their blood-supplementing effects. The dosage must be determined on the basis of the pattern identified.

Comparisons

Bái zhǐ (dahurian angelica)[22] tends to treat yáng brightness (*yáng míng*) channel (frontal) wind-damp headache. *Chuān xiōng* tends to treat lesser yáng (*shào yáng*) channel (either side of the head) headaches resulting from blood depression and qì stagnation.

Research

According to modern research, animal experiments have shown that this medicinal has hypotensive effects. Small doses have also been shown to increase uterine contractions in pregnant animals. Nevertheless, large doses have the opposite effect and inhibit contractions.

Dosage

The dosage is generally 1.5–9 g/5 fēn–3 qián.

Caution

This medicinal is inappropriate for effulgent yīn vacuity fire.

2. 丹参 Dān Shēn   Salviae Miltiorrhizae
Salvia   Radix

Bitter in flavor and slightly cold in nature, *dān shēn* (salvia) quickens static blood, engenders new blood, cools the blood, and quiets the spirit.

1. Quickening Static Blood: For any disease due to qì stagnation and blood stasis, this medicinal can be selected and used in accordance with the pattern identified. Examples are given below.

a) Dysmenorrhea or menstrual block: For these conditions, it can be combined with medicinals such as:

dāng guī (当归 Chinese angelica, Angelicae Sinensis Radix)

chì sháo (赤芍 red peony, Paeoniae Radix Rubra)

shú dì huáng (熟地黄 cooked rehmannia, Rehmanniae Radix Praeparata)

chuān xiōng (川芎 chuanxiong, Chuanxiong Rhizoma)

táo rén (桃仁 peach kernel, Persicae Semen)

hóng huā (红花 carthamus, Carthami Flos)

xiāng fù (香附 cyperus, Cyperi Rhizoma)

shēng pú huáng (生蒲黄 raw typha pollen, Typhae Pollen Crudum)

niú xī (牛膝 achyranthes, Achyranthis Bidentatae Radix)

qiàn cǎo (茜草 madder, Rubiae Radix)

b) Concretions, conglomerations, accumulations, and gatherings[544] (癥瘕积聚 *zhēng jiǎ jī jù*): For these conditions, which include hepatosplenomegaly, abdominal cysts, and tumors, *dān shēn* can be combined with medicinals such as:

zhì biē jiǎ (炙鳖甲 mix-fried turtle shell, Trionycis Carapax cum Liquido Frictus)

shēng mǔ lì (生牡蛎 crude oyster shell, Ostreae Concha Cruda)

zhǐ shí (枳实 unripe bitter orange, Aurantii Fructus Immaturus)

dāng guī wěi (当归尾 Chinese angelica tail, Angelicae Sinensis Radicis Extremitas)

táo rén (桃仁 peach kernel, Persicae Semen)

hóng huā (红花 carthamus, Carthami Flos)

bái zhú (白术 white atractylodes, Atractylodis Macrocephalae Rhizoma)

fú líng (茯苓 poria, Poria)

sān léng (三棱 sparganium, Sparganii Rhizoma)

é zhú (莪术 curcuma rhizome, Curcumae Rhizoma)

shān zhā hé (山楂核 crataegus pit, Crataegi Endocarpium et Semen)

cāng zhú (苍术 atractylodes, Atractylodis Rhizoma)

xiāng fù (香附 cyperus, Cyperi Rhizoma)

guì zhī (桂枝 cinnamon twig, Cinnamomi Ramulus)

Some physicians of the past have used *dān shēn* singly and over a long period of time to treat tumors in the abdomen, such as *dān shēn sǎn* (Salvia Powder) from *Shěn Shì Zūn Shēng* (沈氏尊生 "Shěn's Respect for Life").

c) Static blood abdominal pain: This presents as pain with a relatively fixed location, a long course of illness, stasis macules on the tongue, or a history of knocks and falls. For this purpose it is combined with medicinals such as:

dāng guī (当归 Chinese angelica, Angelicae Sinensis Radix)

chì sháo (赤芍 red peony, Paeoniae Radix Rubra)

bái sháo (白芍 white peony, Paeoniae Radix Alba)

hóng huā (红花 carthamus, Carthami Flos)

táo rén (桃仁 peach kernel, Persicae Semen)

mù xiāng (木香 costusroot, Aucklandiae Radix)

wū yào (乌药 lindera, Linderae Radix)

wú yú (吴萸 evodia, Evodiae Fructus)

wǔ líng zhī (五灵脂 squirrel's droppings, Trogopteri Faeces)

shēng pú huáng (生蒲黄 raw typha pollen, Typhae Pollen Crudum)

liú jì nú (刘寄奴 anomalous artemisia, Artemisiae Anomalae Herba)

For stomach duct pain (including pain from ulcers) that has persisted over a long period of time (enduring illness tends to enter the blood aspect) with variable signs of vacuity and repletion that appear together and with cold and heat signs that alternate, I often use the following combination of formulas to quicken stasis and regulate qì:

Dān shēn yǐn 丹参饮   Salvia Beverage

---

dān shēn (丹参 salvia, Salviae Miltiorrhizae Radix) 30 g/2 liǎng

tán xiāng (檀香 sandalwood, Santali Albi Lignum) 6 g/2 qián (add at end)

shā rén (砂仁 amomum, Amomi Fructus) 3 g/1 qián

Liáng fù wán 良附丸   Lesser Galangal and Cyperus Pill

---

gāo liáng jiāng (高良姜 lesser galangal, Alpiniae Officinarum Rhizoma)
    9 g/3 qián

xiāng fù (香附 cyperus, Cyperi Rhizoma) 9 g/3 qián

Bǎi hé tāng 百合汤   Lily Bulb Decoction

---

bǎi hé (百合 lily bulb, Lilii Bulbus) 30 g/1 liǎng

wū yào (乌药 lindera, Linderae Radix) 9 g/3 qián

If there is pronounced blood stasis, one can use *shī xiào sǎn* (Sudden Smile Powder), which contains *wǔ líng zhī* (squirrel's droppings) and *pú huáng* (typha pollen). In most cases, very good results can be achieved by adding or subtracting two or three medicinals from these formulas. For ease of memory, I call this *sān hé tāng* (Three-Combination Decoction) or *sì hé tāng* (Four-Combination Decoction).

d) Painful swollen joints: When wind, cold, and dampness evils obstruct the channels and network vessels, become depressed, and transform into heat, the result is painful, swollen joints that also have signs of redness and heat. To treat this condition, *dān shēn* can be combined with medicinals such as *rěn dōng téng* (lonicera stem and leaf), *qín jiāo* (large gentian), *wēi líng xiān* (clematis), *yǐ mǐ* (coix), *hóng huā* (carthamus), *chì sháo* (red peony), *huáng bǎi* (phellodendron), *qiāng huó* (notopterygium), *dú huó* (pubescent angelica), *sāng zhī* (mulberry twig), and *cán shā* (silkworm droppings).

e) Cinnabar toxin and swollen welling-abscess: For these conditions, *dān shēn* can be combined with medicinals such as *dān pí* (moutan), *chì sháo* (red peony), *tiān huā fěn* (trichosanthes root), *jīn yín huā* (lonicera), *lián qiáo* (forsythia), and *pú gōng yīng* (dandelion).

2. Engendering New Blood: *Dān shēn* specifically moves into the blood aspect and has the effects of dispelling stasis and engendering the new. There is a traditional saying, "The single medicinal *dān shēn* has the effect of *sì wù tāng* (Four Agents Decoction)." This medicinal is most suitable for blood vacuity with slight heat signs; it can engender new blood as well as supplementing blood vacuity. For this purpose it is often combined with medicinals such as *dāng guī* (Chinese angelica), *shēng dì huáng* (dried/fresh rehmannia), *bái sháo* (white peony), *chuān xiōng* (chuanxiong), *dǎng shēn* (codonopsis), *bái zhú* (white atractylodes), and *fú líng* (poria). In recent years this medicinal has been shown to be effective in treating various forms of anemia and thrombocytopenic purpura (when it presents as blood heat). This medicinal is slightly cold in nature; therefore for dual vacuity of qì and blood without heat signs it is better to select *chǎo dān shēn* (stir-fried salvia), because stir-frying corrects its slightly cold nature.

3. Cooling the Blood and Quieting the Spirit: For warm disease heat entering construction-blood and causing blood-heat vexation, marked by calm in the morning and vexation at night (昼静夜躁 *zhòu jìng yè zào*) or maculopapular eruptions, *dān shēn* can be combined with medicinals such as *shēng dì huáng* (dried/fresh rehmannia), *xuán shēn* (scrophularia), *chì sháo* (red peony), *dān pí* (moutan), *dì gǔ pí* (lycium root bark), and *guǎng xī jiǎo* (African rhinoceros horn). For blood vacuity with heat that results in vexation and agitation and in sleeplessness, it is combined with medicinals such as *shēng dì huáng* (dried/fresh rehmannia), *huáng lián* (coptis), *yù jīn* (curcuma), *yuǎn zhì* (polygala), *suān zǎo rén* (spiny jujube), *zhēn zhū mǔ* (mother-of-pearl), and *mài dōng* (ophiopogon).

COMPARISONS

Dāng guī (Chinese angelica)[111] is warm in nature and its blood-supplementing action is stronger than its stasis-dispelling action, whereas *dān shēn* is slightly cold in nature and its stasis-dispelling action is stronger than its blood-supplementing action. Being said to dispel stasis and engender the new, *dān shēn* does have a blood-engendering action, although its supplementing power is not as great as that of *dāng guī*.

Zǐ cǎo (arnebia/lithospermum)[309] breaks blood, frees the channels, frees the nine orifices, disinhibits urine and stool, and tends to enter the liver channel. *Dān shēn* dispels stasis and engenders the new, nourishes the blood and quiets the spirit, and tends to enter the heart channel.

RESEARCH

According to modern research reports, animal experiments have shown that *dān shēn* is hypotensive. Some reports also show that, in patients with hepatosplenomegaly resulting from advanced-stage hepatitis or schistosomiasis, *dān shēn* can promote improvements in liver function and can shrink and soften an enlarged liver. *Dān shēn* contains iodine and is therefore effective in treating thyroid enlargement due to iodine deficiency.

DOSAGE

The dosage is generally 9–30 g/3 qián–1 liǎng.

CAUTION

Use with caution in cases of profuse menstruation, coughing of blood, or blood in the urine.

---

3. 延胡索 Yán Hú Suǒ   Corydalis Rhizoma
Corydalis

Also called *yuán hú* 元胡. Acrid and slightly bitter in flavor and warm in nature, *yán hú suǒ* (corydalis) primarily quickens the blood and moves qì. There is an old saying that it "moves qì stagnation in the blood and blood stagnation in the qì." By quickening the blood and moving qì it treats any type of pain anywhere in the entire body—in the upper body or lower body, inside or outside, in the heart [region] and abdomen, or in the lumbus and the knees.

1. **Treating Pain:** This medicinal is warm, acrid, and mobile[557] (善走 *shàn zǒu*); it quickens the blood and disinhibits qì. When qì and blood are free, there is no pain. For example, heat-type stomach duct pain characterized by dry mouth, yellow tongue fur, pain that comes and goes, a liking for cool food and drinks, and a rapid pulse is treated by combining *yán hú suǒ* with medicinals such as *jīn líng zǐ* (toosendan),[1] *huáng lián* (coptis), *xiāng fù* (cyperus), and *chǎo zhī zǐ* (stir-fried gardenia).

For cold pain in the abdomen (characterized by a liking for warmth, a white tongue fur, a liking for hot foods, and a stringlike pulse), *yán hú suǒ* is combined with medicinals such as *gāo liáng jiāng* (lesser galangal), *ròu guì* (cinnamon bark), *gān jiāng* (dried ginger), and *fù zǐ* (aconite).

For pain due to qì stagnation (characterized by sudden, stabbing pain that increases when the patient is angry), it is combined with medicinals such as *xiāng fù* (cyperus), *qīng pí* (unripe tangerine peel), *mù xiāng* (costusroot), *shā rén* (amomum), and *chén xiāng* (aquilaria).

---

[1] *Yán hú suǒ* (corydalis) and *jīn líng zǐ* (toosendan) combine to form *jīn líng zǐ sǎn* (Toosendan Powder). (Au.)

For pain due to static blood (characterized by pain with a fixed location, a long course of illness, stasis macules on the tongue, or a history of knocks and falls), it is combined with medicinals such as *wǔ líng zhī* (squirrel's droppings), *rǔ xiāng* (frankincense), *mò yào* (myrrh), *táo rén* (peach kernel), and *hóng huā* (carthamus).

In cases of pain and **unilateral sagging of the testicles**[22] (睾丸偏坠 *gāo wán piān zhuì*), or mounting pain that extends to the lesser abdomen, it is combined with medicinals such as:

xiǎo huí xiāng (小茴香 fennel, Foeniculi Fructus)

jú hé (橘核 tangerine pip, Citri Reticulatae Semen)

lì zhī hé (荔枝核 litchee pit, Litchi Semen)

wū yào (乌药 lindera, Linderae Radix)

chuān liàn zǐ (川楝子 toosendan, Toosendan Fructus)

wú zhū yú (吴茱萸 evodia, Evodiae Fructus)

For menstrual pain, *yán hú suǒ* is combined with medicinals such as *xiāng fù* (cyperus), *dāng guī* (Chinese angelica), *bái sháo* (white peony), *chuān xiōng* (chuanxiong), and *shú dì huáng* (cooked rehmannia).

For pain in the upper limbs, it is combined with medicinals such as *guì zhī* (cinnamon twig), *sāng zhī* (mulberry twig), *qiāng huó* (notopterygium), and *piàn jiāng huáng* (sliced turmeric); for pain in the lower limbs, it is combined with medicinals such as *sāng jì shēng* (mistletoe), *niú xī* (achyranthes), *xù duàn* (dipsacus), and *dú huó* (pubescent angelica).

For pain due to knocks and falls (injury or trauma), *yán hú suǒ* is combined with medicinals such as *rǔ xiāng* (frankincense), *mò yào* (myrrh), *xuè jié* (dragon's blood), *sū mù* (sappan), and *gǔ suì bǔ* (drynaria).

Care should be taken to apply the principle of pattern identification as the basis of treatment and to vary formulas in accordance with signs. The suggestions here should not be followed slavishly.

2. **Eliminates Concretions and Conglomerations:** In the abdomen, especially the lower abdomen, blood congealing qì gathering can become strips and lumps. Those that persist over a long period of time and have a fixed location are called concretions[544] (癥 *zhèng*). Those that appear in episodes of illness and disappear when there is no illness, that may be large or small, and that are sometimes present and sometimes not, are called conglomerations (瘕 *jiǎ*).[544] *Yán hú suǒ* moves in the blood aspect and disperses stasis and disinhibits qì, as well as dispersing accumulations and expelling concretions. To treat concretions and conglomerations, it can be combined with medicinals such as:

dāng guī (当归 Chinese angelica, Angelicae Sinensis Radix)

chì sháo (赤芍 red peony, Paeoniae Radix Rubra)

hóng huā (红花 carthamus, Carthami Flos)

táo rén (桃仁 peach kernel, Persicae Semen)

niú xī (牛膝 achyranthes, Achyranthis Bidentatae Radix)

zé lán (泽兰 lycopus, Lycopi Herba)

zhì shān jiǎ (炙山甲 mix-fried pangolin scales, Manis Squama cum Liquido Fricta)

é zhú (莪术 curcuma rhizome, Curcumae Rhizoma)

sān léng (三棱 sparganium, Sparganii Rhizoma)

dà huáng (大黄 rhubarb, Rhei Radix et Rhizoma)

wū yào (乌药 lindera, Linderae Radix)

qīng pí (青皮 unripe tangerine peel, Citri Reticulatae Pericarpium Viride)

COMPARISONS

Hú lú bā (fenugreek)[358] tends to be used for abdominal pain with a liking for heat and pressure. *Yán hú suǒ* tends to be used for abdominal pain with tension of the sinews and aversion to pressure.

Xiāng fù (cyperus)[225] and *yán hú suǒ* are both qì and blood medicinals. Nevertheless, *xiāng fù* mainly enters the qì aspect and rectifies the qì in the twelve channels and eight vessels. By moving qì it also moves stagnant blood in the qì. *Yán hú suǒ* mainly enters the blood aspect and rectifies general body pain, whether in the upper or lower body, in the inside or outside. By moving blood it also moves qì stagnation in the blood.

Xiǎo huí xiāng (fennel)[353] treats painful **mounting-conglomeration**[558] (疝瘕 *shàn jiǎ*) and tends to rectify qì. *Yán hú suǒ* treats painful mounting-conglomeration and tends to quicken the blood.

RESEARCH

According to modern research reports, *yán hú suǒ* contains tetrahydropalmitine and has analgesic, sedative, anti-emetic, and hypnotic effects. It is effective against simple pain due to diseases of the digestive system, peripheral nerve pain, and other body pains. It is also effective against temporary insomnia.

PROCESSING

When used raw, it has stronger blood-quickening effects. When stir-fried with vinegar, it is used to stanch bleeding.

DOSAGE

The dosage is generally 2.5–9 g/8 fēn–3 qián. Today, we often use a fine powder that can be taken drenched with decoction medicine, in which case 0.9–2.5 g/ 3–8 fēn should be taken twice a day.

CAUTION

This medicinal is contraindicated in blood heat with qì vacuity and in pregnant women.

---

4. 姜黄 Jiāng Huáng   Curcumae Longae
Turmeric   Rhizoma

Acrid and bitter in flavor and warm in nature, *jiāng huáng* (turmeric) breaks blood and moves qì.

Jiāng huáng breaks blood and also rectifies qì stagnation in the blood. It enters the liver and spleen channels and has a propensity to break blood stasis and qì-bind in these two channels. Its functions are to quicken the blood and transform stasis and to move qì and relieve pain.

1) For chest and rib-side pain caused by static blood and bound qì, *jiāng huáng* is combined with medicinals such as:

zhǐ qiào (枳壳 bitter orange, Aurantii Fructus)

sū gěng (苏梗 perilla stem, Perillae Caulis)

jié gěng (桔梗 platycodon, Platycodonis Radix)

chuān liàn zǐ (川楝子 toosendan, Toosendan Fructus)

xiāng fù (香附 cyperus, Cyperi Rhizoma)

yán hú suǒ (延胡索 corydalis, Corydalis Rhizoma)

guì xīn (桂心 shaved cinnamon bark, Cinnamomi Cortex Rasus)

2) In treating stomach duct or abdominal pain, *jiāng huáng* is combined with medicinals such as:

gāo liáng jiāng (高良姜 lesser galangal, Alpiniae Officinarum Rhizoma)

xiāng fù (香附 cyperus, Cyperi Rhizoma)

shā rén (砂仁 amomum, Amomi Fructus)

mù xiāng (木香 costusroot, Aucklandiae Radix)

gān jiāng (干姜 dried ginger, Zingiberis Rhizoma)

wū yào (乌药 lindera, Linderae Radix)

yán hú suǒ (延胡索 corydalis, Corydalis Rhizoma)

3) For menstrual pain, *jiāng huáng* is combined with medicinals such as *dāng guī* (Chinese angelica), *bái sháo* (white peony), *ài yè* (mugwort), *xiāng fù* (cyperus), and *wǔ líng zhī* (squirrel's droppings). For hepatitis patients with pronounced pain in the liver region, I often add *jiāng huáng* or *piàn jiāng huáng* (sliced turmeric) as well as *zhǐ qiào* (bitter orange), *bái jí lí* (tribulus), and *chuān liàn zǐ* (toosendan) to an appropriate formula for the pattern. This is helpful for both alleviating pain and improving liver function.

According to modern research reports, *jiāng huáng* (turmeric) has an inhibitory effect on the hepatitis virus and can improve liver function.

COMPARISONS

Piàn jiāng huáng (sliced turmeric) and *jiāng huáng* (turmeric) have primarily the same functions, however, *piàn jiāng huáng* also has a special capacity to enter places on the shoulder, back, arm, and hand to quicken the blood and dispel wind, and thereby treats wind-damp impediment. It is often combined with medicinals such as:

guì zhī (桂枝 cinnamon twig, Cinnamomi Ramulus)

qiāng huó (羌活 notopterygium, Notopterygii Rhizoma et Radix)

dāng guī wěi (当归尾 Chinese angelica tail, Angelicae Sinensis Radicis Extremitas)

hóng huā (红花 carthamus, Carthami Flos)

fáng fēng (防风 saposhnikovia, Saposhnikoviae Radix)

qín jiāo (秦艽 large gentian, Gentianae Macrophyllae Radix)

It is primarily used to treat patients with wind-cold-damp impediment that causes pain in the upper body or shoulder joint.

Yù jīn (curcuma)[386] and *jiāng huáng* both break blood and quicken stasis. While *yù jīn* is bitter and cold, enters the heart, and tends to quicken the blood, *jiāng huáng* is warm and acrid, enters the spleen and liver, and also rectifies the qì in the blood.

É zhú (curcuma rhizome)[389] is bitter and warm and tends to enter the qì aspect of the liver channel. It can also break blood within qì. *Jiāng huáng* is warm and acrid and tends to enter the blood aspect of the liver channel. It moves the qì within the blood.

RESEARCH

According to modern research reports, *jiāng huáng* has an excitatory effect on the uterus and stimulates intermittent contractions. It has also been shown to increase the secretion of bile in anesthetized dogs; this effect is weak, but long-lasting.

DOSAGE

The dosage is generally 2.5–9 g/8 fēn–3 qián.

CAUTION

Use with care in patients without static blood and those in weak health.

---

5. 郁金 Yù Jīn   Curcumae Radix
Curcuma

Yù jīn (curcuma) is acrid and bitter in flavor and cold in nature. Its main functions are to quicken stasis, cool the blood, move qì, and resolve depression.

1. **Blood Ejection; Spontaneous External Bleeding:** When depression and anger damage the liver, there is binding depression of liver qì. Qì depression engenders fire, blood heat, and blood stasis. Liver fire ascends counterflow so that blood invades upward and causes signs such as blood ejection, coughing of blood, nosebleed, stabbing pain in the chest and rib-side, blood ejection with clots, and inverted menstruation[554] (倒经 *dào jīng*, nosebleeds that occur whenever the menstrual period is due). In such cases, *yù jīn* is used to cool the blood, dissipate stasis, resolve depression, and move qì. It is often combined with medicinals such as:

shēng dì huáng (生地黄 dried/fresh rehmannia, Rehmanniae Radix Exsiccata seu Recens)

dān shēn (丹参 salvia, Salviae Miltiorrhizae Radix)

dān pí (丹皮 moutan, Moutan Cortex)

chǎo zhī zǐ (炒栀子 stir-fried gardenia, Gardeniae Fructus Frictus) *sān qī* (三七 notoginseng, Notoginseng Radix)

ǒu jié (藕节 lotus root node, Nelumbinis Rhizomatis Nodus)

niú xī (牛膝 achyranthes, Achyranthis Bidentatae Radix)

zé lán (泽兰 lycopus, Lycopi Herba)

2. Blood-Heat Clouded Spirit, Mania and Withdrawal, Fright, and Epilepsy: In treating evil heat entering the heart and in blood-heat with phlegm-turbidity that clouds the heart and causes unclear spirit-mind, fright mania, epilepsy, and related patterns, *yù jīn* clears heart heat and opens the orifices of the heart, quickens static blood, and transforms phlegm turbidity. For this purpose it is often combined with medicinals such as *zhū shá* (cinnabar), *huáng lián* (coptis), *tiān zhú huáng* (bamboo sugar), *niú huáng* (bovine bezoar), *yuǎn zhì* (polygala), and *chāng pú* (acorus). The combination of this medicinal and *bái fán* (alum) is known as *bái jīn wán* (Alum and Curcuma Pill), which is used to treat epilepsy and fright mania.

I often use *yù jīn* in the following combination, which is varied in accordance with signs, to treat manic agitation, insomnia, and abnormal laughing and cursing in schizophrenia or hysteria. This produces definite results and so I offer this experience for your reference.

shēng bái sháo (生白芍 raw white peony, Paeoniae Radix Alba Cruda)

shēng dài zhě shí (生代赭石 crude hematite, Haematitum Crudum)

zhēn zhū mǔ (珍珠母 mother-of-pearl, Concha Margaritifera)

tiān zhú huáng (天竹黄 bamboo sugar, Bambusae Concretio Silicea)

dǎn xīng (胆星 bile arisaema, Arisaema cum Bile)

yuǎn zhì (远志 polygala, Polygalae Radix)

chāng pú (菖蒲 acorus, Acori Tatarinowii Rhizoma)

bàn xià (半夏 pinellia, Pinelliae Rhizoma)

fú líng (茯苓 poria, Poria)

huáng lián (黄连 coptis, Coptidis Rhizoma)

shēng tiě luò (生铁落 iron flakes, Ferri Frusta)

shēng dà huáng (生大黄 raw rhubarb, Rhei Radix et Rhizoma Crudi)

3. Rib-Side Distention and Oppression; Chest and Abdominal Pain: *Yù jīn* has an acrid-dispersing and bitter-downbearing nature. It enters the liver and lung channels, relieves qì depression, and disperses blood stasis. Therefore, chest and rib-side distention and oppression, stabbing pain, and abdominal pain that are caused by qì stagnation and blood stasis can be treated with *yù jīn* combined with medicinals such as:

chái hú (柴胡 bupleurum, Bupleuri Radix)

chì sháo (赤芍 red peony, Paeoniae Radix Rubra)

xiāng fù (香附 cyperus, Cyperi Rhizoma)

zhǐ qiào (枳壳 bitter orange, Aurantii Fructus)

qīng pí (青皮 unripe tangerine peel, Citri Reticulatae Pericarpium Viride)

chén pí (陈皮 tangerine peel, Citri Reticulatae Pericarpium)

dāng guī (当归 Chinese angelica, Angelicae Sinensis Radix)

bái sháo (白芍 white peony, Paeoniae Radix Alba)

yán hú suǒ (延胡索 corydalis, Corydalis Rhizoma)

táo rén (桃仁 peach kernel, Persicae Semen)

mù xiāng (木香 costusroot, Aucklandiae Radix)

It should be noted that *chén pí* (tangerine peel) is used to treat distending pain in the chest and rib-side, and *mù xiāng* (costusroot) is used to treat abdominal pain.

4. Gallbladder Heat and Jaundice: When owing to depressed liver-gallbladder heat, gallbladder heat causes bile to spill out and give rise to jaundice, *yù jīn* dissipates liver depression, cools liver blood, quickens blood, dissipates stasis, and fortifies the stomach and benefits the gallbladder. According to modern research, this medicinal promotes the excretion of bile. It is often combined with medicinals such as:

yīn chén hāo (茵陈蒿 virgate wormwood, Artemisiae Scopariae Herba)

zhī zǐ (栀子 gardenia, Gardeniae Fructus)

shēng dà huáng (生大黄 raw rhubarb, Rhei Radix et Rhizoma Crudi)

chē qián zǐ (车前子 plantago seed, Plantaginis Semen)

huáng bǎi (黄柏 phellodendron, Phellodendri Cortex)

zé xiè (泽泻 alisma, Alismatis Rhizoma)

jiāo sān xiān (焦三仙 scorch-fried three immortals, Tres Immortales Usti)

zhǐ shí (枳实 unripe bitter orange, Aurantii Fructus Immaturus)

COMPARISONS

Chuān yù jīn (Sìchuān curcuma) quickens the blood and transforms stasis more markedly than it rectifies qì, whereas *guǎng yù jīn* (southern curcuma) moves qì and resolves depression more markedly than it quickens the blood.

Xiāng fù (cyperus)[225] primarily moves qì, but within its action of moving qì it also rectifies the blood; *yù jīn* primarily breaks blood, but within moving the blood it also rectifies qì.

RESEARCH

In modern times, researchers have reported that *yù jīn* contains volatile oils that can soften and dissolve cholesterol, promote the excretion of bile, and promote the contraction of the gallbladder. It can be used to treat biliary calculi, cholecystitis, and jaundice.

DOSAGE

The dosage is generally 3–9 g/1–3 qián.

CAUTION

This medicinal is contraindicated for blood vacuity patients without blood stasis or stagnation and for pregnant women.

6. 莪术 É Zhú   Curcumae Rhizoma
Curcuma Rhizome

Acrid and bitter in flavor and warm in nature, *é zhú* (curcuma rhizome) is a commonly used qì-moving, blood-breaking, accumulation-dispersing medicinal that also aids digestion.

1. **Dispersing Strings, Glomus, Concretions, and Aggregations:** Stasis of blood and qì in the abdomen can accumulate over time until it gathers and binds together to form lumps. When these are in the center of the stomach duct and abdomen, or slightly to the right, they are called "glomus"[551] (痞 *pǐ*). When they are hidden in the rib-side, they are called "aggregations"[542] (癖 *pì*). Those that are below or to either side of the umbilicus are called "strings"[565] (痃 *xián*); they are shaped like a string and may be as taut as a bowstring or may resemble a child's arm. Lumps in the lower abdomen are called "concretions"[544] (癥 *zhēng*); concretions that are not always palpable are called "conglomerations"[545] (瘕 *jiǎ*). *É zhú* treats any of the conditions described above, in combination with medicinals such as:

táo rén (桃仁 peach kernel, Persicae Semen)

hóng huā (红花 carthamus, Carthami Flos)

sān léng (三棱 sparganium, Sparganii Rhizoma)

chì sháo (赤芍 red peony, Paeoniae Radix Rubra)

bīng láng (槟榔 areca, Arecae Semen)

shān zhā hé (山楂核 crataegus pit, Crataegi Endocarpium et Semen)

zhì shān jiǎ (炙山甲 mix-fried pangolin scales, Manis Squama cum Liquido Fricta)

dāng guī (当归 Chinese angelica, Angelicae Sinensis Radix)

Generally speaking, to treat glomus lumps, use *é zhú* with medicinals such as:

shén qū (神曲 medicated leaven, Massa Medicata Fermentata)

mài yá (麦芽 barley sprout, Hordei Fructus Germinatus)

lái fú zǐ (莱菔子 radish seed, Raphani Semen)

bàn xià (半夏 pinellia, Pinelliae Rhizoma)

huáng lián (黄连 coptis, Coptidis Rhizoma)

zhǐ shí (枳实 unripe bitter orange, Aurantii Fructus Immaturus)

For aggregation lumps on the right rib-side, combine it with medicinals such as *chái hú* (bupleurum), *zhǐ qiào* (bitter orange), *shēng mǔ lì* (crude oyster shell), and *piàn jiāng huáng* (sliced turmeric). For aggregations on the left rib-side, combine it with medicinals such as:

chái hú (柴胡 bupleurum, Bupleuri Radix)

zhì biē jiǎ (炙鳖甲 mix-fried turtle shell, Trionycis Carapax cum Liquido Frictus)

gé fěn (蛤粉 mactra clamshell powder, Mactrae Concha Pulverata)

shè gān (射干 belamcanda, Belamcandae Rhizoma)

For strings and accumulations, combine it with medicinals such as:

xiāng fù (香附 cyperus, Cyperi Rhizoma)

qīng pí (青皮 unripe tangerine peel, Citri Reticulatae Pericarpium Viride)

dān shēn (丹参 salvia, Salviae Miltiorrhizae Radix)

yù jīn (郁金 curcuma, Curcumae Radix)

guì zhī (桂枝 cinnamon twig, Cinnamomi Ramulus)

For concretion lumps, combine it with medicinals such as:

yán hú suǒ (延胡索 corydalis, Corydalis Rhizoma)

hēi bái chǒu (黑白丑 morning glory, Pharbitidis Semen)

niú xī (牛膝 achyranthes, Achyranthis Bidentatae Radix)

zé lán (泽兰 lycopus, Lycopi Herba)

wǔ líng zhī (五灵脂 squirrel's droppings, Trogopteri Faeces)

zhè chóng (蟅虫 ground beetle, Eupolyphaga seu Steleophaga)

In sum, it is important determine treatment in accord with patterns identified and modify the formula to fit the pattern. It is especially important to note the relationship between supporting the right and dispelling evil in determining patterns. One cannot simply send in troops to fight the accumulations and lumps; one must consider all aspects of the situation.

2. Aiding Digestion and Dispersing Distending Pain: *É zhú* moves qì and quickens stasis, aids digestion, and disperses accumulation and stagnation. When owing to dietary predilections (饮食偏嗜 *yǐn shí piān shì*) food damage impairs spleen and stomach function, giving rise to distention and pain in the stomach or abdomen, indigestion, and stagnation and accumulation of food and drink that fails to transform, combine *é zhú* with medicinals such as:

gǔ yá (谷芽 millet sprout, Setariae Fructus Germinatus)

bīng láng (槟榔 areca, Arecae Semen)

zhǐ shí (枳实 unripe bitter orange, Aurantii Fructus Immaturus)

mù xiāng (木香 costusroot, Aucklandiae Radix)

chǎo shān zhā (炒山楂 stir-fried crataegus, Crataegi Fructus Frictus)

shā rén (砂仁 amomum, Amomi Fructus)

xiāng fù (香附 cyperus, Cyperi Rhizoma)

dà fù pí (大腹皮 areca husk, Arecae Pericarpium)

COMPARISONS

Sān léng (sparganium)[391] is bitter and neutral and breaks the qì within blood; its ability to break blood is greater than its ability to break qì. *É zhú* is acrid and warm, and breaks the blood within qì; its ability to break qì is greater than its ability to break blood. When the two medicinals are used together, they can dissipate all cases of blood stasis and bound qì.

Xiāng fù (cyperus)[225] moves qì and also quickens the blood, freeing the twelve channels; its primary function is to move qì. *É zhú* moves qì and breaks blood; it primarily enters the liver channel and its primary function is to dissipate qì stagnation and blood bind in the liver channel. *Xiāng fù* is mild in strength; *é zhú* is harsh.

Yán hú suǒ (corydalis),[382] *yù jīn* (curcuma),[386] and *jiāng huáng* (turmeric)[384] are all qì-in-blood medicinals, i.e., they quicken the blood and move qì. *É zhú* is a blood-in-qì medicinal, i.e., it moves qì and breaks blood.

RESEARCH

According to modern research reports, this medicinal has definite anti-cancer effects and has been used by some people in recent years to treat cancer.

When I have added this medicinal to formulas for treating cancer patients, I have often found that the patient will begin feeling pain around the affected area. In such cases, I reduce the dose, and then gradually increase it (from 3 g to 9 g). The patient does not experience pain if this method is used. I therefore do not recommend giving large doses of this medicinal all at once.

DOSAGE

The dosage is generally 3–9 g/1–3 qián.

CAUTION

This medicinal is contraindicated for patients with qì and blood vacuity and for pregnant women.

---

7. 三棱 Sān Léng
Sparganium
Sparganii Rhizoma

Bitter in flavor and neutral in nature, *sān léng* (sparganium) is primarily used to dissipate blood and move qì and to soften hardness and disperse accumulations. It is often used with *é zhú* (curcuma rhizome).

For all cases of blood stasis and qì stagnation that present as hard lumps in the abdomen (including hepatosplenomegaly), food accumulation, phlegm stagnation, or blood stasis menstrual block in women, this medicinal can be used to quicken blood and transform stasis, to move qì and disperse accumulations, and to free the channels and dissipate binds. Generally speaking, for hard lumps in the abdomen, *sān léng* is combined with medicinals such as:

é zhú (莪术 curcuma rhizome, Curcumae Rhizoma)

shēng mǔ lì (生牡蛎 crude oyster shell, Ostreae Concha Cruda)

zhì biē jiǎ (炙鳖甲 mix-fried turtle shell, Trionycis Carapax cum Liquido Frictus)

zhì shān jiǎ (炙山甲 mix-fried pangolin scales, Manis Squama cum Liquido Fricta)

jiāo shān zhā (焦山楂 scorch-fried crataegus, Crataegi Fructus Ustus)

shén qū (神曲 medicated leaven, Massa Medicata Fermentata)

hēi bái chǒu (黑白丑 morning glory, Pharbitidis Semen)

hóng huā (红花 carthamus, Carthami Flos)

táo rén (桃仁 peach kernel, Persicae Semen)

dāng guī (当归 Chinese angelica, Angelicae Sinensis Radix)

For food accumulations and phlegm accumulation with indigestion, *sān léng* is often combined with medicinals such as:

mù xiāng (木香 costusroot, Aucklandiae Radix)

shā rén (砂仁 amomum, Amomi Fructus)

mài yá (麦芽 barley sprout, Hordei Fructus Germinatus)

gǔ yá (谷芽 millet sprout, Setariae Fructus Germinatus)

bàn xià (半夏 pinellia, Pinelliae Rhizoma)

lái fú zǐ (莱菔子 radish seed, Raphani Semen)

chén pí (陈皮 tangerine peel, Citri Reticulatae Pericarpium)

fú líng (茯苓 poria, Poria)

For blood-stasis menstrual block, *sān léng* is often combined with medicinals such as:

dāng guī (当归 Chinese angelica, Angelicae Sinensis Radix)

chì sháo (赤芍 red peony, Paeoniae Radix Rubra)

táo rén (桃仁 peach kernel, Persicae Semen)

hóng huā (红花 carthamus, Carthami Flos)

niú xī (牛膝 achyranthes, Achyranthis Bidentatae Radix)

xiāng fù (香附 cyperus, Cyperi Rhizoma)

qiàn cǎo (茜草 madder, Rubiae Radix)

COMPARISONS

É zhú (curcuma rhizome)[389] is better able to move qì and break blood, dissipate stasis, and disperse accumulations than *sān léng*, but *sān léng* has a more pronounced ability to soften hardness, dissipate binds, and eliminate old lumps.

Sān léng (sparganium) and *é zhú* (curcuma rhizome) are often used to disperse accumulations and eliminate concretions. Nevertheless, they should only be used for repletion patterns. For example, in treating accumulation lumps caused by non-movement of center qì, one should primarily use medicinals that fortify and move the center burner and only secondarily use medicinals that wear away at the accumulation lump and gradually cause it to disperse. One should never forget to take care of the right qì and simply send in soldiers to attack.

DOSAGE

The dosage is generally 3–9 g/1–3 qián.

CAUTION

This medicinal is contraindicated for patients with spleen-stomach vacuity and for pregnant women.

8. 乳香　Rŭ Xiāng
Frankincense
Olibanum

Rŭ xiāng (frankincense) is acrid and bitter in flavor and slightly warm in nature.

1. **Moving Qì and Quickening the Blood:** *Rŭ xiāng* possesses an aromatic qì; it penetrates with aroma to regulate the qì of the body. By its acrid flavor, it dissipates stasis and quickens the blood. By its warm nature, it frees the channels and network vessels. For all cases of qì stagnation and blood stasis with congealing and blockage causing heart [region] and abdomen pain, for swelling and pain due to knocks and falls, and for swollen welling-abscess pain, it is used with the medicinals appropriate to the pattern. For example:

1) For heart [region] and abdominal pain, *rŭ xiāng* is combined with medicinals such as *yán hú suŏ* (corydalis), *wŭ líng zhī* (squirrel's droppings), *căo dòu kòu* (Katsumada's galangal seed), and *mò yào* (myrrh). Take equal proportions of the medicinals listed above and grind them together into a fine powder. Administer 1–2 qián per dose. This can be taken in an alcohol mixture or swallowed with warm water. People in former times called this *shŏu niān săn* (Instant Relief Powder) because it relieves pain quickly.

2) For damage from knocks and falls that appears purplish green-blue, swollen, and painful, *rŭ xiāng* is combined with medicinals such as:

dāng guī wĕi (当归尾 Chinese angelica tail, Angelicae Sinensis Radicis Extremitas)

hóng huā (红花 carthamus, Carthami Flos)

chuān xiōng (川芎 chuanxiong, Chuanxiong Rhizoma)

niú xī (牛膝 achyranthes, Achyranthis Bidentatae Radix)

xù duàn (续断 dipsacus, Dipsaci Radix)

gŭ suì bŭ (骨碎补 drynaria, Drynariae Rhizoma)

mò yào (没药 myrrh, Myrrha)

3) For initial-stage welling-abscesses and sores when they are red, swollen, raised, large, and painful, combine *rŭ xiāng* with medicinals such as *jīn yín huā* (lonicera), *lián qiáo* (forsythia), *chì sháo* (red peony), *hóng huā* (carthamus), *tiān huā fĕn* (trichosanthes root), *zào jiăo cì* (gleditsia thorn), *zhì shān jiă* (mix-fried pangolin scales), *bái zhĭ* (Dahurian angelica), and *fáng fēng* (saposhnikovia). If they have burst leaving an open wound, this formula is inappropriate; *zào jiăo cì* (gleditsia thorn) and *shān jiă* (pangolin scales) should be removed.

If the pus has already drained completely, use *rŭ xiāng* and *mò yào* (myrrh) in combination with medicinals such as *duàn lóng gŭ* (calcined dragon bone), *xuè jié* (dragon's blood), *ér chá* (cutch), and *bīng piàn* (borneol). These medicinals should be ground to a fine powder and applied topically. Use a medicinal plaster to secure it and protect the skin. This has the effects of engendering flesh and closing the wound.

For initial-stage flat-abscesses that are flat or sunken, and are neither red nor painful, combine *rǔ xiāng* with medicinals such as:

dāng guī (当归 Chinese angelica, Angelicae Sinensis Radix)

huáng qí (黄芪 astragalus, Astragali Radix)

lián qiáo (连翘 forsythia, Forsythiae Fructus)

mù xiāng (木香 costusroot, Aucklandiae Radix)

mò yào (没药 myrrh, Myrrha)

guì xīn (桂心 shaved cinnamon bark, Cinnamomi Cortex Rasus)

jié gěng (桔梗 platycodon, Platycodonis Radix)

dǎng shēn (党参 codonopsis, Codonopsis Radix)

gān cǎo (甘草 licorice, Glycyrrhizae Radix)

This combination has the effects of expelling toxin from the interior and freeing the channels, quickening stasis, and dispersing swelling.

Rǔ xiāng has **internal-expression**[553] (托里 *tuō lǐ*) and heart-protecting effects, forcing the toxic qì out of the body so that it does not attack internally. It is a commonly used medicinal in external medicine.

2. **Stretching the Sinews and Soothing the Network Vessels:** *Rǔ xiāng* warms and frees the channels and vessels, and also stretches the sinews and soothes the network vessels. It is used for wind-cold-damp impediment or wind strike with hemilateral withering (偏枯 *piān kū*, i.e., hemiplegia) and hypertonicity of sinews in which it is difficult to stretch the limbs due to impeded flow of qì and blood. It is combined with medicinals such as:

qiāng huó (羌活 notopterygium, Notopterygii Rhizoma et Radix)

dú huó (独活 pubescent angelica, Angelicae Pubescentis Radix)

fáng fēng (防风 saposhnikovia, Saposhnikoviae Radix)

chuān xiōng (川芎 chuanxiong, Chuanxiong Rhizoma)

dāng guī (当归 Chinese angelica, Angelicae Sinensis Radix)

mò yào (没药 myrrh, Myrrha)

hóng huā (红花 carthamus, Carthami Flos)

dì lóng (地龙 earthworm, Pheretima)

zhì shān jiǎ (炙山甲 mix-fried pangolin scales, Manis Squama cum Liquido Fricta)

yǐ mǐ (苡米 coix, Coicis Semen)

In addition, *rǔ xiāng* enters the heart; sometimes it is combined with medicinals such as *zhū shā* (cinnabar), *suān zǎo rén* (spiny jujube), and *yuǎn zhì* (polygala) to treat mania and withdrawal.

DOSAGE

The dosage is generally 1.5–9 g/5 fēn–3 qián.

CAUTION

This medicinal is contraindicated in the absence of qì stagnation and blood stasis and in pregnancy. Do not use internally for patients with welling-abscesses or sores that are ulcerated.

9. 没药 Mò Yào
Myrrh
Myrrha

Bitter and acrid in flavor and neutral in nature, *mò yào* (myrrh) dissipates blood stasis, frees binds and stagnation, disperses swelling, and settles pain.

1. **Toxic Swelling of Welling-Abscesses:** For the onset of red, swollen, hot, and painful welling-abscesses, *mò yào* quickens stasis and dissipates binds, and disperses swelling and settles pain. For this purpose it is often combined with medicinals such as:

jīn yín huā (金银花 lonicera, Lonicerae Flos)

lián qiáo (连翘 forsythia, Forsythiae Fructus)

chì sháo (赤芍 red peony, Paeoniae Radix Rubra)

hóng huā (红花 carthamus, Carthami Flos)

fáng fēng (防风 saposhnikovia, Saposhnikoviae Radix)

bái zhǐ (白芷 Dahurian angelica, Angelicae Dahuricae Radix)

dāng guī wěi (当归尾 Chinese angelica tail, Angelicae Sinensis Radicis Extremitas)

zhì shān jiǎ (炙山甲 mix-fried pangolin scales, Manis Squama cum Liquido Fricta)

zào jiǎo cì (皂角刺 gleditsia thorn, Gleditsiae Spina)

2. **Knocks and Falls:** For bruises (static blood), swelling, and pain of sinew, bone, or flesh, *mò yào* is combined with medicinals such as:

dāng guī (当归 Chinese angelica, Angelicae Sinensis Radix)

chuān xiōng (川芎 chuanxiong, Chuanxiong Rhizoma)

niú xī (牛膝 achyranthes, Achyranthis Bidentatae Radix)

hóng huā (红花 carthamus, Carthami Flos)

xù duàn (续断 dipsacus, Dipsaci Radix)

gǔ suì bǔ (骨碎补 drynaria, Drynariae Rhizoma)

rǔ xiāng (乳香 frankincense, Olibanum)

3. **Menstrual Block with Concretions and Conglomerations; Postpartum Abdominal Pain:** *Mò yào* is used for congealing blood stagnating qì that cause chronic menstrual block with congeals in the abdomen that increases by the day, resembling pregnancy. In such cases, there will be a palpable lump or severe pain that refuses pressure. For this pattern, *mò yào* is used with medicinals such as:

dāng guī (当归 Chinese angelica, Angelicae Sinensis Radix)

táo rén (桃仁 peach kernel, Persicae Semen)

hóng huā (红花 carthamus, Carthami Flos)

chuān xiōng (川芎 chuanxiong, Chuanxiong Rhizoma)

sān léng (三棱 sparganium, Sparganii Rhizoma)

é zhú (莪术 curcuma rhizome, Curcumae Rhizoma)

rǔ xiāng (乳香 frankincense, Olibanum)

yán hú suǒ (延胡索 corydalis, Corydalis Rhizoma)

shuǐ zhì (水蛭 leech, Hirudo)

méng chóng (虻虫 tabanus, Tabanus)

shēng dà huáng (生大黄 raw rhubarb, Rhei Radix et Rhizoma Crudi)

For postpartum abdominal pain due to unresolved blood stasis, it is combined with medicinals such as:

dāng guī (当归 Chinese angelica, Angelicae Sinensis Radix)

hóng huā (红花 carthamus, Carthami Flos)

chuān xiōng (川芎 chuanxiong, Chuanxiong Rhizoma)

yán hú suǒ (延胡索 corydalis, Corydalis Rhizoma)

pào jiāng (炮姜 blast-fried ginger, Zingiberis Rhizoma Praeparatum)

yì mǔ cǎo (益母草 leonurus, Leonuri Herba)

4. Wind-Damp Impediment Pain: This medicinal enters all twelve channels to free static blood, dissipate bound qì, disperse swelling, and settle pain. To treat wind-cold-damp impediment that causes pain in the joints of the limbs, it is combined with medicinals such as:

qiāng huó (羌活 notopterygium, Notopterygii Rhizoma et Radix)

dú huó (独活 pubescent angelica, Angelicae Pubescentis Radix)

fáng fēng (防风 saposhnikovia, Saposhnikoviae Radix)

sāng jì shēng (桑寄生 mistletoe, Taxilli Herba)

wēi líng xiān (威灵仙 clematis, Clematidis Radix)

xì xīn (细辛 asarum, Asari Herba)

dāng guī (当归 Chinese angelica, Angelicae Sinensis Radix)

chì sháo (赤芍 red peony, Paeoniae Radix Rubra)

hóng huā (红花 carthamus, Carthami Flos)

zhì hǔ gǔ (炙虎骨 mix-fried tiger bone, Tigris Os cum Liquido Frictum)

zhì shān jiǎ (炙山甲 mix-fried pangolin scales, Manis Squama cum Liquido Fricta)

zhì fù piàn (制附片 sliced processed aconite, Aconiti Radix Lateralis Praeparata Secta)

COMPARISONS

Rǔ xiāng (frankincense)[393] and *mò yào* both quicken the blood and relieve pain. However, *rǔ xiāng* moves qì to quicken the blood and also stretches the sinews, frees the channels, soothes the network vessels, and relieves pain. *Mò yào*, by contrast, dissipates stasis to quicken the blood and also disperses swelling and settles pain. The former tends to act on qì, while the latter acts on blood. When the two medicinals are used together the benefits of each are mutually enhanced. Therefore, these two medicinals are almost always used together in clinical practice.

When using *rǔ xiāng* and *mò yào* to relieve pain, the cause of the pain should be carefully investigated. If there is wind, one must disperse wind. If there is heat, one must clear heat. Adding *rǔ xiāng* and *mò yào* to formulas to settle pain is fine, but using only these two medicinals to treat pain violates the spirit of determining treatment in accordance with patterns identified.

Both *rǔ xiāng* and *mò yào* are more effective when prepared with vinegar.

DOSAGE

The dosage is generally 1.5–9 g/5 fēn–3 qián.

CAUTION

Rǔ xiāng and *mò yào* are not appropriate for sores that have already burst. Owing to their blood-moving and stasis-dissipating effects, both of these medicinals are contraindicated in pregnancy.

---

10. 红花 **Hóng Huā**   Carthami Flos
Carthamus

Including
  ▷ *Zàng hóng huā* (藏红花 saffron, Croci Stigma)

Also called *nán hóng huā* 南红花 and *cǎo hóng huā* 草红花. Acrid, sweet, and bitter in flavor and warm in nature, *hóng huā* (carthamus) quickens static blood and engenders new blood. When used in small doses, it has the effect of quickening and nourishing the blood. When used in large doses, however, it has the effect of breaking blood and moving stasis.

Hóng huā is the most commonly used medicinal for quickening the blood and transforming stasis. It is used particularly frequently in gynecology, and it is generally used to treat menstrual block due to blood stasis, scant menstrual flow, menstrual blood clots, or delayed menses. For treating these disorders, it is often combined with medicinals such as:

  dāng guī (当归 Chinese angelica, Angelicae Sinensis Radix)
  chuān xiōng (川芎 chuanxiong, Chuanxiong Rhizoma)
  bái sháo (白芍 white peony, Paeoniae Radix Alba)
  shú dì huáng (熟地黄 cooked rehmannia, Rehmanniae Radix Praeparata)
  táo rén (桃仁 peach kernel, Persicae Semen)
  qiàn cǎo (茜草 madder, Rubiae Radix)
  xiāng fù (香附 cyperus, Cyperi Rhizoma)
  niú xī (牛膝 achyranthes, Achyranthis Bidentatae Radix)

To treat abdominal pain during menstruation, add medicinals such as:

  wǔ líng zhī (五灵脂 squirrel's droppings, Trogopteri Faeces)
  yán hú suǒ (延胡索 corydalis, Corydalis Rhizoma)
  pú huáng (蒲黄 typha pollen, Typhae Pollen)
  chuān liàn zǐ (川楝子 toosendan, Toosendan Fructus)
  wú zhū yú (吴茱萸 evodia, Evodiae Fructus)
  xiǎo huí xiāng (小茴香 fennel, Foeniculi Fructus)

For death of the fetus *in utero*, *hóng huā* is combined with medicinals such as *dāng guī* (Chinese angelica), *chuān xiōng* (chuanxiong), *niú xī* (achyranthes), *ròu guì* (cinnamon bark), *chē qián zǐ* (plantago seed), *shēng dà huáng* (raw rhubarb), *máng xiāo* (mirabilite), *guì zhī* (cinnamon twig), and *táo rén* (peach kernel).

In terms of internal diseases, this medicinal can be used for any condition of obstruction and stagnation of static blood that manifests in stomach duct pain, abdominal pain, and accumulation lumps in the abdomen. Three examples of this use follow.

1) For stomach duct pain, *hóng huā* is combined with medicinals such as:

gāo liáng jiāng (高良姜 lesser galangal, Alpiniae Officinarum Rhizoma)

xiāng fù (香附 cyperus, Cyperi Rhizoma)

wǔ líng zhī (五灵脂 squirrel's droppings, Trogopteri Faeces)

pú huáng (蒲黄 typha pollen, Typhae Pollen)

shā rén (砂仁 amomum, Amomi Fructus)

2) For abdominal pain, it is combined with medicinals such as:

dāng guī (当归 Chinese angelica, Angelicae Sinensis Radix)

bái sháo (白芍 white peony, Paeoniae Radix Alba)

dān shēn (丹参 salvia, Salviae Miltiorrhizae Radix)

yán hú suǒ (延胡索 corydalis, Corydalis Rhizoma)

guì zhī (桂枝 cinnamon twig, Cinnamomi Ramulus)

wú yú (吴萸 evodia, Evodiae Fructus)

mù xiāng (木香 costusroot, Aucklandiae Radix)

3) For accumulation lumps in the abdomen, *hóng huā* is combined with medicinals such as:

sān léng (三棱 sparganium, Sparganii Rhizoma)

é zhú (莪术 curcuma rhizome, Curcumae Rhizoma)

zhì biē jiǎ (炙鳖甲 mix-fried turtle shell, Trionycis Carapax cum Liquido Frictus)

shēng mǔ lì (生牡蛎 crude oyster shell, Ostreae Concha Cruda)

táo rén (桃仁 peach kernel, Persicae Semen)

zhì shān jiǎ (炙山甲 mix-fried pangolin scales, Manis Squama cum Liquido Fricta)

hǎi zǎo (海藻 sargassum, Sargassum)

Hóng huā is also used for dual vacuity of qì and blood that is caused by static blood failing to be eliminated and new blood not being engendered. Used in small amounts it dispels static blood and engenders new blood. For this purpose it is used with medicinals such as:

dāng guī (当归 Chinese angelica, Angelicae Sinensis Radix)

dān shēn (丹参 salvia, Salviae Miltiorrhizae Radix)

bái sháo (白芍 white peony, Paeoniae Radix Alba)

shēng dì huáng (生地黄 dried/fresh rehmannia, Rehmanniae Radix Exsiccata seu Recens)

shú dì huáng (熟地黄 cooked rehmannia, Rehmanniae Radix Praeparata)

bái zhú (白术 white atractylodes, Atractylodis Macrocephalae Rhizoma)

dǎng shēn (党参 codonopsis, Codonopsis Radix)

fú líng (茯苓 poria, Poria)

chén pí (陈皮 tangerine peel, Citri Reticulatae Pericarpium)

zhì gān cǎo (炙甘草 mix-fried licorice, Glycyrrhizae Radix cum Liquido Fricta)

This medicinal enters the heart channel and also the lung channel; therefore it treats **chest impediment**[543] (胸痹 *xiōng bì*) heart pain from blood stasis and qì stagnation or from lack of free flowing qì and blood. For this purpose, *hóng huā* is combined with medicinals such as:

guā lóu (瓜蒌 trichosanthes, Trichosanthis Fructus)

xiè bái (薤白 Chinese chive, Allii Macrostemonis Bulbus)

guì zhī (桂枝 cinnamon twig, Cinnamomi Ramulus)

wǔ líng zhī (五灵脂 squirrel's droppings, Trogopteri Faeces)

zhǐ qiào (枳壳 bitter orange, Aurantii Fructus)

sū gěng (苏梗 perilla stem, Perillae Caulis)

tán xiāng (檀香 sandalwood, Santali Albi Lignum)

I myself often use the following formula, modified to fit the presenting pattern, to treat coronary heart disease and angina pectoris. It is invariably effective.

guā lóu (瓜蒌 trichosanthes, Trichosanthis Fructus) 30 g/1 liǎng

xiè bái (薤白 Chinese chive, Allii Macrostemonis Bulbus) 9 g/3 qián

guì zhī (桂枝 cinnamon twig, Cinnamomi Ramulus) 3–6 g/1–2 qián

tán xiāng (檀香 sandalwood, Santali Albi Lignum) 6 g/2 qián (add at end)

zhì rǔ xiāng (制乳香 processed frankincense, Olibanum Praeparatum)
     3 g/1 qián

hóng huā (红花 carthamus, Carthami Flos) 9 g/3 qián

wǔ líng zhī (五灵脂 squirrel's droppings, Trogopteri Faeces) 9–12 g/3–4 qián

pú huáng (蒲黄 typha pollen, Typhae Pollen) 9 g/3 qián

bīng láng (槟榔 areca, Arecae Semen) 6–9 g/2–3 qián

yuǎn zhì (远志 polygala, Polygalae Radix) 6–9 g/2–3 qián

bàn xià (半夏 pinellia, Pinelliae Rhizoma) 9 g/3 qián

fú shén (茯神 root poria, Poria cum Pini Radice) 15 g/5 qián

For infectious hepatitis (with or without hepatomegaly) that produces symptoms recognized as blood stasis and qì stagnation in Chinese medicine, such as rib-side pain, abdominal distention and oppression, a long course of illness, and a tongue with a dark body or stasis macules, I often combine *hóng huā* with medicinals such as:

chái hú (柴胡 bupleurum, Bupleuri Radix)

zào jiǎo cì (皂角刺 gleditsia thorn, Gleditsiae Spina)

bái jí lí (白蒺藜 tribulus, Tribuli Fructus)

qiàn cǎo (茜草 madder, Rubiae Radix)

chuān liàn zǐ (川棟子 toosendan, Toosendan Fructus)

sū mù (苏木 sappan, Sappan Lignum)

zé lán (泽兰 lycopus, Lycopi Herba)

zé xiè (泽泻 alisma, Alismatis Rhizoma)

jiāo sān xiān (焦三仙 scorch-fried three immortals, Tres Immortales Usti)

bīng láng (槟榔 areca, Arecae Semen)

Use six packets per week for six to ten weeks. This is definitely helpful for recovering liver function as well as for softening and shrinking an enlarged liver. For patients with liver cirrhosis, the formula can be varied according to the pattern with the addition of any of the medicinals listed below, and should be taken for a long period of time.

é zhú (莪术 curcuma rhizome, Curcumae Rhizoma) 3–6 g/1–2 qián

zhì shān jiǎ (炙山甲 mix-fried pangolin scales, Manis Squama cum Liquido Fricta) 6 g/2 qián

piàn jiāng huáng (片姜黄 sliced turmeric, Curcumae Longae Rhizoma Sectum) 6–9 g/2–3 qián

shēng mǔ lì (生牡蛎 crude oyster shell, Ostreae Concha Cruda) 30 g/1 liǎng

chǎo lái fú zǐ (炒莱菔子 stir-fried radish seed, Raphani Semen Frictum) 9 g/3 qián

For **wind strike**[568] (中风 *zhòng fēng*) with hemiplegia, *hóng huā* is combined with medicinals such as:

sāng zhī (桑枝 mulberry twig, Mori Ramulus)

dāng guī (当归 Chinese angelica, Angelicae Sinensis Radix)

chì sháo (赤芍 red peony, Paeoniae Radix Rubra)

chuān xiōng (川芎 chuanxiong, Chuanxiong Rhizoma)

táo rén (桃仁 peach kernel, Persicae Semen)

zhì shān jiǎ (炙山甲 mix-fried pangolin scales, Manis Squama cum Liquido Fricta)

dì lóng (地龙 earthworm, Pheretima)

huáng qí (黄芪 astragalus, Astragali Radix)

niú xī (牛膝 achyranthes, Achyranthis Bidentatae Radix)

piàn jiāng huáng (片姜黄 sliced turmeric, Curcumae Longae Rhizoma Sectum)

zhú lì (竹沥 bamboo sap, Bambusae Succus)

In Chinese, *hóng huā* is often called *nán hóng huā* 南红花, "southern *hóng huā*," to distinguish it from *zàng hóng huā* 藏红花, "Tibetan *hóng huā*," which in English is called "saffron." The two are very similar, but *nán hóng huā* (carthamus) has a more pronounced ability to dispel stasis and quicken the blood, whereas its ability to nourish the blood is comparatively weak. *Zàng hóng huā* (saffron), on the other hand, has a stronger moistening nature, a greater ability to nourish the blood, and a lesser ability to dispel stasis. When one merely writes "*hóng huā* 红花" on a prescription, the pharmacy will fill it with *nán hóng huā* 南红花 (which in Chinese is also called *cǎo hóng huā* 草红花). *Zàng hóng huā* is rather expensive and therefore is not normally used in decoction. Physicians often place 0.9–1.5 g/

3 fēn–5 fēn of *zàng hóng huā* in a wine (alcohol) glass and fill the glass slightly more than half full of *huáng jiǔ* (yellow wine). The liquid is then heated by placing the glass in a pan with boiling water around it. The concentrated liquid is then added to a decocted formula.

COMPARISONS

Táo rén (peach kernel)[401] tends to treat static blood that is localized and has form or that is in the lower abdomen, whereas *hóng huā* tends to treat static blood that is generalized and has no specific site. The two complement one another and so are often used together.

DOSAGE

The dosage is generally 2.5–9 g/8 fēn–3 qián.

CAUTION

It has been written, "Excessive use [of *hóng huā*] causes the blood to flow without ceasing." Therefore we should be careful not to use too much of this medicinal. It is contraindicated for patients without static blood conditions and for pregnant women.

RESEARCH

According to modern research reports, decoctions of *hóng huā* have been shown to have an excitatory effect on the uterus in animal experiments. This effect has been observed in both the uterus of live animals and on the dissected uteri of dead animals. The excitatory effects are even more pronounced on pregnant uteri.

Animal experiments have also shown that this medicinal lowers blood pressure. In experiments with dogs, *hóng huā* was shown to increase both contraction and dilatation in the heart. It also causes contraction of smooth muscle in the bronchii of experimental animals.

---

11. 桃仁 Táo Rén   Persicae Semen
Peach Kernel

Bitter and sweet in flavor and neutral in nature, *táo rén* (peach kernel) primarily breaks blood and dissipates stasis, and moistens dryness and lubricates the intestines.

1. **Breaking Blood and Dissipating Stasis:** For all conditions of static blood or blood amassment, use *táo rén* in combination with other medicinals appropriate to the pattern, as follows.

a) **Blood stasis menstrual block:** Vary the following formula in accordance with the signs identified.

Táo hóng sì wù tāng 桃红四物汤	Peach Kernel and Carthamus Four Agents Decoction

táo rén (桃仁 peach kernel, Persicae Semen)
hóng huā (红花 carthamus, Carthami Flos)
dāng guī (当归 Chinese angelica, Angelicae Sinensis Radix)
chuān xiōng (川芎 chuanxiong, Chuanxiong Rhizoma)
shú dì huáng (熟地黄 cooked rehmannia, Rehmanniae Radix Praeparata)
chì sháo (赤芍 red peony, Paeoniae Radix Rubra)

b) **Blood amassment in the bladder**: In cold damage disease, heat evil and static blood amass and bind in the lower abdomen causing symptoms of fullness and distention in the smaller abdomen, dark stool, uninhibited urine, vexation and agitation, delirious speech, and heat effusion (fever) resembling mania, which is called "**blood amassment in the bladder**."[542] For this pattern modify the following formula in accordance with the signs.

Táo rén chéng qì tāng 桃仁承气汤	Peach Kernel Qì-Coordinating Decoction

táo rén (桃仁 peach kernel, Persicae Semen)
dà huáng (大黄 rhubarb, Rhei Radix et Rhizoma)
máng xiāo (芒硝 mirabilite, Natrii Sulfas)
gān cǎo (甘草 licorice, Glycyrrhizae Radix)
guì zhī (桂枝 cinnamon twig, Cinnamomi Ramulus)

c) **Pulmonary welling-abscess**: Usually caused by internal depression of heat toxin and by blockage and stagnation of qì and blood, **pulmonary welling-abscess** 肺臃 *fèi yōng*)[560] can be treated with the following formula varied according to signs.

Qiān jīn wěi jīng tāng 千金韦茎汤	Thousand Gold Pieces Phragmites Decoction

táo rén (桃仁 peach kernel, Persicae Semen)
dōng guā zǐ (冬瓜子 wax gourd seed, Benincasae Semen)
shēng yǐ mǐ (生苡米 raw coix seed, Coicis Semen Crudum)
lú gēn (芦根 phragmites, Phragmitis Rhizoma)

d) **Intestinal welling-abscess**: Heat toxin gathering internally causing stagnation of qì and congealing of blood and inhibiting conveyance through the intestinal tract results in blocked qì and blood brewing and binding into an **intestinal welling-abscess**[554] (肠痈 *cháng yōng*). The initial symptoms are aversion to cold with heat effusion (fever), lumbar pain that refuses pressure, and a tendency for the legs to curl up [in fetal position]. This pattern includes the Western diagnosis of acute appendicitis. For this pattern, modify the following formula in accordance with the signs.

Dà huáng mǔ dān pí tāng 大黄牡丹皮汤   Rhubarb and Moutan Decoction

---

dà huáng (大黄 rhubarb, Rhei Radix et Rhizoma)

dān pí (丹皮 moutan, Moutan Cortex)

táo rén (桃仁 peach kernel, Persicae Semen)

dōng guā zǐ (冬瓜子 wax gourd seed, Benincasae Semen)

máng xiāo (芒硝 mirabilite, Natrii Sulfas)

e) **Knocks and falls:** For injuries due to knocks and falls, combine *táo rén* with medicinals such as the following.

dāng guī wěi (当归尾 Chinese angelica tail, Angelicae Sinensis Radicis Extremitas)

chì sháo (赤芍 red peony, Paeoniae Radix Rubra)

sū mù (苏木 sappan, Sappan Lignum)

jiāng huáng (姜黄 turmeric, Curcumae Longae Rhizoma)

hóng huā (红花 carthamus, Carthami Flos)

rǔ xiāng (乳香 frankincense, Olibanum)

mò yào (没药 myrrh, Myrrha)

f) **Welling abscesses:** At the onset of welling-abscess swellings and toxin sores, combine *táo rén* with medicinals such as the following.

jīn yín huā (金银花 lonicera, Lonicerae Flos)

lián qiáo (连翘 forsythia, Forsythiae Fructus)

chì sháo (赤芍 red peony, Paeoniae Radix Rubra)

hóng huā (红花 carthamus, Carthami Flos)

tiān huā fěn (天花粉 trichosanthes root, Trichosanthis Radix)

zhì shān jiǎ (炙山甲 mix-fried pangolin scales, Manis Squama cum Liquido Fricta)

rǔ xiāng (乳香 frankincense, Olibanum)

mò yào (没药 myrrh, Myrrha)

2. **Moistening Dryness and Freeing the Intestines:** For insufficient blood, dry intestines, bound stool, and constipation due to debility in old age, blood vacuity and insufficient fluids in enduring illness, or excessive loss of blood in postpartum women, use the following formula.

Wǔ rén wán 五仁丸   Five Kernels Pill

---

táo rén ní (桃仁泥 crushed peach kernel, Persicae Semen Tusum)

xìng rén ní (杏仁泥 crushed apricot kernel, Armeniacae Semen Tusum)

huǒ má rén (火麻仁 cannabis fruit, Cannabis Fructus)

yù lǐ rén (郁李仁 bush cherry kernel, Pruni Semen)

bǎi zǐ rén (柏子仁 arborvitae seed, Platycladi Semen)

Combine this formula with medicinals such as:

dāng guī (当归 Chinese angelica, Angelicae Sinensis Radix)

guā lóu (瓜蒌 trichosanthes, Trichosanthis Fructus)

dì huáng (地黄 rehmannia, Rehmanniae Radix)

COMPARISONS

Xìng rén ní (crushed apricot kernel) enters the qì aspect and is used for constipation due to qì constipation in the large intestine, whereas *táo rén ní* enters the blood aspect and is used for constipation due to blood constipation in the large intestine. These two medicinals are often used together.

DOSAGE

The dosage is generally 2.5–9 g/8 fēn–3 qián.

CAUTION

Contraindicated in the absence of static blood and for pregnant women.

RESEARCH

According to modern research reports, *táo rén* extract has a pronounced anti-coagulant effect.

---

12. 五灵脂 Wǔ Líng Zhī   Trogopteri Faeces
Squirrel's Droppings

Sweet in flavor and warm in nature, *wǔ líng zhī* (squirrel's droppings) quickens the blood and dissipates stasis, and frees the blood vessels. When char-fried (炒炭 *chǎo tàn*), it is used to stanch bleeding. It primarily enters the blood aspect of the liver channel. On the basis of their experience, physicians of the past believed that this medicinal "frees blocked blood [and] stanches copious menstrual [bleeding]." It treats "any pain in the heart, abdomen, ribs, and rib-side in men and women." In clinical practice, it is frequently used to treat any kind of pain due to blood stasis with symptoms such as relatively fixed location of pain, a long course of illness, and stasis macules on the tongue. Examples are given below.

1. For stomach duct pain, *wǔ líng zhī* is combined with medicinals such as:

pú huáng (蒲黄 typha pollen, Typhae Pollen)

rǔ xiāng (乳香 frankincense, Olibanum)

yán hú suǒ (延胡索 corydalis, Corydalis Rhizoma)

gāo liáng jiāng (高良姜 lesser galangal, Alpiniae Officinarum Rhizoma)

xiāng fù (香附 cyperus, Cyperi Rhizoma)

2. For abdominal pain, *wǔ líng zhī* (squirrel's droppings) is combined with medicinals such as *dāng guī* (Chinese angelica), *bái sháo* (white peony), *chuān xiōng* (chuanxiong), *guì zhī* (cinnamon twig), *wú yú* (evodia), *dān shēn* (salvia), and *pào jiāng* (blast-fried ginger). For lesser-abdominal pain, add medicinals such as *chuān liàn zǐ* (toosendan), *xiǎo huí xiāng* (fennel), and *hú lú bā* (fenugreek).

3. For rib-side pain, it is combined with medicinals such as *chái hú* (bupleurum), *zhǐ qiào* (bitter orange), *qīng pí* (unripe tangerine peel), *bái jí lí* (tribulus), *piàn jiāng huáng* (sliced turmeric), *zào jiǎo cì* (gleditsia thorn), and *chì sháo* (red peony).

4. For joint pain, *wǔ líng zhī* is combined with medicinals such as:

jī xuè téng (鸡血藤 spatholobus, Spatholobi Caulis)

sāng zhī (桑枝 mulberry twig, Mori Ramulus)

guì zhī (桂枝 cinnamon twig, Cinnamomi Ramulus)

fù zǐ (附子 aconite, Aconiti Radix Lateralis Praeparata)

sōng jié (松节 knotty pine wood, Pini Nodi Lignum)

wēi líng xiān (威灵仙 clematis, Clematidis Radix)

dāng guī (当归 Chinese angelica, Angelicae Sinensis Radix)

hóng huā (红花 carthamus, Carthami Flos)

qiāng huó (羌活 notopterygium, Notopterygii Rhizoma et Radix)

dú huó (独活 pubescent angelica, Angelicae Pubescentis Radix)

zhì shān jiǎ (炙山甲 mix-fried pangolin scales, Manis Squama cum Liquido Fricta)

5. For menstrual pain, *wǔ líng zhī* (squirrel's droppings) is combined with medicinals such as:

dāng guī (当归 Chinese angelica, Angelicae Sinensis Radix)

chuān xiōng (川芎 chuanxiong, Chuanxiong Rhizoma)

shú dì huáng (熟地黄 cooked rehmannia, Rehmanniae Radix Praeparata)

bái sháo (白芍 white peony, Paeoniae Radix Alba)

táo rén (桃仁 peach kernel, Persicae Semen)

hóng huā (红花 carthamus, Carthami Flos)

pú huáng (蒲黄 typha pollen, Typhae Pollen)

xiāng fù (香附 cyperus, Cyperi Rhizoma)

chuān liàn zǐ (川楝子 toosendan, Toosendan Fructus)

For postpartum abdominal pain, it is combined with medicinals such as:

pú huáng (蒲黄 typha pollen, Typhae Pollen)

zé lán (泽兰 lycopus, Lycopi Herba)

niú xī (牛膝 achyranthes, Achyranthis Bidentatae Radix)

yì mǔ cǎo (益母草 leonurus, Leonuri Herba)

yán hú suǒ (延胡索 corydalis, Corydalis Rhizoma)

pào jiāng (炮姜 blast-fried ginger, Zingiberis Rhizoma Praeparatum)

chuān xiōng (川芎 chuanxiong, Chuanxiong Rhizoma)

hóng huā (红花 carthamus, Carthami Flos)

táo rén (桃仁 peach kernel, Persicae Semen)

dāng guī (当归 Chinese angelica, Angelicae Sinensis Radix)

COMPARISONS

It should be noted that *wǔ líng zhī* is mainly used to quicken blood and dissipate static blood; unlike other blood-quickening medicinals, such as *dān shēn* (salvia),[379] *dāng guī wěi* (Chinese angelica tail),[111] and *hóng huā* (carthamus),[397] it has no blood-engendering effect. This should be taken into account when combining medicinals to fit the pattern at hand.

RESEARCH

According to modern research reports, this medicinal relieves smooth muscle spasms.

Wǔ líng zhī chǎo tàn (五灵脂炒炭, char-fried squirrel's droppings) treats conditions of static blood concurrent with excessive bleeding. For example, it is used to treat women with flooding and spotting or bleeding from hemorrhoids.

It has been noted that *chǎo wǔ líng zhī* (炒五灵脂, stir-fried squirrel's droppings) is used to treat phlegm-drool with bound blood giving rise to intermittent cough with blood-flecked phlegm that cannot be cured over many years. In Western medicine, this condition indicates that a cyst has formed in the lung. I myself have successfully treated bronchiectasis with coughing of blood by adding *chǎo wǔ líng zhī* to formulas devised to treat the pattern identified.

DOSAGE

The dosage is generally 3–9 g/1–3 qián.

CAUTION

Contraindicated for blood vacuity without stasis. This medicinal should not be used with *rén shēn* (ginseng) because they have a fear relationship.

---

13. 蒲黄 Pú Huáng   Typhae Pollen
Typha Pollen

Pú huáng (typha pollen) is sweet in flavor and neutral in nature. Used raw, it has a slippery nature, and it quickens the blood and dispels stasis, cools the blood, and disinhibits urine. Char-fried, it has an astringent nature and stanches bleeding.

1. Bleeding Due to Blood Stasis Transforming into Heat: *Pú huáng* can be used for any case of blood stasis transforming into heat and causing various forms of bleeding. Examples are given below.

a) For blood ejection, *pú huáng* is combined with medicinals such as *shēng dì huáng* (dried/fresh rehmannia), *ē jiāo* (ass hide glue), *cè bǎi yè* (arborvitae leaf), and *bái jí* (bletilla).

b) For nosebleed, it is combined with medicinals such as *dà xiǎo jì* (Japanese/field thistle), *lú gēn* (phragmites), *xuán shēn* (scrophularia), *qīng dài* (indigo), and *shēng dì huáng* (dried/fresh rehmannia).

c) For bloody urine, *pú huáng* is combined with medicinals such as *bái máo gēn* (imperata), *shēng dì huáng* (dried/fresh rehmannia), *dōng kuí zǐ* (mallow seed), and *huáng bǎi tàn* (charred phellodendron).

d) For bloody stool, it is combined with medicinals such as:

huái huā tàn (槐花炭 charred sophora flower, Sophorae Flos Carbonisatus)

fáng fēng (防风 saposhnikovia, Saposhnikoviae Radix)

dì yú tàn (地榆炭 charred sanguisorba, Sanguisorbae Radix Carbonisata)

huái jiǎo (槐角 sophora fruit, Sophorae Fructus)

2. Painful Urination and Bloody Urine: *Pú huáng* disinhibits urine and frees strangury; therefore it is used for difficult, painful urination and bloody urine. For this purpose it is combined with medicinals such as:

huá shí (滑石 talcum, Talcum)

zhū líng (猪苓 polyporus, Polyporus)

huáng bǎi (黄柏 phellodendron, Phellodendri Cortex)

chē qián zǐ (车前子 plantago seed, Plantaginis Semen)

zé xiè (泽泻 alisma, Alismatis Rhizoma)

biǎn xù (萹蓄 knotgrass, Polygoni Avicularis Herba)

qū mài (瞿麦 dianthus, Dianthi Herba)

dà xiǎo jì (大小蓟 Japanese/field thistle, Cirsii Japonici/Cirsii Herba)

bái máo gēn (白茅根 imperata, Imperatae Rhizoma)

3. Stasis Pain: *Pú huáng* relieves pain by quickening the blood and transforming stasis. It is used to treat pain caused by static blood. Examples are given below.

a) For menstrual pain, it is combined with medicinals such as:

dāng guī (当归 Chinese angelica, Angelicae Sinensis Radix)

chuān xiōng (川芎 chuanxiong, Chuanxiong Rhizoma)

wǔ líng zhī (五灵脂 squirrel's droppings, Trogopteri Faeces)

hóng huā (红花 carthamus, Carthami Flos)

bái sháo (白芍 white peony, Paeoniae Radix Alba)

xiāng fù (香附 cyperus, Cyperi Rhizoma)

yán hú suǒ (延胡索 corydalis, Corydalis Rhizoma)

b) For postpartum attacking pain in the lower abdomen with a stasis lump that can be felt when pressure is applied, a condition known as infant's-pillow pain[552] (儿枕痛 *ér zhěn tòng*), it is combined with medicinals such as:

dāng guī (当归 Chinese angelica, Angelicae Sinensis Radix)

chuān xiōng (川芎 chuanxiong, Chuanxiong Rhizoma)

hóng huā (红花 carthamus, Carthami Flos)

pào jiāng (炮姜 blast-fried ginger, Zingiberis Rhizoma Praeparatum)

táo rén (桃仁 peach kernel, Persicae Semen)

wǔ líng zhī (五灵脂 squirrel's droppings, Trogopteri Faeces)

c) For heart and abdominal pain it is combined with medicinals such as *wǔ líng zhī* (squirrel's droppings), *gāo liáng jiāng* (lesser galangal), *xiāng fù* (cyperus), *yán hú suǒ* (corydalis), *rǔ xiāng* (frankincense), and *mò yào* (myrrh).

RESEARCH

According to modern reports of animal experiments, *pú huáng* causes uterine contractions.

Pú huáng takes the form of a yellow powder. Therefore, for bleeding due to external injury the powder can be applied directly to the wound to stanch bleeding. For mouth and tongue sores or eczema, directly apply to the affected area *wǔ líng zhī* (squirrel's droppings) that has been mixed into a paste using refined *zhū yóu* (pork lard) or *mì* (honey). This [paste] has the effects of moistening and enriching, cooling the blood, and dispersing swelling.

Comparisons

Wǔ líng zhī (squirrel's droppings)[404] quickens blood and dissipates stasis, and it has a tendency to warm and dissipate. In contrast, *pú huáng* quickens the blood and transforms stasis and also cools the blood and stanches bleeding.

Dosage

The dosage is generally 3–9 g/1–3 qián.

Caution

Use with care in blood vacuity without stasis or stagnation.

---

14. 穿山甲 Chuān Shān Jiǎ   Manis Squama
Pangolin Scales

Chuān shān jiǎ (pangolin scales) is often written in prescriptions as *zhì shān jiǎ* (炙山甲, mix-fried pangolin scales), *pào jiǎ zhū* (炮甲珠, blast-fried pangolin scales), or *chǎo jiǎ piàn* (炒甲片, stir-fried pangolin scales). It is salty in flavor and slightly cold in nature. Its main actions are freeing the channels and network vessels, quickening static blood, dispersing swollen welling-abscess, and freeing milk. Mobile and penetrating in nature, it is able to reach the site of disease directly.

For rib-side pain caused by blood stasis and qì stagnation, *chuān shān jiǎ* is combined with medicinals such as *bái jí lí* (tribulus), *piàn jiāng huáng* (sliced turmeric), *yán hú suǒ* (corydalis), *xiāng fù* (cyperus), and *chuān liàn zǐ* (toosendan). For blood stasis causing menstrual block, it is combined with medicinals such as:

táo rén (桃仁 peach kernel, Persicae Semen)

hóng huā (红花 carthamus, Carthami Flos)

dāng guī (当归 Chinese angelica, Angelicae Sinensis Radix)

bái sháo (白芍 white peony, Paeoniae Radix Alba)

chuān xiōng (川芎 chuanxiong, Chuanxiong Rhizoma)

qiàn cǎo (茜草 madder, Rubiae Radix)

niú xī (牛膝 achyranthes, Achyranthis Bidentatae Radix)

zé lán (泽兰 lycopus, Lycopi Herba)

To treat wind-cold-damp impediment that causes numbness and tingling in the hands and feet, pain in the limbs, and hypertonicity, use *chuān shān jiǎ* to free the channels and network vessels, and to quicken qì and blood. For this purpose, it is often combined with medicinals such as:

qiāng huó (羌活 notopterygium, Notopterygii Rhizoma et Radix)

fáng fēng (防风 saposhnikovia, Saposhnikoviae Radix)

tiān má (天麻 gastrodia, Gastrodiae Rhizoma)

chuān xiōng (川芎 chuanxiong, Chuanxiong Rhizoma)

dāng guī (当归 Chinese angelica, Angelicae Sinensis Radix)

dú huó (独活 pubescent angelica, Angelicae Pubescentis Radix)

guì zhī (桂枝 cinnamon twig, Cinnamomi Ramulus)

shēn jīn cǎo (伸筋草 ground pine, Lycopodii Herba)

wēi líng xiān (威灵仙 clematis, Clematidis Radix)

luò shí téng (络石藤 star jasmine stem, Trachelospermi Caulis)

The onset of welling-abscess swellings and toxin sores is usually due to qì and blood congealing and gathering that blocks the blood vessels and affects the circulation of qì and blood, thereby causing heat toxin to gather internally. For this pattern, use the following formula from *Wài Kē Zhèng Zōng* (外科正宗 "Orthodox External Medicine").

Xiān fāng huó mìng yǐn 仙方活命饮   Immortal Formula Life-Giving Beverage

---

zào jiǎo cì (皂角刺 gleditsia thorn, Gleditsiae Spina)

dāng guī wěi (当归尾 Chinese angelica tail, Angelicae Sinensis Radicis Extremitas)

chì sháo (赤芍 red peony, Paeoniae Radix Rubra)

hóng huā (红花 carthamus, Carthami Flos)

rǔ xiāng (乳香 frankincense, Olibanum)

mò yào (没药 myrrh, Myrrha)

jīn yín huā (金银花 lonicera, Lonicerae Flos)

tiān huā fěn (天花粉 trichosanthes root, Trichosanthis Radix)

bèi mǔ (贝母 fritillaria, Fritillariae Bulbus)

fáng fēng (防风 saposhnikovia, Saposhnikoviae Radix)

bái zhǐ (白芷 Dahurian angelica, Angelicae Dahuricae Radix)

chén pí (陈皮 tangerine peel, Citri Reticulatae Pericarpium)

CAUTION

Chuān shān jiǎ treats the swelling and toxicity of welling-abscesses and sores. It disperses and dissipates those that have not yet formed pus, and causes those that have already formed pus to burst. It is, however, not suitable for welling-abscesses that have already broken.

For postpartum women with hard, distended breasts and breast milk stoppage due to qì stagnation and blood stasis, use *chuān shān jiǎ* combined with medicinals such as *wáng bù liú xíng* (vaccaria), *tōng cǎo* (rice-paper plant pith), and *lù lù tōng* (liquidambar fruit). I often use the following decoction to treat postpartum women with **scant breast milk**[561] (乳汁少 *rǔ zhī shǎo*) or **breast milk stoppage**[543] (乳汁不通 *rǔ zhī bù tōng*).

dāng guī (当归 Chinese angelica, Angelicae Sinensis Radix) 9–12 g/3–4 qián

tiān huā fěn (天花粉 trichosanthes root, Trichosanthis Radix) 12 g/4 qián *dǎng shēn* (党参 codonopsis, Codonopsis Radix) 9 g/3 qián

zhì shān jiǎ (炙山甲 mix-fried pangolin scales, Manis Squama cum Liquido Fricta) 9 g/3 qián

wáng bù liú xíng (王不留行 vaccaria, Vaccariae Semen) 12 g/4 qián

tōng cǎo (通草 rice-paper plant pith, Tetrapanacis Medulla) 9 g/3 qián

lù lù tōng (路路通 liquidambar fruit, Liquidambaris Fructus) 9 g/3 qián

If the breasts are distended, painful, and hard and have breast milk stoppage (not scant breast milk, but a blockage of flow), then eliminate *dǎng shēn* (codonopsis) and *tiān huā fěn* (trichosanthes root) and add *lòu lú* (rhaponticum) 9–12 g/ 3–4 qián. The dosage of *zhì shān jiǎ* (mix-fried pangolin scales) and *wáng bù liú xíng* (vaccaria) can also be increased, depending on the situation.

If the breasts are soft and there is scant breast milk as well as breast milk stoppage, increase the dosage of *dǎng shēn* (codonopsis), *tiān huā fěn* (trichosanthes root), and *dāng guī* (Chinese angelica) to suit the situation. *Shēng bái zhú* (raw white atractylodes) and *huáng qí* (astragalus) can also be added. Moreover, one can give the patient *zhū tí tāng* (Pig's Trotter Soup).

When I am treating enduring and severe illnesses such as arthritis, wind strike with hemiplegia, or rheumatoid arthritis, I often add this medicinal to the formula prescribed for the pattern, whether it be in pill, powder, or other form. Adding an appropriate amount of *chuān shān jiǎ* not only increases the formula's ability to quicken the blood and channels, it also guides the medicinals "directly to the site of disease," which definitely increases the effectiveness of the formula.

Comparisons

Dì lóng (earthworm)[472] frees the channels and quickens the network vessels. It tends to move downwards and so is effective in treating the lumbus, knees, legs, and feet. *Chuān shān jiǎ* frees the channels and quickens the network vessels. It is powerful enough to reach the entire body and is used when there is stoppage and pain anywhere in the body.[2]

Wáng bù liú xíng (vaccaria)[411] tends to treat breast milk stoppage due to blockage of the blood vessels, whereas *chuān shān jiǎ* tends to treat breast milk stoppage due to obstruction of channels and network vessels.

Zào jiǎo cì (gleditsia thorn) and *chuān shān jiǎ* both break open ulcerated welling-abscess swellings and sores. However, *zào jiǎo cì* also tracks down wind and disperses bound phlegm. *Chuān shān jiǎ* tends to free the channels and quicken the network vessels, and to disperse swelling and expel pus.

Dosage

The dosage is generally 1.5–9 g/5 fēn–3 qián.

Caution

This medicinal is inappropriate for patients without stasis in the channels and

---

[2]Pain is understood as being a stoppage of qì and blood, reflected in the saying: "When there is stoppage, there is pain" (不通则痛 *bù tōng zé tòng*). (Ed.)

network vessels and for those with welling-abscesses and sores that have already broken.

---

15. 王不留行 Wáng Bù Liú Xíng   Vaccariae Semen
Vaccaria

Wáng bù liú xíng (vaccaria) is also called 王不留 *wáng bù liú* in Chinese. The name literally means "the king does not linger." This medicinal is called "non-lingering" because it is said to "move without stopping." Bitter and sweet in flavor and neutral in nature, it frees the blood vessels, expels wind impediment, and frees milk.

For menstrual block or sores and welling-abscesses due to blockage of the vessels and stoppage of qì and blood, one can use this medicinal in formulas tailored to the pattern. For example, to treat menstrual block combine *wáng bù liú xíng* with medicinals such as:

táo rén (桃仁 peach kernel, Persicae Semen)

hóng huā (红花 carthamus, Carthami Flos)

dāng guī (当归 Chinese angelica, Angelicae Sinensis Radix)

chuān xiōng (川芎 chuanxiong, Chuanxiong Rhizoma)

shú dì huáng (熟地黄 cooked rehmannia, Rehmanniae Radix Praeparata)

bái sháo (白芍 white peony, Paeoniae Radix Alba)

qiàn cǎo (茜草 madder, Rubiae Radix)

niú xī (牛膝 achyranthes, Achyranthis Bidentatae Radix)

zé lán (泽兰 lycopus, Lycopi Herba)

xiāng fù (香附 cyperus, Cyperi Rhizoma)

For swollen welling-abscess, it is combined with medicinals such as *dāng guī wěi* (Chinese angelica tail), *chì sháo* (red peony), *lián qiáo* (forsythia), *zào jiǎo cì* (gleditsia thorn), *zhì shān jiǎ* (mix-fried pangolin scales), and *hóng huā* (carthamus).

Based on their experience, physicians of former times formulated the following principle: "To treat wind, first treat the blood; when blood moves, the wind naturally disappears." This medicinal frees the channels and quickens the blood, causing it to flow smoothly; when blood moves, wind naturally disappears. Therefore, it is used to treat generalized and joint pain due to wind-cold-damp impediment. If wind evil is more intense, the pain wanders more, sometimes moving to the upper limbs, and sometimes moving to the lower limbs, sometimes affecting the large joints, and sometimes affecting the small joints. Swelling follows the movement of the pain and it arises and disappears unpredictably. For this pattern, *wáng bù liú xíng* is combined with medicinals such as:

qiāng huó (羌活 notopterygium, Notopterygii Rhizoma et Radix)

dú huó (独活 pubescent angelica, Angelicae Pubescentis Radix)

fáng fēng (防风 saposhnikovia, Saposhnikoviae Radix)

guì zhī (桂枝 cinnamon twig, Cinnamomi Ramulus)

hóng huā (红花 carthamus, Carthami Flos)

wēi líng xiān (威灵仙 clematis, Clematidis Radix)

chì sháo (赤芍 red peony, Paeoniae Radix Rubra)

zhì shān jiǎ (炙山甲 mix-fried pangolin scales, Manis Squama cum Liquido Fricta)

jī xuè téng (鸡血藤 spatholobus, Spatholobi Caulis)

Wáng bù liú xíng is most commonly used to free milk. There is a saying amongst the working people, "When women take *chuān shān jiǎ* and *wáng bù liú xíng*, their breasts grow and flow (with milk)." For postpartum women with breast milk stoppage, *wáng bù liú xíng* is used with medicinals such as *chuān shān jiǎ* (pangolin scales), *lù lù tōng* (liquidambar fruit), *shā shēn* (adenophora/glehnia), *mài dōng* (ophiopogon), and *tōng cǎo* (rice-paper plant pith). See the preceeding item, *chuān shān jiǎ* (pangolin scales) on page 408, for more details.

COMPARISONS

Tōng cǎo (rice-paper plant pith)[57] and *wáng bù liú xíng* both free milk. Nevertheless, *tōng cǎo* (rice-paper plant pith) is bland and lightweight; it upbears and effuses the essential qì of the yáng brightness channel upward and frees milk. *Wáng bù liú xíng* enters the blood aspect of the yáng brightness, thoroughfare, and conception channels; it frees milk by freeing the blood vessels.

DOSAGE

The dosage is generally 1.5–9 g/5 fēn–3 qián. For treating especially serious cases, one can sometimes use up to 15–30 g/5 qián–1 liǎng.

CAUTION

This medicinal is contraindicated for pregnant women and for patients without blood vessel stasis.

---

16. 泽兰 Zé Lán
Lycopus   Lycopi Herba

Acrid, sweet, and bitter in flavor and slightly warm in nature, *zé lán* (lycopus) primarily moves blood and disinhibits water. It supplements without causing stagnation, moves without being harsh, and is neutral and harmonizing in nature.

1. Menstrual Irregularities: For delayed menstruation or menses that only come every two or three months due to abiding stagnant blood, *zé lán* breaks contracted blood and regulates menstruation. For this purpose it is often combined with medicinals such as:

dāng guī (当归 Chinese angelica, Angelicae Sinensis Radix)

chuān xiōng (川芎 chuanxiong, Chuanxiong Rhizoma)

niú xī (牛膝 achyranthes, Achyranthis Bidentatae Radix)

chì sháo (赤芍 red peony, Paeoniae Radix Rubra)

hóng huā (红花 carthamus, Carthami Flos)

táo rén (桃仁 peach kernel, Persicae Semen)

xiāng fù (香附 cyperus, Cyperi Rhizoma)

2. Postpartum Abdominal Pain: For abdominal pain due to unresolved postpartum blood stasis, it is combined with medicinals such as *dāng guī* (Chinese angelica), *chuān xiōng* (chuanxiong), *táo rén* (peach kernel), *pào jiāng* (blast-fried ginger), *hóng huā* (carthamus), and *yì mǔ cǎo* (leonurus).

3. Postpartum Water Swelling: *Zé lán* disinhibits urine and disperses water swelling. For this purpose it is often combined with medicinals such as *fáng jǐ* (fangji), *fú líng* (poria), *zé xiè* (alisma), *chē qián zǐ* (plantago seed), and *chuān xiōng* (chuanxiong).

I have often successfully used *zé lán* in combination with *niú xī* (achyranthes) in addition to a pattern-appropriate decoction medicine for the pattern at hand to treat lumbar pain due to static blood (with symptoms such as pain with a fixed location, sometimes with a history of trauma, and stasis macules on the tongue). The experience of physicians before us is that the combination of *niú xī* and *zé lán* disinhibits dead blood in the knees and lumbus. Clinical experience has proven that this is indeed effective.

I have found *zé lán* effective for treating early-stage cirrhosis of the liver accompanied by a small degree of ascites when combined with medicinals such as *shuǐ hóng huā zǐ* (prince's-feather), *fáng jǐ* (fangji), and *hú lú* (bottle gourd) in addition to a decoction medicine for the pattern identified in order to disperse swelling.

Comparisons

Yì mǔ cǎo (leonurus)[413] and *zé lán* both move blood and disinhibit water. Nevertheless, *yì mǔ cǎo* has a more outstanding ability to move blood and regulate menstruation. *Zé lán*, in addition to moving blood and freeing the channels, also disperses water swelling. It is especially effective for water swelling that is related to the blood aspect. For example, it is often used to treat ascites due to blood drum.

Dosage

The dosage is generally 3–9 g/1–3 qián. More can be used for serious conditions.

---

17. 益母草 Yì Mǔ Cǎo   Leonuri Herba
Leonurus

Including

▷ *chōng wèi zǐ* (茺蔚子 leonurus fruit, Leonuri Fructus)

Acrid and bitter in flavor and slightly cold in nature, *yì mǔ cǎo* (leonurus) specifically enters the blood aspect, and it moves static blood and engenders new blood. It moves static blood without harming new blood, and nourishes new blood without causing further stagnation of static blood. Moreover, it also disinhibits water and disperses swelling.

This medicinal is the most commonly used medicinal in obstetrics. It is used both antepartum and postpartum; therefore an old saying describes it as an "excellent medicinal for menstruation and childbirth."[3] For example, it is often used for menstrual irregularities, as in *yì mǔ shèng jīn dān* (Leonurus Metal-Overcoming Elixir), in combination with the following medicinals:

chuān xiōng (川芎 chuanxiong, Chuanxiong Rhizoma)

dāng guī (当归 Chinese angelica, Angelicae Sinensis Radix)

bái sháo (白芍 white peony, Paeoniae Radix Alba)

dān shēn (丹参 salvia, Salviae Miltiorrhizae Radix)

bái zhú (白术 white atractylodes, Atractylodis Macrocephalae Rhizoma)

xiāng fù (香附 cyperus, Cyperi Rhizoma)

chōng wèi zǐ (茺蔚子 leonurus fruit, Leonuri Fructus)

For difficult delivery or retention of the placenta, it is combined with medicinals such as *shè xiāng* (musk), *dāng guī* (Chinese angelica), *chuān xiōng* (chuanxiong), *rǔ xiāng* (frankincense), *mò yào* (myrrh), and *hēi jīng jiè* (charred schizonepeta) (also called *jīng jiè tàn* 荆芥炭).

One can also use the formula given below to harmonize the blood, normalize qì, nourish the liver, boost the heart, and regulate menstruation. This formula can also be used for both antepartum and postpartum diseases. It should be thoroughly decocted in water and refined with honey into a paste. Note that some versions of this formula also contain *mù xiāng* (costusroot). It is sold as a ready-made product at pharmacies.

Yì mǔ cǎo gāo 益母草膏   Leonurus Paste

yì mǔ cǎo (益母草 leonurus, Leonuri Herba) 2500 g/80 liǎng

shēng dì huáng (生地黄 dried/fresh rehmannia, Rehmanniae Radix Exsiccata seu Recens) 62.5 g/2 liǎng

bái sháo (白芍 white peony, Paeoniae Radix Alba) 47 g/1.5 liǎng

dāng guī (当归 Chinese angelica, Angelicae Sinensis Radix) 62.5 g/2 liǎng

chuān xiōng (川芎 chuanxiong, Chuanxiong Rhizoma) 47 g/1.5 liǎng

Yì mǔ cǎo also disinhibits water and is used to treat kidney vacuity and inhibited qì transformation with symptoms such as scant urine, chronic water swelling, heaviness and pain in the legs and lumbus, distention and oppression in the abdomen after eating, a somber yellow facial complexion, difficulty in moving, and lassitude of spirit. For such conditions, it is combined with medicinals such as *fú líng pí* (poria skin), *dōng guā pí* (wax gourd rind), *chē qián zǐ* (plantago seed), *fú líng* (poria), *zé xiè* (alisma), *guì zhī* (cinnamon twig), and *yín yáng huò* (epimedium). Alternatively, decoct 125 g/4 liǎng of *yì mǔ cǎo* (leonurus) into 300 ml of decoction that can then be divided into three doses for one day.

---

[3]Note that the Chinese name 益母草 *yì mǔ cǎo*, literally "mother-benefiting herb," reflects its clinical use, as does the common English name motherwort.

RESEARCH

In recent years there have been reports that this medicinal has a diuretic effect and that it treats acute and chronic nephritis with water swelling.

According to modern research and experimentation reports, *yì mǔ cǎo* strengthens uterine contractions and is similar in effect to posterior pituitary hormone and *mài jiǎo* (ergot).

Yì mǔ cǎo and *chōng wèi zǐ* (leonurus fruit) (also called *yì mǔ cǎo zǐ* 益母草子 in Chinese) both have a hypotensive effect. *Chōng wèi zǐ* contains vitamin A substances.

DOSAGE

The dosage is generally 6–9 g/2–3 qián. Under special circumstances, one can use up to 30–60 g/1–2 liǎng.

COMPARISON

The fruit of *yì mǔ cǎo* is called *chōng wèi zǐ* (leonurus fruit), and its action is similar to that of *yì mǔ cǎo*. Nevertheless, it also brightens the eyes and boosts essence, thereby providing supplementation within movement. It is often used for liver heat causing red sore swollen eyes, clouded vision, dizziness, headache, and vexation. The dosage is generally 3–6 g/1–2 qián. This medicinal is contraindicated for patients with dilated pupils.

---

18. 骨碎补 Gǔ Suì Bǔ   Drynariae Rhizoma
Drynaria

Bitter in flavor and warm in nature, *gǔ suì bǔ* (drynaria) quickens the blood, stanches bleeding, supplements the kidney, and joins the bones. It also dispels bone-wind and treats toothache. It is often used for patterns such as bone fractures due to trauma, kidney vacuity enduring diarrhea, bone pain, and toothache.

1. **External Damage Bone Fracture:** This medicinal enters the liver and kidney channels to quicken the blood and dispel stasis, stanch bleeding, and join sinew and bone. For treating bone fractures due to trauma, it is often combined with medicinals such as:

dāng guī (当归 Chinese angelica, Angelicae Sinensis Radix)

hóng huā (红花 carthamus, Carthami Flos)

táo rén (桃仁 peach kernel, Persicae Semen)

sū mù (苏木 sappan, Sappan Lignum)

xù duàn (续断 dipsacus, Dipsaci Radix)

zì rán tóng (自然铜 pyrite, Pyritum)

zhè chóng (蟅虫 ground beetle, Eupolyphaga seu Steleophaga)

rǔ xiāng (乳香 frankincense, Olibanum)

mò yào (没药 myrrh, Myrrha)

2. Kidney Vacuity Enduring Diarrhea: *Gǔ suì bǔ* enters the kidney channel, and the kidney controls urine and stool. Enduring diarrhea is often ascribed to kidney vacuity; one cannot blame only the spleen and stomach. For this pattern, it is combined with medicinals such as:

bǔ gǔ zhī (补骨脂 psoralea, Psoraleae Fructus)

ròu dòu kòu (肉豆蔻 nutmeg, Myristicae Semen)

wú zhū yú (吴茱萸 evodia, Evodiae Fructus)

wǔ wèi zǐ (五味子 schisandra, Schisandrae Fructus)

chǎo shān yào (炒山药 stir-fried dioscorea, Dioscoreae Rhizoma Frictum)

fú líng (茯苓 poria, Poria)

chì shí zhī (赤石脂 halloysite, Halloysitum Rubrum)

zhì fù piàn (制附片 sliced processed aconite, Aconiti Radix Lateralis
    Praeparata Secta)

3. Kidney Vacuity Toothache: The teeth are the surplus of bone and belong to the kidney channel. Therefore, when there is kidney vacuity and kidney yáng moves and floats upward causing toothache, combine *gǔ suì bǔ* with medicinals such as:

dì huáng (地黄 rehmannia, Rehmanniae Radix)

shān yú (山萸 cornus, Corni Fructus)

shān yào (山药 dioscorea, Dioscoreae Rhizoma)

fú líng (茯苓 poria, Poria)

zé xiè (泽泻 alisma, Alismatis Rhizoma)

dān pí (丹皮 moutan, Moutan Cortex)

niú xī (牛膝 achyranthes, Achyranthis Bidentatae Radix)

xì xīn (细辛 asarum, Asari Herba)

dú huó (独活 pubescent angelica, Angelicae Pubescentis Radix)

Comparisons

Bǔ gǔ zhī (psoralea)[149] and *gǔ suì bǔ* both supplement the kidney. Nevertheless, *bǔ gǔ zhī* tends to warm and supplement kidney yáng and to treat fifth-watch diarrhea. *Gǔ suì bǔ* tends to dispel toxic wind in the bone. It treats wilting[568] (痿 *bì*), impediment[552] (痹 *bì*), and bone fractures, and it consolidates the kidney and secures the teeth.

Xù duàn (dipsacus) heals fractures and is indicated for sinew damage, whereas *gǔ suì bǔ* heals fractures and is indicated for bone damage.

Xún gǔ fēng (mollissima) treats bone pain due to wind-cold-damp impediment, whereas *gǔ suì bǔ* treats bone pain due to wind-toxin and static blood.

Dosage

The dosage is generally 3–9 g/1–3 qián.

Caution

Gǔ suì bǔ is contraindicated for toothache due to stomach fire.

19. 刘寄奴 Liú Jì Nú
Anomalous Artemisia

Artemisiae Anomalae Herba

Bitter in flavor and warm in nature, *liú jì nú* (anomalous artemisia) specifically enters the blood aspect and acts to free, move, penetrate, and dissipate. It mainly breaks blood and frees the channels. It can be taken internally for blood stasis menstrual block, pain due to postpartum blood stasis, and knocks and falls. It is often combined with medicinals such as:

dāng guī (当归 Chinese angelica, Angelicae Sinensis Radix)

chuān xiōng (川芎 chuanxiong, Chuanxiong Rhizoma)

táo rén (桃仁 peach kernel, Persicae Semen)

hóng huā (红花 carthamus, Carthami Flos)

niú xī (牛膝 achyranthes, Achyranthis Bidentatae Radix)

zé lán (泽兰 lycopus, Lycopi Herba)

rǔ xiāng (乳香 frankincense, Olibanum)

mò yào (没药 myrrh, Myrrha)

yán hú suǒ (延胡索 corydalis, Corydalis Rhizoma)

It can also be applied topically to treat knocks and falls, or knife wounds. In treating external injuries, it quickens stasis and stanches bleeding.

I often employ the freeing, moving, penetrating, and dissipating effects of *liú jì nú* to treat chronic hepatitis. This is definitely helpful in recovering liver function, eliminating symptoms, and resolving hepatomegaly. For this purpose it is combined with medicinals such as:

chái hú (柴胡 bupleurum, Bupleuri Radix)

huáng qín (黄芩 scutellaria, Scutellariae Radix)

zào jiǎo cì (皂角刺 gleditsia thorn, Gleditsiae Spina)

bái jí lí (白蒺藜 tribulus, Tribuli Fructus)

hóng huā (红花 carthamus, Carthami Flos)

zé xiè (泽泻 alisma, Alismatis Rhizoma)

jiāo sān xiān (焦三仙 scorch-fried three immortals, Tres Immortales Usti)

bīng láng (槟榔 areca, Arecae Semen)

qiàn cǎo (茜草 madder, Rubiae Radix)

COMPARISONS

Gǔ suì bǔ (drynaria)[415] breaks blood and also supplements the kidney; it is effective in treating bone fractures. *Liú jì nú* (anomalous artemisia) breaks blood and frees, moves, penetrates, and dissipates. It has no supplementing power, yet when applied topically it quickens stasis and stanches bleeding. It is effective in treating incised wounds and lacerations.

DOSAGE

The dosage is generally 3–9 g/1–3 qián.

Caution

Use with care in the absence of static blood.

---

20. 苏木 Sū Mù   Sappan Lignum
Sappan

Sweet and salty in flavor and neutral in nature, *sū mù* (sappan) enters the blood aspect of the three yīn channels (lesser yīn, greater yīn, and reverting yīn). Its major functions are to quicken the blood and transform stasis, move blood, and dispel wind.

1. **Wind Strike:** In regards to treating wind strike with hemiplegia and loss of speech, this is an old saying that was derived from experience and principles: "To treat wind, first treat the blood; when blood moves, the wind naturally disappears." This medicinal moves blood as well as dispelling exterior and interior wind evil, perfectly matching the spirit of that saying ("...when blood moves, the wind naturally disappears"). Therefore, for wind strike it is often used in combination with medicinals such as the following.

fáng fēng (防风 saposhnikovia, Saposhnikoviae Radix)

sāng zhī (桑枝 mulberry twig, Mori Ramulus)

hóng huā (红花 carthamus, Carthami Flos)

chì sháo (赤芍 red peony, Paeoniae Radix Rubra)

táo rén (桃仁 peach kernel, Persicae Semen)

dì lóng (地龙 earthworm, Pheretima)

piàn jiāng huáng (片姜黄 sliced turmeric, Curcumae Longae Rhizoma Sectum)

dǎn xīng (胆星 bile arisaema, Arisaema cum Bile)

fú líng (茯苓 poria, Poria)

bàn xià (半夏 pinellia, Pinelliae Rhizoma)

zhú lì (竹沥 bamboo sap, Bambusae Succus)

2. **Pain in the Heart [Region] and Abdomen due to Static Blood:** For static blood causing stomach duct pain, *sū mù* is combined with medicinals such as *wǔ líng zhī* (squirrel's droppings), *pú huáng* (typha pollen), *xiāng fù* (cyperus), *gāo liáng jiāng* (lesser galangal), and *sū gěng* (perilla stem).

For gripping or stabbing pain in the abdomen, it is combined with medicinals such as:

dāng guī (当归 Chinese angelica, Angelicae Sinensis Radix)

chì sháo (赤芍 red peony, Paeoniae Radix Rubra)

bái sháo (白芍 white peony, Paeoniae Radix Alba)

dān shēn (丹参 salvia, Salviae Miltiorrhizae Radix)

yán hú suǒ (延胡索 corydalis, Corydalis Rhizoma)

wú yú (吴萸 evodia, Evodiae Fructus)

wǔ líng zhī (五灵脂 squirrel's droppings, Trogopteri Faeces)

wū yào (乌药 lindera, Linderae Radix)

mù xiāng (木香 costusroot, Aucklandiae Radix)

3. **Postpartum Abdominal Pain, Distention, and Oppression:** When unresolved postpartum blood stasis causes abdominal pain, abdominal distention, and oppression and pain so severe the patient feels on the verge of death, *sū mù* is combined with medicinals such as:

dāng guī (当归 Chinese angelica, Angelicae Sinensis Radix)

hóng huā (红花 carthamus, Carthami Flos)

táo rén (桃仁 peach kernel, Persicae Semen)

pào jiāng (炮姜 blast-fried ginger, Zingiberis Rhizoma Praeparatum)

chuān xiōng (川芎 chuanxiong, Chuanxiong Rhizoma)

yì mǔ cǎo (益母草 leonurus, Leonuri Herba)

yán hú suǒ (延胡索 corydalis, Corydalis Rhizoma)

zǐ sū (紫苏 perilla, Perillae Folium, Caulis et Calyx)

4. **Knocks and Falls:** For this, it is combined with medicinals such as:

rǔ xiāng (乳香 frankincense, Olibanum)

mò yào (没药 myrrh, Myrrha)

gǔ suì bǔ (骨碎补 drynaria, Drynariae Rhizoma)

xù duàn (续断 dipsacus, Dipsaci Radix)

dāng guī (当归 Chinese angelica, Angelicae Sinensis Radix)

hóng huā (红花 carthamus, Carthami Flos)

niú xī (牛膝 achyranthes, Achyranthis Bidentatae Radix)

There is an old saying, based on experience, that *sū mù* treats "gripping pain in the heart [region] and abdomen." On the basis of this experience, I often use the following formula (modified in accordance with signs) to treat angina pectoris; it is invariably effective.

sū mù (苏木 sappan, Sappan Lignum) 15–30 g/5 qián–1 liǎng

guā lóu (瓜蒌 trichosanthes, Trichosanthis Fructus) 30 g/1 liǎng

xiè bái (薤白 Chinese chive, Allii Macrostemonis Bulbus) 9 g/3 qián

tán xiāng (檀香 sandalwood, Santali Albi Lignum) 6 g/2 qián (add at end)

wǔ líng zhī (五灵脂 squirrel's droppings, Trogopteri Faeces) 9 g/3 qián

hóng huā (红花 carthamus, Carthami Flos) 9 g/3 qián

pú huáng (蒲黄 typha pollen, Typhae Pollen) 9 g/3 qián

bīng láng (槟榔 areca, Arecae Semen) 9 g/3 qián

yuǎn zhì (远志 polygala, Polygalae Radix) 9 g/3 qián

fú shén mù (茯神木 pine root in poria, Poriae Pini Radix) 15 g/5 qián

COMPARISONS

Hóng huā (carthamus)[397] moves blood and is effective in breaking stasis; it is most often used to break blood and is seldom used to nourish the blood. *Sū mù* moves blood and is effective in dispelling wind; it is most often used to break blood and is seldom used to harmonize the blood. It also dispels wind.

Qiàn cǎo (madder)[420] moves blood and frees the channels, while it also stanches bleeding (when mix-fried). *Sū mù* moves blood and frees the channels, while it also disperses swelling and relieves pain.

DOSAGE

The dosage is generally 3–9 g/1–3 qián. In special circumstances, one can use 15–30 g/5 qián–1 liǎng.

---

21. 茜草 Qiàn Cǎo   Rubiae Radix
Madder

Qiàn cǎo (madder) is also called *hóng qiàn cǎo* 红茜草 in Chinese. It is bitter and slightly sour in flavor and slightly cold in nature. When used raw it moves and quickens the blood, disperses stasis and frees the channels. When char-fried, it stanches bleeding.

1. Menstrual Block: For absence of menses, use 31 g/1 liǎng of *qiàn cǎo* decocted with *huáng jiǔ* (yellow wine) to move blood and free menstruation.

The *Nèi Jīng* (内经 "The Inner Canon") records a formula called *sì wū zéi yī lú rú wán* (Four of Cuttlefish to One of Madder Pill). The two medicinals in the formula (125 g/4 liǎng of *hǎi piāo xiāo* and 31 g/1 liǎng of *qiàn cǎo*) should be ground into a fine powder and made into pills by mixing the powder with sparrow eggs. Each dose should be 3–6 g/1–2 qián and two doses should be taken per day. Swallow the pills with abalone soup. This treats women for blood dessication and absence of menses from debility.

I myself once used this formula to treat a young woman who had suffered from menstrual block for about one and a half years. Her symptoms were steaming bone and night sweating, emaciation, reddening of the cheeks, shortness of breath, fatigue, and general lack of strength in her movements. She was examined at several hospitals, but no cause for her illness was found. I prescribed a decoction medicine appropriate to her pattern to enrich yīn, clear heat, nourish the blood, and soothe depression. At the same time, I gave her the pill described above. After about three months of treatment, her menses gradually began to return. All of her symptoms eventually disappeared and she was cured. The woman at the time of this writing was almost forty years old; she was healthy and was working in a factory.

2. Knocks and Falls; Static Blood Pain and Swelling: For this pattern, *qiàn cǎo* is combined with medicinals such as *hóng huā* (carthamus), *chì sháo* (red peony), *sū mù* (sappan), *rǔ xiāng* (frankincense), *mò yào* (myrrh), and *gǔ suì bǔ* (drynaria).

3. Blood Ejection and Coughing of Blood: For blood heat or blood stasis causing blood ejection, coughing of blood, nosebleed, and other symptoms involving blood loss, *qiàn cǎo* is used char-fried to stanch bleeding. Moreover, it stanches bleeding without causing static blood. For this purpose it is often combined with medicinals such as:

shēng dì huáng (生地黄 dried/fresh rehmannia, Rehmanniae Radix Exsiccata seu Recens)

ē jiāo (阿胶 ass hide glue, Asini Corii Colla)

sān qī (三七 notoginseng, Notoginseng Radix)

ǒu jié (藕节 lotus root node, Nelumbinis Rhizomatis Nodus)

bái jí (白及 bletilla, Bletillae Rhizoma)

RESEARCH

According to modern research reports, *qiàn cǎo tàn* (茜草炭, charred madder) shortens bleeding and coagulation time in rabbits.

4. Flooding and Spotting: *Qiàn cǎo* treats uterine bleeding. In Chinese medicine, sudden uterine bleeding with large amounts of blood is called flooding (*bēng*); constant bleeding with small amounts of blood is called spotting (*lòu*). For treating these conditions, it is combined with medicinals such as:

sāng jì shēng (桑寄生 mistletoe, Taxilli Herba)

xù duàn tàn (续断炭 charred dipsacus, Dipsaci Radix Carbonisata)

chǎo bái zhú (炒白术 stir-fried white atractylodes, Atractylodis Macrocephalae Rhizoma Frictum)

ē jiāo zhū (阿胶珠 ass hide glue pellets, Asini Corii Gelatini Pilula)

zōng lǘ tàn (棕榈炭 charred trachycarpus, Trachycarpi Petiolus Carbonisatus)

ài yè tàn (艾叶炭 charred mugwort, Artemisiae Argyi Folium Carbonisatum)

dāng guī (当归 Chinese angelica, Angelicae Sinensis Radix)

yì mǔ cǎo (益母草 leonurus, Leonuri Herba)

tù sī zǐ (菟丝子 cuscuta, Cuscutae Semen)

chì shí zhī (赤石脂 halloysite, Halloysitum Rubrum)

In addition, because it also has the function of "treating wind impediment and jaundice," it treats joint pain due to arthritis in combination with medicinals such as *qiāng huó* (notopterygium), *dú huó* (pubescent angelica), *fáng fēng* (saposhnikovia), *wēi líng xiān* (clematis), and *chuān shān lóng* (Japanese dioscorea). For jaundice due to icteric infectious hepatitis or blockage of the biliary duct, combine it with medicinals such as *yīn chén* (virgate wormwood), *zhī zǐ* (gardenia), *huáng bǎi* (phellodendron), *chē qián zǐ* (plantago seed), and *zé xiè* (alisma).

COMPARISONS

Zǐ cǎo (arnebia/lithospermum)[309] and *qiàn cǎo* both move and quicken the blood. Nevertheless, *zǐ cǎo* tends to outthrust maculopapular eruptions, while it also frees the stool and urine. *Qiàn cǎo* tends to free the channels and quicken the blood, while it also treats flooding and spotting, and bloody stool. When it is mix-fried, it stanches bleeding more effectively than *zǐ cǎo*.

DOSAGE

The dosage is generally 6–9 g/2–3 qián. In special circumstances, one can use up to 30 g/1 liǎng.

CAUTION

Inappropriate in blood vacuity.

22. 赤芍 Chì Sháo
Red Peony

Paeoniae Radix
Rubra

Acrid and bitter in flavor and slightly cold in nature, *chì sháo* (red peony) is similar in action to *bái sháo* (white peony), but tends to quicken the blood, cool the blood, and disperse swollen welling-abscesses.

1. **Blood Heat Vomiting and Spontaneous Bleeding:** For these conditions, it is combined with medicinals such as:

> *shēng dì huáng* (生地黄 dried/fresh rehmannia, Rehmanniae Radix Exsiccata seu Recens)
>
> *dān pí* (丹皮 moutan, Moutan Cortex)
>
> *xī jiǎo* (犀角 rhinoceros horn, Rhinocerotis Cornu)
>
> *xuán shēn* (玄参 scrophularia, Scrophulariae Radix)
>
> *bái máo gēn* (白茅根 imperata, Imperatae Rhizoma)

2. **Blood Stasis Menstrual Block:** For this pattern, it is combined with medicinals such as:

> *dāng guī* (当归 Chinese angelica, Angelicae Sinensis Radix)
>
> *chuān xiōng* (川芎 chuanxiong, Chuanxiong Rhizoma)
>
> *táo rén* (桃仁 peach kernel, Persicae Semen)
>
> *hóng huā* (红花 carthamus, Carthami Flos)
>
> *xiāng fù* (香附 cyperus, Cyperi Rhizoma)
>
> *niú xī* (牛膝 achyranthes, Achyranthis Bidentatae Radix)
>
> *qiàn cǎo* (茜草 madder, Rubiae Radix)

3. **Damage from Knocks and Falls; Blood Stasis Pain:** For these conditions, it is combined with medicinals such as *táo rén* (peach kernel), *hóng huā* (carthamus), *rǔ xiāng* (frankincense), *mò yào* (myrrh), *xù duàn* (dipsacus), and *gǔ suì bǔ* (drynaria).

4. **Rib-Side Pain:** The rib-side region belongs to the liver channel. *Chì sháo* enters the liver channel, quickens the blood, frees the network vessels, cools the liver, and clears heat. For rib-side pain, it is combined with medicinals such as:

> *chái hú* (柴胡 bupleurum, Bupleuri Radix)
>
> *xiāng fù* (香附 cyperus, Cyperi Rhizoma)
>
> *yù jīn* (郁金 curcuma, Curcumae Radix)
>
> *zhǐ qiào* (枳壳 bitter orange, Aurantii Fructus)
>
> *piàn jiāng huáng* (片姜黄 sliced turmeric, Curcumae Longae Rhizoma Sectum)
>
> *chuān liàn zǐ* (川楝子 toosendan, Toosendan Fructus)

5. **Swelling and Toxin of Welling-Abscesses and Sores:** For heat-toxin in the blood that becomes depressed and static, creating swollen and toxic welling-abscesses and sores, *chì sháo* cools and quickens the blood, dissipates stasis, and disperses swelling, to thereby relieve pain. It is combined with medicinals such as:

jīn yín huā (金银花 lonicera, Lonicerae Flos)

lián qiáo (连翘 forsythia, Forsythiae Fructus)

bái zhǐ (白芷 Dahurian angelica, Angelicae Dahuricae Radix)

tiān huā fěn (天花粉 trichosanthes root, Trichosanthis Radix)

pú gōng yīng (蒲公英 dandelion, Taraxaci Herba)

yě jú huā (野菊花 wild chrysanthemum flower, Chrysanthemi Indici Flos)

dì dīng (地丁 violet, Violae Herba)

zhì shān jiǎ (炙山甲 mix-fried pangolin scales, Manis Squama cum Liquido Fricta)

In sum, one can select this medicinal (in accordance with the symptoms) for all cases of pain, redness, swelling, bleeding, or maculopapular eruptions that result from blood stasis or blood heat.

COMPARISONS

Bái sháo (white peony)[113] tends to nourish the blood and emolliate the liver. Its nature is to contract and supplement and it is effective in treating blood vacuity pain. *Chì sháo* tends to move and quicken the blood. It is dissipating and draining in nature, and effectively treats blood stasis pain.

Dān pí (moutan) drains fire in the heart channel; it eliminates deep-lying heat in the blood and also cools and harmonizes the blood. *Chì sháo* drains fire in the liver channel; it moves stasis in the blood and also quickens the blood and dissipates stasis.

DOSAGE

The dosage is generally 4.5–10 g/1.5 qián–3 qián.

CAUTION

This medicinal is contraindicated for cold pain in the abdomen, diarrhea, and in the absence of blood stasis. It should not be used with *lí lú* (veratrum).

---

23. 血竭 **Xuè Jié**   Daemonoropis Resina
Dragon's Blood

Xuè jié (dragon's blood) is sweet and salty in flavor and neutral in nature. Taken internally, it quickens blood, dissipates stasis, and expels blood impediment. Applied topically, it eliminates rotten flesh, engenders new flesh, and closes sores.

Xuè jié is used for any case of blood stasis and blood gathering that causes pain and stasis swelling. For static blood heart pain, it is combined with medicinals such as *guā lóu* (trichosanthes), *xiè bái* (Chinese chive), *wǔ líng zhī* (squirrel's droppings), *hóng huā* (carthamus), *xì xīn* (asarum), and *guì zhī* (cinnamon twig).

For abdominal pain due to static blood accumulation and stagnation, *xuè jié* is combined with medicinals such as *dāng guī* (Chinese angelica), *hóng huā* (carthamus), *yán hú suǒ* (corydalis), and *pào jiāng* (blast-fried ginger).

For damage from knocks and bone fractures with static blood pain, it is combined with medicinals such as *sū mù* (sappan), *xù duàn* (dipsacus), *rŭ xiāng* (frankincense), *mò yào* (myrrh), and *gŭ suì bŭ* (drynaria). In treating pain and damage due to knocks and falls, the most commonly used ready-prepared medicine is *qī lí sǎn* (Seven Pinches Powder), which contains *xuè jié*.

Qī lí sǎn 七厘散	Seven Pinches Powder

xuè jié (血竭 dragon's blood, Daemonoropis Resina)

rŭ xiāng (乳香 frankincense, Olibanum)

mò yào (没药 myrrh, Myrrha)

hóng huā (红花 carthamus, Carthami Flos)

ér chá (儿茶 cutch, Catechu)

shè xiāng (麝香 musk, Moschus)

bīng piàn (冰片 borneol, Borneolum)

zhū shā (朱砂 cinnabar, Cinnabaris)

When I treat pain in angina pectoris or myocardial infarction that manifests as blood stasis pattern (the signs include pain that is relatively fixed, stabbing pain, a tongue body that is purplish green-blue or that has pronounced stasis macules, and a rough pulse), I often use 0.6–1.5 g/2–5 fēn of *xuè jié fěn* (dragon's blood powder) in capsules. This can be swallowed along with a decoction. I also sometimes add 0.3–0.6 g/1–2 fēn of *sān qī fěn* (notoginseng powder) to quicken the blood and relieve pain. This is definitely helpful. This method can also be used for other conditions with pronounced symptoms of blood stasis. For instance, one can use *qī lí sǎn* (Seven Pinches Powder) (as described above) for an even better effect.

In external medicine, *xuè jié* is usually applied topically and is often combined with medicinals such as those in *shēng jī sǎn* (Flesh-Engendering Powder).

DOSAGE

The dosage for internal use is generally 0.6–2.5 g/2–8 fēn; two doses per day in pill preparation or packed in capsules. These are swallowed with decoction. When applied topically, a suitable amount should be used.

CAUTION

Xuè jié has a rapid, violent nature and should not be used in excess or for long periods of time.

---

24. 水蛭 Shuǐ Zhì   Hirudo
Leech

Bitter and salty in flavor, neutral in nature, and toxic, *shuǐ zhì* (leech) mainly breaks blood, quickens stasis, and dissipates binds.

For blood stasis that causes menstrual block or concretions and conglomerations, *shuǐ zhì* is often combined with medicinals such as:

dāng guī (当归 Chinese angelica, Angelicae Sinensis Radix)

táo rén (桃仁 peach kernel, Persicae Semen)

hóng huā (红花 carthamus, Carthami Flos)

sān léng (三棱 sparganium, Sparganii Rhizoma)

é zhú (莪术 curcuma rhizome, Curcumae Rhizoma)

huáng qí (黄芪 astragalus, Astragali Radix)

zhī mǔ (知母 anemarrhena, Anemarrhenae Rhizoma)

zé lán (泽兰 lycopus, Lycopi Herba)

niú xī (牛膝 achyranthes, Achyranthis Bidentatae Radix)

In cold damage disease that has lasted for six or seven days, the exterior pattern may still be present (with symptoms such as aversion to cold, heat effusion (fever), and headache) or the exterior pattern may have already resolved. If one observes a deep pulse, hardness and fullness in the smaller abdomen that refuses pressure, uninhibited urination (note that if the urination is inhibited, this is not a blood amassment pattern), forgetfulness, manic agitation, and black stool, then it is a blood amassment pattern. The following formula can be used to precipitate static blood and thereby cure the disease.

Dǐ dàng tāng 抵当汤   Dead-On Decoction

---

shuǐ zhì (水蛭 leech, Hirudo) (20 pieces), stir-fry until black with *zhū zhī* (pork lard)

méng chóng (虻虫 tabanus, Tabanus) (20 pieces)

táo rén (桃仁 peach kernel, Persicae Semen) (15 pieces)

dà huáng (大黄 rhubarb, Rhei Radix et Rhizoma) 9 g/3 qián

The exact doses should be determined in accordance with the specific conditions. Decoct the formula with water and divide into two doses.

RESEARCH

According to modern research reports, *shuǐ zhì* contains hirudin, which inhibits blood coagulation. It is therefore used as an anti-coagulant.

DOSAGE

The dosage is generally 1.5–3 g/5 fēn–1 qián for water decoctions. When the powder is encapsulated, the dosage is 0.6–1.8 g/2 fēn–3 fēn.

CAUTION

This medicinal breaks blood in a fierce manner. Therefore it is contraindicated in pregnancy and for those without serious blood stasis.

25. 虻虫 Méng Chóng   Tabanus
Tabanus

Bitter in flavor, slightly cold in nature, and toxic, *méng chóng* (tabanus) breaks blood, expels stasis, disperses concretions, and frees the channels. *Méng chóng* "can attack the blood that is not reached by true qì." It is often used with *shuǐ zhì* (leech).

For static blood and accumulation lumps (concretion lumps) in the abdomen or for menstrual block, combine it with medicinals such as:

shuǐ zhì (水蛭 leech, Hirudo)

táo rén (桃仁 peach kernel, Persicae Semen)

hóng huā (红花 carthamus, Carthami Flos)

chuān xiōng (川芎 chuanxiong, Chuanxiong Rhizoma)

sān léng (三棱 sparganium, Sparganii Rhizoma)

é zhú (莪术 curcuma rhizome, Curcumae Rhizoma)

dāng guī (当归 Chinese angelica, Angelicae Sinensis Radix)

chì sháo (赤芍 red peony, Paeoniae Radix Rubra)

For damage from knocks and falls and for static blood swelling and pain, combine it with medicinals such as *dān pí* (moutan), *gǔ suì bǔ* (drynaria), *xù duàn* (dipsacus), *rǔ xiāng* (frankincense), and *mò yào* (myrrh).

Although *shuǐ zhì* (leech) and *méng chóng* both break blood and expel stasis, *shuǐ zhì* has a milder medicinal strength and longer-lasting effects. It tends to enter the liver and bladder channels and has a superior stasis-expelling effect. The strength of *méng chóng* to break blood is much fiercer than *shuǐ zhì*. It tends to move the channels and network vessels and free the blood vessels. It may cause diarrhea after it is taken. (This will cease after the medicinal action ends.) Its ability to expel stasis is not as reliable as that of *shuǐ zhì* (leech); thus the two medicinals are often used together to enhance their medicinal effects.

DOSAGE

The dosage is generally 1–3 g/3 fēn–1 qián. Take decocted with water or grind into a powder.

CAUTION

This medicinal is contraindicated in pregnancy and in patients without static blood. Use with care in patients with weak health.

26. 蟅虫 Zhè Chóng
Ground Beetle

Eupolyphaga seu Steleophaga

Also called *tǔ biē chóng* (ground beetle) and *dì biē chóng* (ground beetle).[4] Salty in flavor and cold in nature, *zhè chóng* (ground beetle) breaks static blood, disperses concretions and conglomerations, and joins bones and sinews.

In clinical practice, it is used to quicken the blood and free the channels and to disperse concretions and conglomerations. The following formula, which is available as a ready-made pill, is an example of this. Each pill should be slightly more than 3 g/1 qián.

Dà huáng zhè chóng wán 大黄蟅虫丸   Rhubarb and Ground Beetle Pill

---

dà huáng (大黄 rhubarb, Rhei Radix et Rhizoma)

zhè chóng (蟅虫 ground beetle, Eupolyphaga seu Steleophaga)

gān qī (干漆 lacquer, Toxicodendri Resina)

qí cáo (蛴螬 June beetle grub, Holotrichiae Vermiculus)

chì sháo (赤芍 red peony, Paeoniae Radix Rubra)

gān cǎo (甘草 licorice, Glycyrrhizae Radix)

táo rén (桃仁 peach kernel, Persicae Semen)

shēng dì huáng (生地黄 dried/fresh rehmannia, Rehmanniae Radix Exsiccata seu Recens)

méng chóng (虻虫 tabanus, Tabanus)

shuǐ zhì (水蛭 leech, Hirudo)

huáng qín (黄芩 scutellaria, Scutellariae Radix)

xìng rén (杏仁 apricot kernel, Armeniacae Semen)

Mix with honey and form into pills of 3 g/1 qián each.

This formula is indicated for blood stasis that causes irregular menstruation, menstrual block, accumulations, gatherings, lumps, and glomus, blood-stasis abdominal pain, general weakness, postmeridian heat effusion (fever), **encrusted skin**[548] (肌肤甲错 *jī fū jiǎ cuò*), and **dry-blood consumption**[547] (干血劳 *gān xuè láo*). When I encounter these signs, I often prescribe one pill twice a day, swallowed with warm water or warmed wine. For severe illnesses, this pill can be combined with a decoction medicine appropriate to the pattern at hand. The effects of this formula are steady and reliable.

This medicinal can be used to treat scarlet fever, cinnabar toxin [sore], or other acute febrile diseases, as well as other conditions with heat toxin and static blood stagnating on the tongue leading to what physicians of former times called "wooden tongue." The symptoms include partial or complete swelling of the tongue, hardness of the tongue, severe pain, drooling, and difficulty chewing and swallowing. For this

---

[4]The word "ground" in the name of this medicinal reflects the fact that this is a type of beetle that lives in the earth, not one that has been ground in a grinder. (Ed.)

pattern, 6 g/2 qián of *zhè chóng* and 3 g/1 qián of *shí yán* (salt) should be ground into a powder and taken twice a day. This combination can also be decocted. In addition, *zhè chóng* is decocted singly and used as mouthwash.

Zhè chóng has the special function of quickening static blood and joining sinews and bones. For all knocks and falls with bone fractures or ruptured sinews, it can be combined with medicinals such as *rŭ xiāng* (frankincense), *mò yào* (myrrh), *lóng gŭ* (dragon bone), *zì rán tóng* (pyrite), *sān qī* (notoginseng), *hăi fēng téng* (kadsura pepper stem), *gŭ suì bŭ* (drynaria), and *xù duàn* (dipsacus). Grind this mixture into a fine powder, add a small amount of *shè xiāng* (musk), and take with warm wine.

Zhè chóng is used in most external medicine formulas for joining the bones. For wrenching of the lumbus, pain in the chest when breathing, and pain that prevents one from rotating, grind to a powder nine *zhè chóng* that have been stone-baked until yellow and take twice a day. Or, combine it with medicinals such as *niú xī* (achyranthes), *zé lán* (lycopus), *xù duàn* (dipsacus), *gŏu jĭ* (cibotium), *táo rén* (peach kernel), and *chì sháo* (red peony) in a decoction.

In the past, *lóng shī* (cybister) was used in markets as *zhè chóng* (ground beetle), in contradistinction to *tŭ biē chóng* (ground beetle). On the basis of textual evidence and the current circumstances in the market, the *tŭ biē chóng* (ground beetle) currently sold is *zhè chóng* (ground beetle), and *lóng shī* is no longer called *zhè chóng* (ground beetle).

Comparisons

Méng chóng (tabanus)[426] breaks blood and tends to move the channels and network vessels. It eliminates static blood in regions that are not reached by the true qì. *Zhè chóng* (ground beetle) breaks blood and tracks and eliminates blood accumulation. It also joins and supplements sinew and bone fractures and is specifically used for this purpose.

Dosage

The dosage is generally 1.5–4.5 g/5 fēn–1.5 qián. Slightly more is used in decoction; slightly less is used in pills.

Caution

This medicinal is contraindicated for pregnant women and for patients without static blood.

Lecture Nine
Miscellaneous Medicinals
其他药物 *Qí Tā Yào Wù*

In the eight previous lectures, I have introduced about 200 medicinals. This lecture discusses a variety of commonly used medicinals that stanch bleeding, dispel wind-damp, or transform phlegm and suppress cough and that do not fit into any of the preceding categories. Because these medicinals differ from each other in nature, flavor, and actions, they cannot be ascribed to one category. They have therefore been grouped together in this lecture.

---

1. 杏仁 **Xìng Rén** — Armeniacae Semen
Apricot Kernel

Xìng rén (apricot kernel) is bitter, acrid, slightly sweet, and warm; it possesses minor toxicity. It mainly enters the lung channel, and it downbears qì and moves phlegm, eliminates wind and dissipates cold, and moistens dryness and frees the intestines.

1. **Treating Cough:** a) When wind-cold invades the lung, the lung's diffusion and depurative downbearing are impaired; this leads to inhibited lung qì and the sign of cough, which is frequently accompanied by [aversion to] cold and heat [effusion], headache, expectoration of phlegm, and oppression in the chest. Use *xìng rén* (apricot kernel) to dissipate wind-cold, downbear lung qì, transform phlegm and disinhibit the lung, and thereby suppress cough and calm panting. It is frequently combined with medicinals such as *jié gěng* (platycodon), *qián hú* (peucedanum), *sū yè* (perilla leaf), *chén pí* (tangerine peel), *bàn xià* (pinellia), and *zhì gān cǎo* (mix-fried licorice), as in *xìng sū sǎn* (Apricot Kernel and Perilla Powder). b) When wind-heat invades the lung and impairs lung depuration, it results in heat effusion (fever), thirst, cough, and absence of aversion to cold. For this pattern *xìng rén* is combined with *sāng yè* (mulberry leaf), *jú huā* (chrysanthemum), *jié gěng* (platycodon), *bò hé* (mint), and *niú bàng zǐ* (arctium) as in *sāng jú yǐn* (Mulberry Leaf and Chrysanthemum Beverage). In cases of discomfort from counterflow ascent of

lung qì, downbearing lung qì is the primary action of this medicinal; therefore, even if there is no external contraction of wind-cold, if there is counterflow ascent of lung qì resulting in cough, *xìng rén* is used. In such circumstances, it is frequently combined with medicinals such as:

xuán fù huā (旋覆花 inula flower, Inulae Flos)

sū zǐ (苏子 perilla fruit, Perillae Fructus)

bái qián (白前 willowleaf swallowwort, Cynanchi Stauntonii Rhizoma)

chǎo lái fú zǐ (炒莱菔子 stir-fried radish seed, Raphani Semen Frictum)

pí pá yè (枇杷叶 loquat leaf, Eriobotryae Folium)

2. Moistening Dryness and Freeing the Intestines: The lung and large intestine stand in interior-exterior relationship. In qì constipation[561] (气秘 *qì bì*) with dry bound stool due to lung qì failing to bear downwards, *xìng rén* can be used to downbear lung qì, moisten intestinal dryness, open qì constipation, moisten the intestines, and free the stool. It is frequently combined with medicinals such as *guā lóu* (trichosanthes), *táo rén ní* (crushed peach kernel), *bīng láng* (areca), and *zhǐ shí* (unripe bitter orange). *Xìng rén* is rich in fatty oils, so for elderly people (or those with weak health due to enduring sickness) with scant liquid in the intestinal tract and dry bound stool that is difficult to pass, *xìng rén* (apricot kernel) is often combined with medicinals such as:

huǒ má rén (火麻仁 cannabis fruit, Cannabis Fructus)

yù lǐ rén (郁李仁 bush cherry kernel, Pruni Semen)

táo rén (桃仁 peach kernel, Persicae Semen)

sōng zǐ rén (松子仁 pine nut, Pini Semen)

bǎi zǐ rén (柏子仁 arborvitae seed, Platycladi Semen)

3. Calming Hasty Panting: The lung is the delicate viscus. Hasty panting can occur whenever there is impairment of the lung's depurative downbearing or inhibition of lung qì owing to an external contraction or internal damage by an evil (such as wind-cold, wind-heat, phlegm, rheum, fire, and heat) that results in counterflow ascent. *Xìng rén* is specifically used to downbear and disinhibit lung qì, and thereby calm panting, especially when combined with *má huáng* (ephedra). (*Má huáng* diffuses the lung, while *xìng rén* downbears qì.) This combination also increases the capacity of *xìng rén* to stabilize panting, so physicians of the past had the saying, "*Xìng rén* is the helping hand of *má huáng*."[1] Commonly used formulas for panting generally include *xìng rén* (apricot kernel) and *má huáng* (ephedra). Examples are given below:

Sān ào tāng 三拗汤   Rough and Ready Three Decoction

---

má huáng (麻黄 ephedra, Ephedrae Herba)

xìng rén (杏仁 apricot kernel, Armeniacae Semen)

---

[1] *Xìng rén* is valued as the helping hand of *má huáng* for two reasons: 1) it downbears qì to help calm panting and cough, and 2) it moistens the lung and helps to offset the drying nature of the pungent and bitter *má huáng*. (Ed.)

gān cǎo (甘草 licorice, Glycyrrhizae Radix)

This formula treats wind-cold panting.

| Má xìng shí gān tāng 麻杏石甘汤 | Ephedra, Apricot Kernel, Gypsum, and Licorice Decoction |

má huáng (麻黄 ephedra, Ephedrae Herba)
xìng rén (杏仁 apricot kernel, Armeniacae Semen)
shēng shí gāo (生石膏 crude gypsum, Gypsum Fibrosum Crudum)
gān cǎo (甘草 licorice, Glycyrrhizae Radix)

This formula treats panting from depressed heat in the lung or external contraction of wind-cold.

| Dìng chuǎn tāng 定喘汤 | Panting-Stabilizing Decoction |

má huáng (麻黄 ephedra, Ephedrae Herba)
xìng rén (杏仁 apricot kernel, Armeniacae Semen)
bái guǒ (白果 ginkgo, Ginkgo Semen)
kuǎn dōng huā (款冬花 coltsfoot, Farfarae Flos)
sāng bái pí (桑白皮 mulberry root bark, Mori Cortex)
sū zǐ (苏子 perilla fruit, Perillae Fructus)
huáng qín (黄芩 scutellaria, Scutellariae Radix)
bàn xià (半夏 pinellia, Pinelliae Rhizoma)
gān cǎo (甘草 licorice, Glycyrrhizae Radix)
shēng jiāng (生姜 fresh ginger, Zingiberis Rhizoma Recens)

This formula treats panting and wheezing due to lung vacuity with cold contraction or due to qì counterflow and diaphragm heat.

COMPARISONS

Táo rén ní (crushed peach kernel)[2] tends to be used for large intestine blood constipation; *xìng rén ní* (crushed apricot kernel) tends to be used for large intestine qì constipation. Both should be used with a small amount of *chén pí* (tangerine peel) to move qì.

When treating cough or panting, use *xìng rén* (apricot kernel); when treating constipation, use *xìng rén ní* (crushed apricot kernel).

There are two kinds of *xìng rén*: *kǔ xìng rén* (苦杏仁, bitter apricot kernel) and *tián xìng rén* (甜杏仁, sweet apricot kernel). If one merely writes "*xìng rén* 杏仁" on a prescription, the pharmacy will give *kǔ xìng rén* (bitter apricot kernel). If one wants to use *tián xìng rén* (sweet apricot kernel), it must be specified clearly. *Kǔ xìng rén* has a more urgent action; thus it is suitable for strong people and repletion patterns. *Tián xìng rén*, sweet in flavor and neutral in nature, has a more moderate

---

[2] *Táo rén ní* (crushed peach kernel): This usually means ground to fine granules. The Chinese 泥 *ní* literally means "mud," but peach kernels are not usually crushed to a paste. (Ed.)

action; thus it is suitable for elderly people, for those with weak constitutions, or for vacuity taxation cough and panting.

CAUTION

Xìng rén (apricot kernel) possesses minor toxicity. When using it with children, note that the dosage must not be excessive, otherwise it can cause poisoning that may result in respiratory paralysis.

In patterns of enduring cough with lung qì vacuity, *xìng rén* should be used with care. In mild cases of *xìng rén* poisoning, use 62.5 g/2 liǎng of *xìng shù pí* (apricot tree bark) in a decoction, but for more severe cases the person must be taken to a hospital for emergency care.

DOSAGE

The dosage is generally 3–9 g/1–3 qián.

---

2. 桔梗 Jié Gěng — Platycodonis Radix
Platycodon

Jié gěng (platycodon) is bitter and acrid in flavor and neutral in nature; it diffuses lung qì, courses wind and resolves the exterior, dispels phlegm and expels pus, disinhibits the throat, and upraises.

1. **Diffusing Lung Qì; Coursing Wind and Resolving the Exterior:**
The lung governs the skin and [body] hair. When externally contracted wind-cold fetters the skin and [body] hair, this can cause nondiffusion of lung qì. The result is external contraction cough with signs such as aversion to cold, heat effusion (fever), headache, nasal congestion, cough, oppression in the chest, and ejection of white phlegm. Use *jié gěng* (platycodon) to diffuse lung qì and to course and dissipate wind-cold. For this it is frequently combined with medicinals such as the following:

xìng rén (杏仁 apricot kernel, Armeniacae Semen)
sū yè (苏叶 perilla leaf, Perillae Folium)
qián hú (前胡 peucedanum, Peucedani Radix)
chén pí (陈皮 tangerine peel, Citri Reticulatae Pericarpium)
jīng jiè (荆芥 schizonepeta, Schizonepetae Herba)
fáng fēng (防风 saposhnikovia, Saposhnikoviae Radix)
zhì gān cǎo (炙甘草 mix-fried licorice, Glycyrrhizae Radix cum Liquido Fricta)

If wind-heat invades the lung through the skin and [body] hair, nose, or mouth, and results in wind-heat cough with signs such as pronounced heat effusion with little or no aversion to cold, headache, thirst, frequent urination, cough, and ejection of yellow-white or yellow phlegm, this medicinal diffuses the lung and courses the exterior to clear wind-heat. For this *jié gěng* is frequently combined with:

sāng yè (桑叶 mulberry leaf, Mori Folium)
jú huā (菊花 chrysanthemum, Chrysanthemi Flos)
xìng rén (杏仁 apricot kernel, Armeniacae Semen)

niú bàng zǐ (牛蒡子 arctium, Arctii Fructus)

lú gēn (芦根 phragmites, Phragmitis Rhizoma)

jīng jiè (荆芥 schizonepeta, Schizonepetae Herba)

bò hé (薄荷 mint, Menthae Herba)

When liver qì depression inhibits the qì dynamic and affects lung qì, impairing diffusion and producing signs such as oppression in the chest, rib-side distention, frequent sighing, a rash and impatient nature, and an increase in the cough when the patient gets angry, this medicinal diffuses and dissipates lung depression; in such cases it is combined with medicinals such as:

hòu pò (厚朴 officinal magnolia bark, Magnoliae Officinalis Cortex)

xìng rén (杏仁 apricot kernel, Armeniacae Semen)

zhǐ qiào (枳壳 bitter orange, Aurantii Fructus)

sū gěng (苏梗 perilla stem, Perillae Caulis)

xiāng fù (香附 cyperus, Cyperi Rhizoma)

2. Dispelling Phlegm and Expelling Pus: In cases where lung diffusion is impaired and the qì dynamic is inhibited, resulting in phlegm congestion in the lung, cough, copious phlegm, or copious phlegm that is not easily expectorated, *jié gěng* diffuses lung qì, dispels phlegm, and suppresses cough. It is often combined with medicinals such as:

bàn xià (半夏 pinellia, Pinelliae Rhizoma)

jú hóng (橘红 red tangerine peel, Citri Reticulatae Exocarpium Rubrum)

fú líng (茯苓 poria, Poria)

sū zǐ (苏子 perilla fruit, Perillae Fructus)

guā lóu (瓜蒌 trichosanthes, Trichosanthis Fructus)

xìng rén (杏仁 apricot kernel, Armeniacae Semen)

If wind-cold fetters the lung and there is internal heat that is not promptly diffused, depressed evil transforms into heat and accumulates to form a pulmonary welling-abscess (characterized by heavy-sounding cough, dull pain in the chest and rib-side, pain around Central Treasury (*zhōng fǔ*, LU-1), coughing and spitting of pus, phlegm with blood, or purulent phlegm like rice gruel, with a foul, fishy odor), this medicinal dispels phlegm and expels pus, and rapidly expels phlegm turbidity and pus from the body. In this situation, *jié gěng* is frequently combined with medicinals such as:

shēng gān cǎo (生甘草 raw licorice, Glycyrrhizae Radix Cruda)

shēng yǐ mǐ (生苡米 raw coix, Coicis Semen Crudum)

dōng guā zǐ (冬瓜子 wax gourd seed, Benincasae Semen)

jīn yín huā (金银花 lonicera, Lonicerae Flos)

bèi mǔ (贝母 fritillaria, Fritillariae Bulbus)

táo rén (桃仁 peach kernel, Persicae Semen)

lú gēn (芦根 phragmites, Phragmitis Rhizoma)

According to modern research on laboratory animals, this medicinal has an expectorant effect.

3. Disinhibiting the Throat: The throat is the gateway of the lung and stomach. When fire-heat in the lung gives rise to sore red swollen throat and thirst with liking for cold drinks, this medicinal diffuses lung heat to disinhibit the throat and relieve pain. For this pattern, *jié gĕng* is frequently combined with medicinals such as:

shēng gān căo (生甘草 raw licorice, Glycyrrhizae Radix Cruda)

shān dòu gēn (山豆根 bushy sophora, Sophorae Tonkinensis Radix)

bò hé (薄荷 mint, Menthae Herba)

shè gān (射干 belamcanda, Belamcandae Rhizoma)

niú bàng zĭ (牛蒡子 arctium, Arctii Fructus)

If effulgent yīn vacuity fire and upflaming of vacuity fire cause symptoms such as throat pain (without pronounced redness or swelling), nighttime thirst, and heat in the (hearts of the) palms and soles, *jié gĕng* is combined with medicinals such as:

mài dōng (麦冬 ophiopogon, Ophiopogonis Radix)

shēng dì huáng (生地黄 dried/fresh rehmannia, Rehmanniae Radix Exsiccata seu Recens)

xuán shēn (玄参 scrophularia, Scrophulariae Radix)

zhì biē jiă (炙鳖甲 mix-fried turtle shell, Trionycis Carapax cum Liquido Frictus)

4. Upraising: *Jié gĕng* (platycodon) conducts medicinals up into the lung; thus it is often used as a channel conductor. It also upraises lung qì. The lung governs regulation of the waterways. If lung qì is unable to perfuse and qì transformation is inhibited, resulting in symptoms such as generalized water swelling and scant urine, *jié gĕng* is added to a pattern-appropriate decoction medicine with medicinals that disinhibit water (such as *sāng pí* (mulberry root bark), *dōng guā pí* (wax gourd rind), *chén pí* (tangerine peel), *dà fù pí* (areca husk), and *fú líng* (poria)) to upraise lung qì and disinhibit urine. In this situation, *jié gĕng* is frequently combined with medicinals such as *sāng pí* (mulberry root bark), *sū yè* (perilla leaf), *xìng rén* (apricot kernel), and *zhĭ qiào* (bitter orange). Furthermore, this medicinal upbears yáng qì when combined with *zhì huáng qí* (mix-fried astragalus), *chái hú* (bupleurum), and *shēng má* (cimicifuga). It is frequently used in combination with appropriate decoction medicines for center qì fall, gastroptosis, prolapse of the uterus, and prolapse of the rectum.

COMPARISONS

Xìng rén (apricot kernel)[429] downbears lung qì and transforms phlegm turbidity; *jié gĕng* upbears and diffuses lung qì, and dispels phlegm and expels pus.

Shēng yĭ mĭ (raw coix)[74] and *jié gĕng* both treat pulmonary welling-abscess, the former by disinhibiting dampness and expelling pus, and the latter by diffusing the lung, dispelling phlegm, and expelling pus.

DOSAGE

The dosage is generally 3–9 g/1–3 qián. To expel pus after a pulmonary welling-abscess has burst, the dosage is increased. Excessive doses can cause vomiting.

Caution

Do not use for vacuity pattern cough or dry cough without phlegm.

3. 白前 Bái Qián
Willowleaf Swallowwort

Cynanchi Stauntonii
Rhizoma

Bái qián (willowleaf swallowwort),[3] acrid and sweet in flavor and slightly cold in nature, precipitates qì and downbears phlegm. It is used for all cases of lung qì failing to downbear or lung qì ascending counterflow that result in counterflow fullness in the chest and diaphragm, congestion of lung qì, and failure of phlegm turbidity to descend. For example, in externally contracted wind-cold that results in lung qì ascending counterflow with cough, panting, and copious phlegm, *bái qián* is combined with medicinals such as:

> *xìng rén* (杏仁 apricot kernel, Armeniacae Semen)
> *sū yè* (苏叶 perilla leaf, Perillae Folium)
> *sū zǐ* (苏子 perilla fruit, Perillae Fructus)
> *jīng jiè* (荆芥 schizonepeta, Schizonepetae Herba)
> *qián hú* (前胡 peucedanum, Peucedani Radix)
> *shēng jiāng* (生姜 fresh ginger, Zingiberis Rhizoma Recens)

For cough, qì counterflow, and copious phlegm resulting from lung heat, it is combined with medicinals such as:

> *sāng bái pí* (桑白皮 mulberry root bark, Mori Cortex)
> *dì gǔ pí* (地骨皮 lycium root bark, Lycii Cortex)
> *huáng qín* (黄芩 scutellaria, Scutellariae Radix)
> *guā lóu* (瓜蒌 trichosanthes, Trichosanthis Fructus)
> *zhī mǔ* (知母 anemarrhena, Anemarrhenae Rhizoma)

For enduring cough with qì ascent, **puffy swelling**[560] (浮肿 *fú zhǒng*), shortness of breath, distention, fullness, and oppression in the chest, inability to lie flat at night, and phlegm rale in the throat, physicians of the past used the following formula varied in accordance with signs.

Bái qián tāng 白前汤   Willowleaf Swallowwort Decoction

> *bái qián* (白前 willowleaf swallowwort, Cynanchi Stauntonii Rhizoma)
> *zǐ wǎn* (紫菀 aster, Asteris Radix)
> *bàn xià* (半夏 pinellia, Pinelliae Rhizoma)
> *dà jǐ* (大戟 euphorbia/knoxia, Euphorbiae seu Knoxiae Radix)

Comparisons

> *Qián hú* (peucedanum) diffuses lung qì, and it tends to be used for external

---

[3] *Bái wēi* (black swallowwort) is often substituted for *bái qián* (willowleaf swallowwort). This is probably because these two medicinals are similar in appearance. (Ed.)

contraction cough. *Bái qián* drains the lung and downbears phlegm, and it tends to be used for cough and panting that result from phlegm repletion qì counterflow.

Xuán fù huā (inula flower)[211] precipitates qì and moves water, and it tends to be used for phlegm bind hard glomus in the chest and diaphragm or phlegm-spittle that is sticky like glue or lacquer. *Bái qián* precipitates qì and downbears phlegm, and it tends to be used for panting and cough from chest and rib-side counterflow qì or for repletion phlegm in the lung.

Dosage

The dosage is generally 3–10 g/1–3 qián.

Caution

Use with caution in vacuity pattern cough and for those with weak constitutions.

---

4. 贝母 Bèi Mǔ   Fritillariae Bulbus
Fritillaria

Including
  ▷ *Zhè bèi mǔ* (浙贝母 Zhejiang fritillaria, Fritillariae Thunbergii Bulbus)
  ▷ *Chuān bèi mǔ* (川贝母 Sìchuān fritillaria, Fritillariae Cirrhosae Bulbus)

A distinction is made between *chuān bèi mǔ* (Sìchuān fritillaria) and *zhè bèi mǔ* (Zhejiang fritillaria).[4] *Chuān bèi mǔ* (Sìchuān fritillaria) is bitter and sweet in flavor and neutral in nature; it moistens the lung and transforms phlegm, and opens depression and quiets the heart. Because it moistens the lung and transforms phlegm, it is often used for cough resulting from yīn vacuity with taxation heat, for which it is combined with medicinals such as:

bǎi hé (百合 lily bulb, Lilii Bulbus)
shā shēn (沙参 adenophora/glehnia, Adenophorae seu Glehniae Radix)
mài dōng (麦冬 ophiopogon, Ophiopogonis Radix)
xuán shēn (玄参 scrophularia, Scrophulariae Radix)
mì zǐ wǎn (蜜紫菀 honey-fried aster, Asteris Radix cum Mele Praeparata)
shí hú (石斛 dendrobium, Dendrobii Herba)
mì pá yè (蜜杷叶 honey-fried loquat leaf, Eriobotryae Folium cum Mele
       Praeparatum)

After a pulmonary welling-abscess has ruptured and the pus has been completely ejected, if there is cough, ejection of phlegm, shortness of breath, postmeridian heat vexation, and dry mouth and throat, *chuān bèi mǔ* is combined with medicinals such as:

jié gěng (platycodon)
dāng guī (当归 Chinese angelica, Angelicae Sinensis Radix)

---

[4]These two items are distinguished in Chinese (and in English, but not Latin) on the basis of their origin: Sìchuān, a Western province of China, and Zhèjiāng, a province of eastern China to the south of the Yangtze. (Ed.)

shēng huáng qí (生黄芪 raw astragalus, Astragali Radix Cruda)

gān cǎo (甘草 licorice, Glycyrrhizae Radix)

mài dōng (麦冬 ophiopogon, Ophiopogonis Radix)

tiān huā fěn (天花粉 trichosanthes root, Trichosanthis Radix)

Because it opens and dissipates qì depression in the heart channel, it is used for binding depression of the qì dynamic in the heart and chest that results in oppression in the chest, chest pain, palpitations, reduced sleep, forgetfulness, and depression. For this pattern, *chuān bèi mǔ* is frequently combined with medicinals such as the following:

yuǎn zhì (远志 polygala, Polygalae Radix)

fú líng (茯苓 poria, Poria)

xiāng fù (香附 cyperus, Cyperi Rhizoma)

hóng huā (红花 carthamus, Carthami Flos)

yù jīn (郁金 curcuma, Curcumae Radix)

chāng pú (菖蒲 acorus, Acori Tatarinowii Rhizoma)

guā lóu (瓜蒌 trichosanthes, Trichosanthis Fructus)

zhǐ qiào (枳壳 bitter orange, Aurantii Fructus)

Zhè bèi mǔ (Zhejiang fritillaria) is acrid and bitter in flavor and slightly cold in nature. It is similar in effect to *chuān bèi mǔ* (Sìchuān fritillaria), but its acrid-dissipating and heat-clearing strength is greater. Thus it is suitable for external contraction cough, for which it is frequently combined with medicinals such as *sāng yè* (mulberry leaf), *jú huā* (chrysanthemum), *xìng rén* (apricot kernel), *jié gěng* (platycodon), *qián hú* (peucedanum), and *niú bàng zǐ* (arctium). For depressed binding phlegm-fire patterns (superabundance of qì that engenders fire), which result in scrofula that is swollen, enlarged, and painful (regardless of whether it is hemilateral, bilateral, single, or in a string), this medicinal dissipates depression and clears heat, as well as dispersing phlegm and dissipating binds. In such cases, *zhè bèi mǔ* is frequently combined with medicinals such as:

shēng mǔ lì (生牡蛎 crude oyster shell, Ostreae Concha Cruda)

xuán shēn (玄参 scrophularia, Scrophulariae Radix)

xià kū cǎo (夏枯草 prunella, Prunellae Spica)

bái sháo (白芍 white peony, Paeoniae Radix Alba)

xiāng fù (香附 cyperus, Cyperi Rhizoma)

hǎi zǎo (海藻 sargassum, Sargassum)

Zhè bèi mǔ and the first two of the above ingredients comprise *xiāo luǒ wán* (Scrofula-Dispersing Pill).

Xiāo luǒ wán 消瘰丸　　　　　　　　　　　　　　　　Scrofula-Dispersing Pill

---

zhè bèi mǔ (浙贝母 Zhejiang fritillaria, Fritillariae Thunbergii Bulbus)

shēng mǔ lì (生牡蛎 crude oyster shell, Ostreae Concha Cruda)

xuán shēn (玄参 scrophularia, Scrophulariae Radix)

At the onset of sores and toxic swellings, when the local area is hard, swollen, and painful, *zhè bèi mǔ* is used to dissipate binds and open depression in order to assist in dispersing sore-toxin. For this, it is frequently combined with medicinals such as:

jīn yín huā (金银花 lonicera, Lonicerae Flos)

lián qiáo (连翘 forsythia, Forsythiae Fructus)

chì sháo (赤芍 red peony, Paeoniae Radix Rubra)

hóng huā (红花 carthamus, Carthami Flos)

zhì shān jiǎ (炙山甲 mix-fried pangolin scales, Manis Squama cum Liquido Fricta)

dì lóng (地龙 earthworm, Pheretima)

tiān huā fěn (天花粉 trichosanthes root, Trichosanthis Radix)

chén pí (陈皮 tangerine peel, Citri Reticulatae Pericarpium)

Comparisons

Tǔ bèi mǔ (土贝母, bolbostemma) dissipates binds and resolves toxin. It is mostly used for external medicine and should not be confused with *chuān bèi mǔ* and *zhè bèi mǔ*.

Bàn xià (pinellia)[359] is warm and drying. It is primarily used for spleen channel damp phlegm. *Bèi mǔ* (fritillaria) is cool and moistening. It is primarily used for lung channel dry phlegm.

Dosage

The dosage is generally 3–9 g/1–3 qián. *Chuān bèi mǔ* (Sìchuān fritillaria) is ground to a fine powder and taken drenched with the decoction at a dosage of 0.9–1.5 g/3–5 fēn each time.

Research

According to modern research reports, fritimine derived from *chuān bèi mǔ* strengthens uterine contraction in vitro and inhibits intestinal peristalsis in vitro. A large dose of fritimine can cause central paralysis and inhibition of respiration. It also causes dilation of peripheral blood vessels, lowering of blood pressure, and deceleration of heart rate. Peimine derived from *zhè bèi mǔ* has been shown to have a marked antitussive effect in experimental animals.

Caution

Bèi mǔ (fritillaria) should be used with caution if there is dampness, food stagnation, or spleen-stomach vacuity cold.

5. 紫菀 **Zǐ Wǎn**   Asteris Radix
Aster

Also called *zǐ yuàn* 紫菀. Bitter, acrid, and slightly warm, *zǐ wǎn* (aster) transforms phlegm and downbears qì, clears the lung and discharges heat, and regulates the waterways. It is commonly used to treat cough, as in the following examples.

Zǐ wǎn tāng 紫菀汤   Aster Decoction

> *zǐ wǎn* (紫菀 aster, Asteris Radix)
>
> *zhī mǔ* (知母 anemarrhena, Anemarrhenae Rhizoma)
>
> *bèi mǔ* (贝母 fritillaria, Fritillariae Bulbus)
>
> *ē jiāo* (阿胶 ass hide glue, Asini Corii Colla)
>
> *dǎng shēn* (党参 codonopsis, Codonopsis Radix) (or *rén shēn* (人参 ginseng, Ginseng Radix))
>
> *fú líng* (茯苓 poria, Poria)
>
> *gān cǎo* (甘草 licorice, Glycyrrhizae Radix)
>
> *jié gěng* (桔梗 platycodon, Platycodonis Radix)
>
> *wǔ wèi zǐ* (五味子 schisandra, Schisandrae Fructus)
>
> *lián zǐ* (莲子 lotus seed, Nelumbinis Semen)

This formula is suitable for patterns such as taxation heat cough, **pulmonary welling-abscess**[560] (肺痈 *fèi yōng*) (final stage), **lung wilting**[556] (肺痿 *fèi wěi*), and blood ejection.

Zǐ wǎn wán 紫菀丸   Aster Pill

> *zǐ wǎn* (紫菀 aster, Asteris Radix)
>
> *wǔ wèi zǐ* (五味子 schisandra, Schisandrae Fructus)

This formula is suitable for enduring cough with blood-flecked phlegm.

Zhǐ sòu sǎn 止嗽散   Cough-Stopping Powder

> *zǐ wǎn* (紫菀 aster, Asteris Radix)
>
> *bái qián* (白前 willowleaf swallowwort, Cynanchi Stauntonii Rhizoma)
>
> *jīng jiè* (荆芥 schizonepeta, Schizonepetae Herba)
>
> *jié gěng* (桔梗 platycodon, Platycodonis Radix)
>
> *bǎi bù* (百部 stemona, Stemonae Radix)
>
> *chén pí* (陈皮 tangerine peel, Citri Reticulatae Pericarpium)
>
> *gān cǎo* (甘草 licorice, Glycyrrhizae Radix)

This formula is suitable for wind damage cough.

Zǐ wàn sǎn 紫菀散   Aster Powder

> *zǐ wǎn* (紫菀 aster, Asteris Radix)
>
> *kuǎn dōng huā* (款冬花 coltsfoot, Farfarae Flos)
>
> *bǎi bù* (百部 stemona, Stemonae Radix)

Grind to a fine powder and take 3 qián at a time with a decoction made from one *wū méi* (mume) and three pieces of *shēng jiāng* (fresh ginger). This formula is suitable for enduring cough that has not responded to treatment.

Zǐ wǎn (aster) treats "blood phlegm"[542] (血痰 *xuè tán*) particularly well. In former times it was believed that *zǐ wǎn* "drains upward flaming fire and dissipates bound stagnant qì."

According to modern research reports, this medicinal has an expectorant effect in experimental animals. It also has a definite antibacterial effect and inhibits contagious viruses.

Zǐ wǎn also precipitates qì and disinhibits urine. Its bitter flavor downbears qì and reaches the lower body, while its acridity boosts the lung. This allows qì transformation to reach down to the bladder and disinhibit urine. When evil in the lung channel congests lung qì so that qì is unable to descend to the bladder, resulting in inhibited urination and scant reddish urine, *zǐ wǎn* is combined with medicinals such as *fú líng* (poria) and *tōng cǎo* (rice-paper plant pith).

Zǐ wǎn that is mix-fried with honey has a stronger lung-moistening and cough-suppressing effect. Thus *zhì zǐ wǎn* (炙紫菀, mix-fried aster) is used for pulmonary consumption with cough and phlegm containing blood, or for lung dryness, itchy throat, and dry cough.

COMPARISON

Kuǎn dōng huā (coltsfoot)[440] tends to warm the lung and is mostly used for cough from cold-natured phlegm-rheum. *Zǐ wǎn* tends to open and dissipate lung qì depression and is mostly used for cough from wind-heat depressing the lung.

Zǐ wǎn is acrid yet not drying, moistening yet not cold, supplementing yet not stagnating. Therefore, it is frequently used to treat cough, regardless of whether a result of internal injury or external contraction, in formulas that are varied according to the signs.

DOSAGE

The dosage is generally 3–10 g/1–3 qián.

CAUTION

When *zǐ wǎn* is used to treat yīn vacuity cough, it must be used with yīn-enriching medicinals.

---

6. 款冬花 **Kuǎn Dōng Huā**   Farfarae Flos
Coltsfoot

Acrid and slightly bitter in flavor and warm in nature, *kuǎn dōng huā* (coltsfoot) warms the lung and transforms phlegm, suppresses cough and calms panting; when mix-fried with honey, it moistens the lung. *Kuǎn dōng huā* is a commonly used medicinal for treating cough. Using a paper tube to inhale the smoke of burning *kuǎn dōng huā* also treats cough.

For cough, panting, and phlegm in the throat causing a frog rale that results from externally contracted wind-cold, this medicinal dissipates cold and transforms phlegm with warmth and acridity, as well as downbearing qì and calming panting with slight bitterness. For this pattern, *kuǎn dōng huā* is combined with medicinals such as:

shè gān (射干 belamcanda, Belamcandae Rhizoma)

má huáng (麻黄 ephedra, Ephedrae Herba)

bàn xià (半夏 pinellia, Pinelliae Rhizoma)

xì xīn (细辛 asarum, Asari Herba)

zǐ wǎn (紫菀 aster, Asteris Radix)

xìng rén (杏仁 apricot kernel, Armeniacae Semen)

gān cǎo (甘草 licorice, Glycyrrhizae Radix)

I often use *kuǎn dōng huā* to moisten the lung and suppress cough for enduring cough or taxation cough, usually in combination with medicinals such as:

chuān bèi mǔ (川贝母 Sìchuān fritillaria, Fritillariae Cirrhosae Bulbus)

tián xìng rén (甜杏仁 sweet apricot kernel, Armeniacae Semen Dulce)

zǐ wǎn (紫菀 aster, Asteris Radix)

mài dōng (麦冬 ophiopogon, Ophiopogonis Radix)

shā shēn (沙参 adenophora/glehnia, Adenophorae seu Glehniae Radix)

xuán shēn (玄参 scrophularia, Scrophulariae Radix)

For patterns of enduring cough with phlegm containing blood, add *bǎi hé* (lily bulb) and *ǒu jié* (lotus root node); if there is heat in the lung, add *sāng pí* (mulberry root bark), *zhī mǔ* (anemarrhena), and *huáng qín* (scutellaria).

COMPARISONS

Kuǎn dōng huā tends to treat cold-natured cough, so for fire-heat cough it is inappropriate; *mǎ dōu líng* (aristolochia fruit)[443] tends to treat fire-heat cough, so for cold-natured cough it is inappropriate.

Bǎi bù (stemona)[442] is used for acute or enduring cough when appropriate for the pattern, whereas *kuǎn dōng huā* tends to be used for enduring cough.

Zǐ wǎn (aster)[438] tends to treat cough by diffusing the lung and transforming phlegm, whereas *kuǎn dōng huā* tends to treat cough by warming the lung and transforming phlegm. These two medicinals are frequently used together in order to increase the capacity to treat cough. According to modern research reports, whereas *zǐ wǎn* (aster) has no significant antitussive effect, but a pronounced expectorant effect, *kuǎn dōng huā* has no significant expectorant action, but a pronounced antitussive action.

DOSAGE

The dosage is generally 3–9 g/1–3 qián.

CAUTION

The use of *kuǎn dōng huā* is contraindicated in fire-heat cough.

7. 百部 **Băi Bù**   Stemonae Radix
Stemona

Băi bù (stemona) is sweet and bitter in flavor, slightly warm in nature, and possesses minor toxicity. It moistens the lung and suppresses cough. Warm but not drying, moistening but not slimy, this medicinal is used for both acute and enduring cough.

1. **Wind Damage Common Cold:** For common cold due to wind damage with cough, *băi bù* is frequently combined with medicinals such as:

jīng jiè (荆芥 schizonepeta, Schizonepetae Herba)

jié gĕng (桔梗 platycodon, Platycodonis Radix)

zĭ wăn (紫菀 aster, Asteris Radix)

bái qián (白前 willowleaf swallowwort, Cynanchi Stauntonii Rhizoma)

chén pí (陈皮 tangerine peel, Citri Reticulatae Pericarpium)

gān căo (甘草 licorice, Glycyrrhizae Radix)

sū yè (苏叶 perilla leaf, Perillae Folium)

xìng rén (杏仁 apricot kernel, Armeniacae Semen)

2. **Pulmonary Consumption Cough:** For pulmonary consumption[560] (肺劳 *fèi láo*) with cough, *băi bù* is frequently combined with medicinals such as:

shā shēn (沙参 adenophora/glehnia, Adenophorae seu Glehniae Radix)

bèi mŭ (贝母 fritillaria, Fritillariae Bulbus)

zhī mŭ (知母 anemarrhena, Anemarrhenae Rhizoma)

mài dōng (麦冬 ophiopogon, Ophiopogonis Radix)

băi hé (百合 lily bulb, Lilii Bulbus)

ē jiāo (阿胶 ass hide glue, Asini Corii Colla)

tián xìng rén (甜杏仁 sweet apricot kernel, Armeniacae Semen Dulce)

If there are also signs such as tidal heat (fever), night sweating, postmeridian reddening of the cheeks, and vexing heat in the five hearts, add the following:

zhì biē jiă (炙鳖甲 mix-fried turtle shell, Trionycis Carapax cum Liquido Frictus)

dān pí (丹皮 moutan, Moutan Cortex)

dì gŭ pí (地骨皮 lycium root bark, Lycii Cortex)

shēng dì huáng (生地黄 dried/fresh rehmannia, Rehmanniae Radix Exsiccata seu Recens)

xuán shēn (玄参 scrophularia, Scrophulariae Radix)

qín jiāo (秦艽 large gentian, Gentianae Macrophyllae Radix)

According to modern research reports, *băi bù* has an inhibitory effect on human tuberculosis bacteria. For all types of pulmonary tuberculosis, it is used in treatments determined in accordance with patterns identified.

Some reports of using this medicinal singly over a long period of time also show it has some effectiveness for treating pulmonary tuberculosis.

For children suffering from the spasmodic cough of whooping cough, *bǎi bù* is frequently combined with medicinals such as *xì xīn* (asarum), *shēng jiāng* (fresh ginger), *wǔ wèi zǐ* (schisandra), *má huáng* (ephedra), *bái zhú* (white atractylodes), and *zǐ wǎn* (aster). As a single medicinal made into a syrup, it is effective in both treating and preventing whooping cough. According to modern research reports, animal studies have demonstrated this medicinal's antitussive effect. It has also been shown to have both preventive and therapeutic effects against experimental influenza.

Bǎi bù is said to kill roundworm (in ancient books these are also called 长虫 *cháng chóng* "longworm"), pinworm, flies, and lice, as well as tree-boring insects. In decoction, powder preparation, or as an enema, it has a definite therapeutic effect against pinworm.[5] *Bǎi bù* can also be combined with *shǐ jūn zǐ* (quisqualis), *dà huáng* (rhubarb), *hè shī* (carpesium seed), *bīng láng* (areca), and *kǔ liàn pí* (chinaberry bark). Decocted and taken internally, this formula has a definite effect against roundworms.

This medicinal, when burned to produce smoke, can destroy lice (hair lice, body lice, or pubic lice). It can also be decocted and used as a wash. For tree-boring insects, it can be used as a fumigant or decocted in water and then mixed with alcohol to form a spray.

This medicinal is also effective for treating scab and lichen when decocted and used as an external wash.

DOSAGE

The dosage is generally 3–9 g/1–3 qián. Apply topically in an appropriate dosage.

CAUTION

Inappropriate for patients with indigestion or diarrhea.

---

8. 马兜铃 Mǎ Dōu Líng   Aristolochiae Fructus
Aristolochia Fruit

Mǎ dōu líng (aristolochia fruit)[6] is bitter and acrid in flavor and cold in nature; it clears lung heat, downbears qì, and suppresses cough. It also drains large intestinal heat and treats painful, swollen hemorrhoids.

Mǎ dōu líng is primarily used for lung heat cough because it cools the lung and downbears qì. For this purpose it is frequently combined with medicinals such

---

[5]The most common method of applying *bǎi bù fěn* (百部粉, stemona powder) when treating pinworm infestation is to mix the powder with sesame oil and apply it nightly around the anus. When the worms exit at night to lay eggs they are killed by the paste. Two to three weeks of application is necessary to ensure the efficacy of this method. Complementing this with an enema of *bǎi bù* and garlic increases the likelihood of success. (Ed.)

[6]The name *mǎ dōu líng* 马兜铃 literally translates as "bells worn by a horse." The name derives from the visual similarity between fruits hanging from an aristolochia vine that wraps around a tree and bells decorating a horse's neck. (Ed.)

as *sāng bái pí* (mulberry root bark), *zhī zǐ* (gardenia), *huáng qín* (scutellaria), *bèi mǔ* (fritillaria), *xìng rén* (apricot kernel), and *gān cǎo* (licorice); if there is also coughing of blood, add *ē jiāo* (ass hide glue), *bái jí* (bletilla), *ǒu jié* (lotus root node), and *bái máo gēn* (imperata).

COMPARISONS

Jié gěng (platycodon) treats cough and tends to open, diffuse, and course; thus it is suitable for newly-contracted cough in external-evil common cold. *Mǎ dōu líng* also treats cough, but tends to clear, downbear, and cool the lung; thus it is suitable for enduring cough that results in a lung heat cough.

Qián hú (peucedanum) diffuses externally contracted wind-heat, dispels phlegm, downbears qì, and suppresses cough. *Mǎ dōu líng* clears and drains lung heat engendered from enduring cough, and cools the lung, downbears qì, and suppresses cough.

APPLICATIONS

The lung and large intestine stand in interior-exterior relationship. When lung heat spreads to the large intestine, it can engender hemorrhoids and fistulae that cause bloody stool. *Mǎ dōu líng* clears and drains large intestine heat evil to treat painful swollen hemorrhoids. It is frequently combined with medicinals such as:

dì yú (地榆 sanguisorba, Sanguisorbae Radix)

huái huā (槐花 sophora flower, Sophorae Flos)

huái jiǎo (槐角 sophora fruit, Sophorae Fructus)

zhǐ qiào (枳壳 bitter orange, Aurantii Fructus)

huáng qín (黄芩 scutellaria, Scutellariae Radix)

lián qiáo (连翘 forsythia, Forsythiae Fructus)

For **plum-pit phlegm**[559] (梅核痰 *méi hé tán*) use 15–30 g/5 qián–1 liǎng of *mǎ dōu líng*, decocted in water. I frequently use it with:

xuán fù huā (旋覆花 inula flower, Inulae Flos) (boiled in a gauze bag)

shēng dài zhě shí (生代赭石 crude hematite, Haematitum Crudum)

huáng qín (黄芩 scutellaria, Scutellariae Radix)

xiāng fù (香附 cyperus, Cyperi Rhizoma)

sū gěng (苏梗 perilla stem, Perillae Caulis)

bàn xià (半夏 pinellia, Pinelliae Rhizoma)

fú líng (茯苓 poria, Poria)

wū méi tàn (乌梅炭 charred mume, Mume Fructus Carbonisatus)

jīn guǒ lǎn (金果榄 tinospora root, Tinosporae Radix)

Physicians of the past have said of *mǎ dōu líng* that "it often causes vomiting when used in decoctions." In clinical practice, I have found that vomiting is common and often severe after taking *shēng mǎ dōu líng* (raw aristolochia fruit), but is comparatively rare when using *zhì mǎ dōu líng* (mix-fried aristolochia fruit).

DOSAGE

The dosage is generally 3–6 g/1–2 qián.

RESEARCH

According to modern research reports, this medicinal shows an expectorant effect in laboratory animals, as well as a bronchodilatory effect.

CAUTION

This medicinal is inappropriate at the onset of wind-cold cough.[7]

COMPARISON

The root of *mǎ dōu líng* (aristolochia fruit) is called *qīng mù xiāng* (aristolochia root). It clears heat and resolves toxin, disperses swelling and relieves pain; thus it is primarily used for external medicine. Nonetheless, it can also be used for chest, abdominal, and stomach pain.

According to modern research reports, both *qīng mù xiāng* and *mǎ dōu líng* have a hypotensive effect; thus, they are used for hypertension.

9. 桑白皮 Sāng Bái Pí — Mori Cortex
Mulberry Root Bark

See also
- ▷ *Sāng shèn* (桑椹 mulberry, Mori Fructus)[140]
- ▷ *Sāng zhī* (桑枝 mulberry twig, Mori Ramulus)[464]
- ▷ *Sāng piāo xiāo* (桑螵蛸 mantis egg-case, Mantidis Oötheca)[190]

Sweet and acrid in flavor and cold in nature, *sāng bái pí* (mulberry root bark) drains lung fire, downbears lung qì, and disinhibits urine.

1. **Draining Lung Fire, Downbearing Lung Qì, Clearing the Lung and Suppressing Cough:** When fire-heat in the lung results in signs such as cough, ejection of yellow or sticky phlegm, thirst, panting, or coughing of blood, *sāng bái pí* can be combined with other medicinals such as:

dì gǔ pí (地骨皮 lycium root bark, Lycii Cortex)

huáng qín (黄芩 scutellaria, Scutellariae Radix)

shēng shí gāo (生石膏 crude gypsum, Gypsum Fibrosum Crudum)

zhī mǔ (知母 anemarrhena, Anemarrhenae Rhizoma)

gān cǎo (甘草 licorice, Glycyrrhizae Radix)

chuān bèi mǔ (川贝母 Sìchuān fritillaria, Fritillariae Cirrhosae Bulbus)

guā lóu (瓜蒌 trichosanthes, Trichosanthis Fructus)

lú gēn (芦根 phragmites, Phragmitis Rhizoma)

2. **Disinhibiting Water and Dispersing Swelling:** When impaired lung depuration affects normal expulsion of water and leads to water collecting in the skin (and flesh) that appears as water swelling, abdominal fullness, hasty panting, swelling of the head, face, and limbs, and inhibited urination, use this medicinal to

---

[7]It should also be noted that *mǎ dōu líng* (aristolochia fruit) is a member of the genus *Aristolochia* and contains aristolochic acid. (Ed.)

clear lung heat and disinhibit water. For this pattern, *sāng bái pí* is often combined with medicinals such as:

dà fù pí (大腹皮 areca husk, Arecae Pericarpium)

fú líng pí (茯苓皮 poria skin, Poriae Cutis)

chén pí (陈皮 tangerine peel, Citri Reticulatae Pericarpium)

shēng jiāng pí (生姜皮 ginger skin, Zingiberis Rhizomatis Cortex)

dōng guā pí (冬瓜皮 wax gourd rind, Benincasae Exocarpium)

chē qián zǐ (车前子 plantago seed, Plantaginis Semen)

Comparisons

Sāng yè (mulberry leaf) cools the blood, dispels wind, and clears heat. *Sāng zhī* (mulberry twig) frees the joints and outthrusts to the limbs, in order to treat wind-damp and impediment pain.

Dì gǔ pí (lycium root bark)[306] and *sāng bái pí* both clear fire-heat from the lung. Nevertheless, *dì gǔ pí* enters the lung channel blood aspect, downbears latent heat in the lung, boosts the kidney, and eliminates vacuity heat. *Sāng bái pí* enters the lung channel qì aspect, drains repletion fire from the lung, disinhibits water, and disperses swelling.

Chē qián zǐ (plantago seed)[64] tends to disinhibit the lower orifices of water, whereas *sāng bái pí* tends to disinhibit the upper source of water (水之上源 *shuǐ zhī shàng yuán*, i.e., the lung).

Processing

Mix-frying with honey reduces the cold nature of *sāng bái pí* and increases its lung-moistening action. To disinhibit water, one must use *shēng sāng pí* (raw mulberry root bark).

Dosage

The dosage is generally 3–9 g/1–3 qián.

Caution

This medicinal should be used with care in cases of lung qì vacuity and wind-cold cough.

Research

According to modern research reports, *sāng bái pí* has been found to have a pronounced diuretic effect in animal studies.

---

10. 枇杷叶 Pí Pá Yè   Eriobotryae Folium
Loquat Leaf

Bitter in flavor and neutral in nature, *pí pá yè* (loquat leaf) drains the lung and downbears fire, clears heat and transforms phlegm, harmonizes the stomach and downbears qì. The most special characteristic of this medicinal is that it "precipitates qì" (bearing qì downward). It is often used for phlegm-heat cough, retching counterflow, and vomiting.

1. **Phlegm-Heat Cough:** When lung qì fails to bear downward, qì becomes depressed and transforms into heat, and lung heat engenders phlegm, which results in phlegm-heat cough (cough and counterflow qì ascent, sticky phlegm that is difficult to expectorate or yellow phlegm, thirst, a slippery rapid pulse, and a slimy yellow tongue fur). For this, *pí pá yè* can be used to clear the lung and downbear qì. When qì descends, fire bears downward; and when fire downbears, phlegm disperses. For this pattern, *pí pá yè* is frequently combined with medicinals such as *huáng qín* (scutellaria), *zhī zǐ* (gardenia), *shā shēn* (adenophora/glehnia), *guā lóu* (trichosanthes), *zhī mǔ* (anemarrhena), and *xìng rén* (apricot kernel). *Pí pá yè* is mix-fried with honey to increase its lung-moistening effect; it is often used this way for cough due to lung heat with damage to liquid or lung dryness qì counterflow.

2. **Retching Counterflow and Vomiting:** For disharmony of stomach qì that results in qì counterflow and retching, or stomach heat-fire counterflow resulting in either dry vomiting or ejection of hot, malodorous, sour, and putrid substances and thirst, *pí pá yè* clears heat and harmonizes the stomach, downbears qì and checks retching. For this purpose, *pí pá yè* is combined with medicinals such as *zhú rú* (bamboo shavings), *fú líng* (poria), *bīng láng* (areca), *shēng jiāng* (fresh ginger), *bàn xià* (pinellia), *pèi lán* (eupatorium), and *sū zǐ* (perilla fruit). Mix-frying this medicinal with *jiāng zhī* (ginger juice) strengthens its ability to downbear counterflow and check vomiting. In this form, it is used for vomiting caused by stomach qì ascending counterflow.

Comparisons

Sāng bái pí (mulberry root bark)[445] and *pí pá yè* both treat lung heat cough, but *sāng bái pí* also drains the lung and moves water, whereas *pí pá yè* also downbears qì and harmonizes the stomach.

Mǎ dōu líng (aristolochia fruit)[443] and *pí pá yè* both clear lung heat, but *mǎ dōu líng* also clears large intestine heat and treats hemorrhoids, whereas *pí pá yè* also clears stomach heat, as well as downbearing counterflow and checking vomiting.

Dosage

The dosage is generally 6–12 g/2–4 qián; fresh, use 15–30 g/5 qián–1 liǎng. Before using this medicinal, brush off the fine hairs.

---

11. 独活 Dú Huó Pubescent Angelica	Angelicae Pubescentis Radix

Acrid in flavor and warm in nature, *dú huó* (pubescent angelica)[8] tracks wind and dispels dampness, and dissipates wind-cold. It is often used for wind damage

---

[8]See more about *dú huó* (pubescent angelica) in Lecture 2, Effusing & Dissipating Medicinals, page 21. (Ed.)

headache and toothache and for lumbar or leg pain that results from wind-cold-damp impediment.

1. Wind Damage Headache and Toothache: *Dú huó* dissipates wind-cold and is effective in tracking deep-lying wind in the kidney channel. For damage from wind-cold resulting in headache that reaches into the teeth and cheeks, indicating that wind evil has affected the kidney channel, *dú huó* is frequently combined with medicinals such as:

xì xīn (细辛 asarum, Asari Herba)

fáng fēng (防风 saposhnikovia, Saposhnikoviae Radix)

bái fù zǐ (白附子 typhonium, Typhonii Rhizoma)

jīng jiè (荆芥 schizonepeta, Schizonepetae Herba)

chuān xiōng (川芎 chuanxiong, Chuanxiong Rhizoma)

2. Wind-Damp Impediment Pain: When wind-cold-damp evils invade, causing poor flow of qi and blood and engendering sinew and bone pain in the lumbus, knee, foot, and lower leg, use this medicinal to track down wind, dispel dampness, and dissipate cold. It is frequently combined with medicinals such as:

sāng jì shēng (桑寄生 mistletoe, Taxilli Herba)

dù zhòng (杜仲 eucommia, Eucommiae Cortex)

xì xīn (细辛 asarum, Asari Herba)

niú xī (牛膝 achyranthes, Achyranthis Bidentatae Radix)

dāng guī (当归 Chinese angelica, Angelicae Sinensis Radix)

wēi líng xiān (威灵仙 clematis, Clematidis Radix)

xù duàn (续断 dipsacus, Dipsaci Radix)

zhì fù piàn (制附片 sliced processed aconite, Aconiti Radix Lateralis Praeparata Secta)

dì lóng (地龙 earthworm, Pheretima)

COMPARISONS

Qiāng huó (notopterygium)[19] and *dú huó* both dispel wind-damp, but *qiāng huó* is greater in medicinal strength; it is more fierce and tends to enter the greater yáng (bladder) channel. It is effective in treating headache due to wind and dampness contending with each other (especially when the pain is more severe in the back of the head), limb pain, and generalized pain. *Dú huó* is moderate in strength, and it tends to enter the lesser yīn (*shào yīn*) kidney channel. It is effective in tracking deep-lying wind in the lesser yīn channel and is used for impediment pain in the sinews and bones of the lumbus, knee, foot, and lower leg. *Qiāng huó* tends to treat **wandering wind**[566] (游风 *yóu fēng*), whereas *dú huó* tends to treat deep-lying wind.

Wēi líng xiān (clematis)[450] dispels wind-damp, outthrusts the twelve channels, dispels phlegm-water accumulations and gatherings, and has an extremely rapid, disinhibiting character. *Dú huó* dispels wind-damp, primarily tracking deep-lying wind evil and cold-damp in the kidney channel, and it treats **running piglet**[561] (奔豚 *bēn tún*) and **mounting-conglomeration**[558] (疝瘕 *shàn jiǎ*).

Xì xīn (asarum) tends to enter the blood aspect of the liver and kidney channels, and it is effective in treating wind-cold and wind-damp and in opening the nine orifices. *Dú huó* tends to enter the qì aspect of the kidney channel, and it is effective in treating deep-lying wind-cold and cold-damp, as well as treating toothache.

DOSAGE

The dosage is generally 3–9 g/1–3 qián.

CAUTION

This medicinal is inappropriate in yīn vacuity patterns.

---

12. 五加皮 Wŭ Jiā Pí   Acanthopanacis Cortex
Acanthopanax

Acrid and bitter in flavor and warm in nature, *wŭ jiā pí* (acanthopanax)[9] mainly dispels wind-damp, strengthens sinew and bone, and disperses water swelling. It is most commonly used for sinew and bone pain of the lumbus and leg and for limp legs.

1. Wind-Damp Impediment Pain, and Limp Lumbus and Knees: In addition to dispelling wind-damp, *wŭ jiā pí* also boosts liver and kidney, strengthens sinew and bone, and strengthens the lumbus and knees. The kidney governs the bones and the liver governs the sinews; in patterns of dual vacuity of liver and kidney, wind-cold-damp invading the sinews and bones results in painful lumbus and legs and in hypertonicity of the joints. *Wŭ jiā pí* is used to dispel wind-damp and to strengthen sinew and bone. For this purpose it is frequently combined with medicinals such as *cāng zhú* (atractylodes), *yĭ mĭ* (coix), *niú xī* (achyranthes), *bì xiè* (fish poison yam), *mù guā* (chaenomeles), *wēi líng xiān* (clematis), and *dú huó* (pubescent angelica).

For children with limp legs and slowness to walk, *wŭ jiā pí* is combined with medicinals such as *niú xī* (achyranthes), *mù guā* (chaenomeles), and *cāng zhú* (atractylodes). According to modern research reports, this medicinal is rich in vitamins A and B, and is effective in treating leg qì[556] (脚气 *jiăo qì*, i.e., beriberi, which is attributed to vitamin B deficiency).

2. Damp Itching of the Genitals and Generalized Water Swelling: When wind-damp evil qì causes damp itching of the genitals, *wŭ jiā pí* is combined with medicinals such as *huáng băi* (phellodendron), *chāng pú* (acorus), *shé chuáng zĭ* (cnidium seed), *kŭ shēn* (flavescent sophora), *fáng fēng* (saposhnikovia), *jīng jiè* (schizonepeta), and *shēng ài yè* (raw mugwort) to make an external wash.

When kidney vacuity results in lumbar pain and generalized puffy swelling, *wŭ jiā pí* is combined with medicinals such as:

---

[9]The southern variety, *nán wŭ jiā pí* 南五加皮, is *Acanthopanax gracilistylus* W.W. SMITH. The northern variety, *běi wŭ jiā pí* 北五加皮, also called *xiāng jiā pí* 香加皮, in its botanical classification is not an *Acanthopanax* but *Periploca sepium* BGE. The latter is toxic and must be used with care. See footnote on page 80. (Ed.)

zhū líng (猪苓 polyporus, Polyporus)

fú líng (茯苓 poria, Poria)

chē qián zǐ (车前子 plantago seed, Plantaginis Semen)

xù duàn (续断 dipsacus, Dipsaci Radix)

dōng guā pí (冬瓜皮 wax gourd rind, Benincasae Exocarpium)

tíng lì zǐ (葶苈子 lepidium/descurainia, Lepidii/Descurainiae Semen)

zé xiè (泽泻 alisma, Alismatis Rhizoma)

dà fù pí (大腹皮 areca husk, Arecae Pericarpium)

Comparisons

Bái xiǎn pí (dictamnus)[318] dispels wind-damp; its qì is cold and it is mobile. It tends to be used for wind sore, scab and lichen, and all kinds of jaundice and wind impediment. *Wǔ jiā pí* dispels wind-damp and also boosts liver and kidney. It tends to be used for weak sinews and bones.

Mù guā (chaenomeles) rectifies diseases of the sinews, and it tends to be used for tension of the sinews or limp sinews. *Wǔ jiā pí* strengthens sinew and bone, and it tends to be used for weak limp legs without strength. For tension of the sinews it is not as effective as *mù guā* (chaenomeles).

Wǔ jiā pí is divided into southern and northern varieties. The southern variety, *nán wǔ jiā pí* (南五加皮, acanthopanax), is stronger at dispelling wind-damp and at strengthening sinew and bone. It tends to be used for limp legs and weak feet. The northern variety, *běi wǔ jiā pí* (北五加皮, periploca), is stronger at dispersing water swelling and tends to be used for puffy swelling of the legs and feet. According to modern research, *nán wǔ jiā pí* is rich in vitamins A and B, as well as volatile oils, while the northern variety is rich in cardiac glycoside and has an effect similar to that of k-strophanthin. *Nán wǔ jiā pí* is generally considered to be more effective for supplementing the liver and kidney, and so it is regarded as the standard product. Furthermore, *běi wǔ jiā pí* has a definite toxicity and cannot be used in large dosages.

Dosage

The dosage of *nán wǔ jiā pí* (acanthopanax) is generally 4.5–9 g/1.5–3 qián, whereas that of *běi wǔ jiā pí* (periploca) is generally 3–6 g/1–2 qián.

Caution

Běi wǔ jiā pí (periploca) in large doses can cause vomiting and lower the heart rate, and therefore calls for special caution.

---

13. 威灵仙 Wēi Líng Xiān   Clematidis Radix
Clematis

Acrid and salty in flavor and warm in nature, *wēi líng xiān* (clematis) mainly dispels wind-damp. Mobile in nature, it reaches all parts of the body, freeing the five viscera and the twelve channels and network vessels. It also eliminates phlegm and disperses accumulations. *Wēi líng xiān* is used for generalized joint pain and for inhibited bending and stretching. Its effect is even better for pain affecting the lumbus, knees, legs, and feet. *Wēi líng xiān* is frequently combined with medicinals such as the following:

qiāng huó (羌活 notopterygium, Notopterygii Rhizoma et Radix)

dú huó (独活 pubescent angelica, Angelicae Pubescentis Radix)

sāng jì shēng (桑寄生 mistletoe, Taxilli Herba)

guì zhī (桂枝 cinnamon twig, Cinnamomi Ramulus)

xù duàn (续断 dipsacus, Dipsaci Radix)

dāng guī (当归 Chinese angelica, Angelicae Sinensis Radix)

hóng huā (红花 carthamus, Carthami Flos)

fáng jǐ (防己 fangji, Stephaniae Tetrandrae Radix)

yǐ mǐ (苡米 coix, Coicis Semen)

zhì shān jiǎ (炙山甲 mix-fried pangolin scales, Manis Squama cum Liquido Fricta)

zhì fù piàn (制附片 sliced processed aconite, Aconiti Radix Lateralis Praeparata Secta)

Comparisons

Xī xiān cǎo (siegesbeckia)[454] tends to be used for joint pain in which dampness is pronounced. *Wēi líng xiān* tends to be used for joint pain in which wind is pronounced.

Qín jiāo (large gentian)[452] treats pain from wind-damp impediment affecting the yáng brightness channel. *Wēi líng xiān* tends to treat pain from wind-damp impediment affecting the greater yáng channel.

Lǎo guàn cǎo (heron's-bill/cranesbill)[461] dispels wind-damp and fortifies sinew and bone. It is primarily used for damage to sinew, bone, and flesh, as well as numbness and pain from wind-damp impediment. *Wēi líng xiān* is primarily used for impediment pain from wind-cold-damp collecting in the channels and network vessels.

Miscellaneous

Furthermore, for concretions, conglomerations, accumulations, and gatherings, jaundice and puffy swelling, wind-damp phlegm qì, and pain from cold qì, *wēi líng xiān* is combined with other appropriate medicinals. Because its nature is mobile, penetrating, rapid, and disinhibiting, *wēi líng xiān* can increase the speed of the therapeutic effect.

Physicians of the past treated fish bones stuck in the throat using 37.5 g/ 1 liǎng 2 qián of *wēi líng xiān*, 31 g/1 liǎng of *shā rén* (amomum), and a spoonful of *shā táng* (granulated sugar) decocted and taken in frequent small doses. Last year one hospital reported the use of *wēi líng xiān* as a treatment for fish bones stuck in the throat that was effective in more than 10 cases.

Dosage

The dosage is generally 3–12 g/1–4 qián.

CAUTION

For patients with constitutional vacuity and weak qì, *wēi líng xiān* should be used with care. It is contraindicated for hypertonicity pain in the sinews and bones resulting from blood vacuity.

14. 秦艽 Qín Jiāo Large Gentian	Gentianae Macrophyllae Radix

Bitter and acrid in flavor and neutral in nature, *qín jiāo* (large gentian) mainly dispels wind, disinhibits dampness, and abates steaming bone taxation heat.

1. Wind-Cold-Damp Impediment, Generalized Impediment[551] (周痹 *zhōu bì*)**, and Pain and Hypertonicity of the Joints:** When the three evil qì—wind, cold, and dampness—invade the body, they combine to cause disease by affecting the normal movement of qì and blood and by congesting qì and blood, which results in generalized muscular pain, generalized joint pain, or hypertonicity pain of the sinews, sometimes with heat effusion (fever) and swollen joints. *Qín jiāo* dispels wind, disinhibits dampness, abates heat, and moderates hypertonicity. It is frequently combined with medicinals such as:

dú huó (独活 pubescent angelica, Angelicae Pubescentis Radix)

sāng jì shēng (桑寄生 mistletoe, Taxilli Herba)

wēi líng xiān (威灵仙 clematis, Clematidis Radix)

dāng guī (当归 Chinese angelica, Angelicae Sinensis Radix)

hóng huā (红花 carthamus, Carthami Flos)

fáng jǐ (防己 fangji, Stephaniae Tetrandrae Radix)

niú xī (牛膝 achyranthes, Achyranthis Bidentatae Radix)

yǐ mǐ (苡米 coix, Coicis Semen)

If the cold is severe, add *zhì fù piàn* (sliced processed aconite) and *guì zhī* (cinnamon twig); if the dampness is severe, add *cāng zhú* (atractylodes) and *bái zhú* (white atractylodes); if the wind is exuberant, add *fáng fēng* (saposhnikovia) and *qiāng huó* (notopterygium); if the sinew hypertonicity is severe, add *mù guā* (chaenomeles), *bái sháo* (white peony), *shēn jīn cǎo* (ground pine), and *zhì shān jiǎ* (mix-fried pangolin scales).

According to modern research reports, an alkaloid of *qín jiāo* increases adrenal gland function through indirect actions on the pituitary gland via the nervous system. Hence, it is effective in treating arthritis.

2. Yīn Vacuity Taxation Heat: *Qín jiāo* abates steaming bone taxation heat due to yīn vacuity, which is characterized by **postmeridian tidal heat [effusion]**[559] (下午潮热 *xià wǔ cháo rè*), reddening of both cheeks, flesh emaciation, night sweating, red tongue, fine rapid pulse, and dry mouth and thirst at night). For this purpose, *qín jiāo* is frequently combined with medicinals such as *yín chái hú* (stellaria), *dì gǔ pí* (lycium root bark), *bái wēi* (black swallowwort), and *qīng hāo* (sweet wormwood). The following formula is an example:

Qín jiāo biē jiǎ sǎn 秦艽鳖甲散   Large Gentian and Turtle Shell Powder

qín jiāo (秦艽 large gentian, Gentianae Macrophyllae Radix) 15 g/5 qián

biē jiǎ (鳖甲 turtle shell, Trionycis Carapax) 30 g/1 liǎng

chái hú (柴胡 bupleurum, Bupleuri Radix) 30 g/1 liǎng

dì gǔ pí (地骨皮 lycium root bark, Lycii Cortex) 30 g/1 liǎng

dāng guī (当归 Chinese angelica, Angelicae Sinensis Radix) 15 g/5 qián

zhī mǔ (知母 anemarrhena, Anemarrhenae Rhizoma) 15 g/5 qián

Grind to a rough powder, and each time use 15 g/5 qián. Add one *wū méi* (mume) and 1.5 g/5 fēn of *qīng hāo* (sweet wormwood); decoct with water, taking the decoction once in the morning and once at night. This is a commonly used prescription for the treatment of steaming bone taxation heat that can be varied in accordance with signs.

3. **Abating Jaundice:** This medicinal also frees the stool, disinhibits water, and abates jaundice. Physicians of the past noted their use of it in treating "jaundice, liquor jaundice," and for "dispelling generalized yellowing that appears [the color of] gold." When depressed dampness evil steams in the interior and gives rise to yellowing, combine *qín jiāo* with medicinals such as:

yīn chén (茵陈 virgate wormwood, Artemisiae Scopariae Herba)

huáng bǎi (黄柏 phellodendron, Phellodendri Cortex)

chē qián zǐ (车前子 plantago seed, Plantaginis Semen)

zhī zǐ (栀子 gardenia, Gardeniae Fructus)

fú líng (茯苓 poria, Poria)

In 1971, I examined a patient with infectious icteric hepatitis. In the hospital, he had been given large dosages of *yīn chén* (virgate wormwood), *zhī zǐ* (gardenia), *huáng bǎi* (phellodendron), *bǎn lán gēn* (isatis root), and *pú gōng yīng* (dandelion). The jaundice would not abate and continued to be a generalized golden color. Since the patient had already been given medication containing *yīn chén* (virgate wormwood) to no avail, I assumed that further use of *yīn chén* (virgate wormwood) formulas would not be effective, and thought of the jaundice-abating effects of *qín jiāo* (large gentian) and *bái xiǎn pí* (dictamnus). In accordance with the principles for identifying patterns and establishing methods of treatment, I added *qín jiāo* and *bái xiǎn pí* to his prescription and the jaundice gradually dispersed. The prescription is given below:

chái hú (柴胡 bupleurum, Bupleuri Radix) 12 g/4 qián

huáng qín (黄芩 scutellaria, Scutellariae Radix) 9 g/3 qián

chē qián zǐ (车前子 plantago seed, Plantaginis Semen) 15 g/5 qián

huáng bǎi (黄柏 phellodendron, Phellodendri Cortex) 12 g/4 qián

qín jiāo (秦艽 large gentian, Gentianae Macrophyllae Radix) 12 g/4 qián

bái xiǎn pí (白藓皮 dictamnus, Dictamni Cortex) 30 g/1 liǎng

fú líng (茯苓 poria, Poria) 12 g/4 qián

zé xiè (泽泻 alisma, Alismatis Rhizoma) 12 g/4 qián

jiāo sān xiān (焦三仙 scorch-fried three immortals, Tres Immortales Usti) each
9 g/3 qián

bīng láng (槟榔 areca, Arecae Semen) 9 g/3 qián

bái jí lí (白蒺藜 tribulus, Tribuli Fructus) 12 g/4 qián

cǎo dòu kòu (草豆蔻 Katsumada's galangal seed, Alpiniae Katsumadai Semen)
9 g/3 qián

I varied the formula in accordance with signs, and after about 20 packets, he was gradually cured. It is clear from this example that *qín jiāo* possesses a jaundice-abating effect.

Finally, *qín jiāo* enters the large intestine channel and frees the stool. It also treats swelling and pain of the lower teeth, and deviated eyes and mouth. It can be used wherever the pattern calls for it.

Comparisons

Yín chái hú (stellaria)[310] treats vacuity taxation, but it tends to be used for alternating cold and heat. *Qín jiāo* also treats vacuity taxation and tends to be used for tidal heat [effusion] (fever) and steaming bone pattern.

Dú huó (pubescent angelica)[447] and *qín jiāo* both treat wind-damp pain in the lower body. Nevertheless, *dú huó* (pubescent angelica) is used for wind-damp cold pain, whereas *qín jiāo* is used for wind-damp heat pain.

Dosage

The dosage is generally 3–9 g/1–3 qián.

Caution

This medicinal should not be used in patterns of spleen-stomach vacuity cold and diarrhea.

Research

According to modern research reports, animal experiments have demonstrated that *qín jiāo* (large gentian) and *biē jiǎ* (turtle shell) have an antirheumatic effect similar to that of cortisone. They have a definite effect on anaphalactic shock and histamines. They have the effects of raising blood sugar in animals and markedly reducing hepatic glycogens.

15. 豨莶草 Xī Xiān Cǎo   Siegesbeckiae Herba
Siegesbeckia

Xī xiān cǎo (siegesbeckia) when raw is bitter and acrid in flavor and cold in nature; when steamed, it has a sweet flavor and a warm nature. It is primarily used raw to dispel wind-damp, whereas steamed it also boosts liver and kidney, and dispels liver and kidney wind qì. *Xī xiān cǎo* is often used for sinew, bone, and joint pain, for paralysis of the limbs, and for lack of strength in the lumbus and legs. I present several frequently used formulas below:

1. *Xī xiān wán* (Siegesbeckia Pill) from *Jì Shēng Fāng* (济生方 "Life-Saver Formulary") treats wind strike with symptoms such as deviated eyes and mouth, drool foaming at the mouth, difficult speech, and limp, forceless extremities.

Xī xiān wán 豨莶丸	Siegesbeckia Pill

xī xiān cǎo (豨莶草 siegesbeckia, Siegesbeckiae Herba) 500 g/1 jīn (wash the fresh plant, mix with honey and liquor, and steam nine times, steaming for half an hour and then sun-drying each time)

chì sháo (赤芍 red peony, Paeoniae Radix Rubra) 31 g/1 liǎng

bái sháo (白芍 white peony, Paeoniae Radix Alba) 31 g/1 liǎng

shú dì huáng (熟地黄 cooked rehmannia, Rehmanniae Radix Praeparata) 62.5 g/2 liǎng

chuān wū (川乌 aconite root, Aconiti Radix) 18 g/6 qián

qiāng huó (羌活 notopterygium, Notopterygii Rhizoma et Radix) 31 g/1 liǎng

fáng fēng (防风 saposhnikovia, Saposhnikoviae Radix) 31 g/1 liǎng

Grind to a fine powder and mix with *liàn mì* (processed honey) to form pills the size of *wú tóng zǐ* (firmiana seed). Take 100 pills each morning on an empty stomach with either warm liquor or *mǐ tāng* (rice decoction). *Xī xiān wán* (Siegesbeckia Pill) is available as a prepared medicine, but it is slightly different from this formula and is used for arthritis and sciatica.

2. *Xī tóng wán* (Siegesbeckia and Clerodendron Pill) treats contraction of wind-damp passing into the channels and network vessels of the limbs, resulting in symptoms such as sore, weak legs and inability to lift the arms.

Xī tóng wán 豨桐丸	Siegesbeckia and Clerodendron Pill

chǎo xī xiān cǎo (炒豨莶草 stir-fried siegesbeckia, Siegesbeckiae Herba Fricta) 250 g/8 liǎng

chòu wú tóng (臭梧桐 clerodendron, Clerodendri Folium) 62.5 g/2 liǎng (flowers, leaves, stems, and seeds are cut, sun dried, and stir-fried before use)

Grind these ingredients to a fine powder, and use *liàn mì* (processed honey) to form pills the size of *wú tóng zǐ* (firmiana seed). Each morning and evening, take 12.5 g/ 4 qián with water. While taking this prescription, do not eat pig's liver or lamb's blood.

Another formula is:

xī xiān cǎo (豨莶草 siegesbeckia, Siegesbeckiae Herba) 31 g/1 liǎng

chòu wú tóng (臭梧桐 clerodendron, Clerodendri Folium) 93 g/3 liǎng

Grind to a fine powder and take 6–9 g/2–3 qián twice a day. The dosage is increased to 12–15 g/4–5 qián.

When dampness evil is relatively severe and results in joint pain, heaviness of the legs, or sore, weak legs, I frequently combine 15–31 g/5 qián–1 liǎng of *xī xiān cǎo* with:

dú huó (独活 pubescent angelica, Angelicae Pubescentis Radix)

sāng jì shēng (桑寄生 mistletoe, Taxilli Herba)

xù duàn (续断 dipsacus, Dipsaci Radix)

nán wǔ jiā pí (南五加皮 acanthopanax, Acanthopanacis Cortex)

niú xī (牛膝 achyranthes, Achyranthis Bidentatae Radix)

wēi líng xiān (威灵仙 clematis, Clematidis Radix)

yǐ mǐ (苡米 coix, Coicis Semen)

fáng jǐ (防己 fangji, Stephaniae Tetrandrae Radix)

If cold is also severe and the pain is pronounced, add *zhì fù piàn* (sliced processed aconite) and *bǔ gǔ zhī* (psoralea). This produces a highly satisfactory result.

RESEARCH

According to modern research, *xī xiān cǎo* (siegesbeckia) also has a hypotensive effect.

DOSAGE

The dosage is generally 6–13 g/2–4 qián. For severe cases, use up to 15–31 g/ 5 qián–1 liǎng.

---

16. 海风藤 Hǎi Fēng Téng
Kadsura Pepper Stem

Piperis Kadsurae Caulis

Hǎi fēng téng (kadsura pepper stem)[10] is bitter and acrid in flavor and slightly warm in nature. It mainly dispels wind-damp and frees the channels and network vessels. It is often used for wind-cold-damp impediment resulting in joint pain, pain in the flesh, inhibited bending and stretching, and hypertonicity and numbness of the limbs, which become more severe during yīn-type (i.e., damp) weather. *Hǎi fēng téng* is combined with the following:

qiāng huó (羌活 notopterygium, Notopterygii Rhizoma et Radix)

dú huó (独活 pubescent angelica, Angelicae Pubescentis Radix)

qín jiāo (秦艽 large gentian, Gentianae Macrophyllae Radix)

dāng guī (当归 Chinese angelica, Angelicae Sinensis Radix)

guì zhī (桂枝 cinnamon twig, Cinnamomi Ramulus)

chuān xiōng (川芎 chuanxiong, Chuanxiong Rhizoma)

sāng zhī (桑枝 mulberry twig, Mori Ramulus)

rǔ xiāng (乳香 frankincense, Olibanum)

mù xiāng (木香 costusroot, Aucklandiae Radix)

---

[10]Members of the genus *Usnea* are frequently used as substitutes for *hǎi fēng téng* (kadsura pepper stem). These substitutes all have very fine stems and leaf structures whereas the vine of *Piper kadsura* (CHOISY) OHWI is approximately 0.3–2 cm thick. In addition, the substitutes are multi-branched structures and the true medicinal is a linear vine. Further complicating matters is the occasional use of the stem of *nán wǔ wèi zǐ* 南五味子, *Kadsura heteroclita* ROXB. Craib, for *hǎi fēng téng*. This substitute is easily discerned since its stem is 1.5–8 cm in diameter. (Ed.)

qīng fēng téng (青风藤 Orient vine, Sinomenii Caulis)

xī xiān cǎo (豨莶草 siegesbeckia, Siegesbeckiae Herba)

COMPARISON

Qīng fēng téng (Orient vine) dispels wind and moves phlegm, and it tends to be used for wind-damp streaming sores, joint running[555] (历节 *lì jié*), and crane's knee[545] (鹤膝 *hè xī*). *Hǎi fēng téng* dispels wind and frees the channels and network vessels, and it tends to be used for wind-cold-damp resulting in pain of the joints and the flesh.

DOSAGE

The dosage is generally 6–15 g/2–5 qián, but for severe patterns, use up to 30 g/ 1 liǎng.

CAUTION

This medicinal is inappropriate for lumbar and leg pain due to blood vacuity, yīn vacuity, and kidney vacuity (i.e., without wind-cold-damp evils).

---

17. 络石藤 Luò Shí Téng   Trachelospermi Caulis
Star Jasmine Stem

Bitter in flavor and slightly cold in nature, *luò shí téng* (star jasmine stem) frees the channels and network vessels, disinhibits the blood vessels, and dispels wind-damp. It is suitable for joint pain, pain in the flesh, tension of the sinews, inhibited bending and stretching, and enduring depression of wind-cold-damp evils in which the depression transforms into heat; it is also suitable for patients with exuberant yáng, when contention between the right and the evil causes a transformation of yáng into heat with heat effusion in the area of joint pain, mild generalized heat, and other heat signs such as not wanting the limbs to be covered at night. *Luò shí téng* is frequently combined with medicinals such as *sāng zhī* (mulberry twig), *fáng fēng* (saposhnikovia), *hóng huā* (carthamus), *chì sháo* (red peony), *rěn dōng téng* (lonicera stem and leaf), *dāng guī* (Chinese angelica), *rǔ xiāng* (frankincense), *mò yào* (myrrh), *xī xiān cǎo* (siegesbeckia), and *shēn jīn cǎo* (ground pine). I often use this for rheumatic arthritis accompanied by fever.

COMPARISONS

Hǎi fēng téng (kadsura pepper stem)[456] treats wind-damp impediment pain, and it tends to be used for relatively severe wind-cold-damp without heat signs. *Luò shí téng* treats wind-damp impediment pain, and it tends to be used when heat signs are present.

Xī xiān cǎo (siegesbeckia)[454] is used when the dampness evil is more severe and when there is lumbar and leg pain and a lack of strength. It also boosts the liver and kidney. *Luò shí téng* is used when wind-damp transforms into heat and there is pain and tension of the sinews. It tends to free the channels and network vessels and has no supplementing effect.

Dosage

The dosage is generally 6–15 g/2–5 qián, but in severe patterns use up to 30 g/ 1 liǎng.

---

18. 海桐皮　Hǎi Tóng Pí　　Erythrinae Cortex
Erythrina

Bitter in flavor and neutral in nature, *hǎi tóng pí* (erythrina) mainly dispels wind-damp to treat lumbar and leg pain, and wind-damp impediment pain affecting the limbs and the flesh. For wind-damp impediment patterns with pronounced pain, adding *hǎi tóng pí*, in accordance with the pattern, frequently relieves pain. It is commonly combined with medicinals such as:

qiāng huó (羌活 notopterygium, Notopterygii Rhizoma et Radix)

dú huó (独活 pubescent angelica, Angelicae Pubescentis Radix)

wēi líng xiān (威灵仙 clematis, Clematidis Radix)

dāng guī (当归 Chinese angelica, Angelicae Sinensis Radix)

fáng fēng (防风 saposhnikovia, Saposhnikoviae Radix)

hǎi fēng téng (海风藤 kadsura pepper stem, Piperis Kadsurae Caulis)

guì zhī (桂枝 cinnamon twig, Cinnamomi Ramulus)

sāng zhī (桑枝 mulberry twig, Mori Ramulus)

hóng huā (红花 carthamus, Carthami Flos)

zhì fù piàn (制附片 sliced processed aconite, Aconiti Radix Lateralis Praeparata Secta)

For stubborn recurrent itchy sores, itchy papules, or urticaria,[11] I frequently use *hǎi tóng pí* to good effect combined, according to the pattern, with medicinals such as:

fáng fēng (防风 saposhnikovia, Saposhnikoviae Radix)

jīng jiè (荆芥 schizonepeta, Schizonepetae Herba)

hóng huā (红花 carthamus, Carthami Flos)

chì sháo (赤芍 red peony, Paeoniae Radix Rubra)

dān shēn (丹参 salvia, Salviae Miltiorrhizae Radix)

---

[11] *Hǎi tóng pí* (erythrina) was traditionally used as a powder in the treatment of scab and lichen. The *Běn Cǎo Gāng Mù* (本草纲目 "The Comprehensive Herbal Foundation") records combining it with equal parts of *shé chuáng zǐ* (cnidium seed), grinding the two medicinals together, and mixing the resulting powder in pork lard to make a paste. This paste was used to treat wind lichen (风癣 *fēng xiǎn*). *Hǎi tóng pí* (erythrina) is also often used as a steam-soak (or compress) in the treatment of traumatic injury. An example of this use is *hǎi tóng pí tāng* (Erythrina Decoction) from the *Yī Zōng Jīn Jiàn* (医宗金鉴 "The Golden Mirror of Medicine"): *hǎi tóng pí* (erythrina) 6 g, *tòu gǔ cǎo* (speranskia/balsam) 6 g, *rǔ xiāng* (frankincense) 6 g, *mò yào* (myrrh) 6 g, *dāng guī* (Chinese angelica) 4.5 g, *huā jiāo* (zanthoxylum) 9 g, *chuān xiōng* (chuanxiong) 3 g, *hóng huā* (carthamus) 3 g, *wēi líng xiān* (clematis) 2.4 g, *gān cǎo* (licorice) 2.4 g, *bái zhǐ* (Dahurian angelica) 2.4 g, *fáng fēng* (saposhnikovia) 2.4 g. This formula treats enduring pain from damage to bones or sinews. (Ed.)

bái xiăn pí (白藓皮 dictamnus, Dictamni Cortex)

zhì shān jiă (炙山甲 mix-fried pangolin scales, Manis Squama cum Liquido Fricta)

zào jiăo cì (皂角刺 gleditsia thorn, Gleditsiae Spina)

kŭ shēn (苦参 flavescent sophora, Sophorae Flavescentis Radix)

lián qiáo (连翘 forsythia, Forsythiae Fructus)

shé tuì (蛇蜕 snake slough, Serpentis Periostracum) 0.3–0.6 g[12]

Steeped in wine and applied topically, *hăi tóng pí* is used as external medicine for patients with skin diseases such as scab[561] (疥 *jiè*) and lichen[556] (癣 *xiăn*).

Comparisons

Wŭ jiā pí (acanthopanax),[449] i.e., *nán wŭ jiā pí* 南五加皮, tends to strengthen bones and soothe the sinews, and it is used for lack of strength in the lumbus and legs and for pain and hypertonicity of the sinews. *Hăi tóng pí* tends to dispel wind-damp and free the channels and network vessels, and it is used for rheumatic pain. Its pain-relieving effect is relatively pronounced, and it can also be applied topically to treat scab and lichen.

Dosage

The dosage taken internally is generally 3–9 g/1–3 qián; when applied topically, a suitable amount is steeped in wine.

Research

According to modern research reports, *hăi tóng pí* contains alkaloids that have a relaxing effect on striated muscle and a tranquilizing effect on the central nervous system.

Caution

This medicinal is cumulative in effect. Its toxicity takes the form of inhibition of the myocardium and cardiovascular system, so that large doses can cause pronounced arrhythmia and hypotension.

---

19. 千年健 Qiān Nián Jiàn
Homalomena
Homalomenae Rhizoma

Acrid, sweet, and bitter in flavor and warm in nature, *qiān nián jiàn* (homalomena) strengthens sinew and bone, dispels wind qì, quickens the blood, and frees the network vessels. It is suitable for elderly people with a lack of strength in the sinews and bones, and numbness in the extremities.[13] It can also be used according to pattern for strong, young people with wind-damp pain, hypertonicity of the limbs, and inhibited bending and stretching of the sinews and bones. For elderly people, *qiān nián jiàn* is combined with medicinals such as:

---

[12]This medicinal should be used within this dosage range; the others are more variable.

[13]The fact that this medicinal is called *qiān nián jiàn* 千年健, literally "one thousand years of health," may be related to its presence in many formulas for the elderly. (Ed.)

shú dì huáng (熟地黄 cooked rehmannia, Rehmanniae Radix Praeparata)

dāng guī (当归 Chinese angelica, Angelicae Sinensis Radix)

gǒu qǐ zǐ (枸杞子 lycium, Lycii Fructus)

nán wǔ jiā pí (南五加皮 acanthopanax, Acanthopanacis Cortex)

xù duàn (续断 dipsacus, Dipsaci Radix)

guì xīn (桂心 shaved cinnamon bark, Cinnamomi Cortex Rasus)

dú huó (独活 pubescent angelica, Angelicae Pubescentis Radix)

qiāng huó (羌活 notopterygium, Notopterygii Rhizoma et Radix)

hóng huā (红花 carthamus, Carthami Flos)

shān yào (山药 dioscorea, Dioscoreae Rhizoma)

dǎng shēn (党参 codonopsis, Codonopsis Radix)

bái zhú (白术 white atractylodes, Atractylodis Macrocephalae Rhizoma)

shān zhū yú (山茱萸 cornus, Corni Fructus)

chuān xiōng (川芎 chuanxiong, Chuanxiong Rhizoma)

Medicinal wines that strengthen sinew and bone frequently contain this medicinal. Clinically, it is frequently combined with medicinals such as:

dāng guī (当归 Chinese angelica, Angelicae Sinensis Radix)

hóng huā (红花 carthamus, Carthami Flos)

dú huó (独活 pubescent angelica, Angelicae Pubescentis Radix)

sāng jì shēng (桑寄生 mistletoe, Taxilli Herba)

xù duàn (续断 dipsacus, Dipsaci Radix)

zhì shān jiǎ (炙山甲 mix-fried pangolin scales, Manis Squama cum Liquido Fricta)

tòu gǔ cǎo (透骨草 speranskia/balsam, Speranskiae seu Impatientis Herba)

gǔ suì bǔ (骨碎补 drynaria, Drynariae Rhizoma)

luò shí téng (络石藤 star jasmine stem, Trachelospermi Caulis)

hǎi tóng pí (海桐皮 erythrina, Erythrinae Cortex)

Qiān nián jiàn has a rich aroma. When used for stomach pain, it is also effective. For this purpose it is generally combined with medicinals such as:

xiāng fù (香附 cyperus, Cyperi Rhizoma)

gāo liáng jiāng (高良姜 lesser galangal, Alpiniae Officinarum Rhizoma)

mù xiāng (木香 costusroot, Aucklandiae Radix)

shā rén (砂仁 amomum, Amomi Fructus)

dān shēn (丹参 salvia, Salviae Miltiorrhizae Radix)

It is especially appropriate for stomach pain in elderly patients.

Comparison

Luò shí téng (star jasmine stem) tends to free the channels and network vessels, whereas *qiān nián jiàn* tends to strengthen sinew and bone.

Xī xiān cǎo (siegesbeckia) tends to dispel dampness evil, whereas *qiān nián jiàn* tends to dispel wind qì (i..e, treat pain due to wind qì).

DOSAGE

The dosage is generally 6–12 g/2–4 qián, but in severe patterns use up to 30 g/1 liǎng.

---

20. 老鹳草 Lǎo Guàn Cǎo   Erodii seu Geranii Herba
Heron's-bill/cranesbill

Bitter and acrid in flavor and warm in nature, *lǎo guàn cǎo* (heron's-bill/cranesbill) dispels wind-damp, frees the channels and network vessels, quickens the blood, and fortifies sinew and bone. When wind, cold, and dampness evils invade the body and result in joint impediment pain, numbness of the limbs, and tingling and itching of the skin, *lǎo guàn cǎo* is combined with medicinals such as:

dāng guī (当归 Chinese angelica, Angelicae Sinensis Radix)

guì zhī (桂枝 cinnamon twig, Cinnamomi Ramulus)

chì sháo (赤芍 red peony, Paeoniae Radix Rubra)

hóng huā (红花 carthamus, Carthami Flos)

qiāng huó (羌活 notopterygium, Notopterygii Rhizoma et Radix)

dú huó (独活 pubescent angelica, Angelicae Pubescentis Radix)

fáng fēng (防风 saposhnikovia, Saposhnikoviae Radix)

hǎi fēng téng (海风藤 kadsura pepper stem, Piperis Kadsurae Caulis)

I frequently use 30 g/1 liǎng of *lǎo guàn cǎo* for rheumatoid arthritis patients who have inhibited bending and stretching, and blood vessel stoppage, and have found this quite effective.

Lǎo guàn cǎo used singly can be steeped in liquor and taken as a medicinal wine. It can also be made into a liquid extract.

DOSAGE

The dosage is generally 9–15 g/3–5 qián, but in special situations, use up to 30 g/1 liǎng.

---

21. 伸筋草 Shēn Jīn Cǎo   Lycopodii Herba
Ground Pine

Bitter and acrid in flavor and warm in nature, *shēn jīn cǎo* (ground pine) soothes the sinews and quickens the network vessels and also dispels wind-damp. In wind-damp impediment with pain, inhibited bending and stretching, and tension of the sinews, add 15–30 g/5 qián–1 liǎng of *shēn jīn cǎo* to an appropriate medicinal decoction to soothe the sinews and quicken the network vessels. It is frequently combined with medicinals such as:

qiāng huó (羌活 notopterygium, Notopterygii Rhizoma et Radix)

dú huó (独活 pubescent angelica, Angelicae Pubescentis Radix)

dāng guī (当归 Chinese angelica, Angelicae Sinensis Radix)

bái sháo (白芍 white peony, Paeoniae Radix Alba)

mù guā (木瓜 chaenomeles, Chaenomelis Fructus)

shēng yǐ mǐ (生苡米 raw coix, Coicis Semen Crudum)

hóng huā (红花 carthamus, Carthami Flos)

táo rén (桃仁 peach kernel, Persicae Semen)

guì zhī (桂枝 cinnamon twig, Cinnamomi Ramulus)

jī xuè téng (鸡血藤 spatholobus, Spatholobi Caulis)

hǎi fēng téng (海风藤 kadsura pepper stem, Piperis Kadsurae Caulis)

When insufficiency of the liver and kidney deprives the sinews of nourishment and results in inhibited bending and stretching of the sinews and bones, *shēn jīn cǎo* is frequently combined with medicinals such as:

shú dì huáng (熟地黄 cooked rehmannia, Rehmanniae Radix Praeparata)

shān yào (山药 dioscorea, Dioscoreae Rhizoma)

shān zhū yú (山茱萸 cornus, Corni Fructus)

gǒu qǐ zǐ (枸杞子 lycium, Lycii Fructus)

tóng jí lí (潼蒺藜 complanate astragalus seed, Astragali Complanati Semen)

dāng guī (当归 Chinese angelica, Angelicae Sinensis Radix)

bái sháo (白芍 white peony, Paeoniae Radix Alba)

qiān nián jiàn (千年健 homalomena, Homalomenae Rhizoma)

hóng huā (红花 carthamus, Carthami Flos)

nán wǔ jiā pí (南五加皮 acanthopanax, Acanthopanacis Cortex)

COMPARISON

Luò shí téng (star jasmine stem) tends to be used to free the channels and quicken the network vessels, whereas *shēn jīn cǎo* tends to be used to soothe the sinews and quicken the blood.

DOSAGE

The dosage is generally 9–15 g/3–5 qián, but in severe patterns use up to 30 g/ 1 liǎng.

---

22. 透骨草 Tòu Gǔ Cǎo
Speranskia/Balsam

Speranskiae seu Impatientis Herba

Acrid in flavor and warm in nature, *tòu gǔ cǎo* (speranskia/balsam) primarily dispels wind-damp, quickens the blood, and relieves pain. In patterns of wind-damp pain with hypertonicity of the sinews and bones and numbness of the limbs, this medicinal is used in combination with medicinals such as:

dú huó (独活 pubescent angelica, Angelicae Pubescentis Radix)

qiāng huó (羌活 notopterygium, Notopterygii Rhizoma et Radix)

fù zǐ (附子 aconite, Aconiti Radix Lateralis Praeparata)

shēn jīn cǎo (伸筋草 ground pine, Lycopodii Herba)

qiān nián jiàn (千年健 homalomena, Homalomenae Rhizoma)

hǎi tóng pí (海桐皮 erythrina, Erythrinae Cortex)

hóng huā (红花 carthamus, Carthami Flos)

Tòu gǔ cǎo can also be decocted singly to make a steam-wash. Used as an external wash, it also conducts medicinals into the channels, network vessels, and blood vessels, in order to dispel wind, quicken the blood, and relieve pain. This is a special characteristic of *tòu gǔ cǎo*.

For the swelling and toxin of sores and scrotal eczema, use *tòu gǔ cǎo* combined with *shēng ài yè* (raw mugwort), *bái xiǎn pí* (dictamnus), *shé chuáng zǐ* (cnidium seed), and *rěn dōng téng* (lonicera stem and leaf); decoct and apply as an external wash.

In cases of stubborn wind-damp pain with hypertonicity of the sinews and bones, and inhibited bending and stretching, I frequently add 15–30 g/5 qián–1 liǎng of *tòu gǔ cǎo*, 6–9 g/2–3 qián of *chuān wū* (aconite root), 25–30 g/8 qián–1 liǎng of *shēn jīn cǎo* (ground pine), and 9–12 g/3–4 qián of *gǔ suì bǔ* (drynaria) to an appropriate decoction medicine; this invariably enhances the therapeutic effect.

DOSAGE

The dosage is generally 9–15 g/3–5 qián, but in special situations use up to 30 g/1 liǎng. For topical application, increase the dosage appropriately.

CAUTION

Because this medicinal quickens the blood, it is contraindicated in pregnancy.

---

23. 追地枫 Zhuī Dì Fēng
Schizophragma Root Bark
Schizophragmatis Radicis Cortex

Zhuī dì fēng (schizophragma root bark) is sour in flavor and astringent and warm in nature. It dispels wind-damp and is often used for wind-damp impediment pain, sinew and bone pain, and weakness and numbness in the legs and knees. *Zhuī dì fēng* is combined with medicinals such as:

dú huó (独活 pubescent angelica, Angelicae Pubescentis Radix)

sāng jì shēng (桑寄生 mistletoe, Taxilli Herba)

xì xīn (细辛 asarum, Asari Herba)

wēi líng xiān (威灵仙 clematis, Clematidis Radix)

zhì fù piàn (制附片 sliced processed aconite, Aconiti Radix Lateralis Praeparata Secta)

hóng huā (红花 carthamus, Carthami Flos)

tòu gǔ cǎo (透骨草 speranskia/balsam, Speranskiae seu Impatientis Herba)

yǐ mǐ (苡米 coix, Coicis Semen)

Besides entering the liver and kidney channels, *zhuī dì fēng* also enters the large intestine channel. If wind-damp transforms into heat and invades the large intestine channel, attacking upward and causing toothache and sore throat, combine *zhuī dì fēng* with medicinals such as *xuán shēn* (scrophularia), *shēng dì huáng* (dried/fresh rehmannia), *dì gǔ pí* (lycium root bark), *dān shēn* (salvia), and *shān dòu gēn* (bushy sophora). If the heat pours downward, causing red-white dysentery or bloody stool, it is combined with medicinals such as *dì yú* (sanguisorba), *huái huā* (sophora flower), *huáng bǎi* (phellodendron), *huáng lián* (coptis), *mù xiāng* (costusroot), and *fáng fēng* (saposhnikovia).

Dosage

The dosage is generally 6–12 g/2–4 qián, but in special situations use up to 15–30 g/5 qián–1 liǎng.

---

24. 桑枝 Sāng Zhī   Mori Ramulus
Mulberry Twig

See also

▷ *Sāng shèn* (桑椹 mulberry, Mori Fructus)[140]

▷ *Sāng bái pí* (桑白皮 mulberry root bark, Mori Cortex)[445]

▷ *Sāng piāo xiāo* (桑螵蛸 mantis egg-case, Mantidis Oötheca)[190]

Bitter in flavor and neutral in nature, *sāng zhī* (mulberry twig) dispels wind, eliminates dampness, and disinhibits the joints. For wind-damp resulting in shoulder, arm, knee, or leg pain, generalized joint pain, or inhibited bending and stretching, combine *sāng zhī* with medicinals such as:

piàn jiāng huáng (片姜黄 sliced turmeric, Curcumae Longae Rhizoma Sectum)

fáng jǐ (防己 fangji, Stephaniae Tetrandrae Radix)

hǎi tóng pí (海桐皮 erythrina, Erythrinae Cortex)

luò shí téng (络石藤 star jasmine stem, Trachelospermi Caulis)

xī xiān cǎo (豨莶草 siegesbeckia, Siegesbeckiae Herba)

dú huó (独活 pubescent angelica, Angelicae Pubescentis Radix)

sāng jì shēng (桑寄生 mistletoe, Taxilli Herba)

xù duàn (续断 dipsacus, Dipsaci Radix)

niú xī (牛膝 achyranthes, Achyranthis Bidentatae Radix)

wēi líng xiān (威灵仙 clematis, Clematidis Radix)

In wind strike patterns with hemiplegia and hypertonicity of the limbs, combine *sāng zhī* with:

fáng fēng (防风 saposhnikovia, Saposhnikoviae Radix)

jú huā (菊花 chrysanthemum, Chrysanthemi Flos)

bái jí lí (白蒺藜 tribulus, Tribuli Fructus)

bàn xià (半夏 pinellia, Pinelliae Rhizoma)

chén pí (陈皮 tangerine peel, Citri Reticulatae Pericarpium) *zhú lì* (竹沥 bamboo sap, Bambusae Succus)

dǎn xīng (胆星 bile arisaema, Arisaema cum Bile)

hóng huā (红花 carthamus, Carthami Flos)

táo rén (桃仁 peach kernel, Persicae Semen)

chì sháo (赤芍 red peony, Paeoniae Radix Rubra)

dì lóng (地龙 earthworm, Pheretima)

Sāng zhī combined with *bì xiè* (fish poison yam), *fú líng* (poria), *yǐ rén* (coix), *niú xī* (achyranthes), *zé xiè* (alisma), *cāng zhú* (atractylodes), and *qín jiāo* (large gentian) is used for **leg qì**[556] (脚气 *jiǎo qì*).

COMPARISON

Guì zhī (cinnamon twig) is acrid and warm; it frees and outthrusts the yáng qì of the limbs and tends to be used for wind-cold impediment pain. *Sāng zhī* is bitter and neutral; it disinhibits the joints of the limbs and dispels wind qì, and it tends to be used for wind evil transforming into heat and causing joint impediment in the limbs and for hemiplegia following wind strike (when there are heat manifestations).

RESEARCH

According to modern research reports, *sāng zhī* has a pronounced hypotensive effect and contains vitamin B_1.

DOSAGE

The dosage is generally 10–30 g/3 qián–1 liǎng.

---

25. 松节 Sōng Jié   Pini Nodi Lignum
Knotty Pine Wood

Bitter in flavor and warm in nature, *sōng jié* (knotty pine wood) dispels wind-damp, quickens the channels and network vessels, and disinhibits the joints. It is often used for enduring wind-damp impediment pain (including rheumatoid arthritis), hypertonicity pain of the joints, bones, and sinews, pain and distention of the joints, and inhibited bending and stretching. It is combined with medicinals such as:

guì zhī (桂枝 cinnamon twig, Cinnamomi Ramulus)

shēn jīn cǎo (伸筋草 ground pine, Lycopodii Herba)

tòu gǔ cǎo (透骨草 speranskia/balsam, Speranskiae seu Impatientis Herba)

mù guā (木瓜 chaenomeles, Chaenomelis Fructus)

fáng jǐ (防己 fangji, Stephaniae Tetrandrae Radix)

hóng huā (红花 carthamus, Carthami Flos)

wēi líng xiān (威灵仙 clematis, Clematidis Radix)

qiāng huó (羌活 notopterygium, Notopterygii Rhizoma et Radix)

dú huó (独活 pubescent angelica, Angelicae Pubescentis Radix)

zhì shān jiǎ (炙山甲 mix-fried pangolin scales, Manis Squama cum Liquido Fricta)

When cold-damp is more severe, add *zhì fù piàn* (sliced processed aconite), *xì xīn* (asarum), and *guì xīn* (shaved cinnamon bark). *Sōng jié* has a particularly good effect for cold-damp pain in the knee. For this purpose it is combined with *niú xī* (achyranthes), *mù guā* (chaenomeles), and *hǎi tóng pí* (erythrina).

Comparison

Shēn jīn cǎo (ground pine)[461] and *tòu gǔ cǎo* (speranskia/balsam)[462] tend to be used for wind-damp impediment pain with hypertonicity of the sinews and bones.

Sōng jié tends to be used for cold-damp impediment pain with inhibited bending and stretching or swollen joints.

Dosage

The dosage is generally 9–15 g/3–5 qián, but in severe cases use up to 30 g/ 1 liǎng.

---

26. 丝瓜络 Sī Guā Luò
Loofah

Luffae
Fructus Retinervus

Sweet in flavor and neutral in nature, *sī guā luò* (loofah) clears heat and cools the blood, rectifies qì, and frees the channels and network vessels.

For pain that lancinates through the chest and rib-side, use this medicinal with *xiāng fù* (cyperus), *yù jīn* (curcuma), and *zhǐ qiào* (bitter orange). For pain in the chest and rib-side from knocks and falls, combine it with *hóng huā* (carthamus), *táo rén* (peach kernel), *jié gěng* (platycodon), and *piàn jiāng huáng* (sliced turmeric). For **wrenched lumbus with acute pain**[568] (闪腰岔气 *shǎn yào chà qì*), combine it with *rǔ xiāng* (frankincense), *mò yào* (myrrh), *lì zhī hé* (litchee pit), and *yán hú suǒ* (corydalis). For joint pain from rheumatic arthritis, combine it with *dú huó* (pubescent angelica), *qiāng huó* (notopterygium), *sōng jié* (knotty pine wood), and *wēi líng xiān* (clematis).

Sī guā luò also cools the blood and stanches bleeding. For women with flooding and spotting, or for bloody stool or bleeding from hemorrhoids, use char-fried *sī guā luò* ground to a powder. Take 3 g/1 qián two or three times a day. It can also be combined with *xù duàn tàn* (charred dipsacus), *ài yè tàn* (charred mugwort), *ē jiāo zhū* (ass hide glue pellets), and *zōng tàn* (charred trachycarpus) for flooding and spotting, or with *dì yú* (sanguisorba), *huái huā tàn* (charred sophora flower), *fáng fēng* (saposhnikovia), *zhì huái jiāo* (mix-fried sophora fruit), and *huáng qín tàn* (charred scutellaria) for bloody stool or bleeding hemorrhoids.

Dosage

The dosage is generally 6–12 g/2–4 qián.

27. 白花蛇 Bái Huā Shé
Krait/Agkistrodon

Bungarus seu
Agkistrodon

Also called *qí shé* 蕲蛇. Sweet and salty in flavor, warm in nature, and toxic, *bái huā shé* (krait/agkistrodon)[14] tracks down wind and quickens the network vessels and it treats various wind patterns. The experience of past physicians with regard to this medicinal is summed up in the saying, "In the interior it penetrates the bowels and viscera and in the exterior it penetrates the skin; it outthrusts from the bone and tracks wind, interrupts fright, and settles convulsions."

1. **Wind Strike, Deviation of the Mouth and Face, and Hemiplegia:** For wind strike in adults, when wind-phlegm and static blood congest the channels and network vessels, inhibiting movement in the blood vessels and resulting in symptoms such as deviated mouth and face and hemiplegia, *bái huā shé* is combined with:

sāng zhī (桑枝 mulberry twig, Mori Ramulus)

fáng fēng (防风 saposhnikovia, Saposhnikoviae Radix)

dǎn xīng (胆星 bile arisaema, Arisaema cum Bile)

tiān zhú huáng (天竹黄 bamboo sugar, Bambusae Concretio Silicea)

zhú lì (竹沥 bamboo sap, Bambusae Succus)

bái jí lí (白蒺藜 tribulus, Tribuli Fructus)

dāng guī (当归 Chinese angelica, Angelicae Sinensis Radix)

hóng huā (红花 carthamus, Carthami Flos)

chì sháo (赤芍 red peony, Paeoniae Radix Rubra)

zhì shān jiǎ (炙山甲 mix-fried pangolin scales, Manis Squama cum Liquido Fricta)

dì lóng (地龙 earthworm, Pheretima)

táo rén (桃仁 peach kernel, Persicae Semen)

2. **Wind-Heat, Acute or Chronic Fright Wind, Convulsions, and Fright Epilepsy in Children:** Children have delicate bowels and viscera. Exuberant wind-heat or sudden fright can easily give rise to convulsions and fright wind, or even paralysis of the legs. This is treated by combining *bái huā shé* with *zhū shā* (cinnabar), *chāng pú* (acorus), *yù jīn* (curcuma), *dǎn xīng* (bile arisaema), *tiān zhú huáng* (bamboo sugar), *yuǎn zhì* (polygala), *quán xiē* (scorpion), *wú gōng* (centipede), *líng yáng jiǎo* (antelope horn), and *niú huáng* (bovine bezoar). This combination is often used as a pill preparation.

3. **Severe Joint Pain and Numbness of the Limbs:** When wind, cold, and damp evils congest the channels and vessels, resulting in joint pain and numbness of the limbs, *bái huā shé* is combined with medicinals such as:

dú huó (独活 pubescent angelica, Angelicae Pubescentis Radix)

qiāng huó (羌活 notopterygium, Notopterygii Rhizoma et Radix)

---

[14]Some species of *Agkistrodon* are on the CITES endangered species list. The snake used in Chinese medicine is not currently among them. (Ed.)

jīng jiè (荆芥 schizonepeta, Schizonepetae Herba)

fáng fēng (防风 saposhnikovia, Saposhnikoviae Radix)

wēi líng xiān (威灵仙 clematis, Clematidis Radix)

yǐ mǐ (苡米 coix, Coicis Semen)

fáng jǐ (防己 fangji, Stephaniae Tetrandrae Radix)

qín jiāo (秦艽 large gentian, Gentianae Macrophyllae Radix)

fù zǐ (附子 aconite, Aconiti Radix Lateralis Præparata)

hóng huā (红花 carthamus, Carthami Flos)

dāng guī (当归 Chinese angelica, Angelicae Sinensis Radix)

4. Generalized Scab, Lài, White Patch Wind[567] (白癜风 *bái diàn fēng*), **Itchy Papules, and Lichen and Sores:** This medicinal tracks wind by penetrating the bowels and viscera in the interior and by penetrating the skin in the exterior. For all skin diseases due to wind, *bái huā shé* can be combined with medicinals such as:

bái xiǎn pí (白藓皮 dictamnus, Dictamni Cortex)

kǔ shēn (苦参 flavescent sophora, Sophorae Flavescentis Radix)

lián qiáo (连翘 forsythia, Forsythiae Fructus)

hǎi tóng pí (海桐皮 erythrina, Erythrinae Cortex)

hóng huā (红花 carthamus, Carthami Flos)

dān shēn (丹参 salvia, Salviae Miltiorrhizae Radix)

chán tuì (蝉蜕 cicada molting, Cicadae Periostracum)

bò hé (薄荷 mint, Menthae Herba)

zào jiǎo cì (皂角刺 gleditsia thorn, Gleditsiae Spina)

COMPARISON

Wū shāo shé (black-striped snake) is sweet, neutral, and free of toxin. It is used similarly to *bái huā shé*. Generally speaking, *wū shāo shé* tends to be used for insensitivity of the skin, **great wind**[551] (大风 *dà fēng*, i.e., leprosy), and scab and lài. *Bái huā shé* tends to be used for wind strike in adults and fright epilepsy in children.

DOSAGE

Bái huā shé is generally used in doses of 0.9–3 g/3 fēn–1 qián, taken decocted with water. When *bái huā shé* is stir-fried, ground to a fine powder, and taken drenched with a decoction, use 0.3–0.9 g/1–3 fēn, swallowed with warm water, two or three times per day.

CAUTION

Contraindicated in the absence of wind evil and in patterns of blood vacuity engendering wind.

28. 白僵蚕 Bái Jiāng Cán   Bombyx Batryticatus
Silkworm

Also called *jiāng cán* 僵蚕. Salty and acrid in flavor and neutral in nature, *bái jiāng cán* (silkworm) mainly dispels wind and resolves tetany (痉 *jìng*), disperses phlegm and dissipates binds.

1. For childhood convulsions, fright epilepsy, and night crying, combine *bái jiāng cán* with the following:

fáng fēng (防风 saposhnikovia, Saposhnikoviae Radix)

quán xiē (全蝎 scorpion, Scorpio)

wú gōng (蜈蚣 centipede, Scolopendra)

dǎn xīng (胆星 bile arisaema, Arisaema cum Bile)

gōu téng (钩藤 uncaria, Uncariae Ramulus cum Uncis)

tiān zhú huáng (天竹黄 bamboo sugar, Bambusae Concretio Silicea)

chán tuì (蝉蜕 cicada molting, Cicadae Periostracum)

jiāo sān xiān (焦三仙 scorch-fried three immortals, Tres Immortales Usti)

2. For liver wind harassing the upper body, causing headache and dizzy head, *bái jiāng cán* can be combined with the following:

tiān má (天麻 gastrodia, Gastrodiae Rhizoma)

jú huā (菊花 chrysanthemum, Chrysanthemi Flos)

gōu téng (钩藤 uncaria, Uncariae Ramulus cum Uncis)

bái jí lí (白蒺藜 tribulus, Tribuli Fructus)

bái sháo (白芍 white peony, Paeoniae Radix Alba)

3. For contraction of wind in the head and face causing deviated mouth and face, *bái jiāng cán* can be combined with:

wú gōng (蜈蚣 centipede, Scolopendra)

quán xiē (全蝎 scorpion, Scorpio)

bái zhǐ (白芷 Dahurian angelica, Angelicae Dahuricae Radix)

bái fù zǐ (白附子 typhonium, Typhonii Rhizoma)

4. *Bái jiāng cán* is used for baby moth (tonsillitis), mumps (paratotis), and scrofula of the neck. For baby moth, it is combined with:

jié gěng (桔梗 platycodon, Platycodonis Radix)

shēng gān cǎo (生甘草 raw licorice, Glycyrrhizae Radix Cruda)

jǐn dēng lóng (锦灯笼 lantern plant calyx, Physalis Calyx seu Fructus)

shān dòu gēn (山豆根 bushy sophora, Sophorae Tonkinensis Radix)

shè gān (射干 belamcanda, Belamcandae Rhizoma)

For mumps, it is combined with:

bǎn lán gēn (板蓝根 isatis root, Isatidis Radix)

niú bàng zǐ (牛蒡子 arctium, Arctii Fructus)

mǎ bó (马勃 puffball, Lasiosphaera seu Calvatia)

qīng dài (青黛 indigo, Indigo Naturalis)

For scrofula, it is combined with *xuán shēn* (scrophularia), *shēng mŭ lì* (crude oyster shell), and *bèi mŭ* (fritillaria).

DOSAGE

The dosage is generally 3–9 g/1–3 qián.

---

29. 全蝎 Quán Xiē   Scorpio
Scorpion

Sweet and acrid in flavor, neutral in nature, and toxic, *quán xiē* (scorpion) extinguishes wind and checks convulsions. It conducts various forms of wind medicinals directly into the disease site. For various forms of convulsions, fright wind, and fright reversal, *quán xiē* is combined with medicinals such as *wú gōng* (centipede), *tiān má* (gastrodia), and *gōu téng* (uncaria). For example, in chronic spleen wind[543] (慢脾风 *màn pí fēng*) in children (chronic fright wind that occurs after retching, vomiting, diarrhea, or dysentery), use the following:

quán xiē (全蝎 scorpion, Scorpio) 9 g/3 qián

bái zhú (白术 white atractylodes, Atractylodis Macrocephalae Rhizoma) 9 g/3 qián

má huáng (麻黄 ephedra, Ephedrae Herba) 9 g/3 qián

Grind the above together to a fine powder. For children under the age of two, use 0.6–0.9 g/2–3 fēn; for age three and above, use 1.5 g/5 fēn. Take the powder with a decoction of *bò hé* (mint). For wind strike in adults, with symptoms such as deviated eyes and mouth, and hemiplegia, it is combined with *bái jiāng cán* (silkworm), *bái fù zĭ* (typhonium) (these three are known as *qiān zhèng sǎn* (Pull Aright Powder), which treats contraction of wind in the face that causes deviated eyes and mouth), *sāng zhī* (mulberry twig), *fáng fēng* (saposhnikovia), *bàn xià* (pinellia), *chén pí* (tangerine peel), *hóng huā* (carthamus), *táo rén* (peach kernel), *chì sháo* (red peony), *zhì shān jiă* (mix-fried pangolin scales), and *dì lóng* (earthworm) (to treat wind strike hemiplegia).

Using *quán xiē* with *fáng fēng* (saposhnikovia) strengthens its ability to extinguish wind, check tetany, and settle convulsions.

COMPARISON

Wú gōng (centipede) dispels wind and settles tetany, treating arched-back rigidity and rigid spasms very effectively. *Quán xiē* extinguishes wind and settles tetany, effectively treating frequent jerking, tremors of the arms and legs, and shaking of the head. Using the two together enhances the therapeutic effect; thus they are frequently combined.

DOSAGE

The dosage is generally 1.5–9 g/5 fēn–3 qián, but in severe cases this dosage is slightly increased. When using *xiē wěi* (scorpion tail) alone, one should generally use 3–8 tails. *Xiē wěi* is best for dispelling wind and checking tetany, and it is usually used for **tugging wind**[566] (抽风 *chōu fēng*) in children.

---

30. 蜈蚣 Wú Gōng   Scolopendra
Centipede

Acrid in flavor, warm in nature, and toxic, *wú gōng* (centipede) mainly checks tetany, extinguishes wind, and resolves toxin, for which purposes it is frequently used with *quán xiē* (scorpion). In the treatment of epilepsy, *wú gōng* is combined with medicinals such as:

tiān má (天麻 gastrodia, Gastrodiae Rhizoma)

gōu téng (钩藤 uncaria, Uncariae Ramulus cum Uncis)

quán xiē (全蝎 scorpion, Scorpio)

tiān zhú huáng (天竹黄 bamboo sugar, Bambusae Concretio Silicea)

dǎn xīng (胆星 bile arisaema, Arisaema cum Bile)

bàn xià (半夏 pinellia, Pinelliae Rhizoma)

zhū shā (朱砂 cinnabar, Cinnabaris)

yuǎn zhì (远志 polygala, Polygalae Radix)

chāng pú (菖蒲 acorus, Acori Tatarinowii Rhizoma)

chuān bèi mǔ (川贝母 Sìchuān fritillaria, Fritillariae Cirrhosae Bulbus)

When high fever stirs wind, manifesting in unclear spirit-mind, spasm of the limbs, rigidity of the neck, convulsions, and clenched jaw, combine *wú gōng* with medicinals such as:

huáng lián (黄连 coptis, Coptidis Rhizoma)

yù jīn (郁金 curcuma, Curcumae Radix)

tiān zhú huáng (天竹黄 bamboo sugar, Bambusae Concretio Silicea)

líng yáng jiǎo (羚羊角 antelope horn, Saigae Tataricae Cornu)

quán xiē (全蝎 scorpion, Scorpio)

bái jiāng cán (白僵蚕 silkworm, Bombyx Batryticatus)

gōu téng (钩藤 uncaria, Uncariae Ramulus cum Uncis)

fáng fēng (防风 saposhnikovia, Saposhnikoviae Radix)

bái jí lí (白蒺藜 tribulus, Tribuli Fructus)

For lockjaw with signs such as clenched jaw, rigidity of the neck, and convulsions of the limbs, *wú gōng* is combined with:

fáng fēng (防风 saposhnikovia, Saposhnikoviae Radix)

tiān nán xīng (天南星 arisaema, Arisaematis Rhizoma)

quán xiē (全蝎 scorpion, Scorpio)

bái fù zǐ (白附子 typhonium, Typhonii Rhizoma)

bái jiāng cán (白僵蚕 silkworm, Bombyx Batryticatus)

gōu téng (钩藤 uncaria, Uncariae Ramulus cum Uncis)

Finally, *wú gōng* is also used for pain of the sinew and flesh, numbness, and stiffness with a lack of flexibility due to wind-cold-damp impediment. For this pattern, it is frequently combined with medicinals such as:

qiāng huó (羌活 notopterygium, Notopterygii Rhizoma et Radix)

dú huó (独活 pubescent angelica, Angelicae Pubescentis Radix)

qín jiāo (秦艽 large gentian, Gentianae Macrophyllae Radix)

fáng fēng (防风 saposhnikovia, Saposhnikoviae Radix)

wēi líng xiān (威灵仙 clematis, Clematidis Radix)

For sore-toxin, burns and scalds, and scrofula, *wú gōng* has a toxin-resolving effect and it is applied topically in combination with:

rǔ xiāng (乳香 frankincense, Olibanum)

mò yào (没药 myrrh, Myrrha)

ér chá (儿茶 cutch, Catechu)

xióng huáng (雄黄 realgar, Realgar)

Comparisons

Wú gōng and *quán xiē* (scorpion)[470] have roughly the same capacity to settle tetany and extinguish wind. But *wú gōng* relieves pain better than *quán xiē*. *Quán xiē* is better than *wú gōng* for treating stiff tongue, inhibited speech, tremors, and convulsions.

Quán xiē is mainly used to stabilize wind, whereas *wú gōng*, aside from extinguishing wind, can also be used to resolve toxin (attacking toxin with toxin).

Dosage

The dosage is generally 1–3 pieces, or 1.5–4.5 g/5 fēn–1.5 qián.

---

31. 地龙 Dì Lóng   Pheretima
Earthworm

Salty in flavor and cold in nature, *dì lóng* (earthworm) clears heat and disinhibits water, and frees the channels and network vessels.

For warm-heat disease with high fever and manic raving, which in severe cases may become convulsions, *dì lóng* clears heat to quiet the spirit and check tetany. It is frequently combined with medicinals such as:

huáng lián (黄连 coptis, Coptidis Rhizoma)

yù jīn (郁金 curcuma, Curcumae Radix)

yuǎn zhì (远志 polygala, Polygalae Radix)

dà qīng yè (大青叶 isatis leaf, Isatidis Folium)

chāng pú (菖蒲 acorus, Acori Tatarinowii Rhizoma)

tiān zhú huáng (天竹黄 bamboo sugar, Bambusae Concretio Silicea)

lián qiáo (连翘 forsythia, Forsythiae Fructus)

gōu téng (钩藤 uncaria, Uncariae Ramulus cum Uncis)

When damp-heat accumulating in the center and lower burners manifests as ascites, puffy swelling of the legs, and inhibited urination, *dì lóng* is used to clear heat and disinhibit water; for this purpose it is combined with medicinals such as:

zhū líng (猪苓 polyporus, Polyporus)

fú líng (茯苓 poria, Poria)

chē qián zǐ (车前子 plantago seed, Plantaginis Semen)

dà fù pí (大腹皮 areca husk, Arecae Pericarpium)

dōng guā pí (冬瓜皮 wax gourd rind, Benincasae Exocarpium)

zé xiè (泽泻 alisma, Alismatis Rhizoma)

mù tōng (木通 trifoliate akebia, Akebiae Trifoliatae Caulis)

Dì lóng by nature moves downward and disinhibits water-damp; thus it is often used for leg qì with puffy swelling on the upper surface of the foot, damp itch between the toes, and stubborn numbness and limpness of the legs. For this pattern, *dì lóng* is frequently combined with medicinals such as:

mù guā (木瓜 chaenomeles, Chaenomelis Fructus)

fáng jǐ (防己 fangji, Stephaniae Tetrandrae Radix)

wú yú (吴萸 evodia, Evodiae Fructus)

bīng láng (槟榔 areca, Arecae Semen)

zǐ sū (紫苏 perilla, Perillae Folium, Caulis et Calyx)

For numbness of the limbs, pain, and inhibited bending and stretching, *dì lóng* is used to free the channels and quicken the network vessels in combination with medicinals such as:

sāng zhī (桑枝 mulberry twig, Mori Ramulus)

guì zhī (桂枝 cinnamon twig, Cinnamomi Ramulus)

luò shí téng (络石藤 star jasmine stem, Trachelospermi Caulis)

hóng huā (红花 carthamus, Carthami Flos)

zhì shān jiǎ (炙山甲 mix-fried pangolin scales, Manis Squama cum Liquido Fricta)

shēn jīn cǎo (伸筋草 ground pine, Lycopodii Herba)

In recent years, *dì lóng* has been found effective in the treatment of bronchial asthma. It is given as a powder preparation or as an injection.

COMPARISON

Chuān shān jiǎ (pangolin scales) and *dì lóng* both free the channels and quicken the network vessels, and conduct medicinals directly into the disease site. *Chuān shān jiǎ*, however, penetrates the whole body and reaches all sites, whereas *dì lóng* moves downward. By virtue of its downward nature, *dì lóng* is often used for leg qì[556] (脚气 jiǎo qì) and for its ability to disinhibit water-damp and disperse water swelling.

DOSAGE

The dosage is generally 3–9 g/1–3 qián.

RESEARCH

According to modern research reports, this medicinal has bronchodilatory and antipyretic effects. It also has both antihistaminic and hypotensive effects.

---

32. 白蒺藜 Bái Jí Lí   Tribuli Fructus
Tribulus

Acrid and bitter in flavor and slightly warm in nature, *bái jí lí* (tribulus) courses liver depression, dissipates liver wind, drains lung qì, and brightens the eyes.

1. Headache, Dizzy Head, and Dizzy Vision: When liver wind harasses the upper body, resulting in dizzy head, headache, dizzy vision, bitter taste in the mouth, and copious eye discharge, *bái jí lí* is used to course liver depression, dissipate liver wind, and calm the liver in order to treat headache and dizziness. *Bái jí lí* is frequently combined with:

jú huā (菊花 chrysanthemum, Chrysanthemi Flos)

sāng yè (桑叶 mulberry leaf, Mori Folium)

tiān má (天麻 gastrodia, Gastrodiae Rhizoma)

gōu téng (钩藤 uncaria, Uncariae Ramulus cum Uncis)

bái sháo (白芍 white peony, Paeoniae Radix Alba)

shēng mŭ lì (生牡蛎 crude oyster shell, Ostreae Concha Cruda)

líng yáng jiǎo (羚羊角 antelope horn, Saigae Tataricae Cornu)

2. Red Eyes, Eye Pain, and Copious Tears: For externally contracted wind-heat or liver depression transforming into heat and engendering wind that results in red eyes, eye pain, tearing, flowery vision, aversion to light, and copious eye discharge, use this medicinal to dissipate wind and clear heat and to calm the liver. For this pattern, *bái jí lí* is combined with medicinals such as:

zhī zǐ (栀子 gardenia, Gardeniae Fructus)

huáng qín (黄芩 scutellaria, Scutellariae Radix)

mù zéi cǎo (木贼草 equisetum, Equiseti Hiemalis Herba)

jīng jiè (荆芥 schizonepeta, Schizonepetae Herba)

sāng yè (桑叶 mulberry leaf, Mori Folium)

jú huā (菊花 chrysanthemum, Chrysanthemi Flos)

cǎo jué míng (草决明 fetid cassia, Cassiae Semen)

shí jué míng (石决明 abalone shell, Haliotidis Concha)

mì méng huā (密蒙花 buddleia, Buddleja Flos)

3. Pain and Distention in the Chest and Rib-Side: For pain and distention in the chest and rib-side that result from binding depression of liver qì or nondiffusion of lung qì, use this medicinal to course and dissipate liver depression, or to diffuse and drain lung depression. For this purpose it is frequently combined with medicinals such as:

chái hú (柴胡 bupleurum, Bupleuri Radix)

zhǐ qiào (枳壳 bitter orange, Aurantii Fructus)

xiāng fù (香附 cyperus, Cyperi Rhizoma)

yù jīn (郁金 curcuma, Curcumae Radix)

piàn jiāng huáng (片姜黄 sliced turmeric, Curcumae Longae Rhizoma Sectum)

chuān liàn zǐ (川楝子 toosendan, Toosendan Fructus)

yán hú suǒ (延胡索 corydalis, Corydalis Rhizoma)

zào jiǎo cì (皂角刺 gleditsia thorn, Gleditsiae Spina)

For rib-side pain in hepatitis patients, I frequently add 9–12 g/3–4 qián of *bái jí lí* as well as 4.5 g/1.5 qián of *zào jiǎo cì* (gleditsia thorn), or 6–9 g/2–3 qián of *piàn jiāng huáng* (sliced turmeric), to an appropriate decoction medicine that is based on pattern identification and treatment differentiation. This consistently produces the best effects.

4. Aggregation lumps, accumulations, and gatherings[542] (癥块积聚 *pǐ kuài jī jù*): When qì stagnation and blood stasis affect the free flow of qì and blood, enduring accumulation can develop into lumps on the right or the left. *Bái jí lí* is used to course liver qì and dissipate liver depression and thereby move blood and dissipate binds; it is frequently combined with medicinals such as the following:

yán hú suǒ (延胡索 corydalis, Corydalis Rhizoma)

dāng guī wěi (当归尾 Chinese angelica tail, Angelicae Sinensis Radicis Extremitas)

hóng huā (红花 carthamus, Carthami Flos)

táo rén (桃仁 peach kernel, Persicae Semen)

zào jiǎo cì (皂角刺 gleditsia thorn, Gleditsiae Spina)

zhì shān jiǎ (炙山甲 mix-fried pangolin scales, Manis Squama cum Liquido Fricta)

zhì biē jiǎ (炙鳖甲 mix-fried turtle shell, Trionycis Carapax cum Liquido Frictus)

shēng mǔ lì (生牡蛎 crude oyster shell, Ostreae Concha Cruda)

Comparisons

Tóng jí lí (complanate astragalus seed)[140] tends to neutrally supplement the liver and kidney, while *bái jí lí* tends to free and dissipate liver depression.

Gōu téng (uncaria)[478] clears liver heat and extinguishes wind, whereas *bái jí lí* dissipates liver depression and extinguishes wind.

Dosage

The dosage is generally 6–9 g/2–3 qián.

Caution

Should be used with care in patients with blood vacuity and weak qì and in pregnant women.

33. 天麻 Tiān Má   Gastrodiae Rhizoma
Gastrodia

Acrid in flavor and neutral in nature, *tiān má* (gastrodia)[15] extinguishes wind, dispels phlegm, and checks tetany. It is most suitable for vacuity wind stirring internally and for wind-phlegm harassing the upper body that result in dizziness, numbness of the limbs, and convulsions.

1. Headache and Dizziness: Acrid in flavor, *tiān má* dissipates external wind, enters the liver channel, and extinguishes internal wind (liver wind). It outthrusts to the exterior and dispels phlegm. Hence, it both extinguishes wind and dispels phlegm. Generally, medicinals that dispel wind and transform phlegm are drying in nature. Only *tiān má* has an acridity that is moistening and not drying, frees and harmonizes the blood vessels, and boosts the sinews and bones. Thus physicians of the past said that *tiān má* is "a moistening agent among the wind medicinals." When liver wind stirs internally and wind-phlegm harasses the upper body, causing headache, dizziness, darkened vision, unsteady gait, and numbness of the extremities, combine *tiān má* with medicinals such as:

> *gōu téng* (钩藤 uncaria, Uncariae Ramulus cum Uncis)
> *bái jí lí* (白蒺藜 tribulus, Tribuli Fructus)
> *jú huā* (菊花 chrysanthemum, Chrysanthemi Flos)
> *chuān xiōng* (川芎 chuanxiong, Chuanxiong Rhizoma)
> *chì sháo* (赤芍 red peony, Paeoniae Radix Rubra)
> *dǎn xīng* (胆星 bile arisaema, Arisaema cum Bile)
> *sāng yè* (桑叶 mulberry leaf, Mori Folium)
> *shēng dì huáng* (生地黄 dried/fresh rehmannia, Rehmanniae Radix Exsiccata seu Recens)
> *zé xiè* (泽泻 alisma, Alismatis Rhizoma)

For wind strike with deviated eyes and mouth and drooling from the corners of the mouth, combine *tiān má* with:

> *bái jiāng cán* (白僵蚕 silkworm, Bombyx Batryticatus)
> *quán xiē* (全蝎 scorpion, Scorpio)
> *bái fù zǐ* (白附子 typhonium, Typhonii Rhizoma)
> *jīng jiè* (荆芥 schizonepeta, Schizonepetae Herba)
> *bái zhǐ* (白芷 Dahurian angelica, Angelicae Dahuricae Radix)
> *tiān nán xīng* (天南星 arisaema, Arisaematis Rhizoma)
> *bàn xià* (半夏 pinellia, Pinelliae Rhizoma)
> *sū mù* (苏木 sappan, Sappan Lignum)

2. Wind Strike: For wind strike[568] (中风 *zhòng fēng*) with signs such as hemiplegia, inhibited speech, and hemilateral numbness, combine *tiān má* with:

---

[15] *Gastrodia elata* BL. is on the CITES endangered species list and must be accompanied by a Certificate of Cultivation if it is traded internationally. (Ed.)

sāng zhī (桑枝 mulberry twig, Mori Ramulus)

bàn xià (半夏 pinellia, Pinelliae Rhizoma)

zhì nán xīng (制南星 processed arisaema, Arisaematis Rhizoma Praeparatum)

hóng huā (红花 carthamus, Carthami Flos)

fáng fēng (防风 saposhnikovia, Saposhnikoviae Radix)

táo rén (桃仁 peach kernel, Persicae Semen)

chì sháo (赤芍 red peony, Paeoniae Radix Rubra)

dì lóng (地龙 earthworm, Pheretima)

bái jí lí (白蒺藜 tribulus, Tribuli Fructus)

gōu téng (钩藤 uncaria, Uncariae Ramulus cum Uncis)

jī xuè téng (鸡血藤 spatholobus, Spatholobi Caulis)

chuān xiōng (川芎 chuanxiong, Chuanxiong Rhizoma)

3. **Fright Wind and Epilepsy:** For convulsions, clenched jaw, hoisted eyes, and vexation and agitation in child fright wind or adult epilepsy, combine *tiān má* with the following:

quán xiē (全蝎 scorpion, Scorpio)

wú gōng (蜈蚣 centipede, Scolopendra)

gōu téng (钩藤 uncaria, Uncariae Ramulus cum Uncis)

tiān zhú huáng (天竹黄 bamboo sugar, Bambusae Concretio Silicea)

huáng lián (黄连 coptis, Coptidis Rhizoma)

huáng qín (黄芩 scutellaria, Scutellariae Radix)

yù jīn (郁金 curcuma, Curcumae Radix)

chāng pú (菖蒲 acorus, Acori Tatarinowii Rhizoma)

yuǎn zhì (远志 polygala, Polygalae Radix)

xiāng fù (香附 cyperus, Cyperi Rhizoma)

chén pí (陈皮 tangerine peel, Citri Reticulatae Pericarpium)

According to modern research reports, *tiān má* has an ability to control epileptic responses in animals with experimentally induced epilepsy.

In addition, this medicinal combined with *qiāng huó* (notopterygium), *dú huó* (pubescent angelica), *fáng fēng* (saposhnikovia), *qín jiāo* (large gentian), *wēi líng xiān* (clematis), *sāng zhī* (mulberry twig), *dāng guī* (Chinese angelica), and *chén pí* (tangerine peel) is also used for wind-damp impediment pain (including rheumatoid arthritis and rheumatic pain) and numbness of the limbs.

COMPARISONS

Cāng ěr zǐ (xanthium)[27] promotes sweating and dissipates wind-damp; it treats headache and dizzy head, and also tracks external wind. *Tiān má*, on the other hand, dispels phlegm, extinguishes wind, and settles fright epilepsy; it treats dizziness and headache and also internal wind.

Màn jīng zǐ (vitex)[34] dissipates wind-heat in the upper body and tends to treat headache that results from external contraction of repletion evil. In patterns of headache from internal injury with a vacuity nature, it should be used with care.

Tiān má tends to treat headache and dizziness due to internal wind with phlegm. It is not usually used in headache due to external wind.

DOSAGE

The dosage is generally 3–9 g/1–3 qián.

CAUTION

This medicinal should be used with care in patterns of blood vacuity.

---

34. 钩藤 Gōu Téng
Uncaria

Uncariae
Ramulus cum Uncis

Sweet in flavor and slightly cold in nature, *gōu téng* (uncaria) clears heart heat, extinguishes liver wind, stabilizes fright epilepsy, and stops convulsions. It is effective in treating spinning head and dizzy vision in adults, and tugging and slackening (瘈瘲 *jì zòng*, i.e., jerking of the extremities) due to fright wind in children.

1. Heavy-Headedness and Dizziness: Liver wind stirring internally may result in symptoms such as spinning head, dizzy vision, tinnitus, insomnia, heavy head and light feet, and jerking sinews and twitching flesh (a twitching sensation of the sinews and flesh of unfixed location). For such conditions, combine *gōu téng* with medicinals such as:

jú huā (菊花 chrysanthemum, Chrysanthemi Flos)
tiān má (天麻 gastrodia, Gastrodiae Rhizoma)
fáng fēng (防风 saposhnikovia, Saposhnikoviae Radix)
bàn xià (半夏 pinellia, Pinelliae Rhizoma)
fú líng (茯苓 poria, Poria)
bái jí lí (白蒺藜 tribulus, Tribuli Fructus)
zé xiè (泽泻 alisma, Alismatis Rhizoma)
shēng shí jué míng (生石决明 crude abalone shell, Haliotidis Concha Cruda)
shēng dài zhě shí (生代赭石 crude hematite, Haematitum Crudum)

According to modern research reports, this medicinal has a hypotensive effect, so it can be used to treat hypertension.

2. Convulsions in Children with Fever: In children with unabating high fever, extreme heat can engender wind, resulting in grinding of the teeth, stiff neck, drooping of the eyes, convulsions of the limbs, and vexation and agitation. *Gōu téng* clears heart heat and extinguishes liver wind to resolve tetany and tranquilize. For this purpose it is combined with medicinals such as:

jú huā (菊花 chrysanthemum, Chrysanthemi Flos)
quán xiē (全蝎 scorpion, Scorpio)
wú gōng (蜈蚣 centipede, Scolopendra)
huáng lián (黄连 coptis, Coptidis Rhizoma)
yù jīn (郁金 curcuma, Curcumae Radix)
tiān zhú huáng (天竹黄 bamboo sugar, Bambusae Concretio Silicea)

sāng yè (桑叶 mulberry leaf, Mori Folium)

lián qiáo (连翘 forsythia, Forsythiae Fructus)

dǎn xīng (胆星 bile arisaema, Arisaema cum Bile)

3. Wind Strike: When liver wind stirs internally with wind-phlegm harassing the upper body giving rise to sudden clouding collapse, deviated mouth and face, hemiplegia, and inhibited speech, this is **wind strike**[568] (中风 *zhòng fēng*). *Gōu téng* treats wind strike by extinguishing liver wind, and it has a definite ability to soothe the sinews and quicken the network vessels. It is frequently combined with medicinals such as:

bàn xià (半夏 pinellia, Pinelliae Rhizoma)

chén pí (陈皮 tangerine peel, Citri Reticulatae Pericarpium)

fú líng (茯苓 poria, Poria)

jú huā (菊花 chrysanthemum, Chrysanthemi Flos)

sāng zhī (桑枝 mulberry twig, Mori Ramulus)

sāng yè (桑叶 mulberry leaf, Mori Folium)

bái jí lí (白蒺藜 tribulus, Tribuli Fructus)

hóng huā (红花 carthamus, Carthami Flos)

chì sháo (赤芍 red peony, Paeoniae Radix Rubra)

dì lóng (地龙 earthworm, Pheretima)

zhì shān jiǎ (炙山甲 mix-fried pangolin scales, Manis Squama cum Liquido Fricta)

COMPARISONS

Rěn dōng téng (lonicera stem and leaf) clears wind-heat from the channels and network vessels and is used to treat pain of the channels and network vessels. *Gōu téng* extinguishes liver wind and clears liver heat, and is used to treat jerking sinews, twitching flesh, and convulsions of the limbs.

Luò shí téng (star jasmine stem)[457] soothes the sinews and quickens the network vessels and thereby treats sinew hypertonicity and difficulty bending and stretching. *Gōu téng* extinguishes wind and settles tetany; it treats tugging and slackening of the sinews (spasmodic jerking) and hypertonicity of the limbs.

Bái jiāng cán (silkworm)[469] dispels wind and tends to treat fright epilepsy and wind strike, as well as transforming phlegm and dissipating binds. *Gōu téng* extinguishes wind and tends to check spinning dizziness and convulsions; it also clears liver and heart heat evil.

RESEARCH

According to modern research reports, *gōu téng*, besides its hypotensive property, also has a sedative effect, but has no somniferous effect.

When physicians of the past used *gōu téng* to extinguish wind, they emphasized that it should be "added at the end" of the decoction. They believed that the strength of *gōu téng* was greater when added at the end and reduced when decocted for a long time. Modern researchers have demonstrated that when *gōu téng* is decocted for more than 20 minutes the constituent that lowers blood pressure is partially destroyed.

DOSAGE

The dosage is generally 6–15 g/2–5 qián, but in particularly severe patterns up to 30 g/1 liǎng can be used.

---

35. 大薊 Dà Jì
Japanese Thistle

Cirsii Japonici Herba seu Radix

Including

▷ *Xiǎo jì* (小薊 field thistle, Cirsii Herba)

Sweet and sour in flavor and cool in nature, *dà jì* (Japanese thistle) mainly cools the blood and stanches bleeding. It also dissipates stasis and disperses swelling.

1. Nosebleed, Coughing of Blood, Vomiting, and Bloody Urine: These conditions of bleeding are often related to frenetic movement of hot blood. *Dà jì* cools the blood and clears heat so as to stanch bleeding. It is frequently combined with medicinals such as:

cè bǎi yè (側柏叶 arborvitae leaf, Platycladi Cacumen)

qiàn cǎo (茜草 madder, Rubiae Radix)

xiǎo jì (小薊 field thistle, Cirsii Herba)

bái máo gēn (白茅根 imperata, Imperatae Rhizoma)

zhī zǐ (栀子 gardenia, Gardeniae Fructus)

dà huáng (大黄 rhubarb, Rhei Radix et Rhizoma)

mǔ dān pí (牡丹皮 moutan, Moutan Cortex)

zōng lǘ pí (棕榈皮 trachycarpus, Trachycarpi Petiolus)

bò hé (薄荷 mint, Menthae Herba)

These medicinals should be charred (then wrapped in paper and set on the ground overnight to allow the fire toxin to issue), ground to a fine powder, and taken in a 6–9 g/2–3 qián dosage each time. One should take the powder with either *xiān ǒu zhī* (lotus root juice) or *mò zhī* (ink). This formula is called *shí huī sǎn* (Ten Cinders Powder) and is used for coughing of blood and vomiting of blood.

2. Metrorrhagia: In Chinese medicine, metrorrhagia (uterine bleeding) is called 崩漏 *bēng lòu*, "flooding and spotting." "Flooding" is a heavy flow of blood, while "spotting" is a light, persistent amount of bleeding. For flooding and spotting, *dà jì* is frequently combined with medicinals such as:

zōng lǘ tàn (棕榈炭 charred trachycarpus, Trachycarpi Petiolus Carbonisatus)

ài yè tàn (艾叶炭 charred mugwort, Artemisiae Argyi Folium Carbonisatum)

ē jiāo (阿胶 ass hide glue, Asini Corii Colla)

sāng jì shēng (桑寄生 mistletoe, Taxilli Herba)

xù duàn tàn (续断炭 charred dipsacus, Dipsaci Radix Carbonisata)

bái zhú (白术 white atractylodes, Atractylodis Macrocephalae Rhizoma)

xiān hè cǎo (仙鹤草 agrimony, Agrimoniae Herba)

dāng guī tàn (当归炭 charred Chinese angelica, Angelicae Sinensis Radix Carbonisata)

pú huáng tàn (蒲黄炭 charred typha pollen, Typhae Pollen Carbonisatum)

3. Sore-Toxin and Swollen Welling-Abscesses: Sore-toxin that causes swelling and the development of welling-abscesses mostly stems from blood heat and toxin-fire that congest and fail to dissipate. *Dà jì* cools the blood and dissipates stasis, so as to disperse swelling; it is frequently combined with medicinals such as *jīn yín huā* (lonicera), *lián qiáo* (forsythia), *chì sháo* (red peony), *pú gōng yīng* (dandelion), *hóng huā* (carthamus), *yě jú huā* (wild chrysanthemum flower), and *dān pí* (moutan). One to two spoonfuls of fresh juice squeezed from *xiān dà jì* (fresh Japanese thistle) taken once or twice a day is used for intestinal welling-abscess (including acute appendicitis).

There is also *xiǎo jì* (field thistle),[16] which has basically the same nature, flavors, and functions as *dà jì*.[17] Moreover, the two are frequently used together. Nevertheless, careful analysis reveals some differences between the two. The two are very similar in terms of their blood-cooling and blood-stanching effects, but *dà jì* also dissipates stasis and disperses swelling. Whether taken internally or applied topically, it is effective for clove-sore toxin, welling-abscesses, and sores. *Xiǎo jì* does not have this effect. *Xiǎo jì* is relatively effective in treating bloody urine. For example, *xiǎo jì yǐn* (Field Thistle Drink), given below, is a well-known formula for treating bound heat in the lower burner that becomes blood strangury.

Xiǎo jì yǐn 小蓟饮   Field Thistle Drink

xiǎo jì (小蓟 field thistle, Cirsii Herba) 15–30 g/5 qián–1 liǎng

shēng dì huáng (生地黄 dried/fresh rehmannia, Rehmanniae Radix Exsiccata seu Recens) 30–60 g/1–2 liǎng

huá shí (滑石 talcum, Talcum) 15 g/5 qián

tōng cǎo (通草 rice-paper plant pith, Tetrapanacis Medulla) 6 g/2 qián

pú huáng (蒲黄 typha pollen, Typhae Pollen) 9 g/3 qián

ǒu jié (藕节 lotus root node, Nelumbinis Rhizomatis Nodus) 9–15 g/3–5 qián

zhú yè (竹叶 lophatherum, Lophatheri Herba) 6 g/2 qián

dāng guī (当归 Chinese angelica, Angelicae Sinensis Radix) 6 g/2 qián

shēng zhī zǐ (生栀子 raw gardenia, Gardeniae Fructus Crudus) 9 g/3 qián

gān cǎo (甘草 licorice, Glycyrrhizae Radix) 4.5 g/1.5 qián

---

[16]Note that the Chinese names *dà jì* 大蓟 and *xiǎo jì* 小蓟 mean "large thistle" and "small thistle," respectively. (Ed.)

[17]There is much confusion in the marketplace about *dà jì* and its sister medicinal, *xiǎo jì*. *Cirsium japonicum* is the preferred plant for *dà jì*, either the above-ground portion or the root being used. Currently, a product called *dà xiǎo jì* is offered in the West. This name would imply that it is a combination of *dà jì* and *xiǎo jì*, and in a strange way it is. It is the root of *Cirsium japonicum*, which in southern China is used for *xiǎo jì* instead of the correct medicinal (*Cirsium setosum* (WILLD.)) and which in northern China is sometimes used as *dà jì*. True *xiǎo jì* is seldom seen in southern China or in the West at the present time. (Ed.)

The addition of *mù tōng* (trifoliate akebia), *chē qián cǎo* (plantago), *zhū líng* (polyporus), and *biǎn xù* (knotgrass) to this formula enables it to be used to treat acute urinary infection.

RESEARCH

According to modern research reports, char-fried *dà jì* produces its hemostatic effect by decreasing bleeding time; it also lowers blood pressure. *Xiǎo jì* (field thistle), when used raw, produces good hemostatic and vasodilatory effects, decreasing blood coagulation time and prothrombin time, but these effects are reduced by char-frying. *Xiǎo jì* is also a cholagogue; it furthermore decreases blood cholesterol and lowers blood pressure.

DOSAGE

The dosage is generally 3–15 g/1–5 qián; fresh, it is often used in dosages of 60–90 g/2–3 liǎng; in severe diseases, use up to 30 g/1 liǎng of the dried medicinal; when using it char-fried, the dosage is reduced slightly.

---

36. 地榆 Dì Yú   Sanguisorbae Radix
Sanguisorba

Sour and bitter in flavor and slightly cold in nature, *dì yú* (sanguisorba) clears lower burner blood heat and treats blood in the urine and stool. Because it has an astringent nature, it also checks diarrhea. When used raw, the effect of cooling the blood and clearing heat is better, and when used char-fried, the blood-stanching effect is better.

Dì yú clears heat, cools the blood, and stanches bleeding. It is used for all forms of bleeding and is excellent for bleeding in the lower body. To treat bloody stool it is combined with medicinals such as:

huáng qín (黄芩 scutellaria, Scutellariae Radix)

huái jiǎo (槐角 sophora fruit, Sophorae Fructus)

huái huā tàn (槐花炭 charred sophora flower, Sophorae Flos Carbonisatus)

dāng guī (当归 Chinese angelica, Angelicae Sinensis Radix)

bái sháo (白芍 white peony, Paeoniae Radix Alba)

ē jiāo (阿胶 ass hide glue, Asini Corii Colla)

huáng bǎi tàn (黄柏炭 charred phellodendron, Phellodendri Cortex Carbonisatus)

To treat bloody urine, it is combined with medicinals such as:

mù tōng (木通 trifoliate akebia, Akebiae Trifoliatae Caulis)

shēng dì huáng (生地黄 dried/fresh rehmannia, Rehmanniae Radix Exsiccata seu Recens)

zé xiè (泽泻 alisma, Alismatis Rhizoma)

zhū líng (猪苓 polyporus, Polyporus)

fú líng (茯苓 poria, Poria)

qū mài (瞿麦 dianthus, Dianthi Herba)

huáng băi tàn (黄柏炭 charred phellodendron, Phellodendri Cortex
    Carbonisatus)

máo gēn tàn (茅根炭 charred imperata, Imperatae Rhizoma Carbonisatum)

xiăo jì (小蓟 field thistle, Cirsii Herba)

Dì yú cools the blood with sourness and cold. It is applied topically for welling-abscess swellings, sores, and burns and scalds. *Dì yú* is ground to a fine powder and used with *xiāng yóu* (sesame oil). Applied to the affected area, it relieves pain and speeds healing. One can also use *shēng dì yú* (raw sanguisorba) 62.5 g/2 liăng, *bīng piàn* (borneol) 0.6 g/2 fēn, and a small amount of *shè xiāng* (musk), ground to a fine powder. If the skin has ruptured, sprinkle this powder on the affected area; if the skin has not yet broken, apply it mixed with *xiāng yóu* (sesame oil). Also, *dì yú* and berberine are ground to a fine powder and applied to scalds and burns. This combination has an excellent effect.

COMPARISONS

Bái jí (bletilla)[491] stanches bleeding, and it tends to be used for upper burner bleeding. *Dì yú* also stanches bleeding, but it tends to be used for lower burner bleeding.

Zōng lǘ tàn (charred trachycarpus)[487] and *dì yú tàn* (地榆炭, charred sanguisorba) both stanch bleeding, but *zōng lǘ tàn* is used for both cold- and heat-type bleeding, whereas *dì yú tàn* tends to be used for bloody stool from lower burner damp-heat.

RESEARCH

According to modern research reports, *dì yú* has an antibacterial effect, but after high-pressure disinfection, this effect is diminished or lost completely. This medicinal reduces bleeding time and it stanches bleeding in arterioles, especially when using a dilute solution. *Dì yú* is quite effective for ulcers with major bleeding and also for burns. It also controls infection so as to prevent toxemia, reduce exudation, and promote the formation of new skin.

DOSAGE

The dosage is generally 6–15 g/2–5 qián. To stanch bleeding, use *dì yú tàn* (charred sanguisorba). For swollen welling-abscesses and for burns, use 60 g/2 liăng of *shēng dì yú* (raw sanguisorba). For severe disease, the dosage is increased slightly.

CAUTION

Use with care in vacuity cold bleeding.

---

37. 侧柏叶 Cè Băi Yè   Platycladi Cacumen
Biota Leaf

Cè băi yè (arborvitae leaf) is bitter and astringent in flavor and slightly cold in nature. It mainly boosts yīn, cools the blood, and stanches bleeding.

All forms of bleeding can be treated with *cè bǎi yè*. Since this medicinal is slightly cold in nature, it is often used for bleeding of a hot nature. For example, to treat nosebleed, *cè bǎi yè* is combined with medicinals such as *shēng dì huáng* (dried/fresh rehmannia), *dà jì* (Japanese thistle), *xiǎo jì* (field thistle), and *bái máo gēn* (imperata); for coughing of blood, it is combined with *shēng ǒu jié* (raw lotus root node), *bái jí* (bletilla), *xìng rén* (apricot kernel), and *chǎo zhī zǐ* (stir-fried gardenia); for vomiting of blood, it is combined with:

> *bái jí* (白及 bletilla, Bletillae Rhizoma)
> *dì yú* (地榆 sanguisorba, Sanguisorbae Radix)
> *shēng dài zhě shí* (生代赭石 crude hematite, Haematitum Crudum)
> *xuán fù huā* (旋覆花 inula flower, Inulae Flos)
> *hǎi piāo xiāo* (海螵蛸 cuttlefish bone, Sepiae Endoconcha)
> *qiàn cǎo tàn* (茜草炭 charred madder, Rubiae Radix Carbonisata)

For bloody urine, it is combined with:

> *shēng dì huáng* (生地黄 dried/fresh rehmannia, Rehmanniae Radix Exsiccata seu Recens)
> *mù tōng* (木通 trifoliate akebia, Akebiae Trifoliatae Caulis)
> *xiǎo jì* (小薊 field thistle, Cirsii Herba)
> *huáng bǎi* (黄柏 phellodendron, Phellodendri Cortex)
> *zhī mǔ* (知母 anemarrhena, Anemarrhenae Rhizoma)
> *bái máo gēn* (白茅根 imperata, Imperatae Rhizoma)

For flooding and spotting, it is combined with medicinals such as:

> *sāng jì shēng* (桑寄生 mistletoe, Taxilli Herba)
> *xù duàn tàn* (续断炭 charred dipsacus, Dipsaci Radix Carbonisata)
> *yì mǔ cǎo* (益母草 leonurus, Leonuri Herba)
> *xiān hè cǎo* (仙鹤草 agrimony, Agrimoniae Herba)
> *ài yè tàn* (艾叶炭 charred mugwort, Artemisiae Argyi Folium Carbonisatum)
> *zōng tàn* (棕炭 charred trachycarpus, Trachycarpi Petiolus Carbonisatus)

Combined with *pào jiāng tàn* (blast-fried ginger) and *ài yè* (mugwort), *cè bǎi yè* is also used for cold pattern bleeding.

When *cè bǎi yè* is used raw, it not only cools the blood and stanches bleeding, but also boosts yīn and clears heat. Char-fried, it is only used to stanch bleeding. In practice, it is most commonly used to cool the blood and stanch bleeding, so there are more opportunities to use it raw. For example, *sì shēng wán* (Four Fresh Agents Pill), which contains *shēng cè bǎi* (raw biota leaf), *shēng dì huáng* (dried/fresh rehmannia), *shēng ài yè* (raw mugwort), and *shēng hé yè* (raw lotus leaf), is often used for all forms of hot-natured bleeding. This represents the customary use and experience of past physicians. According to the findings of modern research, *shēng cè bǎi* reduces bleeding and coagulation time, while char-frying reduces the effect on coagulation. For women with **inverted menstruation**[554] (倒经 *dào jīng*), I frequently get good results enhancing an appropriate decoction with 15–30 g/5 qián–1 liǎng of *shēng cè bǎi* (raw biota leaf) and 15 g/5 qián each of *dà jì* (Japanese thistle) and *xiǎo jì* (field thistle).

Because *cè bǎi yè* has a relatively cold nature, if it is taken over a long period of time or taken in large doses, it can affect the warming and moving actions of the center burner and give rise to symptoms such as stomach discomfort or reduced appetite. When using this medicinal, therefore, one should also use medicinals that strengthen and fortify the center burner, such as *chén pí* (tangerine peel), *shēng jiāng* (fresh ginger), *jiāo shén qū* (scorch-fried medicated leaven), *chǎo gǔ yá* (stir-fried rice sprout), and *chǎo mài yá* (stir-fried barley sprout).

COMPARISONS

Bái máo gēn (imperata)[485] is sweet and cold; it cools the blood and stanches bleeding, and also drains fire. *Cè bǎi yè* is bitter, astringent, and slightly cold; it cools the blood and stanches bleeding, and in addition nourishes yīn. (It is effective for lung yīn vacuity cough with phlegm containing blood.)

Dì yú (sanguisorba)[482] is sour and cold; it stanches bleeding and tends to treat bleeding in the lower body. *Cè bǎi yè* is bitter, astringent, and slightly cold; it boosts yīn, cools the blood, and stanches bleeding, especially bleeding in the upper body.

Ài yè (mugwort)[357] warms, frees, and rectifies the blood, and it stanches bleeding. *Cè bǎi yè* clears damp-heat in the blood and stanches bleeding.

DOSAGE

The dosage is generally 6–12 g/2–4 qián, but in severe patterns use 15–30 g/ 5 qián–1 liǎng.

---

38. 白茅根 Bái Máo Gēn   Imperatae Rhizoma
Imperata

Including
  ▷ *Máo zhēn* (茅针 imperata tips, Imperatae Rhizomatis Extremitas)
  ▷ *Máo huā* (茅花 imperata flower, Imperatae Flos)

Also called *máo gēn* 茅根. Sweet in flavor and cold in nature, *bái máo gēn* (imperata) mainly cools the blood and stanches bleeding, clears heat and disinhibits water. Though sweet in flavor, it is not slimy and does not clog the stomach; though cold in nature, it does not damage the stomach; although it disinhibits water, it does not damage yīn liquid. *Bái máo gēn* is a commonly used heat-clearing blood-stanching medicinal.

For nosebleed, coughing of blood, vomiting of blood, bloody urine, or other diseases characterized by bleeding, *bái máo gēn* is frequently combined with medicinals such as *xiǎo jì* (field thistle), *ǒu jié* (lotus root node), *lú gēn* (phragmites), *huáng bǎi tàn* (charred phellodendron), *dān pí tàn* (charred moutan), and *shēng dì tàn* (charred dried/fresh rehmannia). *Bái máo gēn* treats bloody urine especially well, and this is considered one of its special characteristics.

Bái máo gēn clears heat and disinhibits water. For damp-heat strangury (including urinary infection) or water swelling, it is combined with medicinals such as:

chē qián zǐ (车前子 plantago seed, Plantaginis Semen)

mù tōng (木通 trifoliate akebia, Akebiae Trifoliatae Caulis)

biǎn xù (萹蓄 knotgrass, Polygoni Avicularis Herba)

qū mài (瞿麦 dianthus, Dianthi Herba)

zhū líng (猪苓 polyporus, Polyporus)

fú líng (茯苓 poria, Poria)

huáng bǎi (黄柏 phellodendron, Phellodendri Cortex)

I frequently achieve a satisfactory effect by enhancing a pattern-appropriate decoction with 30 g/1 liǎng of *máo gēn tàn* (charred imperata), 12 g/4 qián of *huáng bǎi tàn* (charred phellodendron), and 15 g/5 qián of *xiǎo jì* (field thistle) to treat red blood cells appearing in the urine for a long time. When enduring illness results in vacuity and lumbar pain, judiciously add *xù duàn* (dipsacus) or *xù duàn tàn* (charred dipsacus) and *sāng jì shēng* (mistletoe).

Comparisons

Cè bǎi yè (arborvitae leaf)[483] and *bái máo gēn* (imperata) both stanch bleeding. The former clears damp-heat from the blood and is bitter and astringent; the latter clears latent heat in the blood and is sweet and cold.

Máo gēn tàn (charred imperata)[485] tends to be used to stanch bleeding; *shēng máo gēn* (raw imperata) tends to be used to clear heat, disinhibit urine, and cool the blood; *xiān máo gēn* (fresh imperata) has an even better capacity to clear heat and cool the blood.

Máo zhēn (imperata tips) are the new tips of *máo gēn* (imperata) just after it is pulled out of the ground. These are used in external medicine to open sores and expel pus and to break swelling.

Máo huā, the flower of *bái máo gēn*, treats blood ejection, nosebleed, and bleeding due to blood heat in the upper burner better than *máo gēn*.[18] *Bái máo gēn* treats bloody urine better than *máo huā*.

Lú gēn (phragmites) and *bái máo gēn* both clear heat. Nonetheless, *lú gēn* tends to clear qì-aspect heat, engender liquid, and allay thirst, whereas *bái máo gēn* tends to clear blood-aspect heat, boost the stomach, and allay thirst.

Research

According to modern research reports, *bái máo gēn* has a pronounced diuretic effect. *Máo huā* (imperata flower) reduces bleeding, coagulation time, and blood vessel permeability, and thus possesses a hemostatic effect.

---

[18] *Máo huā* (imperata flower) is sweet and balanced. In addition to being used for blood ejection and nosebleed, it is also sometimes applied as a powder to stop bleeding wounds. The dosage for internal use is 10–15 g in decoctions. (Ed.)

Dosage

The dosage is generally 6–18 g/2–6 qián or 30–60 g/1–2 liǎng if using the fresh form. *Máo gēn* as a single medicinal is used in doses of 100 g/3 liǎng or in severe cases 200 g/6 liǎng. The dosage for *máo huā* (imperata flower) and *máo zhēn* (imperata tips) is generally 3–9 g/1–3 qián.

---

39. 棕榈炭 Zōng Lǘ Tàn   Trachycarpi
Charred Trachycarpus   Petiolous Carbonisatus

Also called *zōng tàn* 棕炭. Bitter in flavor and astringent and neutral in nature, *zōng lǘ tàn* (charred trachycarpus) astringes and stanches bleeding.

For nosebleed, coughing of blood, vomiting of blood, bloody urine, bloody stool, flooding, and various other forms of bleeding, *zōng lǘ tàn* astringes and stanches bleeding. It is frequently combined with:

cè bǎi yè (侧柏叶 arborvitae leaf, Platycladi Cacumen)

dà jì (大蓟 Japanese thistle, Cirsii Japonici Herba seu Radix)

xiǎo jì (小蓟 field thistle, Cirsii Herba)

bái máo gēn (白茅根 imperata, Imperatae Rhizoma)

qiàn cǎo tàn (茜草炭 charred madder, Rubiae Radix Carbonisata)

dān pí tàn (丹皮炭 charred moutan, Moutan Cortex Carbonisatus)

hé yè tàn (荷叶炭 charred lotus leaf, Nelumbinis Folium Carbonisatum)

ē jiāo (阿胶 ass hide glue, Asini Corii Colla)

Comparisons

Aì yè tàn (charred mugwort) and *zōng tàn* (charred trachycarpus) are frequently used together to stanch bleeding. *Aì yè tàn*, however, warms the uterus, expels cold-damp, rectifies qì, stanches bleeding and tends to be used for uterine bleeding, flooding and spotting, and vaginal discharge. In contrast, *zōng tàn*, which is bitter and astringent, stanches bleeding and tends to be used for heavy bleeding in the lower body; it works by the law that "astringency can stem desertion." *Aì yè tàn* does not have the drawback of causing stasis and stagnation by astringing. *Zōng tàn* is unsuitable for static blood or stasis obstruction that has not yet been eliminated.

Cè bǎi yè (arborvitae leaf) boosts yīn and cools the blood to stanch bleeding; it is used in the beginning, middle, and end stages of blood patterns. *Zōng tàn* astringes to stanch bleeding; thus it is not appropriate at the onset of bleeding when the stasis has not yet been eliminated.

Huā ruǐ shí (ophicalcite) astringes and stanches bleeding, but it also transforms static blood and aborts a dead fetus. *Zōng tàn* has no ability to transform static blood.

Dosage

The dosage is generally 6–12 g/2–4 qián, but in severe cases use 30–60 g/ 1–2 liǎng.

Caution

At the onset of bleeding, avoid premature use of *zōng tàn* since it can prevent the elimination of static blood.

---

40. 三七 **Sān Qī**   Notoginseng Radix
Notoginseng

Sweet and slightly bitter in flavor and warm in nature, *sān qī* (notoginseng) has two main actions: 1) stanching bleeding and 2) dissipating stasis, dispersing swelling, and settling pain.

Sān qī is often used for various forms of bleeding. The following are examples of medicinals with which it is combined for different kinds of bleeding.

Coughing of blood

shā shēn (沙参 adenophora/glehnia, Adenophorae seu Glehniae Radix)

chǎo zhī zǐ (炒栀子 stir-fried gardenia, Gardeniae Fructus Frictus)

huáng qín (黄芩 scutellaria, Scutellariae Radix)

bái jí (白及 bletilla, Bletillae Rhizoma)

xìng rén (杏仁 apricot kernel, Armeniacae Semen)

shēng ǒu jié (生藕节 raw lotus root node, Nelumbinis Rhizomatis Nodus Crudus)

pí pá yè (枇杷叶 loquat leaf, Eriobotryae Folium)

Vomiting of blood

shēng dài zhě shí (生代赭石 crude hematite, Haematitum Crudum)

zhú rú (竹茹 bamboo shavings, Bambusae Caulis in Taenia)

huáng qín tàn (黄芩炭 charred scutellaria, Scutellariae Radix Carbonisata)

bái jí (白及 bletilla, Bletillae Rhizoma)

jiāo shén qū (焦神曲 scorch-fried medicated leaven, Massa Medicata Fermentata Usta)

hǎi piāo xiāo (海螵蛸 cuttlefish bone, Sepiae Endoconcha)

xiān hè cǎo (仙鹤草 agrimony, Agrimoniae Herba)

zào xīn tǔ (灶心土 oven earth, Terra Flava Usta)

Nosebleed

bái máo gēn (白茅根 imperata, Imperatae Rhizoma)

dà jì (大蓟 Japanese thistle, Cirsii Japonici Herba seu Radix)

xiǎo jì (小蓟 field thistle, Cirsii Herba)

chǎo zhī zǐ (炒栀子 stir-fried gardenia, Gardeniae Fructus Frictus)

hé yè tàn (荷叶炭 charred lotus leaf, Nelumbinis Folium Carbonisatum) *xuè yú tàn* (血余炭 charred hair, Crinis Carbonisatus)

jīn yín huā tàn (金银花炭 charred lonicera, Lonicerae Flos Carbonisatus)

Bloody urine

huáng bǎi tàn (黄柏炭 charred phellodendron, Phellodendri Cortex Carbonisatus)

qū mài (瞿麦 dianthus, Dianthi Herba)

máo gēn tàn (茅根炭 charred imperata, Imperatae Rhizoma Carbonisatum)

xiǎo jì tàn (小蓟炭 charred field thistle, Cirsii Herba Carbonisata)

dēng xīn tàn (灯心炭 charred juncus, Junci Medulla Carbonisata)

shēng dì huáng (生地黄 dried/fresh rehmannia, Rehmanniae Radix Exsiccata seu Recens)

Bloody stool

fáng fēng (防风 saposhnikovia, Saposhnikoviae Radix)

dì yú tàn (地榆炭 charred sanguisorba, Sanguisorbae Radix Carbonisata)

chì shí zhī (赤石脂 halloysite, Halloysitum Rubrum)

huái huā tàn (槐花炭 charred sophora flower, Sophorae Flos Carbonisatus)

Uterine bleeding and profuse menstruation

ē jiāo (阿胶 ass hide glue, Asini Corii Colla)

ài yè tàn (艾叶炭 charred mugwort, Artemisiae Argyi Folium Carbonisatum)

zōng tàn (棕炭 charred trachycarpus, Trachycarpi Petiolus Carbonisatus)

lián fáng tàn (莲房炭 charred lotus receptacle, Nelumbinis Receptaculum Carbonisatum)

dāng guī tàn (当归炭 charred Chinese angelica, Angelicae Sinensis Radix Carbonisata)

xù duàn tàn (续断炭 charred dipsacus, Dipsaci Radix Carbonisata)

sāng jì shēng (桑寄生 mistletoe, Taxilli Herba)

As a single medicinal *sān qī* can be used to stanch bleeding when ground to a fine powder and taken two to three times per day with warm water in doses of 0.9–2.5 g/ 3–8 fēn each time, but it is far more effective when combined with an appropriate decoction medicine.

Sān qī stanches bleeding, as well as dissipates static blood, disperses swelling, and settles pain. It is frequently combined with medicinals such as *rǔ xiāng* (frankincense), *mò yào* (myrrh), *gǔ suì bǔ* (drynaria), *xù duàn* (dipsacus), and *xuè jié* (dragon's blood) for bruises (static blood) from knocks and falls. It is taken internally or applied topically. Grind *sān qī* to a powder for direct use in a wound or pound it to a pulp and apply it to the affected area to stanch bleeding, dissipate stasis, disperse swelling, and settle pain.

Sān qī is combined with *jīn yín huā* (lonicera), *lián qiáo* (forsythia), *chì sháo* (red peony), *hóng huā* (carthamus), *dāng guī wěi* (Chinese angelica tail), *tiān huā fěn* (trichosanthes root), *rǔ xiāng* (frankincense), and *mò yào* (myrrh) for swelling and pain in welling-abscesses and sores.

In recent years, this medicinal has frequently been used as a blood-quickening, stasis-transforming medicinal for various patterns of static blood, as well as blood stasis and qì stagnation, such as purpura, myocardial infarction, and chronic perforated ulcers.

For myocardial infarction with dark purple tongue or stasis macules on the tongue and fixed pain, aside from using a decoction medicine on the basis of pattern identification and treatment determination, one can also use *sān qī* in powder form (0.9–1.5 g/3–5 fēn) with *rén shēn* (ginseng) in powder form (0.9–1.5 g/3–5 fēn) taken with warm water, twice a day. If taken for 2–4 weeks or even longer, this is quite helpful. It can also be used for angina pectoris patients with frequent recurrences, but the dosage should be reduced slightly.

Comparisons

Bái jí (bletilla)[491] and *sān qī* both stanch bleeding, but *bái jí* tends to be used for lung and stomach bleeding, such as coughing of blood and vomiting of blood, whereas *sān qī* tends to be used for all types of bleeding.

Hǎi piāo xiāo (cuttlefish bone),[178] ground to a powder and applied to wounds, also stanches bleeding, but it does this by astringing. *Sān qī*, ground to a powder and applied externally (or pounded to a pulp and applied externally), closes wounds, dissipates stasis, disperses swelling, and stanches bleeding, as well as having an important pain-relieving effect.

Research

In modern reports of animal experiments, notoginsenoside contained in *sān qī* was shown to have a cardiotonic effect, and the liquid extract of *sān qī* was shown to reduce blood congealing time in rabbits and to have a hemostatic effect.

Dosage

Generally, *sān qī* should not be decocted. It is frequently used as a powder and swallowed with warm water or taken with a decoction medicine. Taken in this way, the dosage is 0.6–3 g/2 fēn–1 qián twice a day to stanch bleeding or 3–6 g/1–2 qián to treat external injuries or fractures. According to traditional experience, using *sān qī* in small or medium dosages stanches bleeding and quickens stasis; used in large dosages, it breaks the blood.

According to modern research reports, low concentrations of the notoginsenoside contained in *sān qī* have a vasoconstrictive effect, while high concentrations have a vasodilating effect. This seems to confirm the different use of high and low dosages of this medicinal in traditional practice. Nevertheless, further research and observation are necessary.

41. 白及 Bái Jí
Bletilla
Bletillae Rhizoma

Bitter, sweet, and astringent in flavor and slightly cold in nature, *bái jí* (bletilla)[19] stanches bleeding, disperses swelling, eliminates putrefaction, engenders flesh, supplements the lung, and astringes.

Bái jí is most commonly used for lung and stomach bleeding. For example, for coughing of blood, it is combined with the following:

shēng ǒu jié (生藕节 raw lotus root node, Nelumbinis Rhizomatis Nodus Crudus)

hēi shān zhī (黑山栀 charred gardenia, Gardeniae Fructus Carbonisatus)

xìng rén (杏仁 apricot kernel, Armeniacae Semen)

shā shēn (沙参 adenophora/glehnia, Adenophorae seu Glehniae Radix)

shēng dì huáng (生地黄 dried/fresh rehmannia, Rehmanniae Radix Exsiccata seu Recens)

bǎi hé (百合 lily bulb, Lilii Bulbus)

For blood ejection, it is combined with the following:

chǎo huáng qín (炒黄芩 stir-fried scutellaria, Scutellariae Radix Fricta),

zhī mǔ (知母 anemarrhena, Anemarrhenae Rhizoma)

hǎi piāo xiāo (海螵蛸 cuttlefish bone, Sepiae Endoconcha)

pú huáng tàn (蒲黄炭 charred typha pollen, Typhae Pollen Carbonisatum)

qiàn cǎo tàn (茜草炭 charred madder, Rubiae Radix Carbonisata)

In recent years, frequent successes in the treatment of bleeding ulcers have been achieved by combining *bái jí* with *hǎi piāo xiāo* (cuttlefish bone), *bèi mǔ* (fritillaria), and *gān cǎo* (licorice), ground to a fine powder, and taken two or three times a day with warm water, 3–6 g/1–2 qián each time. 3 g/1 qián of *bái jí* powder can also be combined with 0.9–1.5 g/3–5 fēn of *sān qī* (notoginseng) powder and taken two or three times a day for the same disease. I often achieve excellent results treating pulmonary tuberculosis with coughing of blood by combining *bái jí* with:

xìng rén (杏仁 apricot kernel, Armeniacae Semen)

bǎi bù (百部 stemona, Stemonae Radix)

zǐ wǎn (紫菀 aster, Asteris Radix)

mài dōng (麦冬 ophiopogon, Ophiopogonis Radix)

bǎi hé (百合 lily bulb, Lilii Bulbus)

guā lóu (瓜蒌 trichosanthes, Trichosanthis Fructus)

shēng dì huáng (生地黄 dried/fresh rehmannia, Rehmanniae Radix Exsiccata seu Recens)

huáng qín (黄芩 scutellaria, Scutellariae Radix)

---

[19]*Bletilla striata* (Thunb.) Reichb. is a member of the orchid family and thus is included on the CITES endangered species list. International trade requires a Certificate of Cultivation for this medicinal. (Ed.)

shēng ǒu jié (生藕节 raw lotus root node, Nelumbinis Rhizomatis Nodus Crudus)

According to traditional experience with medicinals, it is believed that *bái jí* has a lung-supplementing effect. For cavernous pulmonary tuberculosis I usually get good results using *bái jí fěn* (白及粉, bletilla powder), in a dosage of 3–6 g/1–2 qián, taken three times a day, after eating, drenched with a decoction of *zǐ cài* (laver) (about 1.5–3 g/5 fēn–1 qián). The *zǐ cài* should also be eaten. When there are numerous clinical symptoms, combine this treatment with a formula devised on the basis of the pattern identified. When clinical symptoms are few, combine it with *yān jiāo* (tannery tar) and take orally. According to modern research reports, this medicinal has a pronounced inhibitory effect on the growth of human tuberculosis bacteria in vitro.

Bái jí also expels stasis and engenders the new, eliminates putrefaction and engenders flesh, and closes sores. Thus it is often used in external medicine for swollen welling-abscess, clove-sore toxin, or sores, and it is effective either taken internally or applied topically.

Comparisons

Hé yè tàn (charred lotus leaf), *zōng tàn* (charred trachycarpus), and other medicinals that stanch bleeding can be too constricting and give rise to blood stasis. *Bái jí* stanches bleeding and at the same time dispels stasis and engenders the new. Even if it is used for a long time, it does not engender static blood.

Sān qī (notoginseng) stanches any type of bleeding, whereas *bái jí* tends to stanch bleeding from the lung or stomach. *Sān qī* dissipates stasis and settles pain, whereas *bái jí* eliminates putrefaction and engenders flesh.

Within stanching bleeding, *shēng ǒu jié* (raw lotus root node) also nourishes yīn and engenders liquid. *Bái jí* within stanching bleeding also supplements the lung and astringes. Neither of these blood-stanching medicinals engenders static blood.

Dosage

The dosage is generally 3–9 g/1–3 qián when taken decocted with water; if swallowed as a powder, use 1.5–4.5 g/5 fēn–2 qián each time, two or three times per day.

Caution

This medicinal cannot be used with *fù zǐ* (aconite) or *wū tóu* (wild aconite).

---

42. 仙鹤草 Xiān Hè Cǎo   Agrimoniae Herba
Agrimony

Bitter in flavor and cool in nature, *xiān hè cǎo* (agrimony) is primarily a blood-stanching medicinal. It also treats heat dysentery.

For coughing of blood, *xiān hè cǎo* is frequently combined with medicinals such as:

bái jí (白及 bletilla, Bletillae Rhizoma)

shēng ǒu jié (生藕节 raw lotus root node, Nelumbinis Rhizomatis Nodus Crudus)

huáng qín (黄芩 scutellaria, Scutellariae Radix)

chǎo zhī zǐ (炒栀子 stir-fried gardenia, Gardeniae Fructus Frictus)

ē jiāo zhū (阿胶珠 ass hide glue pellets, Asini Corii Gelatini Pilula)

For blood ejection, it is frequently combined with:

chǎo huáng qín (炒黄芩 stir-fried scutellaria, Scutellariae Radix Fricta)

zhī mǔ (知母 anemarrhena, Anemarrhenae Rhizoma)

bái jí (白及 bletilla, Bletillae Rhizoma)

hǎi piāo xiāo (海螵蛸 cuttlefish bone, Sepiae Endoconcha)

jiāo sān xiān (焦三仙 scorch-fried three immortals, Tres Immortales Usti)

jiāo bīng láng (焦槟榔 scorch-fried areca, Arecae Semen Ustum)

qiàn cǎo tàn (茜草炭 charred madder, Rubiae Radix Carbonisata)

For uterine bleeding, it is combined with:

yì mǔ cǎo (益母草 leonurus, Leonuri Herba)

sāng jì shēng (桑寄生 mistletoe, Taxilli Herba)

dāng guī tàn (当归炭 charred Chinese angelica, Angelicae Sinensis Radix Carbonisata)

shēng dì tàn (生地炭 charred dried/fresh rehmannia, Rehmanniae Radix Exsiccata seu Recens Carbonisata)

bái sháo (白芍 white peony, Paeoniae Radix Alba)

ē jiāo (阿胶 ass hide glue, Asini Corii Colla)

For heat dysentery with bloody stool, *xiān hè cǎo* is combined with:

dì yú (地榆 sanguisorba, Sanguisorbae Radix)

huái huā tàn (槐花炭 charred sophora flower, Sophorae Flos Carbonisatus)

bái sháo (白芍 white peony, Paeoniae Radix Alba)

mù xiāng (木香 costusroot, Aucklandiae Radix)

huáng lián (黄连 coptis, Coptidis Rhizoma)

huáng bǎi (黄柏 phellodendron, Phellodendri Cortex)

bái tóu wēng (白头翁 pulsatilla, Pulsatillae Radix)

mǎ chǐ xiàn (马齿苋 purslane, Portulacae Herba)

COMPARISON

Yì mǔ cǎo (leonurus)[413] is used for uterine bleeding, but it also quickens the blood and dispels stasis. *Xiān hè cǎo* can also be used for uterine bleeding, but it does not quicken stasis; thus it must be combined with other medicinals that quicken stasis.

RESEARCH

According to modern research reports, *xiān hè cǎo* contains agrimonine and vitamin K; agrimonine increases blood platelets and reduces congealing time. I have treated thrombocyotopenic purpura using 30–60 g/1–2 liǎng of *xiān hè cǎo* in combinations with the following medicinals, varied in accordance with the signs:

> *shēng dì huáng* (生地黄 dried/fresh rehmannia, Rehmanniae Radix Exsiccata seu Recens)
>
> *xuán shēn* (玄参 scrophularia, Scrophulariae Radix)
>
> *bái sháo* (白芍 white peony, Paeoniae Radix Alba)
>
> *dāng guī* (当归 Chinese angelica, Angelicae Sinensis Radix)
>
> *bái máo gēn* (白茅根 imperata, Imperatae Rhizoma)
>
> *ē jiāo* (阿胶 ass hide glue, Asini Corii Colla)
>
> *qiàn cǎo tàn* (茜草炭 charred madder, Rubiae Radix Carbonisata)
>
> *guǐ jiàn yǔ* (鬼箭羽 spindle tree wings, Euonymi Ramulus)
>
> *dān pí tàn* (丹皮炭 charred moutan, Moutan Cortex Carbonisatus)

DOSAGE

The dosage is generally 15–30 g/5 qián–1 liǎng.

---

43. 藕节 Oǔ Jié
Lotus Root Node

Nelumbinis
Rhizomatis Nodus

Oǔ jié (lotus root node) is sweet and astringent in flavor and neutral in nature. Fresh, it cools the blood and stanches bleeding; sun-dried, it astringes and stanches bleeding; when char-fried, it stanches bleeding even more effectively.

Within astringing and stanching bleeding, *ǒu jié* also quickens static blood; thus it stanches bleeding without causing stasis. It is an excellent assistant medicinal for various forms of bleeding. It is often used for coughing of blood, blood ejection, and nosebleed in combination with *bái jí* (bletilla), *cè bǎi yè* (arborvitae leaf), *dà jì* (Japanese thistle), *qiàn cǎo tàn* (charred madder), and *zōng tàn* (charred trachycarpus). For heat pattern bleeding, it should be used raw; for an even better effect, use the juice squeezed from fresh nodes. For cold pattern bleeding, use the char-fried form. Modern research shows that this medicinal reduces bleeding time, especially after it has been char-fried.

COMPARISON

Zōng tàn (charred trachycarpus) astringes and stanches bleeding, and it is specifically used to treat the tip in emergency cases. If it is used too early, in excessive quantities, or singly, it can cause blood stasis to be retained. *Oǔ jié*, by contrast, also has the effect of quickening the blood and transforming stasis. It is either used singly or in combination with *zōng tàn* to reduce the latter's tendency to create blood stasis.

DOSAGE

The dosage is generally 9–15 g/3–5 qián. *Xiān ǒu jié* (fresh lotus root node) is used in doses up to 30–60 g/1–2 liǎng.

44. 菖蒲 Chāng Pú
Acorus

Acori Tatarinowii
Rhizoma

Chāng pú (acorus),[20] acrid in flavor and warm in nature, opens and frees the orifices of the heart, diffuses qì and eliminates phlegm, sharpens hearing and vision, and enhances the voice.

1. Opening and Freeing the Orifices of the Heart, and Diffusing Qì and Eliminating Phlegm: For heat entering the pericardium or phlegm confounding the orifices of the heart that result in coma, clouding, inability to speak, and, in severe cases, convulsions, *chāng pú* is frequently used to open and free the orifices of the heart, diffuse qì, and eliminate phlegm, thereby arousing the brain and clearing the spirit. It is combined with:

yuǎn zhì (远志 polygala, Polygalae Radix)

dǎn xīng (胆星 bile arisaema, Arisaema cum Bile)

tiān má (天麻 gastrodia, Gastrodiae Rhizoma)

quán xiē (全蝎 scorpion, Scorpio)

wú gōng (蜈蚣 centipede, Scolopendra)

tiān zhú huáng (天竹黄 bamboo sugar, Bambusae Concretio Silicea)

yù jīn (郁金 curcuma, Curcumae Radix)

fú líng (茯苓 poria, Poria)

zhū shā (朱砂 cinnabar, Cinnabaris)

chuān bèi mǔ (川贝母 Sìchuān fritillaria, Fritillariae Cirrhosae Bulbus)

When phlegm turbidity and qì depression affect the heart spirit and result in palpitations, forgetfulness, fright and fear, and disquieted essence-spirit, which in severe cases can manifest as epilepsy or mania and withdrawal, *chāng pú* is used to diffuse qì and eliminate phlegm and to open the orifices of the heart in order to quiet the heart spirit. It is frequently combined with:

yuǎn zhì (远志 polygala, Polygalae Radix)

xiāng fù (香附 cyperus, Cyperi Rhizoma)

yù jīn (郁金 curcuma, Curcumae Radix)

hǔ pò (琥珀 amber, Succinum)

zhū shā (朱砂 cinnabar, Cinnabaris)

bái jiāng cán (白僵蚕 silkworm, Bombyx Batryticatus)

quán xiē (全蝎 scorpion, Scorpio)

dǎn xīng (胆星 bile arisaema, Arisaema cum Bile)

fáng fēng (防风 saposhnikovia, Saposhnikoviae Radix)

---

[20]There are two types of *chāng pú* 菖蒲 currently in trade: *shí chāng pú* 石菖蒲 (*Acorus tatarinowii* SCHOTT) and *jiǔ jié chāng pú* 九节菖蒲 (*Anemone altaica* FISCH). The former is the standard variety. The latter is warm and acrid; it opens the orifices, eliminates phlegm, dispels wind and dampness, and fortifies the stomach. The dosage is 2–4.5 grams in decoction. Note that in ancient times *shí chāng pú* 石菖蒲 was sometimes called *jiǔ jié chāng pú* 九节菖蒲. Only in recent times has the name *jiǔ jié chāng pú* 九节菖蒲 been applied to the root of *Anemone altaica* FISCH. (Ed.)

lóng chǐ (龙齿 dragon tooth, Mastodi Dentis Fossilia)

fú líng (茯苓 poria, Poria)

2. Sharpening Hearing, Brightening the Eyes, and Enhancing the Voice: When phlegm qì surges upward and confounds the orifices of the heart or results in sudden collapse from wind strike, producing deafness, distorted vision (inability to see objects), flowery vision, and sluggish tongue that prevents or inhibits speech, *chāng pú* opens the nine orifices and allows speech to issue. It is combined with:

yuǎn zhì (远志 polygala, Polygalae Radix)

tiān zhú huáng (天竹黄 bamboo sugar, Bambusae Concretio Silicea)

bàn xià (半夏 pinellia, Pinelliae Rhizoma)

chán tuì (蝉蜕 cicada molting, Cicadae Periostracum)

xì xīn (细辛 asarum, Asari Herba)

chén pí (陈皮 tangerine peel, Citri Reticulatae Pericarpium)

fú líng (茯苓 poria, Poria)

xiāng fù (香附 cyperus, Cyperi Rhizoma)

shēng dài zhě shí (生代赭石 crude hematite, Haematitum Crudum)

bīng láng (槟榔 areca, Arecae Semen)

cí shí (磁石 loadstone, Magnetitum)

In addition, for center burner damp turbidity obstruction or qì depression impeding the center burner, which result in distention and oppression in the chest and abdomen, abdominal pain, vomiting and diarrhea, and poor appetite, *chāng pú* is frequently combined with:

huò xiāng (藿香 agastache, Agastaches Herba)

hòu pò (厚朴 officinal magnolia bark, Magnoliae Officinalis Cortex)

zǐ sū (紫苏 perilla, Perillae Folium, Caulis et Calyx)

bàn xià (半夏 pinellia, Pinelliae Rhizoma)

chén pí (陈皮 tangerine peel, Citri Reticulatae Pericarpium)

fú líng (茯苓 poria, Poria)

jiāo shén qū (焦神曲 scorch-fried medicated leaven, Massa Medicata
   Fermentata Usta)

This has the effect of warming the intestines and stomach and of diffusing qì and dispersing distention to treat pain in the heart [region] and abdomen.

Comparisons

Yuǎn zhì (polygala) and *chāng pú* both enter the heart and open the orifices. Nevertheless, *yuǎn zhì* promotes heart-kidney interaction, supplements the heart and boosts the kidney, and tends to be used for fright palpitations, forgetfulness, insomnia, and **spiritlessness**[564] (失神 *shī shén*). *Chāng pú* opens the orifices, diffuses qì, eliminates phlegm, and boosts the heart and liver; it tends to be used for phlegm qì confounding the heart (clouded spirit), deafness, distorted vision, and loss of voice.

For qì block[560] (气闭 *qì bì*) in the chest and diaphragm, which manifests in oppression in the chest with distending pain, using *chāng pú* to free and open is very effective. On the basis of this experience, when treating angina pectoris that takes the form of qì block, I often add 6–9 g/2–3 qián of *chāng pú* to an appropriate decoction medicine to help eliminate oppression and relieve pain.

When using medicinals such as *dì huáng* (rehmannia), *yù zhú* (Solomon's seal), *mài dōng* (ophiopogon), or *shān yào* (dioscorea), add a little *chāng pú* to diffuse and abduct without engendering stagnation.

DOSAGE

The dosage is generally 3–9 g/1–3 qián.

CAUTION

Contraindicated in patients with dissipated heart qì.

---

45. 麝香 Shè Xiāng
Musk
Moschus

Acrid in flavor and warm in nature, *shè xiāng* (musk)[21] opens the orifices of the heart, frees the channels and network vessels, frees the twelve channels above and below, and penetrates in to the bone and marrow and out to the skin and [body] hair. As an aromatic, mobile, and penetrating substance, it opens the gates (i.e., frees the jaws) and disinhibits the orifices.

1. Clouded Spirit: For coma and clenched jaw that result from wind strike, heat entering the pericardium, or phlegm confounding the orifices of the heart, this medicinal opens the orifices of the heart and arouses the heart spirit. *Shè xiāng* is frequently combined with medicinals such as:

sū hé xiāng (苏合香 storax, Styrax)

tán xiāng (檀香 sandalwood, Santali Albi Lignum)

dīng xiāng (丁香 clove, Caryophylli Flos)

chāng pú (菖蒲 acorus, Acori Tatarinowii Rhizoma)

zhū shā (朱砂 cinnabar, Cinnabaris)

yù jīn (郁金 curcuma, Curcumae Radix)

niú huáng (牛黄 bovine bezoar, Bovis Calculus)

zhēn zhū (珍珠 pearl, Margarita)

Sū hé xiāng wán/sǎn (Storax Pill/Powder) and *ān gōng niú huáng wán/sǎn* (Peaceful Palace Bovine Bezoar Pill/Powder), two examples of this use, are both available as ready-prepared medicines.

2. Qì and Blood Obstruction of the Channels and Network Vessels: Obstructed qì and blood of the channels and network vessels gives rise to pain, swollen welling-abscesses, nodes, concretions and conglomerations, and strings and

---

[21] The deer from which musk is derived is on the CITES endangered species list. It is also listed as endangered by the United States Fish and Wildlife Service. (Ed.)

aggregations[565] (痃癖 *xián pì*). When writing prescriptions to free qì and quicken blood, the addition of a small amount of *shè xiāng* to strengthen the power to free the channels and quicken the network vessels helps to enhance the ability to relieve pain, dissipate swollen welling-abscesses, and eliminate concretions and conglomerations. Pill medicines that are frequently used for this purpose, such as *xī huáng wán* (Rhinoceros Bezoar Pill), *xǐng xiāo wán* (Awake to Dispersion Pill), *xiǎo jīn dān* (Minor Golden Elixir), and *huà zhēng huí shēng dān* (Concretion-Transforming Return-to-Life Elixir), all contain *shè xiāng*. Generally, this medicinal is used in pills or powders.

3. Knocks and Falls: To treat bruises and pain due to local blood stasis and qì stagnation after external injury, formulas used to quicken the blood and transform stasis can be enhanced by the addition of *shè xiāng*, which moves qì and frees the channels and network vessels, thereby strengthening the ability to disperse swelling and relieve pain. An example is *qī lí sǎn* (Seven Pinches Powder), which treats knocks and falls.

Qī lí sǎn 七厘散   Seven Pinches Powder

> *xuè jié* (血竭 dragon's blood, Daemonoropis Resina)
> *rǔ xiāng* (乳香 frankincense, Olibanum)
> *mò yào* (没药 myrrh, Myrrha)
> *hóng huā* (红花 carthamus, Carthami Flos)
> *ér chá* (儿茶 cutch, Catechu)
> *shè xiāng* (麝香 musk, Moschus)
> *bīng piàn* (冰片 borneol, Borneolum)
> *zhū shā* (朱砂 cinnabar, Cinnabaris)

This formula is taken internally, 0.2–0.9 g/seven pinches to 3 fēn at a time; it can also be applied topically (provided the skin and flesh are not broken).

Because this medicinal is aromatic, mobile, and penetrating, if used inappropriately or in excessive doses it can consume and dissipate the right qì. This medicinal's strength to diffuse qì and blood is rapid and fierce; hence it is contraindicated in pregnancy. According to modern research reports, *shè xiāng* promotes glandular secretion, accelerates respiration and heart beat, and increases blood corpuscles.

DOSAGE

The dosage is generally 0.06–0.1 g/2–3 pinches or up to 0.6–1 g/2–3 fēn. This medicinal is generally ground and added to pills or powder preparations for internal use. Only under special conditions is it swallowed with a decoction. In pills or powders, although *shè xiāng* is invariably used in very small doses, its volatile, mobile, and penetrating nature helps to make full use of and strengthen the actions of other medicinals.

46. 冰片 Bīng Piàn
Borneol
Borneolum

Also called *lóng nǎo xiāng* 龙脑香, "dragon brain fragrance," and *méi piàn* 梅片, "plum flakes."[22] Acrid and bitter in flavor and slightly cold in nature, *bīng piàn* (borneol) is aromatic, penetrating, and mobile; there is nowhere it does not reach. It dissipates depressed fire and frees all the orifices, clears the heart and arouses the brain, and dispels eye redness and nebulous eye screens (云翳 *yún yì*).

1. **Acute Wind-Phlegm Block or Fright Epilepsy with Sudden Collapse:** For all symptoms such as coma, hoisted eyes[552] (吊眼 *diào yǎn*), convulsions, and loss of speech that result from wind-phlegm harassing the upper body, or phlegm-heat confounding the heart, acute childhood fright wind due to febrile disease, epilepsy, or sudden collapse from wind strike, use *bīng piàn* to open the orifices of the heart and clear heart heat and to arouse the brain and quiet the spirit. *Bīng piàn* is frequently combined with the following medicinals in pill preparations.

niú huáng (牛黄 bovine bezoar, Bovis Calculus)

dǎn xīng (胆星 bile arisaema, Arisaema cum Bile)

xióng huáng (雄黄 realgar, Realgar)

shè xiāng (麝香 musk, Moschus)

tiān zhú huáng (天竹黄 bamboo sugar, Bambusae Concretio Silicea)

quán xiē (全蝎 scorpion, Scorpio)

wú gōng (蜈蚣 centipede, Scolopendra)

fáng fēng (防风 saposhnikovia, Saposhnikoviae Radix)

huáng lián (黄连 coptis, Coptidis Rhizoma)

yù jīn (郁金 curcuma, Curcumae Radix)

chāng pú (菖蒲 acorus, Acori Tatarinowii Rhizoma)

yuǎn zhì (远志 polygala, Polygalae Radix)

For example, *niú huáng qīng xīn wán* (Bovine Bezoar Heart-Clearing Pill) and *zhèn jīng wán* (Fright-Settling Pill) are both available as ready-prepared medicines.

2. **Sore Swollen Throat, Mouth Sores, and Toothache:** When depressed and blocked fire-heat attacks upward and causes throat pain, mouth and tongue sores, and swelling and pain of the gums, *bīng piàn* can be combined with:

huáng lián (黄连 coptis, Coptidis Rhizoma)

huáng qín (黄芩 scutellaria, Scutellariae Radix)

niú huáng (牛黄 bovine bezoar, Bovis Calculus)

shēng dà huáng (生大黄 raw rhubarb, Rhei Radix et Rhizoma Crudi)

---

[22]The traditional method of deriving this medicinal is to steam the wood of *Dryobalanops aromatica* and collect the gray and translucent crystals that form as the wood cools. The crystals are called 梅片 *méi piàn* or 老梅片 *lǎo méi piàn*. Nowadays, *bīng piàn* (borneol) is synthesized and the resulting crystals are pure white. Most books suggest that the synthesized material should only be used externally and that *méi piàn* should be used for application to the oral cavity. *Méi piàn* is usually sold by the liǎng and is expensive. Synthesized *bīng piàn* (borneol) is sold by the pound and is inexpensive. (Ed.)

xuán shēn (玄参 scrophularia, Scrophulariae Radix)

shēng dì huáng (生地黄 dried/fresh rehmannia, Rehmanniae Radix Exsiccata seu Recens)

lián qiáo (连翘 forsythia, Forsythiae Fructus)

fáng fēng (防风 saposhnikovia, Saposhnikoviae Radix)

shān dòu gēn (山豆根 bushy sophora, Sophorae Tonkinensis Radix)

Bīng piàn is often used in ready-prepared medicines, such as *niú huáng shàng qīng wán* (Bovine Bezoar Upper-Body-Clearing Pill). It can also be used topically, as in the following example:

dēng xīn (灯心 juncus, Junci Medulla) 3 g/1 qián

huáng bǎi (黄柏 phellodendron, Phellodendri Cortex) 1.5 g/5 fēn

These ingredients are subjected to **nature-preservative burning**[558] (烧存性 *shāo cún xìng*) and ground to a fine powder. Next, the following are ground into this mixture:

kū fán (枯矾 calcined alum, Alumen Dehydratum) 2 g/7 fēn

bīng piàn (冰片 borneol, Borneolum) 0.9 g/3 fēn.

Use 0.3–0.6 g/1–2 fēn each time as a **laryngeal insufflation**[556] (吹喉 *chuī hòu*). This formula is used for wind-heat congesting the upper burner, resulting in sore swollen throat and throat block phlegm congestion. Another example is *bīng piàn* (borneol) 3 g/1 qián and *zhū shā* (cinnabar) 3 g/1 qián ground to a fine powder and applied to toothache; this mixture has a pain-relieving effect.

3. Sore Swollen Welling-Abscesses; Red Eyes and Nebulous Eye Screens: For swelling and toxin related to various forms of sores, *bīng piàn* is applied topically to disperse swelling and relieve pain. For sores that have already ruptured, it also dispels toxin, engenders flesh, and eliminates malodor. The formula *shēng jī sǎn* (Flesh-Engendering Powder) from the *Zhòng Lóu Yù Yuè* (重楼玉钥 "Jade Key to the Secluded Chamber") is an example of this use.

Shēng jī sǎn 生肌散   Flesh-Engendering Powder

---

chì shí zhī (赤石脂 halloysite, Halloysitum Rubrum)

rǔ xiāng (乳香 frankincense, Olibanum)

mò yào (没药 myrrh, Myrrha)

qīng fěn (轻粉 calomel, Calomelas)[23]

péng shā (硼砂 borax, Borax)

duàn lóng gǔ (煅龙骨 calcined dragon bone, Mastodi Ossis Fossilia Calcinata)

hái ér chá (孩儿茶 cutch, Catechu)

méi huā (梅花 mume flower, Mume Flos)

bīng piàn (冰片 borneol, Borneolum)

When wind-fire attacks upward and affects the head and eyes, resulting in painful, red eyes and nebulous eye screens, use this medicinal with *lú gān shí*

---

[23] *Qīng fěn* (calomel) is a lead compound and can be omitted from the formula to avoid the danger to the health now know to be posed by heavy metals. (Ed.)

(calamine), *zhū shā* (cinnabar), *náo shā* (sal ammoniac), *shè xiāng* (musk), *zhēn zhū* (pearl), and *xióng dǎn* (bear's gall). (This preparation must be carefully refined.) Made into a topical eye medication and applied, it will abate redness and eliminate eye screens to brighten the eyes and relieve pain. The commonly used eye-brightening medicines and pastes all contain *bīng piàn*.

Comparisons

Zhāng nǎo (camphor) is acrid and hot. It eliminates dampness and is not very mobile or penetrating. It is commonly used topically to kill worms and prevent putrefaction. *Bīng piàn* is acrid, bitter, and slightly cold. Mobile, penetrating, and very quick, there is nowhere it does not reach; it penetrates into the bone and marrow and dissipates evil to the exterior.

When disease is in the deep regions of the body, *bīng piàn* conducts the other medicinals into the diseased area. When the disease evil is still in the superficial regions of the body, using *bīng piàn* can potentially conduct the evil deeper into the body.

Shè xiāng (musk)[497] is mobile, penetrating, volatile, and warm in nature. It frees the channels and quickens the network vessels more strongly than *bīng piàn*. It is contraindicated for pregnant women. *Bīng piàn* is mobile and penetrating, opens the orifices, and is cool in nature. It clears heat and resolves toxin more strongly than *shè xiāng* (musk), and also arouses the brain and raises the spirit[561] (提神 *tí shén*). There is no contraindication for pregnant women.

Dosage

The dosage is generally 0.09–0.3 g/3 pinches to 1 fēn. It is only rarely used in decoction medicine, more commonly being used in pills or powders.

---

47. 神曲 Shén Qū   Massa Medicata
Medicated Leaven   Fermentata

Sweet and acrid in flavor and warm in nature, *shén qū* (medicated leaven)[24] primarily aids digestion. It opens the stomach and fortifies the spleen, transforms food and disperses accumulations.

For food accumulation with stomach distention, abdominal pain, and poor appetite, *shén qū* is combined with medicinals such as:

mài yá (麦芽 barley sprout, Hordei Fructus Germinatus)

shān zhā (山楂 crataegus, Crataegi Fructus)

---

[24] *Shén qū* (medicated leaven) is a leavened cube of six medicinals. For this reason it is sometimes called *liù qū* 六曲 or *liù shén qū* 六神曲 (六 *liù* means six). The ingredients are *xìng rén* (apricot kernel), *cāng ěr zǐ* (xanthium), *qīng hāo* (sweet wormwood), *chì xiǎo dòu* (rice bean), wheat flour, and bran. There is another product that contains *shén qū chá* with the addition of 11 or more other ingredients; it is called *shén qū chá* (神曲茶, medicated leaven tea) (茶 *chá* means tea) of *jiàn shén qū* (建神曲, Fújiàn medicated leaven). The function of *shén qū chá* 神曲茶 is similar to *shén qū*, but it is more commonly used to address wind-cold patterns that cause digestive stagnation. In the West, *shén qū chá* is often sold as *shén qū*. (Ed.)

chǎo lái fú zǐ (炒莱菔子 stir-fried radish seed, Raphani Semen Frictum)

huò xiāng (藿香 agastache, Agastaches Herba)

chén pí (陈皮 tangerine peel, Citri Reticulatae Pericarpium)

zhǐ shí (枳实 unripe bitter orange, Aurantii Fructus Immaturus)

When food and drink accumulate over a period of time and phlegm and food bind together to engender aggregations, lumps, concretions, or conglomerations, combine *shén qū* with:

shān zhā hé (山楂核 crataegus pit, Crataegi Endocarpium et Semen)

cāng zhú (苍术 atractylodes, Atractylodis Rhizoma)

bái zhú (白术 white atractylodes, Atractylodis Macrocephalae Rhizoma)

sān léng (三棱 sparganium, Sparganii Rhizoma)

é zhú (莪术 curcuma rhizome, Curcumae Rhizoma)

mài yá (麦芽 barley sprout, Hordei Fructus Germinatus)

hóng huā (红花 carthamus, Carthami Flos)

táo rén (桃仁 peach kernel, Persicae Semen)

shēng mǔ lì (生牡蛎 crude oyster shell, Ostreae Concha Cruda)

zhì biē jiǎ (炙鳖甲 mix-fried turtle shell, Trionycis Carapax cum Liquido Frictus)

For conditions such as spleen-stomach vacuity, poor appetite, and indigestion, *shén qū* is combined with:

dǎng shēn (党参 codonopsis, Codonopsis Radix)

bái zhú (白术 white atractylodes, Atractylodis Macrocephalae Rhizoma)

fú líng (茯苓 poria, Poria)

zhì gān cǎo (炙甘草 mix-fried licorice, Glycyrrhizae Radix cum Liquido Fricta)

chén pí (陈皮 tangerine peel, Citri Reticulatae Pericarpium)

gǔ yá (谷芽 millet sprout, Setariae Fructus Germinatus)

mài yá (麦芽 barley sprout, Hordei Fructus Germinatus)

Scorch-frying this medicinal strengthens its food-dispersing action; therefore, *jiāo shén qū* (scorch-fried medicated leaven) is often used with other **abductive dispersion medicinals**[541] (消导药 *xiāo dǎo yào*). Used raw, it not only fortifies the spleen and opens the stomach, but also effuses and dissipates; therefore for food accumulation with concurrent external contraction and heat effusion, it is appropriate to use the raw form.

Shén qū also helps the digestion and absorption of metal and stone medicinals. Thus, when using medicinals such as *cí shí* (loadstone) and *dài zhě shí* (hematite), use a little *shén qū* as an assistant. This addition helps movement, transformation, and absorption, and it also protects digestive function. For example, in the ancient formula *cí zhū wán* (Loadstone and Cinnabar Pill), *cí shí* (loadstone) and *zhū shā* (cinnabar) are ground to a fine powder and made into pills using *shén qū hú* (medicated leaven paste).[25] This is an excellent method of combination.

---

[25] *Shén qū hú*: *Shén qū* ground to a powder and mixed with water.

Dosage

The dosage is generally 3–9 g/1–3 qián.

---

48. 麦芽 Mài Yá
Barley Sprout

Hordei Fructus
Germinatus

Sweet in flavor and slightly warm in nature, *mài yá* (barley sprout) disperses food and opens the stomach. It transforms accumulation and stagnation due to consumption of grain, flour, or fruit. It helps upward movement of stomach qì, promotes the spleen, and fortifies splenic movement, allowing turbid qì to descend, eliminating distention, and loosening the intestines. In large doses, it can terminate lactation.

For food accumulation (especially accumulation and stagnation due to grain, flour, and starch) *mài yá* is combined with:

shén qū (神曲 medicated leaven, Massa Medicata Fermentata)

bàn xià (半夏 pinellia, Pinelliae Rhizoma)

chǎo lái fú zǐ (炒莱菔子 stir-fried radish seed, Raphani Semen Frictum)

chǎo jī nèi jīn (炒鸡内金 stir-fried gizzard lining, Galli Gigeriae Endothelium Corneum Frictum)

jiāo shān zhā (焦山楂 scorch-fried crataegus, Crataegi Fructus Ustus)

bīng láng (槟榔 areca, Arecae Semen)

zhǐ shí (枳实 unripe bitter orange, Aurantii Fructus Immaturus)

cāng zhú (苍术 atractylodes, Atractylodis Rhizoma)

For a woman who wishes to terminate lactation, use 60 g/2 liǎng of *chǎo mài yá* (stir-fried barley sprout), decocted in water and taken once a day, continuously over a period of days. The breast milk will decrease and then terminate.

Using raw *mài yá* enhances stomach qì, aids digestion, and opens the stomach. It is used for reduced eating or food stagnation with the presence of stomach heat. It also has a liver-soothing, qì-regulating effect. Stir fried, it is used for food stagnation with stomach cold; scorch fried, it has the strongest capacity to disperse food and transform accumulation. Select the appropriate form of *mài yá* on the basis of presenting conditions.

Dosage

The dosage is generally 3–9 g/1–3 qián.

Caution

In the absence of accumulation and if taken over a long period of time, it can damage the right qì.

49. 山楂 Shān Zhā   Crataegi Fructus
Crataegus

Sweet and sour in flavor and slightly warm in nature, *shān zhā* (crataegus) disperses accumulations and transforms phlegm, moves qì and quickens stasis. It also outthrusts pox papules in children.

1. **Dispersing Accumulations and Transforming Phlegm:** *Shān zhā* is best for meat-type food accumulation for which it is commonly combined with medicinals such as *chǎo jī nèi jīn* (stir-fried gizzard lining), *shén qū* (medicated leaven), *mài yá* (barley sprout), *chǎo bīng láng* (stir-fried areca), and *lái fú zǐ* (radish seed). In center burner phlegm-damp obstruction that endures and engenders lumps, use this medicinal to transform phlegm and disperse accumulations; it is combined with:

> *bái zhú* (白术 white atractylodes, Atractylodis Macrocephalae Rhizoma)
> *zhǐ shí* (枳实 unripe bitter orange, Aurantii Fructus Immaturus)
> *bàn xià* (半夏 pinellia, Pinelliae Rhizoma)
> *chén pí* (陈皮 tangerine peel, Citri Reticulatae Pericarpium)
> *shén qū* (神曲 medicated leaven, Massa Medicata Fermentata)
> *mài yá* (麦芽 barley sprout, Hordei Fructus Germinatus)
> *sān léng* (三棱 sparganium, Sparganii Rhizoma)
> *é zhú* (莪术 curcuma rhizome, Curcumae Rhizoma)
> *hóng huā* (红花 carthamus, Carthami Flos)
> *táo rén* (桃仁 peach kernel, Persicae Semen)
> *zhì shān jiǎ* (炙山甲 mix-fried pangolin scales, Manis Squama cum Liquido Fricta)

2. **Moving Qì and Quickening Stasis:** *Shān zhā* enters the blood aspect, so it moves qì and quickens stasis. For postpartum women with static blood pain in the lower abdominal area (commonly known as **infant's-pillow pain**[552] 儿枕痛 *ér zhěn tòng*) and persistent flow of lochia, it is combined with medicinals such as *táo rén* (peach kernel), *hóng huā* (carthamus), *pào jiāng* (blast-fried ginger), *chuān xiōng* (chuanxiong), and *dāng guī* (Chinese angelica). When treating chest impediment pain (which includes angina pectoris), I frequently add about 15 g/5 qián of *shēng shān zhā* to an appropriate decoction medicine for its blood-quickening and pain-relieving action.

3. **Outhrusting Pox Papules in Children:** When pox papules are not outthrusting easily, use 6–9 g/2–3 qián of this medicinal decocted in water and taken by mouth.

COMPARISONS

Used raw, *shān zhā* opens the stomach and disperses food, as well as quickens the blood and transforms stasis; used scorch-fried, it disperses food and abducts stagnation; *shān zhā tàn* (charred crataegus) disperses food and checks diarrhea.

Shén qū (medicated leaven) is effective in dispersing grain-type accumulations, and moreover it transforms phlegm and abducts stagnation. It is used to ease digestion of metals and stones. *Mài yá* (barley sprout) is effective in dispersing flour- or noodle-type accumulations, and moreover it assists stomach qì. *Shān zhā* is effective for dispersing meat-type food accumulations and concretion lumps, and it also moves qì and quickens the blood.

Shān zhā hé (crataegus pit) disperses food and grinds accumulations, and it also treats **mounting qì pain**[558] (疝气痛 *shàn qì tòng*).

Wū méi (mume)[183] and *shān zhā* (crataegus) are both sour, but *wū méi* is sour and promotes astriction, constrains the lung, and astringes the intestines, whereas *shān zhā* is sour and breaks and drains, disperses accumulations, and dissipates stasis.

The combination of *jiāo shén qū* (scorch-fried medicated leaven), *jiāo mài yá* (scorch-fried barley sprout), and *jiāo shān zhā* (scorch-fried crataegus) is known as *jiāo sān xiān* (焦三仙, scorch-fried three immortals). They are used together to increase food-dispersing and stagnation-abducting effects. If *jiāo bīng láng* (scorch-fried areca) is added, it is called *jiāo sì xiān* (焦四仙, scorch-fried four immortals). This combination precipitates qì and disperses accumulations with a stronger action. These medicinals are frequently used in combination.

RESEARCH

According to modern reports, a 50% *shān zhā* wine, taken 10–20 ml each time, can relieve angina pectoris.

DOSAGE

The dosage is generally 3–15 g/1–5 qián.

CAUTION

If *shān zhā* is taken in excess or taken over a long period of time, it can quell the qì engendered by the spleen and stomach. Thus, in patterns of spleen-stomach vacuity without accumulation, it should be used with care.

---

50. 鸡内金 Jī Nèi Jīn
Gizzard Lining
Galli Gigeriae
Endothelium
Corneum

Jī nèi jīn (gizzard lining), sweet in flavor and neutral in nature, primarily disperses food and opens the stomach, but it also frees strangury and transforms stones, and checks childhood enuresis.

1. **Dispersing Food and Opening the Stomach:** For adults or children with poor digestion that results in stagnation of food and drink, distention of the stomach duct and abdomen, vomiting, diarrhea, and **nontransformation of food**[558] (食不消化 *shí bù xiāo huà*), *jī nèi jīn* is used to fortify the spleen and open the stomach, disperse water and grain, and assist movement and transformation. *Jī nèi jīn* is frequently combined with medicinals such as:

huò xiāng (藿香 agastache, Agastaches Herba)

zǐ sū (紫苏 perilla, Perillae Folium, Caulis et Calyx)

jiāo shén qū (焦神曲 scorch-fried medicated leaven, Massa Medicata
Fermentata Usta)

jiāo shān zhā (焦山楂 scorch-fried crataegus, Crataegi Fructus Ustus)

jiāo mài yá (焦麦芽 scorch-fried barley sprout, Hordei Fructus Germinatus
Ustus)

zhǐ shí (枳实 unripe bitter orange, Aurantii Fructus Immaturus)

bàn xià (半夏 pinellia, Pinelliae Rhizoma)

chén pí (陈皮 tangerine peel, Citri Reticulatae Pericarpium)

For childhood gān accumulation with indigestion, yellow face, emaciated flesh, and postmeridian low-grade fever, remove *huò xiāng* (agastache) and add *hú huáng lián* (picrorhiza), *yín chái hú* (stellaria), *shǐ jūn zǐ* (quisqualis), and *jiāo bīng láng* (scorch-fried areca).

2. Freeing Strangury and Dispersing Stones: For dribbling urine and pain, with sand and stones in the urine (urinary calculus), which in former times was called "sand and stone strangury" (砂石淋 *shā shí lín*), this medicinal is used in combination with:

dōng kuí zǐ (冬葵子 mallow seed, Malvae Semen)

chē qián zǐ (车前子 plantago seed, Plantaginis Semen)

qū mài (瞿麦 dianthus, Dianthi Herba)

biǎn xù (萹蓄 knotgrass, Polygoni Avicularis Herba)

fú líng (茯苓 poria, Poria)

zhū líng (猪苓 polyporus, Polyporus)

niú xī (牛膝 achyranthes, Achyranthis Bidentatae Radix)

zé lán (泽兰 lycopus, Lycopi Herba)

jīn qián cǎo (金钱草 moneywort, Lysimachiae Herba)

mù tōng (木通 trifoliate akebia, Akebiae Trifoliatae Caulis)

For biliary calculus pain, it is combined with:

zhǐ shí (枳实 unripe bitter orange, Aurantii Fructus Immaturus)

bàn xià (半夏 pinellia, Pinelliae Rhizoma)

chuān liàn zǐ (川楝子 toosendan, Toosendan Fructus)

chái hú (柴胡 bupleurum, Bupleuri Radix)

bái sháo (白芍 white peony, Paeoniae Radix Alba)

yù jīn (郁金 curcuma, Curcumae Radix)

mù tōng (木通 trifoliate akebia, Akebiae Trifoliatae Caulis)

shēng dà huáng (生大黄 raw rhubarb, Rhei Radix et Rhizoma Crudi)

jīn qián cǎo (金钱草 moneywort, Lysimachiae Herba)

3. Checking Enuresis: In child enuresis or adult bedwetting, *jī nèi jīn* checks enuresis and astringes urine, and can be added for this purpose to a pattern-appropriate decoction medicine.

Used raw, *jī nèi jīn* frees strangury and transforms stones; stir-fried, it disperses food and opens the stomach.

DOSAGE

The dosage is generally 3–9 g/1–3 qián.

---

51. 常山 Cháng Shān   Dichroae Radix
Dichroa

Cháng shān (dichroa) is bitter, acrid, and cold; it disperses phlegm, induces ejection, and interrupts malaria.

This medicinal has a strong tendency to cause vomiting. Physicians of the past sometimes used *cháng shān* to eject collected and bound phlegm-turbidity or phlegm-rheum from the chest and diaphragm. *Cháng shān* and *gān cǎo* (licorice) taken internally can cause a patient to vomit phlegm-drool or water-rheum, allowing the chest and diaphragm to feel loose and uninhibited. Ejection (emesis) is rarely applied nowadays, so this medicinal is mainly used to treat malaria.

Cháng shān treats malaria, and physicians of the past said that it could "interrupt malaria" (截疟 *jié nüè*), which means that it powerfully checks the progression of malaria. Nonetheless, one must still follow the spirit of pattern identification and treatment determination and use other medicinals to thoroughly regulate the body and eliminate other disease-causing factors. Thus, when using *cháng shān* to interrupt malaria, the first step is to harmonize the exterior and interior, raise the evil to the outer body, dissipate the exterior evil, eliminate phlegm and disperse accumulations, clear and resolve the liver and gallbladder, and regulate the intestines and stomach. After several days of this treatment, *cháng shān* can then be added to pattern-appropriate decoctions to interrupt malaria. This is the experience of past physicians. When I use *cháng shān* to treat malaria, I frequently use the following ingredients:

> *chái hú* (柴胡 bupleurum, Bupleuri Radix) 9–30 g/3 qián–1 liǎng
>
> *huáng qín* (黃芩 scutellaria, Scutellariae Radix) 9–12 g/3–4 qián
>
> *bàn xià* (半夏 pinellia, Pinelliae Rhizoma) 10 g/3 qián
>
> *cháng shān* (常山 dichroa, Dichroae Radix) 6–9 g/2–3 qián
>
> *cǎo guǒ* (草果 tsaoko, Tsaoko Fructus) 9 g/3 qián
>
> *bīng láng* (槟榔 areca, Arecae Semen) 9 g/3 qián
>
> *wū méi* (乌梅 mume, Mume Fructus) 3–4.5 g/1–1.5 qián
>
> *shēng jiāng* (生姜 fresh ginger, Zingiberis Rhizoma Recens) 3 pieces
>
> *dà zǎo* (大枣 jujube, Jujubae Fructus) 3–5 pieces
>
> *zhì gān cǎo* (炙甘草 mix-fried licorice, Glycyrrhizae Radix cum Liquido Fricta) 3–6 g/1–2 qián

This should be decocted with water and taken 3–4 hours before an episode; thus one should determine the times for taking the formula on the basis of the specific situation. For dry stool, add 3–9 g/1–3 qián of *shēng dà huáng* (raw rhubarb). If during a malarial episode heat effusion (fever) is more pronounced than aversion to cold (chills) or unaccompanied by any feeling of cold, there is great sweating, and thirst with desire to drink, add 30–60 g/1–2 liǎng of *shēng shí gāo* (crude gypsum) and 9–12 g/3–4 qián of *zhī mǔ* (anemarrhena). If during an episode there is primarily aversion to cold and no heat effusion, or if the aversion to cold lasts longer while the heat effusion is very short and mild, add 9–15 g/3–5 qián of *guì zhī* (cinnamon twig), 9–15 g/3–5 qián of *bái sháo* (white peony), and 6–9 g/ 2–3 qián of *wú yú* (evodia). If the disease has persisted for a long time, numerous treatments have been given to no avail, and the patient's condition is characterized by vacuity, or if the patient is elderly with a weak constititution, add 15–30 g/ 5 qián–1 liǎng of *dǎng shēn* (codonopsis) and 15–30 g/5 qián–1 liǎng of *hé shǒu wū* (flowery knotweed).

Cháng shān can cause counterflow ascent of the chest and stomach qì and give rise to vomiting. To prevent this side-effect, combine it with qì-downbearing *bīng láng* (areca) and stomach-harmonizing *bàn xià* (pinellia).

Comparisons

Cǎo guǒ (tsaoko) eliminates miasma, pestilence, and damp qì, and tends to be used for miasmic malaria (this is a type of malaria caused by contraction of mountain forest miasmic qì; it is similar to pernicious malaria[26]). *Cháng shān* dispels phlegm accumulation and tends to be used for tertian malaria[27] or enduring malaria. Added to appropriate decoction medicines, it is used for all forms of malaria.

Research

According to modern research reports, *cháng shān* is more effective than quinine for tertian malaria. Some reports suggest that it has an antipyretic effect.

Dosage

The dosage is generally 3–6 g/1–2 qián. In severe cases, use 9 g/3 qián.

Caution

Should be used with care for vacuous patients.

---

52. 草果 Cǎo Guǒ Tsaoko	Tsao-Ko Fructus

Acrid in flavor and warm in nature, *cǎo guǒ* (tsaoko) dries dampness with aroma and dispels cold with warmth and acridity. It also interrupts malaria.

---

[26]Pernicious malaria, 恶性疟 *è xìng nüè*: A Western medical concept denoting malaria that is caused by *Plasmodium falciparum* and that is characterized by severe symptoms accompanied by cerebral, hemorrhagic, or gastroenteric complications. (Ed.)

[27]Tertian malaria, 间日疟 *jiān rì nüè*: A Western medical term denoting malaria characterized by episodes that recur every 48 hours. Tertian malaria is either vivax malaria, attributed to *Plasmodium vivax*, the most common and widespread form of malaria, or a benign malaria called ovale malaria, attributed to *Plasmodium ovale*. (Ed.)

When cold-damp evil collecting in the stomach and intestines affects movement and transformation in the center burner and results in pathoconditions such as stomach pain, abdominal distention, abdominal pain, vomiting, diarrhea, fullness and oppression, and poor appetite, use this medicinal to dry dampness with aroma, dispel cold, and warm the center. *Cǎo guǒ* is frequently combined with:

huò xiāng (藿香 agastache, Agastaches Herba)

shā rén (砂仁 amomum, Amomi Fructus)

mù xiāng (木香 costusroot, Aucklandiae Radix)

shēng jiāng (生姜 fresh ginger, Zingiberis Rhizoma Recens)

bàn xià (半夏 pinellia, Pinelliae Rhizoma)

wú yú (吴萸 evodia, Evodiae Fructus)

gāo liáng jiāng (高良姜 lesser galangal, Alpiniae Officinarum Rhizoma)

xiāng fù (香附 cyperus, Cyperi Rhizoma)

For great exuberance of cold-damp in the center burner that results in glomus and oppression in the chest and stomach duct, and in poor appetite, *cǎo guǒ* is combined with *hòu pò* (officinal magnolia bark), *chén pí* (tangerine peel), *cǎo dòu kòu* (Katsumada's galangal seed), *mài yá* (barley sprout), *fú líng* (poria), *cāng zhú* (atractylodes), and *shā rén* (amomum).

In exuberant dampness evil that results in malaria, or malaria with concurrent center burner cold-damp obstruction, *cǎo guǒ* is combined with:

chái hú (柴胡 bupleurum, Bupleuri Radix)

huáng qín (黄芩 scutellaria, Scutellariae Radix)

bàn xià (半夏 pinellia, Pinelliae Rhizoma)

cāng zhú (苍术 atractylodes, Atractylodis Rhizoma)

pèi lán (佩兰 eupatorium, Eupatorii Herba)

cǎo dòu kòu (草豆蔻 Katsumada's galangal seed, Alpiniae Katsumadai Semen)

bīng láng (槟榔 areca, Arecae Semen)

cháng shān (常山 dichroa, Dichroae Radix)

hòu pò (厚朴 officinal magnolia bark, Magnoliae Officinalis Cortex)

The effect is relatively good for miasmic malaria caused by mountain forest miasmic qì or foul turbidity dampness evil.

COMPARISONS

Cǎo dòu kòu (Katsumada's galangal seed)[217] tends to warm the center and regulate the stomach, check retching and disperse distention. *Cǎo guǒ* tends to dry dampness and dispel cold, eliminate miasma and interrupt malaria.

DOSAGE

The dosage is generally 2–6 g/7 fēn–2 qián. For severe cases, use up to 9 g/ 3 qián.

CAUTION

Contraindicated in the absence of cold-damp in the spleen and stomach.

53. 使君子 Shǐ Jūn Zǐ   Quisqualis Fructus
Quisqualis

Sweet in flavor and warm in nature, *shǐ jūn zǐ* (quisqualis) fortifies the spleen and stomach, eliminates vacuity heat, disperses accumulations, and kills worms. It is often used for various diseases in children that are caused by weakness in the spleen and stomach.

Children with spleen-stomach vacuity easily suffer from breast milk stagnation, food stagnation, damp-heat depression, and indigestion, which can result in gān disease, worm accumulation, or glomus. Frequently observed manifestations include: yellow face and emaciated flesh, dry and brittle hair, indigestion, diarrhea, an enlarged abdominal vein, low-grade fever, poor appetite, appetite for eating mud and earth, enlargement of the liver and spleen, fatigue, and a tendency to fright crying. *Shǐ jūn zǐ* fortifies the spleen and stomach, eliminates vacuity heat, disperses accumulations, and kills worms. It is frequently combined with medicinals such as *hú huáng lián* (picrorhiza), *jiāo sān xiān* (scorch-fried three immortals), *jī nèi jīn* (gizzard lining), *bīng láng* (areca), *bái zhú* (white atractylodes), and *fú líng* (poria). Two examples of this use follow.

Jiā wèi féi ér wán 加味肥儿丸   Supplemented Chubby Child Pill

---

mài yá (麦芽 barley sprout, Hordei Fructus Germinatus)
shén qū (神曲 medicated leaven, Massa Medicata Fermentata)
bái zhú (白术 white atractylodes, Atractylodis Macrocephalae Rhizoma)
shān zhā (山楂 crataegus, Crataegi Fructus)
shǐ jūn zǐ (使君子 quisqualis, Quisqualis Fructus)
hú huáng lián (胡黄连 picrorhiza, Picrorhizae Rhizoma)
bīng láng (槟榔 areca, Arecae Semen)
mù xiāng (木香 costusroot, Aucklandiae Radix)
zhǐ shí (枳实 unripe bitter orange, Aurantii Fructus Immaturus)
jī nèi jīn (鸡内金 gizzard lining, Galli Gigeriae Endothelium Corneum)
chén pí (陈皮 tangerine peel, Citri Reticulatae Pericarpium)

Grind these ingredients to a powder and form into a honey pill.

Jiàn pí féi ér sǎn 健脾肥儿散   Spleen-Fortifying Chubby Child Powder

---

shǐ jūn zǐ (使君子 quisqualis, Quisqualis Fructus)
jī nèi jīn (鸡内金 gizzard lining, Galli Gigeriae Endothelium Corneum)
bái zhú (白术 white atractylodes, Atractylodis Macrocephalae Rhizoma)
shān yào (山药 dioscorea, Dioscoreae Rhizoma)
gān cǎo (甘草 licorice, Glycyrrhizae Radix)
fú líng (茯苓 poria, Poria)

shān zhā (山楂 crataegus, Crataegi Fructus)

Grind these ingredients to a fine powder.

Shǐ jūn zǐ expels roundworm. Experiments have demonstrated that the water-soluble constituent of *shǐ jūn zǐ* (potassium salt of quisqualic acid) was able to cause paralysis of the head portion of roundworm in pork, allowing it to be expelled. Used alone, *shǐ jūn zǐ* is taken decocted with water at a dosage of 3–15 g/1–5 qián per day; alternatively, remove the outer shell, roast the kernel until it is cooked, and chew it. It can also be combined with medicinals such as:

kǔ liàn zǐ (苦楝子 chinaberry seed, Meliae Semen),

wú yí (芜荑 elm cake, Ulmi Fructus Praeparatio)

gān cǎo (甘草 licorice, Glycyrrhizae Radix)

zhū dǎn zhī (猪胆汁 pig's bile, Suis Bilis)

In addition, *shǐ jūn zǐ* is effective against hookworm and pinworm. For hookworm, it is combined with *fěi zǐ* (torreya). To treat pinworm, it is used together with *bǎi bù* (stemona) and *dà huáng* (rhubarb) (decoct *shǐ jūn zǐ* and *dà huáng* in water, then add *bǎi bù*, and continue decocting to make a retention enema).

DOSAGE

The dosage is generally 3–9 g/1–3 qián.

CAUTION

A large dose can cause hiccup, abdominal distention, dizzy head, and nausea or other side-effects.

---

54. 苦楝根皮 Kǔ Liàn Gēn Pí   Meliae
Chinaberry Root Bark   Radicis Cortex

Aslo called *kǔ liàn pí* 苦楝皮. Bitter in flavor, cold in nature, and toxic, *kǔ liàn gēn pí* (chinaberry root bark) is mainly used to expel roundworm. Being bitter and cold, it also drains damp-heat.

Generally, decoctions are used to expel roundworm. Use a 100% concentrated decoction of *kǔ liàn gēn pí* taken internally. (Adults can take 5–15 ml each day.) One can also use dry powder made into pills.

I have used a 50% concentrated decoction of *kǔ liàn gēn pí*, in doses of 5–10 ml a day, for more than thirty 6–12-year-old children with roundworm. In most cases this causes the roundworms to descend and one does not need to use draining medicinals.

This medicinal is used singly or with *wú yí* (elm cake), *léi wán* (omphalia), and *hè shī* (carpesium seed).

DOSAGE

The dosage is generally 3–9 g/1–3 qián. Use up to 25 g/8 qián of fresh root bark.

RESEARCH

According to the findings of modern research, the effect of *kǔ liàn gēn pí* is similar to that of santonin, although it is slower acting and less toxic.

Toxic reactions associated with this medicinal include dizzy head, headache, nausea, vomiting, red facial complexion, abdominal pain, diarrhea, and numbness of the limbs. In severe cases, *kǔ liàn gēn pí* can give rise to convulsions and arrythmia.

CAUTION

Use with care in patients with weak health, heart disease, and active pulmonary tuberculosis. Do not use in pregnancy.

---

55. 芜荑 Wú Yí   Ulmi Fructus
Elm Cake   Praeparatio

Acrid and bitter in flavor and warm in nature, *wú yí* (elm cake)[28] is mainly used to treat parasitic diseases of the intestines. It also dries dampness and transforms food accumulation.

In cases of roundworm or tapeworm that result in yellow face, emaciated flesh, abdominal pain, abdominal distention, diarrhea, and low-grade fever, use this medicinal with:

dà huáng (大黄 rhubarb, Rhei Radix et Rhizoma)

hè shī (鹤虱 carpesium seed, Carpesii Fructus)

bīng láng (槟榔 areca, Arecae Semen)

hē zǐ (诃子 chebule, Chebulae Fructus)

mù xiāng (木香 costusroot, Aucklandiae Radix)

gān jiāng (干姜 dried ginger, Zingiberis Rhizoma)

fù zǐ (附子 aconite, Aconiti Radix Lateralis Praeparata)

wū méi (乌梅 mume, Mume Fructus)

shén qū (神曲 medicated leaven, Massa Medicata Fermentata)

mài yá (麦芽 barley sprout, Hordei Fructus Germinatus)

In addition, it is used for cold-damp pain in the heart [region] and abdomen and for cold dysentery. It is frequently combined with medicinals such as *ròu dòu kòu* (nutmeg), *gāo liáng jiāng* (lesser galangal), *shā rén* (amomum), and *hē zǐ* (chebule).

DOSAGE

The dosage is generally 4.5–6 g/1.5–2 qián.

CAUTION

Contraindicated for spleen-stomach vacuity.

---

[28]This medicinal is the fermented seeds of *Ulmus macrocarpa* HANCE. The seeds are soaked in water and fermented and then mixed with elm bark, red earth, powdered *jú huā* (chrysanthemum) and water to make a thick paste. The paste is cut into small cubes and then sun-dried to its final form. This medicinal is generally taken in pill or powder form and not in decoction. For external use it is powdered and mixed with honey to treat scabs and lichen. (Ed.)

56. 鹤虱 Hè Shī
Carpesium Seed
Carpesii Fructus

Hè shī (carpesium seed) is bitter and acrid in flavor and neutral in nature. It is mainly used for various forms of intestinal parasitic infestations. It possesses minor toxicity.

For intestinal parasites with signs such as abdominal pain and abdominal distention (white macules on the face, worm macules on the lips, intermittent abdominal pain, and craving for raw rice, mud, or dirt), use this medicinal alone, ground to a powder, and taken with a meat broth. Alternatively, *hè shī* is also used with *kŭ liàn pí* (chinaberry bark), *bīng láng* (areca), and *shǐ jūn zǐ* (quisqualis). An example of this use is as follows:

Huà chóng wán 化虫丸 | Worm-Transforming Pill

> *wú yí* (芜荑 elm cake, Ulmi Fructus Praeparatio)
> *hè shī* (鹤虱 carpesium seed, Carpesii Fructus)
> *kŭ liàn pí* (苦楝皮 chinaberry bark, Meliae Cortex)
> *bīng láng* (槟榔 areca, Arecae Semen)
> *kū fán* (枯矾 calcined alum, Alumen Dehydratum)
> *shǐ jūn zǐ* (使君子 quisqualis, Quisqualis Fructus)
> *mù xiāng* (木香 costusroot, Aucklandiae Radix)
> *léi wán* (雷丸 omphalia, Omphalia)

Grind these ingredients to a powder and form into pills with *liàn mì* (processed honey).

These pills are used for worm accumulation, food accumulation, and milk accumulation causing bloating and distention of the abdomen, pain, vomiting, clamoring stomach, and low food intake.

DOSAGE

The dosage is generally 2.5–6 g/8 fēn–2 qián.

57. 雷丸 Léi Wán
Omphalia
Omphalia

Léi wán (omphalia) is bitter in flavor, cold in nature, and possesses minor toxicity. It is primarily used as a worm-expelling medicinal to treat tapeworm, hookworm, roundworm, and filaria.

It is most commonly used for tapeworm and cysticercus (bladder worm), which is the result of eating improperly cooked pork or beef that contains worm eggs, or other unclean food. The clinical symptoms can include diarrhea, abdominal pain, abdominal distention, poor appetite, nausea, vomiting, and stool that contains pieces of the worm bodies. In cysticercosis, it is possible to observe small nodules the size of yellow beans (biopsy can reveal the presence of cysticercus). If cysticercus reproduce in the brain there can be symptoms similar to those of epilepsy. *Léi wán* is able to destroy tapeworm segments and cysticercus in the intestines, and thereby expel worms. When used as a single medicinal, it is taken internally at a dosage of 60 g/2 liǎng for two consecutive days.

According to modern reports, using *léi wán* with *gān qī* (lacquer), *xióng huáng* (realgar), and *zhì shān jiǎ* (mix-fried pangolin scales) in pill preparation over an extended period of time has a definite effect on cysticercus in the brain. *Léi wán* is also effective against filiaria when taken as a decoction at a dosage of 30 g/ 1 liǎng a day for seven days. It is ineffective against roundworm.

Some people use 125 g/4 liǎng of *léi wán* ground to a powder and divided into three packets. The patient takes one pack a day for three days in one course of treatment. This method is effective against hookworm.

DOSAGE

The dosage is generally 9–20 g/3–7 qián. It is best used in powder preparation or in pills.

RESEARCH

According to modern research reports, when this medicinal is heated to 60°C for half an hour, it loses the majority of its effects. After an hour, it loses all its effects. Thus it is not suitable for use in decoction.

---

58. 紫硇砂 Zǐ Náo Shā   Sal Ammoniacum
Purple Sal Ammoniac   Purpureum

Zǐ náo shā (purple sal ammoniac) is salty, acrid, and bitter in flavor, hot in nature, and toxic. It disperses accumulations, breaks binds, softens hardness, dissipates stasis, and disperses swelling.

1. **Dispersing Meat-Type Food Accumulation:** When overconsumption of meat damages the spleen and stomach and affects movement and transformation in the center burner, there is qì stagnation and blood stasis, and binding of phlegm and food, and gradual engendering of strings, aggregations, and concretions. In this situation, use *zǐ náo shā* combined with the following medicinals to make pills.

> *ē wèi* (阿魏 asafetida, Ferulae Resina)
> *jiāo shān zhā* (焦山楂 scorch-fried crataegus, Crataegi Fructus Ustus)
> *jiāo shén qū* (焦神曲 scorch-fried medicated leaven, Massa Medicata Fermentata Usta)
> *bái zhú* (白术 white atractylodes, Atractylodis Macrocephalae Rhizoma)
> *hēi bái chǒu* (黑白丑 morning glory, Pharbitidis Semen)
> *dān shēn* (丹参 salvia, Salviae Miltiorrhizae Radix)

zhì biē jiǎ (炙鳖甲 mix-fried turtle shell, Trionycis Carapax cum Liquido Frictus)

é zhú (莪术 curcuma rhizome, Curcumae Rhizoma)

2. Dysphagia-Occlusion: Physicians of the past used *zǐ náo shā* combined in pill or powder preparation with *bīng láng* (areca), *dīng xiāng* (clove), *hòu pò* (officinal magnolia bark), *cāng zhú* (atractylodes), and *huáng dān* (minium) to treat **dysphagia-occlusion**[548] (噎膈 *yē gé*) and **stomach reflux**[564] (反胃 *fǎn wèi*). According to modern research reports, this medicinal has a definite inhibitory effect on sarcoma 180, carcinoma 256, and ascites carcinoma in mice. On the basis of the experience of past physicians, I have used this medicinal to treat dysphagia-occlusion. Combining this experience with modern research that shows this medicinal has an anti-cancer effect, I have given it internally to several patients with esophageal cancer (verified by X-ray). After the treatment some of these patients were able to swallow noodles and dumplings (饺子 *jiǎo zǐ*),[29] and their essence-spirit, strength, and food intake all showed pronounced improvement. These patients felt that many of the symptoms were relieved, and there seems to be a definite therapeutic effect. Below, I present the treatment method that I used.

Use 12 g/4 qián of *zǐ náo shā* and as much *qiáo mài miàn* (buckwheat flour) as is needed. Take *qiáo mài miàn* and mix it with water to form a dough like that used to wrap dumplings. Wrap the *zǐ náo shā* in the dough. Make it about the size of large Lantern Festival soup dumplings (元宵 *yuán xiāo*)[30] with skins about 1–1.3 cm thick. Using a large charcoal fire, calcine until it becomes a scorched yellow color. Wait until it has cooled and then cut it open. Take the damp *zǐ náo shā* from the center and dry it over a slow flame. Take 6 g and grind into it 12 g/ 4 qián of *bīng láng* (areca) and 4 pieces of *gōng dīng xiāng* (clove) (some also add 3 g of *chén xiāng fěn* (aquilaria powder)). Grind together and mix into a fine powder. Take 0.2–0.3 g each time with warm water or warm yellow wine, three times a day. This should be taken one hour before meals and at the same time the patient should be taking a pattern-appropriate decoction. I frequently use the formula below with variations:

shēng dài zhě shí (生代赭石 crude hematite, Haematitum Crudum) 30 g/1 liǎng (precook)

xuán fù huā (旋覆花 inula flower, Inulae Flos) 10 g/3 qián (wrap)

bàn xià (半夏 pinellia, Pinelliae Rhizoma) 10 g/3 qián

dǎng shēn (党参 codonopsis, Codonopsis Radix) 10 g/3 qián

shā shēn (沙参 adenophora/glehnia, Adenophorae seu Glehniae Radix) 10 g/3 qián

dān shēn (丹参 salvia, Salviae Miltiorrhizae Radix) 15 g/5 qián

---

[29]Dumplings, 饺子 *jiǎo zǐ*: A wrapping of flour and water dough enclosing ground meat and sometimes vegetables. Dumplings are similar to Italian ravioli, but each dough wrapping is rolled individually. *Jiǎo zi* are easily chewed and swallowed. (Ed.)

[30]Lantern Festival soup dumplings, 元宵 *yuán xiāo*: Glutinous rice flour dumplings (汤圆 *tāng yuán*), usually with a sweet filling such as of ground sesame seed, traditionally eaten at the Lantern Festival on the 15th day of the first lunar month. They are usually about 3–4 cm in diameter. (Ed.)

chuān bèi mǔ (川贝母 Sìchuān fritillaria, Fritillariae Cirrhosae Bulbus)
6 g/2 qián

jiāo sān xiān (焦三仙 scorch-fried three immortals, Tres Immortales Usti)
9 g/3 qián each

shēng dà huáng (生大黄 raw rhubarb, Rhei Radix et Rhizoma Crudi)
2–10 g/6 fēn–3 qián

gān cǎo (甘草 licorice, Glycyrrhizae Radix) 2–6 g/6 fēn–2 qián

dāo dòu zǐ (刀豆子 sword bean, Canavaliae Semen) 10 g/3 qián

chǔ tóu kāng (杵头糠 rice husk, Oryzae Testa) ("fine husk") 1 scoop

guā lóu (瓜蒌 trichosanthes, Trichosanthis Fructus) 30 g/1 liǎng

Take decocted with water. Use one packet a day, divided into two doses. Unfortunately, the duration of my survey was not long, only 3–5 months, and I was unable to continue the survey or draw any conclusion from it. I merely present my experience.

Zǐ náo shā is also used as a topically applied medicinal to consume **malign flesh**[556] (恶肉 *è ròu*). In modern times, it is also used for skin cancer. In ophthalmology, it is applied in topical eye medications to treat eye screens and excrescences. Nevertheless, it must only be used after proper processing and those without experience in its use should not use it lightly.

COMPARISON

White *bái náo shā* (sal ammoniac) transforms phlegm; thus it is used for cough with copious, thick, sticky phlegm that is not easy to expectorate. It is not used as an anti-cancer medicinal. If, when writing a prescription, one only writes *náo shā* (sal ammoniac), most pharmacies will give *zǐ náo shā* (purple sal ammoniac). It is best to specify clearly when writing prescriptions.

The dosage is generally 0.2–1 g/0.6–3 fēn. When taking this medicinal, the patient should not eat goat's or sheep's blood.

---

59. 山慈菇 Shān Cí Gū
Cremastra/Pleione

Cremastrae seu
Pleiones
Pseudobulbus

Sweet and slightly acrid in flavor, cold in nature, with minor toxicity, *shān cí gū* (cremastra/pleione)[31] clears heat and resolves toxin, disperses welling-abscesses, and dissipates binds.

Shān cí gū is mainly used to treat clove sores, welling-abscesses, malign sores, scrofula nodes, scorpion stings, and insect bites. *Shān cí gū* is combined with:

jīn yín huā (金银花 lonicera, Lonicerae Flos)

---

[31] This medicinal is the bulb of *Cremastra appendiculata* (D. Don) Mak., *Pleione bulbocodioides* (Franch.) Rolfe, or *Pleione yunanensis* (Rolfe) Rolfe. Because substitutes are commonly used, careful identification is necessary. (Ed.)

lián qiáo (连翘 forsythia, Forsythiae Fructus)

pú gōng yīng (蒲公英 dandelion, Taraxaci Herba)

dì dīng (地丁 violet, Violae Herba)

cāng ěr zǐ (苍耳子 xanthium, Xanthii Fructus) (which can include the stems and leaves)

wǔ bèi zǐ (五倍子 sumac gallnut, Galla Chinensis)

zhū shā (朱砂 cinnabar, Cinnabaris)

The most commonly used clinical prescription is *zǐ jīn dìng* (Purple Gold Tablet) and its formulation and processing is described below.

---

zǐ jīn dìng 紫金锭   Purple Gold Tablet

---

shān cí gū (山慈菇 cremastra/pleione, Cremastrae seu Pleiones Pseudobulbus) 60 g/2 liǎng

hóng yá dà jǐ (红芽大戟 knoxia, Knoxiae Radix) (mix-fry with vinegar) 45 g/1.5 liǎng

qiān jīn zǐ shuāng (千金子霜 caper spurge seed frost, Euphorbiae Semen Pulveratum) 30 g/1 liǎng

wǔ bèi zǐ (五倍子 sumac gallnut, Galla Chinensis) 30 g/1 liǎng.

Grind into a fine powder and mix together. Add:

zhū shā fěn (朱砂粉 cinnabar powder, Cinnabaris Pulverata) 9 g/3 qián

xióng huáng fěn (雄黄粉 realgar powder, Realgar Pulveratus) 9 g/3 qián

shè xiāng (麝香 musk, Moschus) 9 g/3 qián

Separately, take 96 g/3 liǎng of *nuò mǐ miàn* (glutinous rice flour) and mix it with enough water to make it into a paste. Steam the paste, then mix the powder from above into this paste until thoroughly mixed. Form the resulting mixture into 3 g/ 1 qián tablets. The damp mixture will weigh about 3.5 g/1.2 qián before drying. Take internally at a dosage of 1.5 g/5 fēn twice a day. Divide each tablet in half, grind, and take with warm water. At the same time, this mixture is ground up with vinegar and applied to the affected area. The indications include all types of toxic heat in the bowels and viscera, seasonal epidemic scourge evil, red swelling of the cheek and neck, clove-sore toxin and malign sores, scrofula nodes, insect bites, scorpion stings, and innominate toxin swelling. The medicinal powder above, when not made into a tablet, is called *yù shū dān* (Jade Pivot Elixir). It is usually taken drenched with a decoction.

Yù shū dān (Jade Pivot Elixir) resolves toxin and checks retching. For nephritis and uremia with pronounced nausea and vomiting, I sometimes add 2 g/6 fēn of *yù shū dān* (Jade Pivot Elixir) to an appropriate decoction medicine, divided into 1 g doses and taken drenched with the decoction.

According to modern research reports, *shān cí gū* has a definite anti-cancer effect. When I am treating esophageal cancer, stomach cancer, liver cancer, and pancreatic cancer, I will have patients take 0.7–1.5 g of *yù shū dān* (Jade Pivot Elixir) twice a day with an appropriate decoction medicine devised in accordance with the principle of pattern identification as the basis of determining treatment. Alternatively, I add 6–9 g/2–3 qián of *shān cí gū* to the prescription or use *zǐ náo shā* (purple sal ammoniac) in powder preparation, taken drenched. (See *zǐ náo shā*.[514]) This therapeutic approach succeeded in reducing symptoms and bringing about an improvement in the spirit and strength of patients. Nevertheless, because most of my patients are in the advanced stages of illness or outpatients, I have not been able to perform a systematic observation over a sufficiently large number of cases. Hence it is difficult to draw a definite conclusion about these therapeutic effects.

DOSAGE

The dosage is 3–9 g/1–3 qián.

---

60. 半枝莲 Bàn Zhī Lián   Scutellariae Barbatae
Bearded Scutellaria   Herba

Acrid in flavor and cool in nature, *bàn zhī lián* (bearded scutellaria) clears heat and resolves toxin, quickens stasis and disperses swelling. In modern times, it has been commonly used as an anti-cancer medicinal.

In recent years, there have been reports of using *bàn zhī lián* (bearded scutellaria) 60 g/2 liǎng, *shān dòu gēn* (bushy sophora) 30 g/1 liǎng, *lù fēng fáng* (hornet's nest) 30 g/1 liǎng, and *shān cí gū* (cremastra/pleione) 30 g/1 liǎng, ground to a fine powder, and made into water pills the size of *lù dòu* (mung bean). These pills are taken with warm water after eating, fifteen at a time, 2–3 times a day. They are used to treat various forms of tumor. Also, there is *fù fāng bàn zhī lián kàng ái zhù shè yè* (Compound Bearded Scutellaria Anti-Cancer Injectable Fluid), which comprises:

bàn zhī lián (半枝莲 bearded scutellaria, Scutellariae Barbatae Herba)
bái huā shé shé cǎo (白花蛇舌草 oldenlandia, Oldenlandiae Diffusae Herba)
bàn biān lián (半边莲 Chinese lobelia, Lobeliae Chinensis Herba)
zhū yāng yāng (猪殃殃 galium, Galii Herba)
bái yīng (白英 climbing nightshade, Solani Lyrati Herba)
lóng kuí (龙葵 black nightshade, Solani Nigri Herba)

This is injected in doses of 2–4 ml in the flesh or in specific acupuncture points. This injection has a definite therapeutic effect on rectal carcinoma, stomach cancer, esophageal cancer, and cervical cancer.

When treating various forms of cancer, I frequently add 15–30 g/5 qián–1 liǎng of *bàn zhī lián* or *bàn biān lián* (Chinese lobelia) and *shān cí gū* (cremastra/pleione) to an appropriate decoction chosen on the basis of pattern identification and treatment determination.

DOSAGE

The dosage is generally 15–50 g/5 qián–1.5 liǎng.

<table>
<tr><td>

61. 白花蛇舌草
Bái Huā Shé Shé Cǎo
Oldenlandia

</td><td>

Oldenlandiae
Diffusae Herba

</td></tr>
</table>

Sweet and bland in flavor and cool in nature, *bái huā shé shé cǎo* (oldenlandia)[32] clears heat and resolves toxin, quickens the blood and disperses swelling, and disinhibits urine. In recent years, it has been used as an anti-cancer medicinal.

This medicinal combined with *zǐ huā dì dīng* (violet), *yě jú huā* (wild chrysanthemum flower), and *pú gōng yīng* (dandelion) is used for acute appendicitis. Combined with *bái máo gēn* (imperata), *hǎi jīn shā* (lygodium spore), and *chuān huáng bǎi* (Sìchuān phellodendron), it is used for damp-heat strangury (including acute urinary infection). Combined with *xuán shēn* (scrophularia), *jīn dēng lóng* (lantern plant calyx), *jīn yín huā* (lonicera), *huáng qín* (scutellaria), and *shè gān* (belamcanda), it is used for sore swollen throat and acute tonsillitis.

When treating various forms of cancer, I frequently add about 30–40 g/1–1.3 liǎng of this medicinal to an appropriate decoction medicine devised according to the principle of pattern identification as the basis of determining treatment. I may also add other Chinese medicinals and herbal medicines that are known to have anti-cancer effects, such as *shān cí gū* (cremastra/pleione), *bàn zhī lián* (bearded scutellaria), *é zhú* (curcuma rhizome), and *shān dòu gēn* (bushy sophora). The essential point is that this must be done in a formula that is varied in accordance with the signs; these medicinals are rarely used alone.

Dosage

The dosage is generally 20–50 g/7 qián–1.5 liǎng.

Anti-Cancer Agents

According to modern research reports, the following medicinals all have anti-cancer effects.

guā lóu (瓜蒌 trichosanthes, Trichosanthis Fructus)

shè gān (射干 belamcanda, Belamcandae Rhizoma)

zhū líng (猪苓 polyporus, Polyporus)

xià kū cǎo (夏枯草 prunella, Prunellae Spica)

huáng yào zǐ (黄药子 air potato, Dioscoreae Bulbiferae Rhizoma)

zhè chóng (蟅虫 ground beetle, Eupolyphaga seu Steleophaga)

quán chóng (全虫 scorpion, Scorpio)

wú gōng (蜈蚣 centipede, Scolopendra)

shuǐ zhì (水蛭 leech, Hirudo)

chán sū (蟾酥 toad venom, Bufonis Venenum)

---

[32] *Oldenlandia corymbosa* L. is often substituted for the correct species of *Oldenlandia diffusa* (Willd.) Roxb. The substitute is easily discerned by observing the number of flowers per leaf pair. The correct species has a single flower stemming from a leaf pair and *Oldenlandia corymbosa* has three or four flowers sprouting as a group from a leaf pair. (Ed.)

dān shēn (丹参 salvia, Salviae Miltiorrhizae Radix)

chì sháo (赤芍 red peony, Paeoniae Radix Rubra)

sān qī (三七 notoginseng, Notoginseng Radix)

dà xiǎo jì (大小蓟 Japanese/field thistle, Cirsii Japonici/Cirsii Herba)

yā dǎn zǐ (鸦胆子 brucea, Bruceae Fructus)

zǐ cǎo (紫草 arnebia/lithospermum, Arnebiae/Lithospermi Radix)

bǔ gǔ zhī (补骨脂 psoralea, Psoraleae Fructus)

bái zhú (白术 white atractylodes, Atractylodis Macrocephalae Rhizoma)

xióng huáng (雄黄 realgar, Realgar)

shān zhū yú (山茱萸 cornus, Corni Fructus) 9 g/3 qián

yín yáng huò (淫羊藿 epimedium, Epimedii Herba)

zào jiǎo cì (皂角刺 gleditsia thorn, Gleditsiae Spina)

xìng rén (杏仁 apricot kernel, Armeniacae Semen)

zhè bèi mǔ (浙贝母 Zhejiang fritillaria, Fritillariae Thunbergii Bulbus)

lái fú zǐ (莱菔子 radish seed, Raphani Semen)

é zhú (莪术 curcuma rhizome, Curcumae Rhizoma)

hǎi zǎo (海藻 sargassum, Sargassum)

kūn bù (昆布 kelp, Laminariae/Eckloniae Thallus)

shè xiāng (麝香 musk, Moschus)

wēi líng xiān (威灵仙 clematis, Clematidis Radix)

wū tóu (乌头 wild aconite, Aconiti Kusnezoffii Radix)

On the foundation created through proper application of the principle of pattern identification as the basis for treatment, it is possible to integrate medicinal natures with any special disease characteristics and patterns, and logically create an appropriate formula that can be varied according to the signs.

Lecture Ten
Composing Formulas
谈谈组织药方 *Tán Tán Zŭ Zhī Yào Fāng*

The composing of a medicinal formula (方剂 *fāng jì*), loosely referred to as 开方儿 *kāi fāngr* in Chinese, and "writing a medicinal prescription" in English, is what the physician does after identifying the pattern (辨证 *biàn zhèng*) and establishing the method (立法 *lì fă*). It involves choosing suitable medicinals on the basis of the requirements of the chosen method of treatment and on the requirement of the patient's specific condition. It also involves following the principles of formula composition, being aware of the interactions that occur when combining medicinals, and, on the basis of these considerations, determining the appropriate dosage. Formula composition is the practical application of treatment principles and is one of the important tasks the physican has to perform in treating illness. It is an essential element in the process of determining principles, methods, formulas, and medicinals (理、法、方、药 *lĭ, fă, fāng, yào*) within traditional Chinese medicine's system of determining treatment on the basis of pattern identification.

Through years of medical practice and the continuous process of drawing together experience in the fight against disease, physicians of the past gradually realized that by combining many single medicinals into a prescription they could focus the strengths of the medicinals and bring into play effects derived from the interaction between the ingredients of a formula, and thereby achieve an overall new medicinal strength to produce the best therapeutic result. Furthermore, well composed combinations allow each medicinal to assert its strengths while diminishing its weaknesses. After a prescription is formed, it can be varied according to pattern and flexibly transformed so that the range of application can become quite broad. Thereupon, they gradually began using composed medicinal prescriptions, and during the course of many years of practice, they accumulated a bountiful reservoir of methodologies and experience. One can say that the emergence of prescriptions is one of the great developments and advancements in the use of medicinals. Below, I have tried to use my personal experience to discuss the formation of prescriptions through a series of relevant issues.

1. **Compositional Principles for Prescriptions:** For a prescription to produce the best therapeutic effect, each medicinal must be allowed to exhibit its effects

to the greatest degree. Furthermore, we must use the interactions between medicinals, such as mutual reinforcing, fearing, mutual need, and empowering. In this way we can supplement what is insufficient, control what is excessive, and strengthen the therapeutic use of the formula. Thus, when composing a prescription, medicinals are not simply combined in equal proportions. They must be carefully gauged according to requirements of the treatment method and the priorities of the needs posed by the specific condition. It is generally said that a prescription should contain medicines in the roles of chief (sovereign), support (minister), assistant, and conductor (courier).[1]

1) **Chief medicinal** (主药 *zhǔ yào*): The chief medicinal directly addresses the condition or the cause of the disease. It treats the governing pattern and should resolve the primary contradictions in that pattern. It is the substance with the most ample medicinal strength directed at the governing pattern.

2) **Support medicinal** (辅药 *fǔ yào*): The support medicinal reinforces or controls the chief medicinal in a way that allows for the therapeutic effect to be brought into play even more effectively.

3) **Assistant medicinal** (佐药 *zuǒ yào*): The assistant medicinal treats concurrent patterns. It may also allow for even better utilization of medicinal strengths to develop beneficial conditions. The assistant strengthens the therapeutic effect of the chief and support medicinals.

4) **Conductor medicinal** (引药 *yǐn yào*): The conductor conducts the strength of the medicinals directly into the locus of the disease. It can also conduct medicinals upward, downward, to the exterior, or to the interior. The conductor harmonizes all the other medicinals, corrects the flavors, or may act as an excipient (a relatively inert substance that acts as a diluent or vehicle for other medicinals).

In addition, there is also a category known as "paradoxical assistant" (反佐药 *fǎn zuò yào*).[2] This refers to a small amount of cold medicinals added to a primarily hot formula or a small amount of hot medicinals added to a primarily cold formula, in order to enhance the treatment. Cases calling for paradoxical assistants are comparatively rare.

The general principles of prescription composition are described above. To give an example, consider *má huáng tāng* (Ephedra Decoction), which contains *má huáng* (ephedra), *guì zhī* (cinnamon twig), *xìng rén* (apricot kernel), and *gān cǎo* (licorice). This is the governing formula for greater yáng disease cold damage

---

[1]This book was written during the period in the People's Republic of China when socialist activists considered the names 君臣佐使 *jūn chén zuǒ shǐ* (sovereign, minister, assistant, and courier) to have a feudal ring and attempted to replace them with the neutral-sounding terms 主辅佐引 *zhǔ fǔ zuǒ yǐn* (chief, support, assistant, and conductor). The attempt failed, probably because of the weight of classical literature and because socialist activism soon went out of fashion. Consequently, the traditional terms 君臣佐使 *jūn chén zuǒ shǐ* are still used today. In the Chinese text of this book, Professor Jiāo uses the terms 主辅佐使 *zhǔ fǔ zuǒ shǐ* (chief, support, assistant and courier), idiosyncratically retaining two of the traditional terms. (Ed.)

[2]The concept of paradoxical assistant derives from the distinction between straight treatment (正治 *zhèng zhì*), i.e., treating cold with heat and treating heat with cold, and paradoxical treatment (反治 *fǎn zhì*), treating heat with heat and treating cold with cold. (Ed.)

and exterior repletion patterns (headache, aversion to cold, heat effusion (fever), absence of sweating, panting, generalized soreness and pain, and a floating, tight pulse). Within this formula, *má huáng*, the chief medicinal, promotes sweating with warmth and acridity and resolves the exterior and dissipates cold; *guì zhī*, the support medicinal, frees yáng with warmth and acridity, and strengthens the effect of *má huáng* to promote sweating and dissipate cold; *xìng rén*, the assistant medicinal, disinhibits the lung qì with bitterness and balance and also treats the concurrent pattern of panting. At the same time, the bitter downbearing nature of *xìng rén* prevents excessive dissipation due to the acridity of the chief medicinal. *Gān cǎo*, the conductor medicinal, harmonizes the center with sweetness and moderation, and it regulates the rest of the medicinals. The combination of these four medicinals promotes sweating with warmth and acridity, and it resolves the exterior and dissipates cold.

The example above describes the broad lines of formula composition. In a complicated or severe condition, it is acceptable to use two or three chief medicinals, two to four support medicinals, and three to five assistant and conductor medicinals, or even six or seven assistant and conductor medicinals. Sometimes a prescription is composed by using one chief and two or three supporting medicinals; sometimes it may have no supporting medicinals, but only two or three assistants or conductors. It is even possible that a prescription can be composed solely of a chief and a conductor. Thus, not every prescription will have medicinals serving as chief, support, assistant, conductor, and paradoxical assistant. Such decisions must be made according to the requirements of the method of treatment and the needs of the specific condition; one should not make them inflexibly.

2. Varying Prescriptions Flexibly: A prescription must reflect a definite composing principle, but the formula must also be flexibly varied to accord with changes in the signs. The frequently used methods for varying prescriptions are summarized below.

a) Variation by adding or removing medicinals: As an example, let us use *sì wèi bǔ qì tāng* (Four-Ingredient Qì-Supplementing Decoction) (this used to be called *sì jūn zǐ tāng* (Four Gentlemen Decoction)), which is composed of the four medicinals *dǎng shēn* (codonopsis) (or *rén shēn* (ginseng)) *bái zhú* (white atractylodes), *fú líng* (poria), and *gān cǎo* (licorice). When encountering a patient who has spleen-stomach vacuity yet is unable to receive supplementation (while taking this formula they experience symptoms such as stomach distention, oppression in the chest, abdominal distention, and poor appetite), adding *chén pí* (tangerine peel) to the formula will move qì and regulate the stomach and thereby avoid the problems described above. This formula, called *wǔ wèi yì gōng sǎn* (Five-Ingredient Special Achievement Powder), is a commonly used prescription for spleen qì vacuity. If the patient exhibits more severe phlegm-damp signs, such as a thick slimy white tongue fur, nausea, and retching counterflow, *bàn xià* (pinellia) and *chén pí* (tangerine peel) can be added to form *liù jūn zǐ tāng* (Six Gentlemen Decoction).[3] If there is also center burner qì stagnation with fullness in the stomach and abdominal distention, *mù xiāng* (costusroot) and *shā rén* (amomum) can be added to move qì, disperse distention, and harmonize the center. The formula is then called *xiāng xià liù jūn zǐ tāng* (Costusroot and Amomum Six Gentlemen Decoction).[4]

Another example of this is *xiǎo chái hú tāng* (Minor Bupleurum Decoction).

Xiǎo chái hú tāng 小柴胡汤　　　　　　　　　　Minor Bupleurum Decoction

---

chái hú (柴胡 bupleurum, Bupleuri Radix)

huáng qín (黄芩 scutellaria, Scutellariae Radix)

bàn xià (半夏 pinellia, Pinelliae Rhizoma)

gān cǎo (甘草 licorice, Glycyrrhizae Radix)

dǎng shēn (党参 codonopsis, Codonopsis Radix)

shēng jiāng (生姜 fresh ginger, Zingiberis Rhizoma Recens)

dà zǎo (大枣 jujube, Jujubae Fructus)

If the patient is extremely thirsty, remove *bàn xià* and add *tiān huā fěn* (trichosanthes root). If the patient has a strong constitution, the disease is new, and the right qì is not vacuous, remove *dǎng shēn*.

b) Varying the dosage: Let us consider *zhǐ zhú tāng* (Unripe Bitter Orange and White Atractylodes Decoction), which contains 24 g/8 qián of *zhǐ shí* (unripe bitter orange) and 12 g/4 qián of *bái zhú* (white atractylodes). The dosage of *zhǐ shí* is greater than that of *bái zhú*. The indications are accumulation and stagnation in the stomach duct and abdomen, hard fullness, and lumps. On the other hand, in *zhǐ zhú wán* (Unripe Bitter Orange and White Atractylodes Pill), which contains 30 g/1 liǎng of *zhǐ shí* (unripe bitter orange) and 60 g/2 liǎng of *bái zhú* (white atractylodes), the dosage of *bái zhú* is greater than that of *zhǐ shí* so that this becomes a formula that fortifies the spleen, harmonizes the center, and assists the center burner. In these two prescriptions, we can see that differences in the relative dosages change the effect of the formula and its relevant indications. (See Lecture One for more on this topic.)

c) Varying the combinations of qì and flavor: In *xiǎo jiàn zhōng tāng* (Minor Center-Fortifying Decoction), for example, which contains *guì zhī* (cinnamon twig), *bái sháo* (white peony), *zhì gān cǎo* (mix-fried licorice), *shēng jiāng* (fresh ginger), *dà zǎo* (jujube), and *yí táng* (malt sugar), a combination of sour and sweet flavors (*bái sháo* and *yí táng*) is chosen to engender yīn, and a combination of acrid and sweet flavors (*guì zhī* and *gān cǎo*) is chosen to engender yáng. The nature and flavor of the entire prescription is primarily sweet, moderate, and warm. This is

---

[3]In the original text, *liù jūn zǐ tāng* (Six Gentlemen Decoction) is called *liù wèi tāng* (Six-Ingredient Decoction). See footnote on page 3 on term changes in the People's Republic of China. (Ed.)

[4]In the original text, *xiāng xià liù jūn zǐ tāng* (Costusroot and Amomum Six Gentlemen Decoction) is called *xiāng xià liù wèi tāng* (Costusroot and Amomum Six-Ingredient Decoction). See footnote on page 3. (Ed.)

an effective formula for the treatment of vacuity taxation abdominal urgency and abdominal pain. Another example is *wū méi wán* (Mume Pill):

Wū méi wán 乌梅丸   Mume Pill

---

wū méi (乌梅 mume, Mume Fructus)

xì xīn (细辛 asarum, Asari Herba)

guì zhī (桂枝 cinnamon twig, Cinnamomi Ramulus)

fù zǐ (附子 aconite, Aconiti Radix Lateralis Praeparata)

dǎng shēn (党参 codonopsis, Codonopsis Radix)

huáng bǎi (黄柏 phellodendron, Phellodendri Cortex)

gān jiāng (干姜 dried ginger, Zingiberis Rhizoma)

huáng lián (黄连 coptis, Coptidis Rhizoma)

chuān jiāo (川椒 zanthoxylum, Zanthoxyli Pericarpium)

dāng guī (当归 Chinese angelica, Angelicae Sinensis Radix)

This formula uses the special characteristics of combining sour, acrid, warm, and bitter characteristics (roundworms soften with sourness, subside with acridity, become tranquil with warmth, and are made to descend by bitterness) to create an effective formula for the treatment of roundworm, especially in patients vomiting up roundworm. In recent years, this formula has frequently been used to treat biliary ascariasis; varied in accordance with the signs, it has an excellent effect. Furthermore, to clear heat and drain fire, one should mostly use bitter, cold ingredients, whereas to enrich yīn and downbear fire one should use sweet, cold ingredients.

d) Variations in function as a result of combinations: *Huáng lián* (coptis), for example, is combined with *wú yú* (evodia) to make *zuǒ jīn wán* (Left-Running Metal Pill), which is indicated for liver depression transforming into heat and invading the stomach causing acid swallowing and clamoring stomach. *Huáng lián* combined with *mù xiāng* (costusroot), makes *xiāng lián wán* (Costusroot and Coptis Pill), is indicated for damp-heat dysentery with tenesmus. *Huáng lián* combined with *ròu guì* (cinnamon bark), which makes *jiāo tài wán* (Peaceful Interaction Pill), is used to treat noninteraction of the heart and kidney causing insomnia. *Huáng lián* combined with *bàn xià* (pinellia) and *guā lóu* (trichosanthes) makes *xiǎo xiàn xiōng tāng* (Minor Chest Bind Decoction), a formula used for glomus, oppression, and pain below the heart. Furthermore, experiments with *sháo yào gān cǎo tāng* (Peony and Licorice Decoction) have shown that *bái sháo yào* (white peony) accelerates and excites intestinal movement while *gān cǎo* (licorice) has the opposite effect of inhibiting intestinal movement. A combination of the two medicinals creates a marked inhibitory effect, especially in diseases characterized by abnormal intestinal excitation. In addition, recent research reports of animal experiments with *bǔ zhōng yì qì tāng* (Center-Supplementing Qì-Boosting Decoction), which comprises *huáng qí* (astragalus), *dǎng shēn* (codonopsis), *bái zhú* (white atractylodes), *dāng guī* (Chinese angelica), *chén pí* (tangerine peel), *gān cǎo* (licorice), *shēng má* (cimicifuga), and *chái hú* (bupleurum), revealed that *shēng má* and *chái hú* have a pronounced cooperative effect. They strengthen the effect of the other medicinals, particularly with regards to their effect on peristalsis. If these two medicinals are removed, the effect on peristalsis is weakened. If only *shēng má* (cimicifuga) or *chái hú* (bupleurum) is used, the effects mentioned above are completely absent. Thus we can see that variations in function as a result of combinations has an important role in composing formulas. (See Lecture One for further discussion of this issue.)

e) Variations due to differences in preparation form: Differences in preparation create differences in therapeutic effect that naturally influence formula composition. Generally, acute diseases and severe diseases are treated using decoctions. Decoction prescriptions should not include too many different medicinals. Normally, the number of ingredients should not exceed nine to twelve. Examples include:

Dāng guī bǔ xuè tāng 当归补血汤   Chinese Angelica Blood-Supplementing Decoction

---

huáng qí (黄芪 astragalus, Astragali Radix)
dāng guī (当归 Chinese angelica, Angelicae Sinensis Radix)

Sì wù tāng 四物汤   Four Agents Decoction

---

shú dì huáng (熟地黄 cooked rehmannia, Rehmanniae Radix Praeparata)
dāng guī (当归 Chinese angelica, Angelicae Sinensis Radix)
bái sháo (白芍 white peony, Paeoniae Radix Alba)
chuān xiōng (川芎 chuanxiong, Chuanxiong Rhizoma)

Bā zhēn tāng 八珍汤   Eight-Gem Decoction

---

dǎng shēn (党参 codonopsis, Codonopsis Radix)
bái zhú (白术 white atractylodes, Atractylodis Macrocephalae Rhizoma)
fú líng (茯苓 poria, Poria)
gān cǎo (甘草 licorice, Glycyrrhizae Radix)
shú dì huáng (熟地黄 cooked rehmannia, Rehmanniae Radix Praeparata)
dāng guī (当归 Chinese angelica, Angelicae Sinensis Radix)
bái sháo (白芍 white peony, Paeoniae Radix Alba)
chuān xiōng (川芎 chuanxiong, Chuanxiong Rhizoma)

Shí quán dà bǔ tāng 十全大补汤   Perfect Major Supplementation Decoction

---

Eight-Gem Decoction (八珍汤 *bā zhēn tāng*) plus
huáng qí (黄芪 astragalus, Astragali Radix)
ròu guì (肉桂 cinnamon bark, Cinnamomi Cortex)

Pills tend to be used in chronic diseases and during recovery from illness. In general, pill preparations are commonly taken with more frequency; thus prescriptions for pills can contain a larger variety of medicinals. For example, *rén shēn zài zào wán* (Ginseng Renewal Powder), *biē jiǎ jiān wán* (Turtle Shell Decocted Pill), and *ān kūn zàn yù wán* (Female-Quieting Procreation Pill). Some pills contain thirty or forty medicinals.

In vacuity patterns, paste preparations can also be used. In prescriptions for paste preparations, generally we choose medicinals that have abundant juice, such as *shēng dì huáng* (dried/fresh rehmannia), *mài dōng* (ophiopogon), *tiān dōng* (asparagus), *xiān shí hú* (fresh dendrobium), *lí zhī* (pear juice), *fēng mì* (honey), and *bīng táng* (rock candy). These are easy to make into a paste. In depression patterns and acute patterns, we may also use powders. Examples are given below.

Xiāo yáo sǎn 逍遥散   Free Wanderer Powder

---

chái hú (柴胡 bupleurum, Bupleuri Radix)

bái sháo (白芍 white peony, Paeoniae Radix Alba)

dāng guī (当归 Chinese angelica, Angelicae Sinensis Radix)

chén pí (陈皮 tangerine peel, Citri Reticulatae Pericarpium)

bái zhú (白术 white atractylodes, Atractylodis Macrocephalae Rhizoma)

wēi jiāng (煨姜 roasted ginger, Zingiberis Rhizoma Tostum)

fú líng (茯苓 poria, Poria)

gān cǎo (甘草 licorice, Glycyrrhizae Radix)

bò hé (薄荷 mint, Menthae Herba)

Sì nì sǎn 四逆散   Counterflow Cold Powder

---

chái hú (柴胡 bupleurum, Bupleuri Radix)

zhǐ shí (枳实 unripe bitter orange, Aurantii Fructus Immaturus)

bái sháo (白芍 white peony, Paeoniae Radix Alba)

gān cǎo (甘草 licorice, Glycyrrhizae Radix)

Liù yī sǎn 六一散   Six-to-One Powder

---

huá shí (滑石 talcum, Talcum)

gān cǎo (甘草 licorice, Glycyrrhizae Radix)

Kāi guān sǎn 开关散   Gate-Opening Powder

---

zào jiǎo (皂角 gleditsia, Gleditsiae Fructus)

xì xīn (细辛 asarum, Asari Herba)

In addition, powder formulas can also be used. The ingredients are ground to a rough powder and decocted in water (a preparation known as a "boiled powder") or ground to a fine powder and taken directly with warm water or wine. Other preparations include washes and gargles. When writing a prescription, it is important to pay attention to the special characteristics of each of these.

This is a description of the general situation with regards to variations due to differences in preparation. Because this discussion is focused on decoctions and their variations in medicinal composition, the other preparation methods are not discussed further. Given all of the points that I have made above, we can see the importance of flexibly varying prescriptions.

3. The Relationship Between Prescription and Treatment Method: The formulation of a prescription must be guided by the requirements of the method of treatment. Physicians of the past described this process as "using the method to unite the prescription" (以法统方 *yǐ fǎ tǒng fāng*). The idea is that the effect of the prescription should accord with the requirements of the treatment method; there should be a union between the method and the prescription. For example, if the method of treatment is to supplement qì, one forms a prescription using a formula like *sì wèi bǔ qì tāng* (Four-Ingredient Qì-Supplementing Decoction) (formerly called *sì jūn zǐ tāng* (Four Gentlemen Decoction)) or *bǔ zhōng yì qì tāng* (Center-Supplementing Qì-Boosting Decoction), and varying it according to signs; if the method of treatment is to supplement the blood, one uses a formula like *sì wù tāng* (Four Agents Decoction) or *rén shēn yǎng róng tāng* (Ginseng Construction-Nourishing Decoction), varied in accordance with signs; if the method of treatment is to supplement kidney yīn, one uses a formula like *liù wèi dì huáng tāng* (Six-Ingredient Rehmannia Decoction), varied according to signs; if the method of treatment is to supplement kidney yáng, one uses a formula like *guì fù dì huáng tāng* (Cinnamon, Aconite, and Rehmanniae Decoction), also known as *shèn qì wán* (Kidney Qì Pill), varied with the signs; if the method of treatment is draining precipitation, one uses a formula like *dà chéng qì tāng* (Major Qì-Coordinating Decoction) or *xiǎo chéng qì tāng* (Minor Qì-Coordinating Decoction), varied with the signs. Nevertheless, one must also be aware of the reciprocal relationship that there are "many formulas within one method and many methods within one formula" (一法之中可有数方，一方之中可有数法 *yī fǎ zhī zhōng kě yǒu shù fāng, yī fāng zhī zhōng kě yǒu shù fǎ*). For example, within the method of precipitation, there is *dà chéng qì tāng* (Major Qì-Coordinating Decoction) (urgent precipitation), *tiáo wèi chéng qì tāng* (Stomach-Regulating Qì-Coordinating Decoction) (moderate precipitation), *zēng yè chéng qì tāng* (Humor-Increasing Qì-Coordinating Decoction) (moistening precipitation), and *dà huáng fù zǐ tāng* (Rhubarb and Aconite Decoction) (warming precipitation). Thus we can see "many formulas within one method." Furthermore, in the formula *fáng fēng tōng shèng sǎn* (Saposhnikovia Sage-Inspired Powder) we can see the methods of sweating (resolving the exterior), clearing (clearing heat), and precipitation (draining fire) as well as quickening stasis. This is an example of "many methods within one formula."

Fáng fēng tōng shèng sǎn 防风通圣散   Saposhnikovia Sage-Inspired Powder

---

fáng fēng (防风 saposhnikovia, Saposhnikoviae Radix)

chuān xiōng (川芎 chuanxiong, Chuanxiong Rhizoma)

dāng guī (当归 Chinese angelica, Angelicae Sinensis Radix)

chì sháo (赤芍 red peony, Paeoniae Radix Rubra)

dà huáng (大黄 rhubarb, Rhei Radix et Rhizoma)

bò hé (薄荷 mint, Menthae Herba)

má huáng (麻黄 ephedra, Ephedrae Herba)

lián qiáo (连翘 forsythia, Forsythiae Fructus)

máng xiāo (芒硝 mirabilite, Natrii Sulfas)

shēng shí gāo (生石膏 crude gypsum, Gypsum Fibrosum Crudum)

huáng qín (黄芩 scutellaria, Scutellariae Radix)

jié gěng (桔梗 platycodon, Platycodonis Radix)

huá shí (滑石 talcum, Talcum)

gān cǎo (甘草 licorice, Glycyrrhizae Radix)

jīng jiè (荆芥 schizonepeta, Schizonepetae Herba)

bái zhú (白术 white atractylodes, Atractylodis Macrocephalae Rhizoma)

zhī zǐ (栀子 gardenia, Gardeniae Fructus)

shēng jiāng (生姜 fresh ginger, Zingiberis Rhizoma Recens)

When composing a prescription, therefore, we must pay attention to using the method to unite the prescription, but at the same time, we must also be aware of the formulas within the method and the methods within the formula. The most important point is the unity between the prescription and the method of treatment.

4. Drawing Upon and Using Effective Formulas: When composing a prescription, it is important to bear in mind effective formulas, both ancient and modern. Taking such formulas as a basis for treatment, their ingredients can be varied in accordance with the condition and age of the patient, the weather, and any relevant geographical features. For example, if the pattern identified is warm disease qì-aspect intense heat, the required method of treatment is to clear qì-aspect heat, for which *shí gāo zhī mǔ tāng* (Gypsum and Anemarrhena Decoction) (formerly called *bái hǔ tāng* (White Tiger Decoction)) can be chosen and varied in accordance with signs.

Shí gāo zhī mǔ tāng 石膏知母汤   Gypsum and Anemarrhena Decoction

---

shēng shí gāo (生石膏 crude gypsum, Gypsum Fibrosum Crudum)

zhī mǔ (知母 anemarrhena, Anemarrhenae Rhizoma)

gān cǎo (甘草 licorice, Glycyrrhizae Radix)

gēng mǐ (粳米 non-glutinous rice, Oryzae Semen)

If the patient has had a high fever for many days and the fluids have already been damaged, add *xiān lú gēn* (fresh phragmites), *tiān huā fěn* (trichosanthes root), or other medicinals in this category. If the patient either has a weak constitution, is older, or has already had a high fever for a number of days so that the right qì is insufficient, add medicinals such as *dǎng shēn* (codonopsis), *bái rén shēn* (white ginseng), or other medicinals in this category. If the patient has already had a high fever for several days and originally there was extreme thirst with copious intake, but now the patient is not too thirsty, the tongue body has become red, the fever is worse in the afternoon and the evening, and the pulse has become finer than before, this is evidence that the warm disease evil in the qì aspect is entering the construction aspect. At this time, the method of treatment is to clear qì-aspect heat and clear construction-aspect heat. One can vary *shí gāo zhī mǔ tāng* (Gypsum and Anemarrhena Decoction) by removing *gān cǎo* (licorice) and adding *shēng dì huáng* (dried/fresh rehmannia) and *xuán shēn* (scrophularia), to clear construction-aspect heat. Also add *jīn yín huā* (lonicera) and *lián qiáo* (forsythia) to outthrust construction and clear qì, so that the evil heat is abducted from the construction towards the qì and then outthrusted to the exterior. This prescription uses relevant portions of *shí gāo zhī mǔ tāng* (Gypsum Anemarrhena Decoction) and *qīng yíng tāng* (Construction-Clearing Decoction), but it primarily clears qì-aspect heat.

If warm disease evil is gradually entering the construction aspect and one observes persistent generalized heat [effusion] (fever) that is severe at night and mild in the morning, a crimson red tongue, absence of thirst, indistinct macules and papules beginning to appear on the body, chest, or back, and a fine rapid pulse, then the method of treatment should primarily be to clear construction-aspect heat. Add *dān shēn* (salvia), *mài dōng* (ophiopogon), *huáng lián* (coptis), *zhú yè* (lophatherum), and *xī jiǎo* (rhinoceros horn) to the previous formula in order to strengthen its capacity to clear construction-aspect heat. Because evil heat has already left the qì aspect, remove *shēng shí gāo* (crude gypsum) and *zhī mǔ* (anemarrhena). This prescription employs *qīng yíng tāng* (Construction-Clearing Decoction) from *Wēn Bìng Tiáo Biàn* (温病条辨 "Systematized Identification of Warm Diseases"), varied in accordance with the signs.

If the patient still shows evidence of a qì-aspect pattern, then the method of treatment should be to clear both qì and construction. In that case, do not remove *shēng shí gāo* (crude gypsum) and *zhī mǔ* (anemarrhena). The resultant prescription reflects the spirit of *yù nǚ jiān* (Jade Lady Brew), which can then be varied according to the signs.

If the patient has thick yellow tongue fur with scant liquid, bound stool that has not moved for several days, delirious speech at night, abdominal fullness with inability to eat, and a deep replete and forceful pulse, and is observed picking at bedclothes, this indicates a change to yáng brightness (*yáng míng*) warm disease with heat binding in the intestines and stomach. The method of treatment should then be precipitation. Use the previous formula, but remove *dān shēn* (salvia), *huáng lián* (coptis), *xī jiǎo* (rhinoceros horn), *zhú yè* (lophatherum), *shēng shí gāo* (crude gypsum), and *zhī mǔ* (anemarrhena) and add *shēng dà huáng* (raw rhubarb) and *máng xiāo* (mirabilite), in order to drain bound heat from the stomach and intestines. This new prescription is based on *zēng yè chéng qì tāng* (Humor-Increasing Qì-Coordinating Decoction). If the patient has a Western medical diagnosis of epidemic encephalitis B, we can integrate the results of modern medical research and add *dà qīng yè* (isatis leaf) and *bǎn lán gēn* (isatis root), or inject "clear heat and resolve toxin [injection]," which is *qīng wēn bài dú yǐn* (Scourge-Clearing Toxin-Vanquishing Beverage) processed into an injection fluid. Thus we can see that as the disease pattern changes, the method of treatment must also change. As the method of treatment changes, the composition of the prescription must change accordingly. During the process of transformation in composing prescriptions, we can draw upon and use ancient or modern formulas that are known to be effective by paying attention to varying them in accordance with the signs.

5. Integrating Traditional Experience with the Findings of Modern Research: The experience of past physicians in composing formulas can be integrated with the findings of modern research in order to create formulas. If when composing a prescription one is unable to find a suitable formula amongst ancient or modern prescriptions, one can follow the previously described principles and methods in combination with the findings of modern scientific research and create a new formula.

For example, if the method of treatment is to resolve the exterior with warmth and acridity, choose *jīng jiè* (schizonepeta), *fáng fēng* (saposhnikovia), *sū yè* (perilla leaf), *qiāng huó* (notopterygium), and *shēng jiāng* (fresh ginger) for the prescription; if the method of treatment is resolving the exterior with coolness and acridity, choose *sāng yè* (mulberry leaf), *jú huā* (chrysanthemum), *jīn yín huā* (lonicera), *bò hé* (mint), *lián qiáo* (forsythia), and *dòu chǐ* (fermented soybean) for the prescription; if the method of treatment is to nourish yīn and subdue yáng, choose *shēng dì huáng* (dried/fresh rehmannia), *bái sháo* (white peony), *xuán shēn* (scrophularia), *mài dōng* (ophiopogon), and *shí hú* (dendrobium) to nourish yīn and choose *shēng shí jué míng* (crude abalone shell), *shēng mǔ lì* (crude oyster shell), and *zhēn zhū mǔ* (mother-of-pearl) to subdue yáng; if the method of treatment is to settle the liver and extinguish wind, choose *shēng dài zhě shí* (crude hematite), *huáng qín* (scutellaria), *shēng tiě luò* (iron flakes), *bái jí lí* (tribulus), *gōu téng* (uncaria), *quán xiē* (scorpion), and *líng yáng jiǎo* (antelope horn) for the prescription. The formulas *bǔ yáng huán wǔ tāng* (Yáng-Supplementing Five-Returning Decoction) and *gé xià zhú yū tāng* (Infradiaphragmatic Stasis-Expelling Decoction) from *Yī Lín Gǎi Cuò* (医林改错 "Correction of Errors from Medical Circles") and *zhèn gān xī fēng tāng* (Liver-Settling Wind-Extinguishing Decoction) from *Zhōng Zhōng Cān Xī Lù* (衷中参西录 "Heart of Chinese Tradition with References to Western Knowledge") are all examples of these authors creating effective formulas by applying principles of formula composition, drawing on traditional experience in the use of medicinals, and taking account of their own personal experience.

In order to improve treatment efficacy and advance the development of medical studies, we should draw upon the findings of modern scientific research, while simultaneously drawing upon the experience of physicians of the past in composing medicinal formulas. Examples of this strategy include treating acute appendicitis with *lán wěi huà yū tāng* (Appendix Stasis-Transforming Decoction) or *lán wěi qīng huà tāng* (Appendix Clearing and Transforming Decoction), treating acute pancreatitis with *qīng yí tāng* (Pancreas-Clearing Decoction), treating intestinal obstruction with *gān suì tōng jié tāng* (Kansui Bind-Freeing Decoction), treating ectopic pregnancy with *jiā wèi huó luò xiào líng dān* (Supplemented Network-Quickening Miraculous Effect Elixir), or even *shēn fù jiāng zhù shè yè* (Ginseng, Aconite, and Ginger Injection Fluid), *shēng mài sǎn zhù shè yè* (Pulse-Engendering Powder Injection Fluid), *fù fāng dān shēn zhù shè yè* (Compound Salvia Injection Fluid), *chuān xiōng jiǎn zhù shè yè* (Chuanxiong Alkali Injection Fluid), *shè xiāng pēn wù jì* (Musk Spray), and *rè shēn pēn wù jì* (Hot Ginseng Spray).

Lán wěi huà yū tāng 阑尾化瘀汤   Appendix Stasis-Transforming Decoction

---

chuān liàn zǐ (川楝子 toosendan, Toosendan Fructus)

yán hú suǒ (延胡索 corydalis, Corydalis Rhizoma)

dān pí (丹皮 moutan, Moutan Cortex)

táo rén (桃仁 peach kernel, Persicae Semen)

mù xiāng (木香 costusroot, Aucklandiae Radix)

jīn yín huā (金银花 lonicera, Lonicerae Flos)

shēng dà huáng (生大黄 raw rhubarb, Rhei Radix et Rhizoma Crudi)

Lán wěi qīng huà tāng 阑尾清化汤   Appendix Clearing and Transforming Decoction

---

jīn yín huā (金银花 lonicera, Lonicerae Flos)

pú gōng yīng (蒲公英 dandelion, Taraxaci Herba)

dān pí (丹皮 moutan, Moutan Cortex)

dà huáng (大黄 rhubarb, Rhei Radix et Rhizoma)

chuān liàn zǐ (川楝子 toosendan, Toosendan Fructus)

chì sháo (赤芍 red peony, Paeoniae Radix Rubra)

táo rén (桃仁 peach kernel, Persicae Semen)

shēng gān cǎo (生甘草 raw licorice, Glycyrrhizae Radix Cruda)

Qīng yí tāng 清胰汤   Pancreas-Clearing Decoction

---

chái hú (柴胡 bupleurum, Bupleuri Radix)

huáng qín (黄芩 scutellaria, Scutellariae Radix)

hú huáng lián (胡黄连 picrorhiza, Picrorhizae Rhizoma)

bái sháo (白芍 white peony, Paeoniae Radix Alba)

mù xiāng (木香 costusroot, Aucklandiae Radix)

yán hú suǒ (延胡索 corydalis, Corydalis Rhizoma)

shēng dà huáng (生大黄 raw rhubarb, Rhei Radix et Rhizoma Crudi)

máng xiāo (芒硝 mirabilite, Natrii Sulfas)

Gān suì tōng jié tāng 甘遂通结汤   Kansui Bind-Freeing Decoction

---

gān suì mò (甘遂末 kansui powder, Kansui Radix Pulverata)

táo rén (桃仁 peach kernel, Persicae Semen)

chì sháo (赤芍 red peony, Paeoniae Radix Rubra)

niú xī (牛膝 achyranthes, Achyranthis Bidentatae Radix)

hòu pò (厚朴 officinal magnolia bark, Magnoliae Officinalis Cortex)

dà huáng (大黄 rhubarb, Rhei Radix et Rhizoma)

mù xiāng (木香 costusroot, Aucklandiae Radix)

Jiā wèi huó luó xiào líng dān 加味活络效灵丹   Supplemented Network-Quickening
Miraculous Effect Elixir

---

dān shēn (丹参 salvia, Salviae Miltiorrhizae Radix)

chì sháo (赤芍 red peony, Paeoniae Radix Rubra)

táo rén (桃仁 peach kernel, Persicae Semen)

rǔ xiāng (乳香 frankincense, Olibanum)

mò yào (没药 myrrh, Myrrha)

All of these formulas absorb the invaluable experience of past physicians in composing prescriptions and integrate this with the findings of modern scientific research, breaking down old restrictions and foreign conventions, daring to create new formulas and enhance therapeutic effects. In time we will absorb and integrate the fruits of modern scientific research, integrating Chinese and Western medicine and creating new formulas.

In the sections above, I have introduced the principles of formula composition and flexible variation in accordance with the signs, as well as how to employ effective formulas. Below, I present some of my own thoughts regarding prescription composition using case histories.

Case 1. Mr. Zhōng. 22 years old. Date of first visit: November 27, 1975.

Brief history: During the previous year, the patient had frequently experienced bleeding from the gums. Each time, he had to go to an oral specialist to stanch the bleeding. This time when the bleeding occurred the physician was unable to stanch it and he was brought into the emergency department observation ward. On 11/19, they removed two front incisors on the left, then used thread to tie off the small blood vessels. After this procedure, however, the bleeding continued. They gave the patient large doses of hemostatic injections, and also had him take a hemostatic powder internally and apply it topically. The patient also took *yún nán bái yào* (Yunnan White) internally, but the bleeding did not stop. On 11/27, I was brought in on the case and treated him with integrated Chinese-Western medicine.

Presenting signs: bleeding gums at the front incisors with fresh red blood, swollen and distended sensation throughout the gums, throbbing of the heart, a sensation of upward rushing movement in the left rear region of the brain that seemed to follow the throbbing of the heart, thirst with ability to drink, bound stool, old yellow tongue fur, rapid pulse (stringlike slippery and forceful on the left; stringlike fine and slightly slippery on the right).

Pattern identification: The yáng brightness (*yáng míng*) channel enters the teeth, and the gums also belong to the yáng brightness channel. Seeing that this patient was young and had a vigorous constitution, and that the pulse was stringlike, slippery and forceful, we knew that this was a repletion pattern. The thirst with ability to drink, gum swelling, yellow tongue fur, and rapid pulse indicate stomach channel repletion heat. The bound stool, old yellow tongue fur, and slippery rapid forceful pulse are manifestations of large intestinal heat bind. The incessant gum bleeding, fresh red blood, and stringlike rapid forceful pulse indicate the frenetic movement of hot blood. Throbbing of the heart and upward-surging pulsation in the back of the head are evidence of heat accumulation transforming into fire, so that the blood follows the qì as it upbears and the qì follows the blood as it ascends. According to the pulse and signs, the diagnosis is intense fire-heat in the yáng brightness channel (stomach and large intestine) with frenetic movement of hot blood giving rise to bleeding gums.

Method of treatment: clear and drain yáng brightness, and cool the blood and stanch bleeding.

According to the requirements of the method of treatment, clearing and draining yáng brightness is the key. The selected formula must enter the yáng brightness channel and clear and drain yáng brightness channel fire-heat. I thought of *bái hǔ tāng* (White Tiger Decoction), [5] which clears evil heat from the qì aspect of the yáng brightness channel, and the various qì-coordinating decoctions that drain fire-heat bind in the yáng brightness channel. From these I selected *shēng shí gāo* (crude gypsum) to clear yáng brightness qì-aspect evil heat and *shēng dà huáng* (raw rhubarb) to drain large intestinal heat bind as the chief medicinals. To this I added the supporting medicinals *zhī mǔ* (anemarrhena) and *huáng qín* (scutellaria), to help clear heat and drain fire. Furthermore, one of the requirements of the method of treatment was to cool the blood, because this patient had exuberant yáng brightness channel fire-heat due to which both the qì and blood were hot, the blood was distressed by heat, and there was frenetic movement of hot blood, causing incessant bleeding gums. Thus, without clearing heat and cooling the blood, I would not be able to reach the goal of stanching bleeding. Therefore, I added *shēng dì huáng* (dried/fresh rehmannia) and *xuán shēn* (scrophularia) to cool the blood and downbear fire. Furthermore, because the disease had already persisted for more than ten days and the bleeding was copious, the resultant constipation reflected not only the heat bind, but also liquid damage. Consequently, I also added *mài dōng* (ophiopogon) to enrich yīn and cool the blood (with *shēng dì huáng* (dried/fresh rehmannia), *xuán shēn* (scrophularia), and *shēng dà huáng* (raw rhubarb); this has an effect like *zēng yè chéng qì tāng* (Humor-Increasing Qì-Co-ordinating Decoction). These were all considered assistant medicinals. Finally, following the principle of "treating the tip in acute patterns," I also added the conductors *bái máo gēn* (imperata), *dà xiǎo jì* (Japanese/field thistle), and *shēng ǒu jié* (raw lotus root node), to cool the blood and stanch bleeding. The full prescription is below:

shēng shí gāo (生石膏 crude gypsum, Gypsum Fibrosum Crudum)
    47 g/1.6 liǎng (precook)

shēng dà huáng (生大黃 raw rhubarb, Rhei Radix et Rhizoma Crudi)
    6 g/2 qián

zhī mǔ (知母 anemarrhena, Anemarrhenae Rhizoma) 9 g/3 qián

huáng qín (黃芩 scutellaria, Scutellariae Radix) 12 g/4 qián

---

[5]In the original text, *bái hǔ tāng* (White Tiger Decoction) is called *shí gāo zhī mǔ tāng* (Gypsum and Anemarrhena Decoction). See footnote on page 3 on term changes in the People's Republic of China. (Ed.)

shēng dì huáng (生地黄 dried/fresh rehmannia, Rehmanniae Radix Exsiccata seu Recens) 25 g/6 qián

xuán shēn (玄参 scrophularia, Scrophulariae Radix) 30 g/1 liǎng

mài dōng (麦冬 ophiopogon, Ophiopogonis Radix) 9 g/3 qián

bái máo gēn (白茅根 imperata, Imperatae Rhizoma) 30 g/1 liǎng

dà xiǎo jì (大小蓟 Japanese/field thistle, Cirsii Japonici/Cirsii Herba) each 15 g/5 qián

shēng ǒu jié (生藕节 raw lotus root node, Nelumbinis Rhizomatis Nodus Crudus) 30 g/1 liǎng

To be decocted with water. Four packets to be taken.

The evening after taking the first packet, the bleeding stopped. The patient continued on the formula with the following modifications varied in accordance with signs: *shēng dài zhě shí* (crude hematite), *dì gǔ pí* (lycium root bark), *yuán míng fěn* (refined mirabilite), *dān pí* (moutan), and *qiàn cǎo tàn* (charred madder). Altogether he took thirteen packets, after which the disease was cured and he left the hospital. He continued on the formula (the above formula with modifications) for more than ten additional packets in order to consolidate the therapeutic effect. On a follow-up visit on January 25, 1977, he reported that since taking the formula, he had been working normally and had not experienced any recurrences of gum bleeding.

Case 2: Mr. Cáo, 18 years old. Date of first visit: June 10, 1970.

Current disease history and current pathomechanism: For more than ten days, the patient had cough and shortness of breath. The cough would cause chest and rib-side pain, which was more pronounced on the left rib-side. When sleeping, he was only able to lie on his side—he could not lie supine. Even small movement would give rise to shortness of breath and panting. He reported dry mouth, but no desire to drink water. He had a poor appetite, yet urination and bowel movements were normal. His tongue fur was thin and light yellow. His pulse was deep, fine, and rapid.

Examination summary: Normal development and nourishment, marked sickly appearance, clear spirit-mind, and shortness of breath when speaking. Chest percussion diagnosis: The upper, middle, and lower areas of the left side of the chest were all flat sounding. The border of cardiac dullness had disappeared. Auscultation: The breath sound on the left side had disappeared. The heart had displaced towards the right side and the heart sounds were only heard on the right side. No murmur was noted. Roentgenoscopic examination: Left-sided exudative pleurisy, mediastinum forced to the right.

Pattern identification: On the basis of the symptoms of cough, chest and rib-side pain, shortness of breath, cough causing pain, dry mouth without desire to drink, and being only able to lie on one side, we know that the qì dynamic of the chest and lung was inhibited, and that water-rheum had collected in the chest and rib-side. In consideration of pulse and signs, the condition was diagnosed as **suspended rheum**[565] (旋饮 *xuán yǐn*).

Method of treatment: Expel water and disperse rheum.

According to the requirements of the method of treatment in combination with the pathomechanism, we considered that the suspended rheum was the result of water-rheum collected in the chest and rib-side. In this patient the collected water-rheum was copious so it was appropriate to urgently disperse rheum. In the *Jīn Guì Yào Lüè* (金匮要略 "Essential Prescriptions of the Golden Coffer"), we find *shí zǎo tāng* (Ten Jujubes Decoction), which, although it treats suspended rheum, contains toxic medicinals and has a harsh attacking action. This patient's disease had already persisted for more than half a month. His food intake was scant, even small movements would cause panting, and the right qì was already vacuous; therefore this formula was not suitable. Thus I chose to treat the suspended rheum using *jiāo mù guā lóu tāng* (Zanthoxylum Seed and Trichosanthes Formula), a formula from *Yī Chún Shèng Yì* (医醇賸义 "Enriching the Meaning of the Wine of Medicine"), varied in accordance with signs. When treating water-rheum, one must use the three channels of lung (abduct water from its high source 导水必自高源 *dǎo shuǐ bì zì gāo yuán*), spleen (build up to create an embankment 筑以防堤 *zhú yǐ fáng tí*), and kidney (allow the water to flow into its gully 使水归壑 *shǐ shuǐ guī hè*).[6] Thus the chief medicinals disinhibit lung qì, i.e., *chuān jiāo mù* (zanthoxylum seed) disperses water swelling and expels rheum, and *guā lóu* (trichosanthes) loosens the chest and transforms phlegm. *Tíng lì zǐ* (lepidium/descurainia), *sāng bái pí* (mulberry root bark), *xìng rén* (apricot kernel), and *zhǐ qiào* (bitter orange) drain phlegm and water from the lung, normalize qì, and downbear counterflow; as supporting medicinals they assist *jiāo mù* and *guā lóu* by increasing the downbearing and draining of phlegm and water. The assistant medicinals, *fú líng* (poria), *zhū líng* (polyporus), and *dōng guā pí* (wax gourd rind), disinhibit dampness to fortify the spleen. Also, the conductors *zé xiè* (alisma) and *chē qián zǐ* (plantago seed) abduct water downward so that it goes out with the urine. In addition, *guì zhī* (cinnamon twig) warms and assists the yáng qì of the kidney and bladder to strengthen bladder qì transformation so that water is disinhibited. The entire prescription is written below:

> *chuān jiāo mù* (川椒目 zanthoxylum seed, Zanthoxyli Semen) 9 g/3 qián
>
> *guā lóu* (瓜蒌 trichosanthes, Trichosanthis Fructus) 30 g/1 liǎng
>
> *sāng bái pí* (桑白皮 mulberry root bark, Mori Cortex) 12 g/4 qián
>
> *tíng lì zǐ* (葶苈子 lepidium/descurainia, Lepidii/Descurainiae Semen)
>   9 g/3 qián
>
> *xìng rén* (杏仁 apricot kernel, Armeniacae Semen) 9 g/3 qián
>
> *zhǐ qiào* (枳壳 bitter orange, Aurantii Fructus) 9 g/3 qián
>
> *zhū líng* (猪苓 polyporus, Polyporus) 30 g/1 liǎng
>
> *fú líng* (茯苓 poria, Poria) 30 g/1 liǎng
>
> *dōng guā pí* (冬瓜皮 wax gourd rind, Benincasae Exocarpium) 30 g/1 liǎng
>
> *zé xiè* (泽泻 alisma, Alismatis Rhizoma) 12 g/4 qián
>
> *chē qián zǐ* (车前子 plantago seed, Plantaginis Semen) 12 g/4 qián (wrap)

---

[6]Professor Jiāo specifically uses terms here that relate to controlling water in the outside environment to represent treatment principles. (Ed.)

guì zhī (桂枝 cinnamon twig, Cinnamomi Ramulus) 4.5 g/1.5 qián

Taken decocted with water, a total of five packets. The patient also took 300 mg of Rimafon and 8 g of PAS each day.

After taking the prescription, the cough, shortness of breath, and pain were significantly relieved, and the urine was significantly increased. After 15 packets, the patient was able to lie on either side freely. The heart had returned to the left side of the chest. After 29 packets of this formula, he was able to return to normal work. At that point there was no accumulated liquid in the chest and he was completely cured.

Case 3: Mr. Chái, 44 years old

Current disease history and current pathocondition: For the previous two days the patient had experienced severe pain on the right side of the lesser abdomen that affected the right low back area and radiated into the urethra. After urinating, he felt scorching pain in the urethra. He had frequent urges to urinate and reported short voidings of reddish urine. In the external medicine department of a local hospital he had been diagnosed with urinary calculus. He was given an injection of morphine and three packets of Chinese medicinals. After returning home, he took one packet of the Chinese medicinals and immediately vomited. Because the abdominal pain was severe, he returned to the hospital where he was admitted to the emergency observation ward. His chief complaint was the same as before, and in addition he had dry mouth with no desire to drink much, dry stool without a bowel movement for two days, and yellow tongue fur. His pulse was stringlike and rapid on the left and slippery and rapid on the right.

Pattern identification: The presence of scorching pain during urination and frequent urge to urinate meant that this was a strangury disease. Given that there was an acute onset, short voidings of reddish urine, a yellow tongue fur, and a slippery rapid pulse, we knew that there was damp-heat amassment in the lower burner. Furthermore, seeing that there was right-side lesser abdominal pain and lumbar pain, and that the pulse was stringlike and rapid, we had to consider that the damp-heat had been brewing for a long time and scorching the fluids, so that the heat bind created a stone. In this pattern of stone strangury, the stone obstructed the channels and network vessels, and the qì and blood stoppage gave rise to periodic pain.

Integrating the hospital diagnosis of urinary calculus with the pulse, signs, and pattern identification, we concluded that this was a pattern of damp-heat strangury and sand/stone strangury.

Treatment method: Clear heat and disinhibit dampness; move qì and quicken the blood; assist with medicinals to transform the stone.

On the basis of the requirements of principle and method, in combination with the pathomechanism and signs of bladder damp-heat and heat bind creating a stone, I chose the chief medicinals (1) *huáng bǎi* (phellodendron), which consolidates the kidney and clears heat, and (2) *fú líng* (poria) and (3) *zhū líng* (polyporus), which disinhibit dampness by bland percolation. The supporting medicinals were a) *huáng*

qín (scutellaria), which clears center burner damp-heat, b) *biǎn xù* (knotgrass) and
c) *qū mài* (dianthus), which disinhibit dampness and free strangury, d) *dōng kuí zǐ*
(mallow seed), which lubricates the orifices, and e) *jīn qián cǎo* (moneywort), which
expels stones. The assistants were 1. *wū yào* (lindera), which normalizes bladder
and kidney counterflow qì, 2. *niú xī* (achyranthes) and 3. *zé lán* (lycopus), which
quicken static blood in the low back and knees, and 4. *yán hú suǒ* (corydalis), which
moves the qì in the blood; these four medicinals move qì, quicken the blood, and
settle pain, and they also help to disinhibit the expulsion of the stone. I further
added *shēng dà huáng* (raw rhubarb) as a conductor to drain heat and quicken
stasis, and flush stagnation downward to assist with expelling stones and clearing
heat. The ingredients in the prescription are listed below:

> *huáng bǎi* (黄柏 phellodendron, Phellodendri Cortex) 12 g/4 qián
>
> *zhū líng* (猪苓 polyporus, Polyporus) 15 g/5 qián
>
> *fú líng* (茯苓 poria, Poria) 15 g/5 qián
>
> *huáng qín* (黄芩 scutellaria, Scutellariae Radix) 9 g/3 qián
>
> *biǎn xù* (萹蓄 knotgrass, Polygoni Avicularis Herba) 12 g/4 qián
>
> *qū mài* (瞿麦 dianthus, Dianthi Herba) 12 g/4 qián
>
> *dōng kuí zǐ* (冬葵子 mallow seed, Malvae Semen) 15 g/5 qián
>
> *jīn qián cǎo* (金钱草 moneywort, Lysimachiae Herba) 30 g/1 liǎng
>
> *wū yào* (乌药 lindera, Linderae Radix) 9 g/3 qián
>
> *zé lán* (泽兰 lycopus, Lycopi Herba) 12 g/4 qián
>
> *niú xī* (牛膝 achyranthes, Achyranthis Bidentatae Radix) 15 g/5 qián
>
> *shēng dà huáng* (生大黄 raw rhubarb, Rhei Radix et Rhizoma Crudi) 9 g/3 qián

The patient took two packets of the above formula (in the second packet, *shēng
dà huáng* was changed to 6 g/2 qián). He expelled three stones in his urine, each
about the size of a small grain of rice. After this, all the symptoms were resolved
and the patient left the hospital.

Let's look at the method used to compose the prescriptions in the three case
examples above. In the first, I used *bái hǔ tāng* (White Tiger Decoction) and *zēng
yè chéng qì tāng* (Humor-Increasing Qì-Coordinating Decoction) with medicinals
to cool the blood and stanch bleeding (varied in accordance with signs). In the
second case, I used the spirit of *jiāo mù guā lóu tāng* (Zanthoxylum Seed and Trichosanthes Formula), combined with the knowledge gained from past physicians'
experience that when treating rheum disease we must "harmonize with warm medicinals." This was then integrated with the specific condition and varied according
to the signs in order to create a new formula, which was even more suited to the
disease condition and thus enhanced the therapeutic efficacy. In the third case,
starting with the requirements of establishing a method, drawing upon the principles of prescription composition from past physicians, and combining this with
the findings of modern laboratory studies (adding medicinals to expel stones), I
was then able to create a new prescription. In all three cases, the therapeutic effect was comparatively good. Thus my personal experience is that no matter if we
are using ancient formulas, modern formulas, or creating new formulas, we must
act in accordance with Comrade Máo Zé-Dōng's teachings of "make the past serve

the present; make foreign things serve China" and "weed through the old to bring forth the new" so as to develop our national medicine. We must use modern scientific methods to systematize and elevate integrated Chinese-Western medicine. It is essential to orient treatment to the specific disease condition and vary formulas flexibly to ensure a definite and intimate connection between theory and reality. All of this then must serve to resolve practical problems. We must never cease to make connections with our experience in order to progress forward and have the courage to create. We must struggle to create a new medicine and a new medicinal therapy so as to make a contribution to speeding the progress toward the realization of the Four Modernizations.

Appendix
Glossary of Terms
词汇表 *Cí Huì Biǎo*

Most terms appearing in this book that are not explained in the text or in this glossary can be found in *A Practical Dictionary of Chinese Medicine*. This glossary explains terms that may be unfamiliar to some readers.

abductive dispersion, 消导 *xiāo dǎo*: Also called dispersing food and abducting stagnation (消食导滞 *xiāo shí dǎo zhì*). A method of treatment used to disperse stagnant food and enable it to be carried through the digestive tract. Dispersing food and abducting stagnation is employed in the treatment of food stagnation that causes oppression in the stomach duct and abdominal distention, poor appetite, putrid belching, swallowing of upflowing acid, nausea and upflow, abdominal pain, constipation, or diarrhea with ungratifying defecation. Commonly used abductive dispersion medicinals include *shān zhā* (crataegus), *shén qū* (medicated leaven), *mài yá* (barley sprout), *jī nèi jīn* (gizzard lining), and *gǔ yá* (millet sprout). *Lái fú zǐ* (radish seed), *zhǐ shí* (unripe bitter orange), and *bīng láng* (areca) may be added to break qì, precipitate phlegm, and free the stool.

acid swallowing, 吞酸 *tūn suān*: The welling up of acid fluid that is swallowed before it can be spat out. Swallowing of upflowing acid occurs in liver qì invading the stomach and is associated with either heat or cold signs: in heat patterns, accompanying signs include vexation, dry throat, bitter taste in the mouth, and yellow tongue fur; in cold patterns, signs include dull pain in the chest and stomach duct, ejection of clear drool, and a pale tongue with white fur.

acid vomiting, 吐酸 *tù suān*: Expulsion through the mouth of sour fluid that flows up from the stomach. Acid vomiting is similar to **acid swallowing**, in which sour water flowing up from the stomach is swallowed before it is ejected, but differs in that the sour water is actually ejected. Acid vomiting is attributed to abiding food (宿食 *sù shí*), phlegm-fire, liver fire invading the stomach, or spleen-stomach vacuity cold.

add at end, 后下 *hòu xià*: Add a medicinal toward the end of the process of decocting the other medicinals in the formula. Some exterior-resolving medicinals, such as *bò hé* (mint), *huò xiāng* (agastache), and *pèi lán* (eupatorium), lose their qì and flavor when boiled for a long time (i.e., they lose their volatile oils). They are therefore added after the other medicinals have boiled for 15 minutes for the final 5–10 minutes. *Gōu téng* (uncaria) is added just a few seconds before the end. *Dà huáng* (rhubarb) may be first soaked in a small amount of water and likewise added a few seconds before the decoction process is complete.

aggregation, 癖 *pì*: See **strings and aggregations**[565] (痃癖 *xián pì*).

alternating heat and cold, 寒热往来 *hán rè wǎng lái*: Aversion to cold and heat effusion (fever) occurring in regular or irregular alternating succession, associated with lesser yáng (*shào yáng*) midstage patterns (half exterior half interior pattern), malaria, or damp-heat obstructing the triple burner.

arched-back rigidity, 角弓反张 *jiǎo gōng fǎn zhāng*: Rigidity of the neck and back causing them to arch or bow backward.

baby moth, 乳蛾 *rǔ é*: Redness, swelling, and soreness of either or both of the throat nodes (tonsils) with a yellowish white discharge visible on their surface. Baby moth is attributable to a) congesting lung-stomach heat with fire toxin steaming upward; b) qì stagnation and congealing blood together with old phlegm and liver fire binding to form malign blood; or c) liver kidney yīn-liquid depletion with vacuity fire flaming upward.

blood amassment in the bladder, 膀胱蓄血 *páng guāng xù xuè*: A greater yáng (*tài yáng*) cold damage pattern in which evil heat enters the interior to contend with the blood, causing stasis heat amassing and binding internally and manifesting in the form of smaller-abdominal pain and distention; heat effusion and aversion to cold; and clear-mindedness in the daytime that gives way to delirious raving, mania, confused speech, and vociferation and violent behavior at night. Blood amassment is treated by offensive precipitation of static blood using *dǐ dàng wán* (Dead-On Pill), *táo hé chéng qì tāng* (Peach Kernel Qi-Co-ordinating Decoction), *gé xià zhú yū tāng* (Infradiaphragmatic Stasis-Expelling Decoction) plus *dà huáng* (rhubarb), or *xī jiǎo dì huáng tāng* (Rhinoceros Horn and Rehmannia Decoction).

blood dizziness, 血晕 *xuè yūn*: Dizziness due to loss of blood.

blood drum, 血臌 *xuè gǔ*: Drum distention[546] (臌胀 *gǔ zhàng*) arising when blood stasis and qì stagnation hamper the movement of water-damp. Blood drum is characterized by enlargement of the abdomen with green-blue prominent vessels (caput medusae), and red-thread marks (红缕赤痕 *hóng lǚ chì hén*, i.e., spider nevi), black stool, short voidings of reddish urine, and a scallion-stalk pulse. In some cases there is spontaneous external bleeding or blood ejection.

blood phlegm, 血痰 *xuè tán*: Phlegm flecked with blood.

boil, 疖 *jié*: A small, round, superficial swelling that is hot and painful, suppurates within a few days, and easily bursts. It is attributable to heat toxin or to summerheat-heat and usually occurs in the summer and autumn.

booming heat [effusion], 轰热 *hōng rè*: Heat effusion[551] (发热 *fā rè*, i.e., fever) that comes in sudden acute episodes and quickly abates.

breast milk stoppage, 乳汁不下 *rǔ zhī bù xià*: Also called 乳汁不通 *rǔ zhī bù xià*. See scant breast milk[561] (乳汁少 *rǔ zhī shǎo*).

brighten the eyes, 明目 *míng mù*: Enhance visual acuity.

chest bind, 结胸 *jié xiōng*: A pattern that arises when evil qì binds in the chest, causing pain below the heart with hard fullness that can be felt under pressure. It occurs when offensive precipitation is administered too early in greater yáng (*tài yáng*) disease and causes exterior heat to fall into the inner body and bind with water-rheum. It may also occur (without inappropriate precipitation) when greater yáng disease passes to yáng brightness (*yáng míng*) and yáng brightness repletion heat combines with preexisting water-rheum.

chest impediment, 胸痹 *xiōng bì*: From *Líng Shū* (灵枢 "The Magic Pivot"). In *Zhǒu Hòu Bèi Jí Fāng* (肘后备急方 "Emergency Standby Remedies") and *Jīn Guì Yào Lüè* (金匮要略 "Essential Prescriptions of the Golden Coffer"), chest impediment is described as a disease pattern characterized by fullness and oppression in the anterior chest, in severe cases with pain stretching to the back, and panting that prevents the patient from lying down. It is caused by yīn evils like phlegm turbidity and static blood that congeal and bind, preventing diffusion of chest yáng. Depending on severity, chest impediment may take the form of fullness in the chest (胸满 *xiōng mǎn*) or chest pain (胸痛 *xiōng tòng*).

child gān accumulation, 小儿疳积 *xiǎo ér gān jī*: A disease of infancy or childhood characterized by emaciation, dry hair, heat effusion of varying degree, abdominal distention with visible superficial veins, yellow face and emaciated flesh, and loss of essence-spirit vitality. Pathomechanically, it essentially involves dryness of the fluids due to damage to the spleen and stomach owing to dietary factors, evils, and in particular, worms.

chronic spleen wind, 慢脾风 *màn pí fēng*: A disease pattern in young children that arises when excessive vomiting or diarrhea weakens right qì, causing closed eyes and shaking head, dark green-blue face and lips, sweating brow, clouded spirit, somnolence, reversal cold of the limbs, and wriggling of the extremities. It is a form of chronic fright wind characterized by spleen yīn vacuity and spleen yáng debilitation.

cinnabar toxin [sore], 丹毒 *dān dú*: A condition characterized by sudden localized reddening of the skin, giving it the appearance of having been smeared with cinnabar. Cinnabar toxin usually affects the face and lower legs, is most common among children and the elderly, and usually occurs in spring and summer. Cinnabar toxin is known by different names according to form and location.

When it affects the head, it is called *head fire cinnabar* (抱头火丹 *bào tóu huǒ dān*). When it assumes a wandering pattern, it is called *wandering cinnabar* (赤游丹 *chì yóu dān*), as is observed in newborns. Cinnabar toxin of the lower legs is called *fire flow* (流火 *liú huǒ*) or *fire cinnabar leg* (火丹脚 *huǒ dān jiǎo*). Cinnabar toxin arises when damaged skin and insecurity of defense qì allow evil toxin to enter the body and give rise to heat in the blood aspect, which becomes trapped in the skin. If the toxin is accompanied by wind, the face is affected; if accompanied by dampness, the lower legs are affected. Thus the facial type tends to be wind-heat, whereas the lower leg type is damp-heat. The disease develops swiftly. The onset of heat effusion and aversion to cold is followed by the rapid outbreak of red patches on the skin. These patches are clearly defined and slightly raised at the edges; they feel painful and are scorching hot to the touch. They quickly spread in all directions, turn from a bright to a darker red, and may scale. In some cases, there are also vesicles that leak yellow fluid on bursting and cause pain and itching. Other signs include vexing thirst, generalized heat [effusion], constipation, reddish urine, and other general heat signs. Development of a vigorous heat [effusion] with vomiting, clouded spirit, delirious speech, or even tetanic reversal (痉厥 *jìng jué*) are signs of the toxin attacking the body's interior. Cinnabar toxin sore mostly corresponds to erysipelas in Western medicine.

clamoring stomach, 嘈杂 *cáo zá*: A sensation of emptiness and burning in the stomach duct or heart [region] described as being like hunger but not hunger, and like pain but not pain, and accompanied by belching, nausea, swallowing of upflowing acid, and fullness.

clear-eye blindness, 青盲 *qīng máng*: Gradual blindness that in severe cases can be total. It is attributable to insufficiency of the liver and kidney and depletion of essence blood, combined with spleen-stomach vacuity preventing essential qì from reaching up to the eyes. Note that in the Chinese term, the character 青 *qīng*, green-blue, also has the meaning of black or any dark color. It appears to be used here to suggest blindness without any white or other pale-colored eye screen; hence it is rendered more clearly in English as "clear-eye."

concretions, conglomerations, accumulations, and gatherings, 癥瘕积聚 *zhēng jiǎ jī jù*: Four kinds of abdominal masses associated with pain and distention. Concretions and accumulations are masses of definite form and fixed location that are associated with pain of fixed location. They stem from disease in the viscera and blood aspect. Conglomerations and gatherings are masses of indefinite form that gather and dissipate at irregular intervals and are attended by pain of unfixed location. They are attributed to disease in the bowels and qì aspect. Accumulations and gatherings chiefly occur in the center burner. Concretions and conglomerations chiefly occur in the lower burner and in many cases are the result of gynecological diseases. In general, concretions, conglomerations, accumulations, and gatherings arise when emotional depression or dietary intemperance causes damage to the liver and spleen. The resultant organ disharmony leads to obstruction and stagnation of qì, which in turn causes static blood to gradually collect. Most often the root cause is insufficiency of right qì. Concretions, conglomerations, accumulations, and gatherings also include other specific masses such as **strings and aggregations**[565] (痃癖 *xián pì*).

conglomeration, 瘕 *jiǎ*: See concretions, conglomerations, accumulations, and gatherings[544] (癥瘕积聚 *zhēng jiǎ jī jù*).

corn, 鸡眼 *jī yǎn*: A local thickening and hardening of the skin of the foot such as at the distal edge of the sole or between the toes and especially at the base joint of the great toe. A corn is called a "chicken's eye" (鸡眼 *jī yǎn*) or "flesh spike" (肉刺 *ròu cì*) in Chinese; it has a deep root and a hard hollow head, is painful when pressed, and affects walking. It is produced by friction and pressure from footwear, occurring especially in cases where the affected part is abnormally protuberant.

crane's knee, 鹤膝 *hè xī*: Also called crane's-knee wind 鹤膝风 *hè xī fēng*. A condition characterized by swelling and pain of the joints, and emaciation of the lower leg, such that it has a shape like a crane's knee.

damp leg qì, 湿脚气 *shī jiǎo qì*: Painfully swollen feet with heaviness and numbness that hinders movement.

damp sore, 湿疮 *shī chuāng*: Any of a variety of skin diseases characterized by itching, ulceration, exudation, crusting, and recurrence. It specifically includes: scrotal wind (肾囊风 *shèn náng fēng*); four bends wind (四弯风 *sì wān fēng*); umbilical damp (脐湿 *qí shī*); nipple wind (乳头风 *rǔ tóu fēng*); and invisible worm sore of the nose (䘌鼻 *nì bí*). Acute forms are ascribed mainly to damp-heat, very often with external wind. Wind is a yáng evil, light and buoyant; it easily invades the interstices of the head, face, and upper body. It is swift and changeable; it often changes location and spreads quickly. Dampness is a yīn evil, it is sticky and stagnating, and is spreading and pervasive. It is heavy and turbid and tends to be found in low places. When it invades the body, it can cause water vesicles, ulceration, and exudation. Wind and dampness easily harbor brewing heat, and the three evils together cause dampness, scorching heat, itching, and soreness of the skin. Chronic damp sores tend to be caused by blood vacuity and wind dryness with damp-heat brewing and accumulating. They are recurrent and persistent, associated with severe itching that prevents the patient from sleeping, and poor stomach intake. Yīn blood depletion engenders wind and dryness, depriving the skin of nourishment, and causing dryness, thickening of the skin, and scaling. Persistent damp sores affecting the chest, abdomen, or genitals are associated with liver channel damp-heat. Damp sores affecting the lower body with prominent green-blue veins (varicose veins) are associated with heat brewing internally owing to liquor consumption. Damp sores with nutritional disturbance are ascribed to spleen vacuity with brewing damp-heat.

damp warm disease, 湿温病 *shī wēn bìng*: Also called damp warmth (湿温 *shī wēn*). A febrile disease occurring in the summer or autumn that is attributed to damp-heat and characterized by persistent heat effusion, heavy-headedness, generalized pain, glomus and oppression in the chest and stomach duct, white or yellow slimy tongue fur, and soggy pulse.

deep-source runny nose, 鼻渊 *bí yuān*: Persistent runny nose with turbid snivel (nasal mucus); it is attributable to wind-cold, wind-heat, or gallbladder heat. Note that this was previously referred to in English as "deep-source nasal congestion."

dispersion-thirst, 消渴 *xiāo kě*: Any disease characterized by thirst, increased fluid intake, and copious urine. Dispersion-thirst is categorized as upper burner, center burner, and lower burner dispersion, depending on the pathomechanism. Includes diabetes mellitus, diabetes insipidus, and hypoadrenocorticism.

disquieted heart spirit, 心神不安 *xīn shén bù ān*: Spirit disturbed as a result of the heart's failure to store it. The spirit is stored by the heart and is often referred to as the heart spirit. Disquieted heart spirit arises in heart disease when the heart fails to store the spirit, and manifests as heart palpitations, fearful throbbing, susceptibility to fright, heart vexation, and insomnia.

dormant papules, 瘾疹 *yǐn zhěn*: Wheals that come and go, so named by their ability to remain latent between eruptions. Being itchy and of unfixed location, they bear the attributes of wind; hence an alternative name is "papular wind lumps" (风疹块 *fēng zhěn kuài*). Dormant papules can arise when wind evil invades owing to looseness of the interstices, or when toxin from insect bites gets trapped in the fleshy exterior and flows into the channels. Another cause is accumulated heat in the stomach and intestines that can neither discharge through the bowels nor thrust out through the exterior and so becomes depressed in the skin. In some cases, they are brought on by eating fish or shrimp. Dormant papules usually start abruptly with itchy skin, which produces raised wheals of different sizes when scratched. They are most commonly observed on the inner face of the arm and usually disappear without trace. Hot red papules accompanied by a red tongue and floating rapid pulse are due to wind-heat. White wheals associated with aversion to cold, thin white tongue fur, and a tight floating pulse are wind-cold. Persistent recurrent eruptions indicate qì-blood depletion.

draining precipitation, 泻下 *xiè xià*: The stimulation of downward flow of waste in the intestines (precipitation) to expel repletion evils (draining) and remove accumulation and stagnation. Often referred to as "purgation."

dribbling urinary block, 癃闭 *lóng bì*: Dribbling urination or, in severe cases, almost complete blockage of urine flow. Distinction is made between a number of vacuity and repletion patterns. Vacuity patterns include insufficiency of center qì and insufficiency of kidney qì. The repletion patterns include lower burner damp-heat, lung qì congestion, binding depression of liver qì, and urinary tract stasis blockage.

drum distention, 臌胀 *gǔ zhàng*: Severe abdominal distention. Drum distention is also called "abdominal distention" or "simple drum," when swelling of the limbs is absent, as is usually the case. Drum distention is associated with a somber yellow coloration of the skin and prominent green-blue veins (caput medusae). Causes include: a) emotional frustration (anger damaging the liver); b) fondness for liquor and sweet fatty food; c) glomus lump; d) enduring illness; e) water toxin qì bind (mentioned in *Zhū Bìng Yuán Hòu Lùn* (诸病源候论 "The Origin and Indicators of Disease") and now understood as blood fluke infestation). Two major pathomechanisms operate. **1. Spleen disease affecting the liver**: Fondness for liquor and sweet fatty food causes damage to the spleen and prevents it from transforming damp turbidity so that damp-heat brews. The damp-heat then obstructs qì dynamic, causing liver depression. On the one hand, prolonged liver depression can cause blood stasis; on the other, it can cause liver qì to invade the spleen and the stomach, impairing movement and transformation of water-damp. Spleen vacuity and water-damp exacerbate each other, and spleen qì vacuity gives way to spleen yáng vacuity, which finally leads to dual vacuity of the spleen and kidney with inhibited urination that prevents the discharge of fluids. Drum distention thus arises as a result of qì stagnation, blood stasis, and water collecting in the abdomen. **2. Liver and spleen disease affecting the kidney**: Spleen vacuity deprives the kidney of nourishment, causing insufficiency of kidney yáng and inhibited bladder qì transformation. Debilitation of the life gate fire (kidney yáng) exacerbates spleen yáng vacuity. Liver depression transforms into heat to damage yīn and causes liver-kidney yīn vacuity. Damp-heat can similarly damage yīn. In former times, distinction was made between qì drum (气臌 *qì gǔ*), blood drum (血臌 *xuè gǔ*), water drum (水臌 *shuǐ gǔ*), and worm drum (虫臌 *chóng gǔ*). However, modern texts suggest that no clearly defined line can be drawn between the first three.

dry blood consumption, 干血痨 *gān xuè láo*: A disease recorded in *Xuè Zhèng Lùn* (血证论 "On Blood Patterns") that in signs and treatment corresponds to what is mentioned in *Jīn Guì Yào Lüè* (金匮要略 "Essential Prescriptions of the Golden Coffer") as "dry blood." Dry blood consumption is mostly seen in women. It results from long steaming of vacuity heat and internal binding of dry blood with stasis and stagnation, stemming from damage by the five taxations. When, in enduring conditions, static blood is not eliminated, new blood is engendered with difficulty, and liquid and blood fail to create luxuriance in the outer body. Signs include absence of menstruation, markedly emaciated body, no desire for food and drink, steaming bone tidal heat [effusion], encrusted skin, and dull black complexion.

dysentery, 痢疾 *lì jí*: A disease characterized by abdominal pain, tenesmus, and stool containing pus and blood (described as mucoid and bloody stool in Western medicine). Dysentery usually occurs in hot weather and arises when gastrointestinal vacuity and eating raw, cold, or unclean food allow damp-heat or other evils to brew in the intestines. It takes the form of vacuity or repletion. Depending on the cause, distinction is made between summerheat dysentery, damp-heat dysentery, cold dysentery, and heat dysentery. Depending on the nature of the stool, distinction is made between red dysentery (blood in the stool), white dysentery (pus in the stool), and red and white dysentery (stool containing pus and blood).

dysphagia-occlusion, 噎膈 *yē gé*: A disease characterized by sensation of blockage on swallowing, difficulty in getting food and drink down, and, in some cases, immediate vomiting of ingested food. The Chinese term is a compound of 噎 *yē*, meaning difficulty in swallowing (dysphagia), and 膈 *gé*, meaning blockage that prevents food from going down (occlusion). Dysphagia and occlusion may occur independently. Dysphagia most commonly but not necessarily develops into occlusion. There are four principal patterns: phlegm and qì obstructing each other, liquid depletion and heat bind, static blood binding internally, and qì vacuity and yáng debilitation.

eighteen clashes, 十八反 *shí bā fǎn*: Eighteen medicinals that clash, i.e., create noxious effects when used together with other medicinals:

Gān cǎo (甘草 licorice, Glycyrrhizae Radix) clashes with:
  dà jǐ (大戟 euphorbia/knoxia, Euphorbiae seu Knoxiae Radix)
  yuán huā (芫花 genkwa, Genkwa Flos)
  gān suì (甘遂 kansui, Kansui Radix)
  hǎi zǎo (海藻 sargassum, Sargassum)

Wū tóu (乌头 wild aconite, Aconiti Kusnezoffii Radix) clashes with:
  bèi mǔ (贝母 fritillaria, Fritillariae Bulbus)
  guā lóu (瓜蒌 trichosanthes, Trichosanthis Fructus)
  bàn xià (半夏 pinellia, Pinelliae Rhizoma)
  bái liǎn (白蔹 ampelopsis, Ampelopsis Radix)
  bái jí (白及 bletilla, Bletillae Rhizoma)

Lí lú (藜芦 veratrum, Veratri Nigri Radix et Rhizoma) clashes with:
  rén shēn (人参 ginseng, Ginseng Radix)
  dān shēn (丹参 salvia, Salviae Miltiorrhizae Radix)
  shā shēn (沙参 adenophora/glehnia, Adenophorae seu Glehniae Radix)
  kǔ shēn (苦参 flavescent sophora, Sophorae Flavescentis Radix)
  xuán shēn (玄参 scrophularia, Scrophulariae Radix)
  xì xīn (细辛 asarum, Asari Herba)
  sháo yào (芍药 peony, Paeoniae Radix)

emolliate the liver, 柔肝 *róu gān*: To treat liver yīn vacuity (or insufficiency of liver blood), which is characterized by loss of visual acuity, dry eyes, night blindness, periodic dizzy head and tinnitus, and pale nails, or poor sleep, profuse dreaming, dry mouth with lack of fluid, and a fine weak pulse.

encrusted skin, 肌肤甲错 *jī fū jiǎ cuò*: Skin with a high degree of dryness and lack of moisture.

excrescence creeping over the eye, 胬肉攀睛 *nǔ ròu pān jīng*: A gray-white fleshy growth at the canthus that progressively grows over the eye, in severe cases partially affecting vision. Excrescence creeping over the eye arises when heat congesting in the heart and lung channel causes qì stagnation and blood stasis. It may also result from effulgent yīn vacuity fire. Corresponds to pterygium in Western medicine.

expiration sweating, 绝汗 *jué hàn*: Sweating in critical conditions where separation of yīn and yáng is imminent; also called desertion sweating. Expiration sweating is characterized by putting forth of pearly sweat that sticks to the body and does not run.

external screen, 外翳 *wài yì*: Eye screen[549] (目翳 *mù yì*). All eye screens belong to the category of external obstructions (which also includes excrescences of the canthi, etc.), hence the term "external screen."

eye screen, 目翳 *mù yì*: Any external obstruction involving murky opacity or deformation of the black of the eye, or any scarring of this area left after disease, e.g., congealed-fat screen (凝脂翳 *níng zhī yì*). Screens may occur in repletion patterns of liver wind-heat and vacuity patterns of liver-kidney depletion and effulgent vacuity fire. Repletion patterns are treated by coursing wind and clearing heat, resolving toxin and draining the liver. Vacuity patterns are treated by enriching the liver and kidney, and nourishing yīn and clearing heat. In addition, screens may arise through external injury.

fearful throbbing, 怔忡 *zhēng chōng*: Severe heart palpitations that are not brought on by emotional stimulus and that occur continually, in contrast to fright palpitations, which are brought on by fright or other emotional stimulus. More severe than fright palpitations, fearful throbbing may be experienced as a violent palpitation not only in the chest, but even as low as the umbilical region. It is observed in patients in a poor state of health and always forms part of vacuity patterns. From the Western medical perspective, it is usually the manifestation of organic rather than nervous disease.

fetal spotting, 胎漏 *tāi lòu*: Also called 包漏 *bāo lòu*. A discharge of bloody fluid via the vagina during pregnancy, unaccompanied by abdominal pain.

fifth-watch diarrhea, 五更泄 *wǔ gēng xiè*: Also called cockcrow diarrhea, 鸡鸣 泄 *jī míng xiè*. Diarrhea that occurs at dawn or very early in the morning. It is attributable to spleen-kidney yáng vacuity.

fire-heat, 火热 *huǒ rè*: Fire as a heat evil.

flavor, 味 *wèi*: There are five principal flavors: acridity, sourness, sweetness, bitterness, and saltiness. Medicinals or foodstuffs of different flavors have different actions. Acridity can dissipate and move; sourness can contract and astringe; sweetness can supplement and relax (i.e., relieve pain and tension); bitterness can drain and dry; saltiness can soften hardness and induce moist precipitation. In addition to the five flavors, there is a sixth, blandness, which has a water-disinhibiting action. According to *Sù Wèn* (素问 "Elementary Questions"), the flavors can be classified as yīn and yáng: "Acrid and sweet effusing (i.e., diaphoretic) and dissipating medicinals are yáng; sour and bitter upwelling (i.e., emetic) and discharging (i.e., draining) medicinals are yīn; salty upwelling and discharging medicinals are yīn; bland percolating and discharging medicinals are yáng." According to *Běn Cǎo Gāng Mù* (本草纲目 "The Comprehensive Herbal Foundation"), there is a relationship between flavor and bearing: "No sour or salty medicinals bear upward; no sweet or acrid ones bear downward. No cold medicinals float; no hot ones sink."

flooding and spotting, 崩漏 *bēng lòu*: Any abnormal discharge of blood via the vagina. Flooding 崩 (*bēng*) (or 血崩 *xuè bēng*) is heavy menstrual flow or abnormal bleeding via the vagina (uterine bleeding); spotting 漏 (*lòu*) (or 漏下 *lòu xià*) is a slight, often continual discharge of blood via the vagina.

free milk, 通乳 *tōng rǔ*: Promote lactation. A method of treatment used to promote the flow of breast milk after delivery. Freeing milk takes one of two forms. **Supplementing qì and blood:** This is used to treat patients with qì and blood vacuity and little or no milk, but without distention or pain in the breasts. General signs include pale complexion and nails, pale tongue without fur, and a fine vacuous pulse. Medicinals used include:

> *dǎng shēn* (党参 codonopsis, Codonopsis Radix)
> *huáng qí* (黄芪 astragalus, Astragali Radix)
> *dāng guī* (当归 Chinese angelica, Angelicae Sinensis Radix)
> *mài mén dōng* (麦门冬 ophiopogon, Ophiopogonis Radix)
> *jié gěng* (桔梗 platycodon, Platycodonis Radix)
> *wáng bù liú xíng* (王不留行 vaccaria, Vaccariae Semen)
> *tōng cǎo* (通草 rice-paper plant pith, Tetrapanacis Medulla)

Moving qì and freeing the network vessels: This is used to treat qì stagnation and breast milk stoppage with distention and fullness of the breasts, thin tongue fur, and stringlike pulse. Medicinals used include:

> *dāng guī* (当归 Chinese angelica, Angelicae Sinensis Radix)
> *chuān xiōng* (川芎 chuanxiong, Chuanxiong Rhizoma)
> *chái hú* (柴胡 bupleurum, Bupleuri Radix)
> *xiāng fù zǐ* (香附子 cyperus, Cyperi Rhizoma)
> *chuān shān jiǎ* (穿山甲 pangolin scales, Manis Squama)
> *wáng bù liú xíng* (王不留行 vaccaria, Vaccariae Semen)

frenetic movement of hot blood, 血热妄行 *xuè rè wàng xíng*: Excessive movement of the blood due to blood heat manifesting in the form of bleeding or maculopapular eruptions.

fright epilepsy, 惊痫 *jīng xián*: Epilepsy caused by fright.

fright wind, 惊风 *jīng fēng*: Also called child fright wind, 小儿惊风 *xiǎo ér jīng fēng*. A disease of infants and children that is characterized by convulsions and loss of consciousness. Fright wind is equivalent to tetany (痉 *jìng*) in adults. Distinction is made between acute and chronic forms.

frog rale in the throat, 喉中有水鸡声 *hóu zhōng yǒu shuǐ jī shēng*: A continuous high-pitched rale produced by phlegm blocking the respiratory tract, so named because of its similarity to the croaking of frogs (in chorus). Frog rale in the throat is characteristic of wheezing patterns.

gān accumulation, 疳积 *gān jī*: See child gān accumulation[543] (小儿疳积 *xiǎo ér gān jī*).

gastrointestinal qì bind, 肠胃结气 *cháng wèi jié qì*: Qì stagnation of the stomach and intestines.

generalized impediment, 周痹 *zhōu bì*: Generalized wandering pain, heaviness, and numbness due to wind-cold-damp evil invading the blood vessels.

glomus, 痞 *pǐ*: A localized subjective feeling of fullness and blockage. Severe glomus in the chest (胸痞 *xiōng pǐ*) can be associated with a feeling of oppression; hence the terms "fullness in the chest," "distention in the chest," "glomus in the chest," and "oppression in the chest" are to some degree synonymous. In the abdomen, glomus is the sensation of a lump that cannot be detected by palpation. Hard glomus below the heart, which can be subjectively felt and objectively palpated, is a sign of evil heat with water collecting in the stomach. Any palpable abdominal mass is referred to as glomus lump although in texts predating *Shāng Hán Lùn* (伤寒论 "On Cold Damage"), these were referred to as "glomus." Glomus lumps in traditional literature are labeled differently, according to shape, behavior, and pathomechanism. See concretions, conglomerations, accumulations, and gatherings[544] (癥瘕积聚 *zhēng jiǎ jī jù*) and Prof. Jiāo's comments on page 389.

great wind, 大风 *dà fēng*: Also called numbing wind 麻风 *má fēng*. Leprosy. A transmissible disease that is characterized by localized numbing and subsequent appearance of red patches which swell and rupture without suppuration and that may spread to other parts of the body, causing loss of the eyes, collapse of the nose, fissuring of the lips, and boring of holes in the soles of the feet. This disease has disappeared in Western countries, but is still observed in China.

head wind, 头风 *tóu fēng*: Persistent, remittent, usually intense headache attributed to wind-cold or wind-heat invasion and obstruction of the channels by phlegm or static blood. Head wind may be accompanied by various other signs such as eye pain and loss of vision, runny nose, nausea, dizziness, numbness of the head, or stiffness of the neck.

heat effusion, 发热 *fā rè*: Abnormal bodily heat that can be detected by palpation or that is experienced subjectively; fever. Heat effusion occurring with aversion to cold or aversion to wind at the onset of illness indicates external evils invading the fleshy exterior. If the aversion to cold is more pronounced than the heat effusion, the pattern is one of wind-cold. Pronounced heat effusion with only aversion to wind suggests wind-heat. Heat effusion without aversion to cold occurs in various patterns. Distinction is made between vigorous heat (壮热 *zhuàng rè*), tidal heat (潮热 *cháo rè*), vexing heat in the five hearts (五心烦热 *wǔ xīn fán rè*), steaming bone tidal heat (骨蒸潮热 *gǔ zhēng cháo rè*), baking heat (烘热 *hōng rè*), and unsurfaced generalized heat (身热不扬 *shēn rè bù yáng*). Dr. Jiāo also speaks of booming heat[543] (轰热 *hōng rè*).

heat reversal, 热厥 *rè jué*: A reversal pattern (i.e., a pattern characterized by a) clouding collapse (fainting) and loss of consciousness and/or b) reversal cold of the limbs) that occurs in generalized heat [effusion] and headache and that is attributable to overexuberant evil depressing yáng qì and preventing its warming force from reaching the extremities. Its features are clouded spirit, reversal cold of the limbs, and a sunken or hidden pulse that is slippery under pressure. There may be aversion to heat, thirst with desire for fluids, flailing of the arms and legs, vexation and agitation, insomnia, scorching (palpable) heat in the chest and abdomen, constipation, and reddish urine.

hemilateral headache, 偏头痛 *piān tóu tòng*: Any headache on one side or one part of the head, as opposed to medial headache (the more common type of headache).

hoisted eyes, 吊眼 *diào yǎn*: Eyes open and turned upward. A critical sign. Also called upward staring eyes (两目上视 *liǎng mù shàng shì*).

impediment, 痹 *bì*: Blockage of the channels that arises when wind, cold, and dampness invade the fleshy exterior and the joints and that manifests in signs such as joint pain, sinew and bone pain, and heaviness or numbness of the limbs. *Sù Wèn* (素问 "Elementary Questions") states, "When wind, cold, and damp evils concur and combine, they give rise to impediment." For this reason it is often called wind-cold-damp impediment. Distinction is made between three pattern types, each of which corresponds to a prevalence of one of the three evils: wind impediment (风痹 *fēng bì*), also called moving impediment (行痹 *xíng bì*), characterized by wandering pain and attributed to a prevalence of wind; cold impediment (寒痹 *hán bì*), also called painful impediment (痛痹 *tòng bì*), associated with acute pain and attributed to a prevalence of cold; and damp impediment (湿痹 *shī bì*), also called fixed impediment (着痹 *zhuó bì*), characterized by heaviness and attributed to a prevalence of dampness. A fourth type, heat impediment (热痹 *rè bì*), occurs when the three evils transform into heat. Impediment is readily complicated by qì vacuity and blood vacuity.

incised wound, 金创 *jīn chuāng*: Wounds caused by metal objects, but also including suppuration and ulcerated sores due to injury.

incontinent intestinal efflux, 肠滑不禁 *cháng huá bù jìn*: Also called intestinal vacuity efflux desertion (肠虚滑脱 *cháng xū huá tuō*). Loss of voluntary control of bowels, sometimes associated with prolapse of the rectum.

infant's-pillow pain, 儿枕痛 *ér zhěn tòng*: Postpartum lower abdominal pain caused by static blood. This pattern may stem from incomplete elimination of the lochia or wind-cold exploiting vacuity to invade the uterine vessels causing a collection of static blood. Both patterns involve stasis, but their pathomechanisms differ.

inhibited urination, 小便不利 *xiǎo biàn bù lì*: Difficult voiding of scant urine. Inhibited urination is ascribed to nondiffusion of lung qì, devitalization of spleen yáng, debilitation of kidney yáng, internal damp-heat obstruction, or qì stagnation with damp obstruction. These patterns all involve reduced flow of urine to the bladder due to yáng qì vacuity or the presence of evil qì. In addition, there are yīn vacuity patterns, which, according to some, should not strictly be considered as inhibited urination patterns because they are essentially attributable to depletion of fluids.

innominate toxin swellings, 无名肿毒 *wú míng zhǒng dú*: Localized pain and swelling that suddenly appears on any part of the body. *Wài Kē Dà Chéng* (外科大成 "The Great Compendium of External Medicine") states, " . . . not a welling-abscess, not a flat-abscess, not a sore, not lichen, resembling a malign sore in form, either healing or worsening; it is called an innominate toxin swelling." It is caused by wind, cold, or heat lodging in the channels. When due to wind evil, there is neither head nor root. When due to qì contending with the blood, there is a head but no root. When due to wind-cold, the swelling is hard and white. When due to heat toxin, the swelling is red and hot.

intermittent dysentery, 休息痢 *xiū xī lì*: Dysentery that goes on for months and years, continually starting and stopping; hence the name. Intermittent dysentery usually arises from inappropriate treatment or stems from such factors as qì-blood vacuity or insufficiency of the spleen and kidney, causing right vacuity and lingering evil, whereby damp-heat lies latent in the stomach and intestines. During periods of remission, the only signs that remain are lassitude of spirit and lack of strength, poor appetite, emaciation, and lack of warmth in the extremities.

internal expression, 托里 *tuō lǐ*: Pushing (toxin) outward from within; one of the three main methods of treating sores. It involves the use of qì and blood-supplementing medicinals to support right qì, express the toxin, and prevent it from falling inward. It includes two forms. **1. Expressing toxin and outthrusting pus** 托毒透脓 *tuó dú tòu nóng*): This method is used for midstage sores when toxin is exuberant but right qì has not yet been damaged and the sore has still not burst. The treatment uses medicinals such as *huáng qí* (astragalus), *dāng guī* (Chinese angelica), *chuān xiōng* (chuanxiong), *chuān shān jiǎ* (pangolin scales), *bái zhǐ* (Dahurian angelica), and *zào jiǎo cì* (gleditsia thorn). **2. Supplemental expression** (补托 *bǔ tuō*): This method is used when right qì vacuity prevents the expulsion of toxin so that the sore becomes flat with a broad root, and either fails to burst or bursts to produce only a thin scant discharge without abatement of swelling and accompanied by generalized heat [effusion], devitalized essence-spirit, yellow facial complexion, and a forceless rapid pulse. Commonly used supplemental-expression medicinals include the following.

> *huáng qí* (黃芪 astragalus, Astragali Radix)
> *bái zhú* (白术 white atractylodes, Atractylodis Macrocephalae Rhizoma)
> *fú líng* (茯苓 poria, Poria)
> *dǎng shēn* (党参 codonopsis, Codonopsis Radix)

    zhì gān cǎo (炙甘草 mix-fried licorice, Glycyrrhizae Radix cum Liquido
      Fricta)

    gān cǎo (甘草 licorice, Glycyrrhizae Radix)

    dāng guī (当归 Chinese angelica, Angelicae Sinensis Radix)

    bái sháo yào (白芍药 white peony, Paeoniae Radix Alba)

    zào jiǎo cì (皂角刺 gleditsia thorn, Gleditsiae Spina)

    bái zhǐ (白芷 Dahurian angelica, Angelicae Dahuricae Radix)

    jīn yín huā (金银花 lonicera, Lonicerae Flos)

    lián qiáo (连翘 forsythia, Forsythiae Fructus)

    jié gěng (桔梗 platycodon, Platycodonis Radix)

    chén pí (陈皮 tangerine peel, Citri Reticulatae Pericarpium)

internal obstruction, 内障 *nèi zhàng*: Any of a number of diseases of the spirit pupil and inner eye that manifest in poor vision. Internal obstructions mostly occur in vacuity patterns and are most commonly attributable to insufficiency of the liver and kidney or dual depletion of qì and blood. Other causes include effulgent yīn vacuity fire, qì stagnation and blood stasis, wind-fire and phlegm-damp harassing the clear orifices, and external injury. Signs include subjective sensations like *mouches volantes,* black floaters, lights and flames appearing to be surrounded by rainbow-like halos, clouded vision, night blindness, or sudden blindness. Very often there are no visible objective signs, although the pupil may be dilated or contracted, deformed, or abnormal in color. Internal obstructions include green-blue wind internal obstruction (青风内胀 *qīng fēng nèi zhàng*) and green wind internal obstruction (绿风内障 *lǜ fēng nèi zhàng*), corresponding to glaucoma in Western medicine.

interstices, 腠理 *còu lǐ*: An anatomical entity of unclear identity, explained in modern dictionaries as being the "grain" of the skin, flesh, and organs or the connective tissue in the skin and flesh. *Sù Wèn* (素问 "Elementary Questions") states: "Clear yáng effuses through the interstices." Usage of the term suggests that the interstices correspond to the sweat ducts in Western medicine.

intestinal welling-abscess, 肠痈 *cháng yōng*: Welling-abscess[567] (痈 *yōng*) of the intestine; attributed to congealing blood that stems from damp-heat or from general qì and blood stagnation. Corresponds to appendicitis or periappendicular abscess in Western medicine.

intractable cold, 痼冷 *gù lěng*: Cold qì lying for a long time in particular channels and network vessels or bowels and viscera, forming a localized cold pattern that persists for a long time. Intractable cold is most often seen in patients with spleen-stomach vacuity, internal cold rheum, or cold-damp enduring impediment.

inverted menstruation, 倒经 *dào jīng*: Spontaneous external bleeding during each menstrual period.

itchy papules, 痒疹 *yǎng zhěn*: Any rash associated with itching.

jaundice, 黄疸 *huáng dǎn*: A condition characterized by the three classic signs of yellow skin, yellow eyes, and yellow urine, i.e., generalized yellowing of the body, yellowing of the whites of the eyes (sclera), and darker-than-normal urine. Jaundice arises when contraction of seasonal evils or dietary irregularities cause damp-heat or cold-damp to obstruct the center burner and prevent bile from flowing according to its normal course. Distinction is made between yáng jaundice and yīn jaundice. **Yáng jaundice** (阳黄 *yáng huáng*) is attributable to contraction of external evils, damp-heat invading the liver and gallbladder, and resultant gallbladder heat causing bile to percolate through to the skin. Yáng jaundice is a vivid yellow described as being like the color of tangerines; it is accompanied by heat effusion, thirst, urine the color of strong tea, constipation, abdominal distention, rib-side pain, slimy yellow tongue fur, and a rapid stringlike pulse. It corresponds to acute infectious hepatitis and obstructive biliary tract diseases in Western medicine. **Yīn jaundice** (阴黄 *yīn huáng*) is characterized by somber withered-yellow facial complexion, torpid stomach, abdominal distention, lassitude of spirit, lack of strength, dull rib-side pain, short voidings of scant urine, unsolid stool, pale tongue with slimy tongue fur, and a sunken slow fine pulse. When this is the result of cold-damp, it is characterized by reduced food intake, oppression in the stomach duct, or even abdominal distention. When due to spleen vacuity and blood depletion, additional signs include dry skin, heart palpitations, and shortness of breath. When due to accumulation of static blood, there is a painful concretion under the left rib-side and red-thread marks (红缕赤痕 *hóng lǚ chì hén*, i.e., spider nevi). Yīn jaundice sometimes develops from yáng jaundice.

jiāo sān xiān (scorch-fried three immortals): *Jiāo shén qū* (scorch-fried medicated leaven), *jiāo mài yá* (scorch-fried barley sprout), and *jiāo shān zhā* (scorch-fried crataegus).

jiāo sì xiān (scorch-fried four immortals): *Jiāo shén qū* (scorch-fried medicated leaven), *jiāo mài yá* (scorch-fried barley sprout), *jiāo shān zhā* (scorch-fried crataegus), and *jiāo bīng láng* (scorch-fried areca).

joint running, 历节 *lì jié*: A disease described in *Jīn Guì Yào Lüè* (金匮要略 "Essential Prescriptions of the Golden Coffer") that is characterized by redness and swelling of the joints, with acute pain and difficulty bending and stretching. Joint-running wind is attributed to transformation of wind-cold-damp into heat in patients suffering from liver-kidney vacuity and falls within the scope of impediment[552] (痹 *bì*).

knocks and falls, 跌打 *dié dǎ*: Blows, collisions, collapses, or falls from heights, especially when resulting in injury; any injury resulting from knocks and falls. Injuries from knocks and falls include stasis swelling (bruises), cuts and grazes, sprains, bone fractures, dislocations, and damage to the bowels and viscera. Treatment methods include dispelling stasis, moving qì, relieving pain, stanching bleeding, soothing the sinews, and strengthening the bones. Commonly used formulas include *qī lí sǎn* (Seven Pinches Powder), *fù yuán huó xuè tāng* (Origin-Restorative Blood-Quickening Decoction), *zhuàng jīn yǎng xuè tāng* (Sinew-Strengthening Blood-Nourishing Decoction), and *zhèng gǔ zǐ jīn dān* (Bone-Righting Purple Gold Elixir).

lài, 癩 *lài*: scab[561] (疥 *jiè*) or lichen[556] (癣 *xuǎn*) that lead to hair loss on the affected area.

laryngeal insufflation, 吹喉 *chuī hòu*: Blowing powdered medicinals into the throat of the patient as a topical application for a sore throat.

leg qì, 脚气 *jiǎo qì*: A disease characterized by numbness, pain, limpness, and in some cases any of a variety of possible signs such as hypertonicity or swelling, withering, redness and swelling of the calf, heat effusion, and in advanced stages by abstraction of spirit-mind, heart palpitations, panting, oppression in the chest, nausea and vomiting, and deranged speech. Leg qì arises when externally contracted damp evil and wind toxin or accumulating dampness due to damage by excessive consumption of rich food engenders heat and pours down into the legs. Chest and abdominal signs are attributed to leg qì surging into the heart. The Western medical correspondence is beriberi (attributed to vitamin B_1 deficiency).

lichen, 癣 *xuǎn*: A skin disease marked by elevation of the skin, serous discharge, scaling, and itching.

lockjaw, 破伤风 *pò shāng fēng*: A disease characterized by clenched jaw and other forms of spasm, which arises when an external injury or mouth sores permit the invasion of wind evil. It is a form of **tetany**[565] (痓 *jìng*). Lockjaw begins with lack of strength in the limbs, headache, pain in the cheeks, clenched jaw, difficulty in turning the neck, and heat effusion and aversion to cold. Subsequently, there is a spasm of the facial muscles that creates the appearance of a strange grimace, tightly clenched jaw, stiff tongue, drooling, intermittent generalized spasm, and **arched-back rigidity**. The pulse is rapid or tight and stringlike. Finally, speech, swallowing, and breathing all become difficult, and, in the worst cases, the patient dies of asphyxiation.

lung wilting, 肺痿 *fèi wěi*: A chronic condition characterized by a dull-sounding cough, ejection of thick turbid foamy drool, panting at the slightest exertion, dry mouth and pharynx, emaciation, red dry tongue, and a vacuous rapid pulse. In some cases, there may be tidal heat [effusion], and, in severe cases, the skin and hair may become dry. It is attributed to dryness-heat and enduring cough damaging the lung, or damage to fluid due to another disease depriving the lung of moisturization.

malaria, 疟疾 *nüè jí*: A recurrent disease characterized by shivering, vigorous heat [effusion], and sweating, and classically attributed to contraction of summer-heat during the hot season, contact with mountain forest miasma, or contraction of cold-damp. Malaria is explained as evil qì latent at midstage (half exterior and half interior). Different forms are distinguished according to signs and causes.

malign blood, 恶血 *è xuè*: Blood that has spilled out of the vessels and accumulated outside the vessels and that manifests in the form of stasis macules, stasis speckles, or blood swelling.

malign flesh, 恶肉 *è ròu*: An unnatural growth on the body surface.

malign obstruction, 恶阻 *è zǔ*: A condition of aversion to food, nausea, and vomiting during pregnancy, not considered untoward unless it severely affects food intake. Malign obstruction is the manifestation of impaired harmonious downbearing of stomach qì.

malign sore, 恶疮 *è chuāng*: Any sore that is burning hot, swollen, and itchy and that continues to spread after bursting and fails to heal.

mammary welling-abscess, 乳痈 *rǔ yōng*: A welling-abscess on the female breast. It is most common after childbirth, but may occur in the later stages of pregnancy. It is characterized by a redness and swelling in the breast, which if left untreated can suppurate and burst.

mania and withdrawal, 癫狂 *diān kuáng*: Mania denotes states of excitement characterized by noisy, unruly, and even aggressive behavior, offensive speech, constant singing and laughter, irascibility, springing walls and climbing roofs, and inability to remain tidily dressed. This is a yáng pattern of the heart spirit straying outward owing to hyperactivity of yáng qì. Withdrawal refers to emotional depression, indifference, deranged speech, taciturnity, and obliviousness to hunger or satiety. It is a yīn pattern caused by binding of depressed qì and phlegm or heart-spleen vacuity.

massive head scourge, 大头瘟 *dà tóu wēn*: A disease that results from invasion of the spleen and stomach channels by seasonal wind-warmth toxin and that is characterized by swelling and redness of the head, and sometimes by painful swelling of the throat, and, in severe cases, signs such as deafness, clenched jaw, clouded spirit, and delirious raving. Massive head scourge usually corresponds to mumps (parotitis) in modern medicine. It is traditionally treated with *pǔ jì xiāo dú yǐn* (Universal Aid Toxin-Dispersing Beverage).

menstrual block, 经闭 *jīng bì*: Amenorrhea. Absence of menstruation. Between menarche and menopause, menstruation normally ceases only in pregnancy. Menstrual block is the continuing absence of menstruation after the age of eighteen or the abnormal cessation of menstrual periods for at least three months in women who are neither pregnant nor lactating. In rare cases, lifelong absence of menstruation is unaccompanied by impairment of reproductive function.

mix-fried, 炙 *zhì*: Stir-fried with liquid adjuvants. The aim of mix-frying is to change medicinal characteristics, improve effectiveness, improve the flavor and smell, resolve toxicity, and prevent rotting. Usually, the adjuvant and materials are first blended, covered, and left to stand for a short time before frying so that the adjuvant soaks well into the materials. The most commonly used adjuvants are honey, vinegar, wine, and brine. *Zhì má huáng* (mix-fried ephedra), *zhì gān cǎo* (mix-fried licorice), and *zhì huáng qí* (mix-fried astragalus) are mix-fried with honey. *Wǔ líng zhī* (squirrel's droppings), *mò yào* (myrrh), and *hóng yá dà jǐ* (knoxia) can be mix-fried with vinegar.

mobile and penetrating, 走窜 *zǒu cuàn*: (Of medicinals) tending to move and penetrate blockages. Mobile and penetrating medicinals are ones that move qì and quicken the blood, free the channels and quicken the network vessels, or free the orifices and free the spirit, such as *mù xiāng* (costusroot), *shè xiāng* (musk), *bīng piàn* (borneol), *zhāng nǎo* (camphor), *xiè bái* (Chinese chive), *chuān shān jiǎ* (pangolin scales), and *zào jiǎo cì* (gleditsia thorn). Such medicinals are generally aromatic, acrid and dissipating, or warm and bitter.

mounting, 疝 *shàn*: Any of various diseases characterized by pain or swelling of the abdomen or scrotum. Traditional literature describes many different diseases and patterns labeled as "mounting." Mounting disease can be divided into three categories: (1) Also called "mounting qì" (疝气 *shàn qì*). Conditions characterized by the protrusion of the abdominal contents through the abdominal wall, the inguen, or base of the abdominal cavity, and usually associated with qì pain (气痛 *qì tòng*). Often called "small intestinal mounting qì" or "small intestinal mounting qì pain." This corresponds to inguinal hernia in Western medicine. (2) Various diseases of the external genitals that correspond to hydrocele, hematoma of testis, traumatic injury of testis, and orchitis. (3) Certain forms of acute abdominal pain associated with urinary and fecal stoppage.

mounting-conglomeration, 疝瘕 *shàn jiǎ*: A swelling of the abdomen that moves under pressure and is associated with abdominal pain stretching into the lumbus and back; attributed to wind-cold binding with qì and blood in the abdomen.

mounting pain, 疝痛 *shàn tòng*: See mounting qì pain[558] (疝气痛 *shàn qì tòng*).

mounting qì, 疝气 *shàn qì*: See mounting[558] (疝 *shàn*).

mounting qì pain, 疝气痛 *shàn qì tòng*: Mounting qì attacking through the abdomen, groin, and lesser abdomen causing pain, or swelling and pain of the testicles.

nature, 性 *xìng*: (Of Chinese medicinals), a basic or essential feature, especially as regards heat and cold. Traditionally, four natures, more commonly called four qì (四气 *sì qì*), are distinguished: cold, heat, warmth, and coolness. Cold medicinals are ones effective in treating heat patterns, whereas hot medicinals are those effective in treating cold patterns. Warm and cool medicinals are medicinals with mildly hot or cold natures. In addition, there is also a neutral nature that is neither predominantly hot nor cold.

nature-preservative burning, 炒存性 *chǎo cún xìng*: Also called char-frying (炒炭 *chǎo tàn*). Stir-frying in a wok over a high flame to make the materials charred and black on the outside, brown on the inside, and brittle. Although a large proportion of the material is charred, the original properties are still present, hence the name "nature-preservative burning."

nebulous eye screen, 目生云翳 *mù shēng yún yì*: A whitish patch on the eye that appears like a cloud. In severe cases, it can cover the pupil and obscure vision.

nontransformation of food, 食不消化 *shí bù xiāo huà*: Failure to digest food properly.

nose piles, 鼻痔 *bí zhì*: Fleshy growths obstructing the nostrils; same as nasal polyps, 鼻息肉 *bí xī ròu*.

numbing wind, 麻风 *má fēng*: See **great wind**[551] (大风 *dà fēng*).

open the stomach, (开胃 *kāi wèi*): Improve the appetite.

outside the membrane within the skin, 皮里膜外 *pí lǐ mó wài*: A membrane that encloses the structures within a given area of the body. This membrane is deeper than the skin, but not as deep as the internal organs.

panting, 喘 *chuǎn*: Hasty, rapid, labored breathing with discontinuity between inhalation and exhalation, in severe cases with gaping mouth, raised shoulders, flaring nostrils, and inability to lie down. When associated with counterflow movement of qì, it is sometimes called "panting counterflow." When breathing is unusually rapid, it is sometimes called "hasty panting." When in severe cases it is associated with raising of the shoulders and flaring nostrils, it is "raised-shoulder breathing." Panting is a manifestation of impaired diffusion and downbearing of lung qì. Since the "lung is the governor of qì" and the "kidney is the root of qì," panting is associated primarily with disease of the lung and/or kidney. Panting occurs in repletion and vacuity. Repletion panting may occur when externally contracted wind-heat or wind-cold invade the lung, when depressed liver qì invades the lung, or when phlegm arising from spleen-lung vacuity obstructs the lung. Vacuity panting occurs in dual vacuity of lung yīn and lung qì, and in failure of the kidney to absorb qì. Kidney vacuity with phlegm obstruction and yáng vacuity water flood are vacuity-repletion complexes that may also give rise to panting.

phlegm nodes, 痰核 *tán hé*: Any lump below the skin that feels soft and slippery under the finger, is associated with no redness, pain, or swelling, and (unlike scrofula) does not suppurate.

phlegm turbidity, 痰浊 *tán zhuó*: Phlegm as a turbid entity that is obstructive to the clear yáng qì of the body. Phlegm turbidity is often said to specifically refer to phlegm-damp or phlegm-rheum. However, phlegm turbidity often implies that the phlegm is thick and sticky, while phlegm-damp often implies that the phlegm is thin.

plum-pit qì, 梅核气 *méi hé qì*: Also called plum-pit phlegm, 梅核痰 *méi hé tán*. A subjective feeling of a lump in the throat like a sticky phlegm node that can be neither coughed up or swallowed, but that does not affect eating and drinking.

postmeridian tidal heat [effusion], 下午潮热 *xià wǔ cháo rè*: Tidal heat effusion occurring any time after midday. Postmeridian tidal heat [effusion] is usually a sign of yīn vacuity, but a vigorous heat that becomes more pronounced at roughly 3–5 P.M., called late afternoon tidal heat (日晡（所）潮热 *rì bū (suǒ) cháo rè*), is associated with yáng brightness (*yáng míng*) interior repletion patterns.

precipitate qì, 下气 *xià qì*: Also called downbear qì (降气 *jiàng qì*). To address counterflow qì ascent that manifests as panting, cough, or hiccup, using medicinals such as *zǐ sū zǐ* (perilla fruit), *xuán fù huā* (inula flower), *bàn xià* (pinellia), *dīng xiāng* (clove), and *dài zhě shí* (hematite). Precipitating qì is one method of rectifying qì.

prickly heat, 痱子 *fèi zi*: A condition characterized by red papules attended with itching and tingling. Prickly heat occurs mostly in hot summer months and is attributed to brewing summerheat-damp that inhibits sweating. It is most commonly observed in infants and obese people, and affects the head, neck, abdomen, back, shoulder, and groin. It appears as red papules the size of millet seeds that quickly turn into water vesicles or pustules and are associated with itching and scorching heat. Scratching can cause the development of a "prickly heat toxin (sore)," equivalent to hidradenitis spoken of in Western medicine.

propping rheum, 支饮 *zhī yǐn*: One of the four rheums (四饮 *sì yǐn*). Water below the heart, causing signs such as cough, copious phlegm, rapid breathing, inability to lie flat, facial swelling, soot black complexion, and dizziness.

puffy swelling, 浮肿 *fú zhǒng*: Water swelling[567] (水肿 *shǐ zhǒng*). A distinction is sometimes made between swelling and puffiness, swelling being repletion and puffiness being vacuity. Puffy swelling is caused by debilitation of the visceral qì of the lung, spleen, and kidney. Lung vacuity deprives water of transformation; spleen vacuity means that water is not dammed; kidney vacuity means that water is not governed. When the spleen is affected, there is puffy swelling of the flesh; when the lung is affected, there is rapid panting.

pulmonary consumption, 肺痨 *fèi láo*: A disease traditionally known by 痨瘵 *láo zhài* and other terms, but popularly referred to since the late Qīng Dynasty as 肺痨 (pulmonary consumption) and identified with pulmonary tuberculosis of Western medicine. Pulmonary consumption is characterized by cough with expectoration of blood, tidal heat, night sweating, and emaciation. The cough is persistent and chronic, producing blood-flecked phlegm or in severe cases mouthfuls of blood. The tidal heat comes in the afternoon and evening and abates in the B1 watch (11 P.M.–1 A.M.). Emaciation develops with reduced food intake as well as fatigue and lack of strength. The pulse is fine and rapid. Consumption begins with yīn depletion, which leads to vacuity fire, and finally, when damage to yīn affects yáng, to dual depletion of yīn and yáng.

pulmonary welling-abscesses, 肺痈 *fèi yōng*: A welling-abscess[567] (痈 *yōng*) in the lung that forms when externally contracted wind evil and heat toxin brew and obstruct the lung, and when the heat causes congestion and blood stasis. In time, it starts to suppurate. The classic signs are coughing up of pus and blood. Pulmonary welling-abscess is associated with heat effusion and shivering, cough, chest pain, rapid respiration, and expectoration of sticky fishy-smelling purulent phlegm. Corresponds to pulmonary abscess and bronchiectasis in Western medicine.

qì block, 气闭 *qì bì*: Blockage and derangement of qì dynamic due to congestion of wind, phlegm, fire, or stasis evil and that manifests in signs such as coma, clenched jaw, clenched fists, or urinary and fecal stoppage. When qì block clouds the clear orifices, there is clouded spirit or loss of consciousness. When it affects the chest, there is fullness in the chest or rough panting.

qì constipation, 气秘 *qì bì*: Constipation attributed to either qì stagnation or qì vacuity. Qì stagnation results from emotional imbalance characterized by fullness in the stomach duct and abdomen, stabbing pain in the chest and rib-side, belching, and the desire but inability to defecate. Constipation due to qì vacuity is attended by lassitude of spirit, laziness to speak, pale tongue, and a weak pulse.

raise the spirit, 提神 *tí shén*: To increase mental vigor.

rectal heaviness, 后重 *hòu zhòng*: Also called abdominal urgency and rectal heaviness, 里急后重 *lǐ jí hòu zhòng*. Tenesmus. The urgent desire to evacuate, with difficulty in defecation characterized by heaviness or pressure in the rectum. Tenesmus with stool containing pus and blood is a major sign of dysentery.

reversal cold of the limbs, 四肢厥冷 *sì zhī jué lěng*: Also called counterflow cold of the extremities (四肢逆冷 *sì zhī nì lěng*). Pronounced cold in the extremities up to the knees and elbows or beyond, as occurs in yáng collapse or internal heat evil block. Reversal cold of the extremities is similar to lack of warmth in the extremities. However, the latter differs in that it is less pronounced, does not reach as far as the knees and elbows, and is observed in general yáng vacuity patterns. Reversal cold of the extremities is called "reversal" because yáng qì recedes away from the extremities.

running piglet, 奔豚 *bēn tún*: Also called running piglet qì disease (奔豚气病 *bēn tún qì bìng*). An ancient disease name that refers to a condition whose manifestations are similar to those of gastrointestinal neurosis. The manifestations include accumulated gas in the intestinal tract, hyperperistalsis, and spasms. It was given this name because the subjective feeling associated with the condition is like a small pig rushing about.

scab, 疥 *jiè*: A skin disease characterized by itching, suppuration, and crusting.

scant breast milk, 乳汁少 *rǔ zhī shǎo*: Insufficient milk to suckle the infant. Scant breast milk is due to postpartum depletion of qì and blood or to liver qì depression. The latter is easily distinguishable by the presence of distention and fullness of the breasts. Qì-blood vacuity results in scant breast milk when it causes insufficiency of the source of milk transformation (i.e., reduced milk production). The chief characteristic is absence of pain and distention in the breasts. Other signs include white lips, low food intake, and fatigue. Treat by the method of supplementing qì and nourishing the blood, assisted by freeing breast milk. Use *tōng rǔ dān* (Lactation Elixir). Scant breast milk due to liver depression and qì stagnation is characterized by fullness, distention, and pain in the breasts, sometimes associated with generalized heat [effusion] and oppression in the chest. It is treated by coursing the liver, resolving depression, and freeing milk. Use *xiāo yáo sǎn* (Free Wanderer Powder)[31] plus *chuān shān jiǎ* (pangolin scales) and *wáng bù liú xíng* (vaccaria).

scrofula, 瘰疬 *luǒ lì*: Lumps beneath the skin down the side of the neck and under the armpits. These are often referred to in older books as saber and pearl-string lumps (马刀侠瘿 *mǎ dāo xiá yǐng*) because of the saber-like formation they can make below the armpit and the necklace-like formation they make on the neck. Scrofula occurs when phlegm gathers in the neck, armpits, or groin. The phlegm is produced by the scorching of fluids by vacuity fire arising in lung-kidney vacuity. In some cases, wind-fire evil toxin is also a factor. Scrofula starts as bean-like lumps, associated with neither pain nor heat. Subsequently the lumps expand and assume a stringlike formation, merge, and even bunch up into heaps. They are hard and do not move under pressure. In the latter stages they may become slightly painful. They can rupture to exude a thin pus and sometimes contain matter that resembles bean curd dregs (residue of ground soybeans in the production of soybean milk and tofu). They can take a long time to heal, old ones healing while new ones arise. In some cases, fistulas may form. In Western medicine scrofula is due to tuberculosis of lymph nodes or lymphadenitis.

seminal cold, 精冷 *jīng lěng*: Also called 精寒 *jīng hán*. A condition characterized by cold, thin, scant semen; a major cause of male sterility. Seminal cold is attributed to insufficiency of kidney qì or to kidney yáng vacuity.

seminal efflux, 滑精 *huá jīng*: Involuntary loss of semen (essence) occurring in sleep without dreaming or when awake, in severe cases several times a day. *Jǐng Yuè Quán Shū* (景岳全书 "Jing-Yue's Complete Compendium") states, "Emission of semen not due to dreaming is called seminal efflux." Seminal efflux results from sexual performance incommensurate with libido and sexual intemperance causing depletion of the kidney origin and insecurity of the essence gate.

seminal emission, 遗精 *yí jīng*: Involuntary loss of semen (essence). In a broad sense, "seminal emission" refers to any involuntary loss of semen (seminal loss); in a narrow sense, it refers to loss of semen during sleep, the most common form. Seminal emission is mildest when it occurs while dreaming (dream emission 梦遗 *mèng yí*). It is more severe if it occurs without dreaming (seminal emission without dreaming 不梦而遗 *bù mèng ér yí*), or while awake in the daytime (seminal efflux 滑精 *huá jīng*) or in great quantity (great seminal discharge 精液大泄 *jīng yè dà xiè*). It is said that "essence [i.e., semen] is moved by the spirit in response to the heart." In dream emission, the disease is mostly in the heart, whereas in seminal emission without dreaming, the disease is usually in the kidney. If evil is involved, the patterns are repletion and heat; if no evil is involved, the patterns are vacuity and cold. Seminal emission at the onset of illness is usually caused by evil fire stirring the essence chamber. In enduring illness it is usually due to internal damage by the seven affects and disharmony of the organs. The main causes are effulgent sovereign and ministerial fire, heart vacuity and liver depression, insecurity of kidney qì, noninteraction of the heart and kidney, and spleen vacuity qì fall.

seven relations, 七情 *qī qíng*: Seven relationships or interactions of medicinals, namely: going alone; mutual need; empowering; fear; aversion; killing; clashing. Going alone (单行 *dān xíng*): The ability of a medicinal to be used alone, as in *gān cǎo tāng* (Licorice Decoction) and *dú shēn tāng* (Pure Ginseng Decoction). **Mutual need** (相须 *xiāng xū*): The combined use of two medicinals of similar action to enhance each other's action. The implication is that the combined use of the two medicinals is greater than the sum of their individual actions. Mutual need medicinals include *zhī mǔ* (anemarrhena) and *huáng bǎi* (phellodendron). **Empowering** (相使 *xiāng shǐ*): The use of one or more medicinals to enhance the action of a main agent. For example, *xìng rén* (apricot kernel) empowers *kuǎn dōng huā* (coltsfoot) to moisten the lung and downbear qì and to suppress cough and transform phlegm. **Fear** (相畏 *xiāng wèi*): Toxicity of a medicinal being counteracted by another. For example, *bàn xià* (pinellia) fears *shēng jiāng* (fresh ginger) because its toxicity is reduced by it. *Huáng qí* (astragalus) was traditionally said to fear *fáng fēng* (saposhnikovia), although in *yù píng fēng sǎn* (Jade Wind-Barrier Powder) *huáng qí* (astragalus) is said to be empowered by *fáng fēng* (saposhnikovia). Note: The Chinese 畏 *wèi* means fear, but in this context the term implies the fear of a benevolent power as the English word "awe." **Aversion** (相恶 *xiāng wù*): The weakening of a medicinal action by another. For example, *huáng qín* (scutellaria) is averse to *shēng jiāng* (fresh ginger), because its action is weakened by it; *rén shēn* (ginseng) is averse to *lái fú* (radish), since its supplementing action is reduced by it. Note: The Chinese 恶 (*wù*) implies dislike, sickening, ailing, hence weakening. **Killing** (相杀 *xiāng shā*): The elimination of side-effects of a medicinal. For example, *lǜ dòu* (mung bean) kills *bā dòu* (croton), i.e., it eliminates the noxious effects of *bā dòu*. **Clashing** (相反 *xiāng fǎn*): The creation of noxious effects when two medicinals are used together. For example, *chuān wū tóu* (aconite root) clashes with *bàn xià* (pinellia), so the two should not be used together.

simple drum distention, 单臌胀 *dān gǔ zhàng*: Pronounced abdominal distention without generalized water swelling.

skin water, 皮水 *pí shuǐ*: Water swelling[567] (水肿 *shuǐ zhǒng*) of gradual onset that engulfs the fingers, associated with drum-like enlargement of the abdomen, with absence of both sweating and thirst, and with a floating pulse. Skin water is attributed to spleen vacuity with severe dampness causing water to spill into the skin.

sloughing flat-abscess, 脱骨疽 *tuō gǔ jū*: A sore of gradual onset appearing on the hands and feet, and more frequently on the toes. It starts as a yellow blister the size of a millet seed. The skin is maroon like the color of boiled jujubes. It gradually putrefies and ulcerates, spreads outward, and penetrates inward to the flesh, sinew, and bone. It gives off a malign smell. On the toes, it can spread up onto the feet, or to other toes. The sore is associated with a burning pain that is usually intermittent and that usually occurs suddenly when walking or at night. It arises when, as a result of rich food, lack of exercise, or excessive consumption of hot kidney-supplementing medicinals, depressed fire toxic evil brews in the bowels and viscera and disperses yīn humor. It may also arise when cold-damp evil toxin causes disharmony of construction and defense and stagnation of qì and blood. A sloughing flat-abscess is difficult to cure, especially if treatment is not administered early in its development.

snivelling nose, 鼻鼽 *bí qiú*: Runny nose with clear snivel.

sore-toxin, 疮毒 *chuāng dú*: The toxin that causes sores and pox.

sparrow-vision night blindness, 雀目夜盲 *què mù yè máng*: Night blindness. Reduced visual acuity in poor lighting. Distinction is made between the earlier heaven type, called high-altitude wind sparrow-vision internal obstruction (高风 雀目内障 *gāo fēng què mù nèi zhàng*), and a later heaven type, called liver vacuity sparrow-vision internal obstruction (肝虚雀目内障 *gān xū què mù nèi zhàng*).

spiritlessness, 失神 *shī shén*: Lack of general vitality as observed in signs such as mental debilitation, apathy, abnormal bearing, torpid expression, dark complexion and dull eyes, low voice, slow, halting speech, and incoherent response to inquiry, indicating a relatively serious condition in which right qì has suffered damage. Although no critical signs may be present, extreme care is necessary in devising treatment.

spontaneous external bleeding, 衄血 *nǜ xuè*: Bleeding visible on the outside of the body that is not due to injury. The Chinese term is often used specifically to mean nosebleed, and in most instances of its appearance in this book we have translated it as nosebleed.

steaming bone tidal heat, 骨蒸劳热 *gǔ zhēng láo rè*: Tidal heat, i.e., heat effusion (fever) occurring at regular intervals, usually in the afternoon or evening (postmeridian tidal heat) that appears to emanate from the bone or marrow. It is attributed to severe yīn vacuity and is accompanied by heart vexation and reduced sleep, heat in the palms, and yellow or reddish urine.

steam-wash, 熏洗 *xūn xǐ*: Exposing the area of the body to be treated to the steam emanating from a decoction of medicinals in a cooking pot, and then when the decoction has cooled sufficiently, using the decoction to wash the area.

stirring fetus, 胎动 *tāi dòng*: Also called 胎动不安 *tāi dòng bù ān*. A disease pattern characterized by movement of the fetus, pain and sagging sensation in the abdomen, and, in severe cases, discharge of blood from the vagina; a sign of possible or impending miscarriage; can be caused by knocks and falls, qì vacuity, blood vacuity, kidney vacuity, or blood heat causing damage to the thoroughfare (*chōng*) and controlling (*rèn*) vessels.

stomach reflux, 反胃 *fǎn wèi*: A disease characterized by distention and fullness after eating, by vomiting in the evening of food ingested in the morning or by vomiting in the morning of food ingested in the evening (i.e., vomiting a long time after eating), untransformed food in the vomitus, lassitude of spirit, and lack of bodily strength. Its principal cause is spleen-stomach vacuity cold, but it may also be due to debilitation of the life gate fire or to dual vacuity of qì and yīn.

strangury, 淋 *lín*: Also called strangury disease (淋病 *lín bìng*). A disease characterized by urinary urgency, frequent short painful rough voidings, and dribbling incontinence. Strangury is attributed to damp-heat gathering and pouring into the bladder. In persistent conditions or in elderly or weak patients, the cause may be center qì fall, kidney vacuity, and impaired qì transformation. Distinction is made between stone strangury (石淋 *shí lín*, which also includes sand strangury 砂淋 *shā lín*), qì strangury (气淋 *qì lín*), blood strangury (血淋 *xuè lín*), unctuous strangury (膏淋 *gāo lín*), and taxation strangury (劳淋 *láo lín*), known collectively as the five stranguries (五淋 *wǔ lín*).

strangury-turbidity, 淋浊 *lín zhuó*: (1) A generic name for strangury and turbidity. (2) A sexually transmissible disease described in *Chì Shuǐ Xuán Zhū* (赤水玄珠 "Mysterious Pearl of Red Water") that is characterized by pain in the penis on urination, with semen dripping down like malodorous rotten pus, and treated by resolving toxin and vanquishing turbidity with *bā zhèng sǎn* (Eight Corrections Powder) plus *bì xiè* (fish poison yam) and *tǔ fú líng* (smooth greenbrier root).

strings and aggregrations, 痃癖 *xián pì*: Strings are elongated masses located at the side of the umbilicus; aggregations are masses located in the rib-side that occur intermittently with pain and at other times are not detectable by palpation. The two conditions belong to the category of **concretions, conglomerations, accumulations, and gatherings**[544] (癥瘕积聚) and are usually referred to together. Both are caused by dietary irregularities damaging the spleen and stomach, the gathering and binding of cold and phlegm, and congealing stagnation of qì and blood. Very often they are associated with emaciation, reduced food intake, and fatigue. Treatment takes the form of dispersing accumulations, dissipating cold, flushing phlegm, rectifying qì, harmonizing the blood, and dispersing stasis.

summerheat stroke, 中暑 *zhòng zhǔ*: Contraction of summerheat evil in the torrid heat of summer. Summerheat stroke is characterized by sudden oppression and collapse, clouding and loss of consciousness, generalized heat [effusion], panting, loss of speech, mild clenching of the jaws or open mouth and dry teeth, great sweating or absence of sweating, and a vacuous rapid pulse. In severe cases, there is coma with convulsions of the limbs.

suspended rheum, 旋饮 *xuán yǐn*: Water in the chest and rib-side that causes local pain and cough with copious phlegm.

take drenched, 冲服 *chōng fú*: To ingest medicinals saturated or dissolved in liquid. Formulas often indicate that dry mineral ingredients such as *máng xiāo* (mirabilite) and *zhū shā* (cinnabar) or sticky medicinals such as *yí táng* (malt sugar) should be taken drenched, which means that they can be mixed with the decoction of the other ingredients or other fluid to facilitate swallowing.

taxation heat, 劳热 *láo rè*: Heat effusion[551] (发热 *fā rè*) in vacuity taxation patterns, attributable to qì-blood depletion or yáng debilitation and yīn vacuity. It takes the form of steaming bone taxation heat [effusion], and vexing heat in the five hearts. Accompanying signs differ according to the nature of the vacuity.

tetany, 痉 *jìng*: Severe spasm such as rigidity in the neck, clenched jaw, convulsions of the limbs, and arched-back rigidity.

throat impediment, 喉痹 *hóu bì*: Critical swelling and soreness of the throat in which the throat becomes severely occluded.

toxin swelling, 肿毒 *zhǒng dú*: Swelling due to the presence of toxin (heat toxin, damp toxin).

treating the unstopped by unstopping, 通因通用 *tōng yīn tōng yòng*: Stopping diarrhea by freeing the bowels. This is an example of paradoxical treatment.

tugging and slackening, 瘛瘲 *jì zòng*: See tugging wind[566] (抽风 *chōu fēng*).

tugging wind, 抽风 *chōu fēng*: Also called tugging and slackening 瘛瘲 *jì zòng*. Alternating tensing and relaxation of the sinews, often observed in externally contracted heat (febrile) disease, epilepsy, and lockjaw. Equivalent to clonic spasm in Western medicine.

turbid unctuous urine, 小便浑浊如膏 *xiǎo biàn hún zhuó rú gāo*: Urine like rice water (water that rice has been washed in), snivel (nasal mucus), or animal fat.

unsurfaced heat [effusion], 身热不扬 *shēn rè bù yáng*: Generalized heat effusion in which heat is felt only by prolonged palpation; mostly due to binding of dampness and heat, where the dampness is blocked on the outside. Since the heat lies deep within the dampness it cannot easily be felt on the surface of the body.

untransformed of food, 完谷不化 *wán gǔ bù huà*: Partially digested food in the stool due to impaired digestion. Nontransformation of food most commonly occurs in spleen vacuity, spleen-kidney yáng vacuity, large intestinal vacuity, or cold accumulation patterns, but may also be observed in heat diarrhea.

vacuity detriment, 虚损 *xū sǔn*: Any form of severe chronic insufficiency of yīn-yáng, qì-blood, or bowels and viscera that arises through internal damage by the seven affects, taxation fatigue, diet, excesses of drink or sex, or enduring illness.

vaginal discharge, 带下 *dài xià*: The emission of a viscid fluid via the vagina, usually white in color, but often tinged with red or yellow (red vaginal discharge, yellow vaginal discharge). Leukorrhea.

wandering wind, 游风 *yóu fēng*: Also called red and white wandering wind, 赤白 游风 *chì bái yóu fēng*. A disease characterized by the sudden appearance, usually on the lips, eyelids, and earlobes, or the chest and abdomen or shoulder and back, of red or white cloud-shaped patches of smooth, puffy skin that feel hard to the touch, associated with burning sensation, numbness, and mild itching. Wandering wind is attributed to spleen-lung dryness-heat or insecurity of exterior qì allowing wind evil to invade the interstices, cause congestion, and disturb construction and defense. When the evil is stagnating in the blood aspect, the patches are red in color (red wandering wind); when stagnating in the qì aspect, the patches are white (white wandering wind).

water drum, 水臌 *shuǐ gǔ*: A disease pattern characterized by abdominal distention which gurgles when the patient moves. Water drum is usually attributable to excessive consumption of liquor that on the one hand causes impairment of free coursing of the liver and consequently liver depression and on the other hand causes impairment of splenic movement and transformation and results in collection of water-damp. Water drum is associated with a withered-yellow facial complexion, rib-side pain, red speckles on the body (spider nevi), and sometimes jaundice. In persistent cases, there is scant urine and generalized swelling that pits when pressed.

water-rheum, 水饮 *shuǐ yǐn*: Fluid exuded by diseased organs. Clear thin fluid is known as "water," whereas thin sticky fluid is known as "rheum." These differ in name and form, but are in essence the same; hence the compound term.

water-rheum intimidating the heart, 水饮凌心 *shuǐ yǐn líng xīn*: Also called water qì intimidating the heart (水气凌心 *shuǐ qì líng xīn*). Upsurge of water qì causing disturbances of the heart. Spleen-yáng vacuity and impairment of qì transformation cause water to be retained in the body and thereby give rise to water qì, which can manifest as phlegm-rheum or water swelling. When the water surges upward and lodges in the chest and diaphragm, it can cause devitalization of heart yáng and disquieting of heart qì that manifests in the form of heart palpitations and hasty breathing. This is what is known as "water qì intimidating the heart." The chief signs are heart palpitations, panting with inability to lie flat, generalized puffy swelling, and a bright white facial complexion. Other signs include flusteredness, lassitude of spirit and fatigue, fear of cold and cold limbs, and short voidings of scant clear urine.

water swelling, 水肿 *shuǐ zhǒng*: Edema. Swelling of the flesh arising when organ dysfunction (spleen, kidney, lung) due to internal or external causes allows water to accumulate. Water swelling stands in contradistinction to toxin swelling, which denotes a localized swelling due to the local presence of toxin, as in the case of sores.

welling-abscess, 痈 *yōng*: A large suppuration in the flesh characterized by a painful swelling and redness that is clearly circumscribed and that before rupturing is soft and characterized by a thin shiny skin. Before suppuration begins, it can be easily dispersed; when pus has formed, it easily ruptures; after rupture, it easily closes and heals. It may be associated with generalized heat [effusion], thirst, yellow tongue fur, and a rapid pulse.

white patch wind, 白癜风 *bái diàn fēng*: White patches on the skin attributed to disharmony of the blood that arises when wind evil assails the exterior, causing the interstices to lose their tightness. White patch wind is most common in youth and the prime of life. Called vitiligo in Western medicine.

white turbidity, 白浊 *bái zhuó*: (1) Murky urine that is white in color, unassociated with inhibited urination or pain on urination. It is attributed to spleen-stomach damp-heat pouring down into the bladder, and is associated with fullness and oppression in the chest and stomach duct, dry mouth and thirst, yellow slimy tongue fur, and a rapid slippery pulse. If the condition persists, it may develop into insufficiency of the heart and spleen and into qì vacuity fall characterized by lassitude of spirit, lack of strength, white complexion, and a soft weak pulse. If there is insufficiency of kidney yīn with vacuity fire, signs include heat vexation, dry pharynx, red tongue, and a fine rapid pulse. If there is insufficiency of kidney yáng and lower origin vacuity cold, signs include white complexion, cold limbs, pale tongue, and a fine sunken pulse. White turbidity with pronounced stinging pain on voiding constitutes "unctuous strangury" (see **strangury**[564] 淋 *lín*). (2) Discharge of a murky white substance from the urethra, associated with inhibited urination and clear urine.

wilting, 痿 *wěi*: Weakness and limpness of the sinews that in severe cases prevents the lifting of the arms and legs and is accompanied by the sensation that the elbow, wrist, knee, and ankle are dislocated. In advanced cases, atrophy sets in. Wilting patterns include withering and paralysis of the limbs in neonates and infants after high fever, which Western medicine attributes to poliomyelitis.

wind papules, 风疹 *fēng zhěn*: (1) dormant papules (瘾疹 *yǐn zhěn*). (2) wind sand (风痧 *fēng shā*). A contagious disease characterized by a papular eruption seen in children under five years of age in the winter and spring; attributed to externally contracted wind-heat lying depressed in the fleshy exterior and manifesting in small pale red papules that appear quickly and disappear without scaling or scarring.

wind strike, 中风 *zhòng fēng*: A disease characterized by the sudden appearance of hemiplegia, deviated eyes and mouth, and impeded speech; wind strike that may or may not start with sudden clouding collapse (loss of consciousness).

wind water, 风水 *fēng shuǐ*: From *Sù Wèn* (素问 "Elementary Questions"). External wind contraction with water swelling. Signs include rapid onset, floating pulse, pain in the joints, heat effusion and aversion to cold, and swelling, particularly of the head and face (the upper part of the body being affected by wind evil). The disease is the result of impairment of lung qì's depurative downbearing by wind evil in patients suffering from spleen-kidney qì vacuity.

wrenched lumbus with acute pain, 闪腰岔气 *shǎn yào chà qì*: Acute sprain or contusion of the lumbus (including slipped disk) with sharp pain that prevents turning or bending forward or backward.

wrenching and contusion, 闪挫 *shǎn cuò*: Damage to the lumbus through lifting heavy weights or due to twisting. Wrenched lumbus pain is characterized by the inability to bend and stretch or difficulty in turning, with any movement exacerbating pain.

yellow-water sore, 黄水疮 *huáng shuǐ chuāng*: A superficial sore that forms pustules, exudes a thick yellow fluid, and then dries into yellow crusts. This disorder primarily affects children and occurs mostly in the warm months. Though this traditional disease name describes a wider disease category than the biomedical terms of impetigo vulgaris or impetigo bullous, which are defined as superficial infections of streptococci or staphylococci, it is now used synonymously with those disease names. Typically *dà huáng* (rhubarb) is combined with *huáng lián* (coptis), *zhī zǐ* (gardenia), and *huáng bǎi* (phellodendron) to treat this disorder. The powdered combination can be daubed onto the moist sores or mixed with water and applied as a paste.

yīn flat-abscess, 阴疽 *yīn jū*: A painful, deep-lying lesion that is white or slightly off-color (darkened), cold or cool to the touch, and diffusely swollen or not swollen at all; attributed to accumulation of heat or toxin deep inside the flesh that is trapped next to the sinews and bones by yīn-cold. Prior to the Sòng dynasty the term referred primarily to collections that do not come to a head, but fester internally. Hence the English translation "flat-abscess." Later, lesions that come to a head and suppurate, but are not red or hot, were also called *jū*. By contrast, hot red sores that come to a head were called 痈 *yōng*, welling-abscesses. Thus *jū* are considered yīn and *yōng* are thought to be yáng. Some books define 阴疽 *yīn jū* as short for 股阴疽 *gǔ yǐn jū*, which is a *jū* on the inner thigh or in the region of the external genitalia.

Index

Terms unique to Western medicine are marked with an asterisk. **Underlined bold** numerals mark the main headings. <u>Underlined</u> numerals indicate entries in the Glossary of Terms.

用药心得十讲
用藥心得十講

TEN LECTURES
ON THE USE OF MEDICINALS

From the Personal Experience of
JIĀO SHÙ-DÉ

After their appearance as a lecture series in the *Barefoot Doctors' Journal*, Jiāo Shù-Dé's *Ten Lectures on the Use of Medicinals* won great acclaim among readers, especially barefoot doctors, on account of their great simplicity and practicality. In response to popular demand, they were subsequently combined into a single volume and published by People's Medical Publishing, Běijīng.

Since its first appearance in book form in 1977, the *Ten Lectures* have enjoyed perennial popularity in the People's Republic of China and Táiwān as the most concise manual of medicinal therapy available.

The present volume presents the lectures in English translation, with the benefit of notes provided by Dr. Jiāo himself.

In the Chinese-speaking world, Dr. Jiāo is widely acclaimed as one of the *míng lǎo zhōng yī* 名老中医, the "Old Master Physicians."

Features

- Introduces 309 Chinese medicinals.

- Explains their use in simple practical terms.

- Contains English and Pīnyīn/Chinese indexes of general terms, names of medicinals, and names of formulas.

JIAO   CLINICAL   CHINESE   MEDICINE   SERIES